PERIODONTICS
REVISITED

PERIODONTICS REVISITED

Shalu Bathla MDS (Gold Medalist)
Reader
Department of Periodontology and Oral Implantology
MM College of Dental Sciences and Research
Mullana, Ambala, Haryana, India

Assisted by

Manish Bathla MD
Assistant Professor
Department of Psychiatry
MM Institute of Medical Sciences and Research
Mullana, Ambala, Haryana, India

Forewords

SG Damle
Thomas E Van Dyke

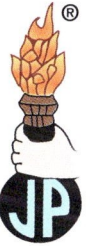

JAYPEE BROTHERS MEDICAL PUBLISHERS (P) LTD

New Delhi • Panama City • London

Published by

Jaypee Brothers Medical Publishers (P) Ltd

Corporate Office

4838/24, Ansari Road, Daryaganj, **New Delhi** 110 002, India
Phone: +91-11-43574357, Fax: +91-11-43574314
Website: www.jaypeebrothers.com

Offices in India

- **Ahmedabad**, e-mail: ahmedabad@jaypeebrothers.com
- **Bengaluru**, e-mail: bangalore@jaypeebrothers.com
- **Chennai**, e-mail: chennai@jaypeebrothers.com
- **Delhi**, e-mail: jaypee@jaypeebrothers.com
- **Hyderabad**, e-mail: hyderabad@jaypeebrothers.com
- **Kochi**, e-mail: kochi@jaypeebrothers.com
- **Kolkata**, e-mail: kolkata@jaypeebrothers.com
- **Lucknow**, e-mail: lucknow@jaypeebrothers.com
- **Mumbai**, e-mail: mumbai@jaypeebrothers.com
- **Nagpur**, e-mail: nagpur@jaypeebrothers.com

Overseas Offices

- **Central America Office, Panama City, Panama**, Ph: 001-507-317-0160
  e-mail: cservice@jphmedical.com, Website: www.jphmedical.com
- **Europe Office, UK**, Ph: +44 (0) 2031708910
  e-mail: info@jpmedpub.com

Periodontics Revisited

This book has been published in good faith that the material provided by contributors is original. Every effort is made to ensure accuracy of material, but the publisher, printer and editor will not be held responsible for any inadvertent error(s). In case of any dispute, all legal matters are to be settled under Delhi jurisdiction only.

First Edition: **2011**

ISBN 978-93-5025-367-0

Typeset at JPBMP typesetting unit

Printed in India

Dedicated to

My Dear Son
Milind

Contributors

Amit Aggarwal
Assistant Professor
Department of Oral Medicine and Radiology
MM College of Dental Sciences and Research
Mullana, Ambala, Haryana, India

Atul Sharma
Assistant Professor
Department of Oral and Maxillofacial Surgery
MM College of Dental Sciences and Research
Mullana, Ambala, Haryana, India

Gayathri S Rao
Assistant Professor
Department of Oral Medicine and Radiology
SDM College of Dental Sciences and Hospital
Dharwad, Karnataka, India

Harpreet Singh Grover
Professor and Head
Department of Periodontology
SGT Dental College and Hospital
Gurgaon, Haryana, India

Jagdish C Bathla
Consultant Psychiatrist
Bathla Psychiatric Hospital
Karnal, Haryana, India

Manish Bathla
Assistant Professor
Department of Psychiatry
MM Institute of Medical Sciences and Research
Mullana, Ambala, Haryana, India

RK Sharma
Professor
Department of Periodontology
PGIMS, Government Dental College
Rohtak, Haryana, India

Sanjay Kalra
Consultant Endocrinologist
Bharti Hospital
Karnal, Haryana, India

Sanjeev Salaria
Professor
Department of Periodontology and Oral Implantology
MM College of Dental Sciences and Research
Mullana, Ambala, Haryana, India

Seema Nayyar
Reader
Department of Conservative Dentistry and Endodontics
MM College of Dental Sciences and Research
Mullana, Ambala, Haryana, India

Shailja Chatterjee
Assistant Professor
Department of Oral and Maxillofacial Pathology
MM College of Dental Sciences and Research
Mullana, Ambala, Haryana, India

Shaveta Sood
Assistant Professor
Department of Periodontology
HS Judge Institute of Dental Sciences
Punjab University
Chandigarh, India

Shashikant Hegde
Professor and Head
Department of Periodontology and Oral Implantology
Yenepoya Dental College
Mangalore, Karnataka, India

Suresh DK
Professor and Head
Department of Periodontology and Oral Implantology
MM College of Dental Sciences and Research
Mullana, Ambala, Haryana, India

Sushant Garg
Professor and Head
Department of Prosthodontics
MM College of Dental Sciences and Research
Mullana, Ambala, Haryana, India

Veenu Madaan Hans
Assistant Professor
Department of Periodontology and Oral Implantology
Kalka Dental College
Meerut, Uttar Pradesh, India

Vikram Jeet Singh Dhingra
Consultant Plastic Surgeon
MM Institute of Medical Sciences and Research
Mullana, Ambala, Haryana, India

Vishnu Das Prabhu
Professor
Department of Oral and Maxillofacial Pathology
Yenepoya Dental College
Mangalore, Karnataka, India

Foreword

Prof. S.G. Damle

Vice Chancellor

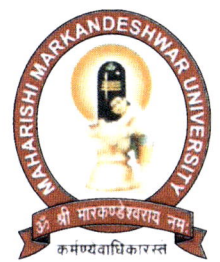

Maharishi Markandeshwar University
Mullana (Ambala)-133203 Haryana, INDIA
Tel. : 0091-1731-304524,
Fax : 0091-1731-274325
E-mail: sgdamle@gmail.com

It is a great pleasure to write foreword for the book of *Periodontics Revisited* by Dr Shalu Bathla, Reader, Department of Periodontology and Oral Implantology, MM College of Dental Sciences and Research, Mullana, Ambala, Haryana, India. The editor is enthusiastic, energetic and possesses amazing potential and competence in teaching. I am aware of her diligent and industrious nature. She has always been curious to keep herself abreast with the latest developments in the profession. She has excellent command and competence in this field and her approach is realistic and unusually supported with novel ideologies propounded and derived out of research. Undoubtedly, this book is a wonderful compilation and fabulous work on Periodontology as she had tried to cover all features and characteristics of the 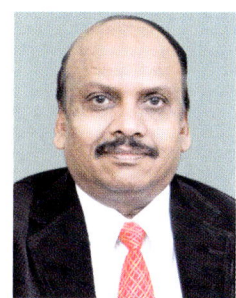 periodontium from the fundamentals to the recent trends in the treatment of periodontal diseases. This is a unique presentation with exhaustive coverage of the relevant issues useful and advantageous to the readers from all angles. In fact, the novelties derived and propounded through latest researches and inventions have completely transformed the standard and pattern of Dental Education. Besides serving as a textbook, this book can also be beneficial for the researchers who are curious to study this subject. In fact, there have been tremendous modifications and amendments which have ultimately affected the teaching patterns.

This work is exceptional outcome of tireless efforts of the editor and is bound to create an impact on the minds of the readers. This is a complete study and deserves applaud and acclamation because of its inherent qualities.

I wish her success in her venture and also mission of life.

SG Damle
Maharishi Markandeshwar University
Mullana (Ambala)-133203 Haryana, INDIA
Tel. : 0091-1731-304524,
Fax : 0091-1731-274325
E-mail: sgdamle@gmail.com

Foreword

Forsyth

The Forsyth Institute
245 First Street
Cambridge, MA 02142

www.forsyth.org

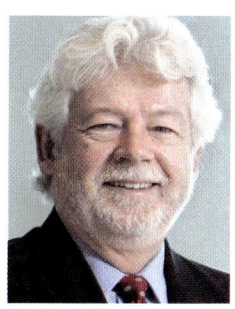

Readers of this book will gain invaluable, practical insights into the science and practice of modern periodontology. Periodontology is a constantly evolving specialty that changes in principle and practice with new discoveries and reinterpretation of available information. Students and practitioners alike must have the most up-to-date information at their fingertips to succeed in a technology driven world. As patient care providers, it is our responsibility to constantly be aware of changes and improvements in our field. By gaining a firm understanding of modern periodontology, practitioners will be more prepared to interact with other specialties of dentistry and offer the highest level of care with the best evidence-based procedures available to them.

One of the few certainties of life is that change will occur. With this in mind, Dr Shalu has focused not only on traditional periodontics but also on emerging technologies and concepts that will drive the periodontology of the future. With clear didactic writing, experienced practitioners and students will be guided in how to provide exceptional care for patients using the most modern methods. Now, more than ever, health practitioners have to keep abreast of new developments and scientific discoveries. This book is a valuable tool that can be used to reinforce and expand the possibilities for learning and teaching.

Thomas E Van Dyke DDS PhD
Vice President, Clinical and Translational Research
Chair of the Department of Periodontology
The Forsyth Institute
Cambridge, Massachusetts, USA

Preface

The support provided to my book *Tips and Tricks in Periodontology* by the students have motivated me to make this effort to write a textbook.

Periodontology is a rapidly changing branch of dentistry with new scientific revelations unveiling many mysteries. Some controversies, still surrounding the basic foundations of etiology, phenomenology, treatment methods, etc. make it very difficult for a student to understand its content.

The book is written in the first place with undergraduate dental students in mind, but is equally helpful for the postgraduate students also. The book is written as per the syllabus of the Dental Council of India.

Organization of the book: The text is organized into eleven sections; and each section is further subdivided into several chapters. With the matter subdivided into these smaller chapters, students will find easier to achieve their learning goals. Starting with the basics in section one, the text flows gradually from epidemiology; etiology; pathology; diagnosis; treatment including non-surgical, surgical and implantology with the inclusion of interdisciplinary approaches onto the recent advances in the field of periodontology.

Learning devices in the book: The effort has been made to learn the subject in a simpler and easier way by the use of tables, easy-to-understand line diagrams, original colored photographs, flow diagrams and points to ponder at the end of each chapter. Key information boxes are color coded to use as navigational aid for readers. Each chapter is supported by bibliography and also the important landmark studies related to the topic. MCQs are also included at the end of the chapter with answers in view of these being included in the exam system.

I do not claim exclusive credit for the book. No doubt there will be errors, few imperfections, omissions and over simplification. Hoping that rest of the material will be enough to stimulate insight and new trains of thoughts into the subject of Periodontics which will be immensely educative and helpful.

My job is not to make peoples' journey through life easier,
It's to let them know that the journey exists and that the destination is worth the travel.

Any suggestions and criticisms are most welcome at **periodonticsrevisited@gmail.com**

Shalu Bathla

Acknowledgments

Respected **Parents and GOD**, I lay this book at your feet.

No one walks alone and when one is walking on the journey of life just where you start to thank those that joined you, walked beside you, and helped you along the way. Over the years, those that I have met and worked with have continuously urged me to write a book, to put my thoughts down on paper, and to share my insights together with the secrets to my continual, positive approach to life and all that life throws at us. So at last, here it is in your hands. So, perhaps this book and its pages will be seen as "thanks" to many people who have helped make my life what it is today. I have poured my heart and soul into these pages, so now I pray that my words touch your heart, soul and mind.

A teacher affects eternity, he can never tell where his influence stops.

— **Henry Brooks Adams**

I am forever grateful to my mentors who have shaped me from human being to a dentist and to a periodontist; Mrs Sangeeta Bhatia, Dr RK Sharma, Dr Rajan Gupta, Dr SC Narula and Dr Shikha Tiwari. I am extremely thankful to my other teachers who have influenced me tremendously; Dr CS Samibi, Dr Ravi Kapur, Dr Sanjay Tiwari, Dr Nageshwar Iyer, Dr Poonam Sikri, Dr Shashikant Hegde, Dr Rajesh Kashyap, Dr Devender Choudhary, Dr Vimal Miglani, Dr Nikhil Srivastava and Dr Neeraj Gugnani.

A teacher I respect for his sincerity, straightforwardness and ability to work hard untiringly is Prof SG Damle; Vice Chancellor, MM University, Mullana, Ambala, Haryana, India. I am highly thankful to this renowned stalwart and icon of Pediatric and Preventive Dentistry for writing the foreword of this book.

I am also grateful to Prof Thomas E Van Dyke; Vice President, Clinical and Translational Research, Chair of the Department of Periodontology, The Forsyth Institute, Cambridge, Massachusetts, USA; for writing the foreword of this book, as no other person in the field of Periodontology is more respected than him. I have been fortunate to obtain his valuable expert guidance and knowledge.

I particularly thank Head of Department, Dr Suresh DK who had been a constant source of helpful ideas concerned with photography. Special thanks to Dr RK Sharma, Dr SK Salaria and Dr Veenu Madaan for their creative comments at every step during the preparation of the book.

I wish to express my gratitude to all the contributors who have helped me in preparing the manuscript of the book and providing their knowledge in the concerned field. I would like to thank the postgraduate students for proofreading of this book—Dr Akanksha, Dr Nitika, Dr Rachna, Dr Anushi, Dr Anish, Dr Rajni, Dr Sugandha, Dr Harveen Singh, Dr Deepak, Dr Jyotsna and Dr Amita. Thanks to Dr Amita, Dr Arvind, departmental colleagues and all of my students, your questions and insights have challenged and strengthened me to present this work in a more friendly way to your desk.

I appreciate the willing help of Dr SK Salaria, Dr Rohit Singal, Dr Tanu Bansal, Dr Ameesha Singla, Dr Siddharth Ahluwalia, Dr Parul Rana, and Dr Megha Verma for helping me to make the figures of the book.

I would like to acknowledge Shri Tarsem Garg, Chancellor, MM University, Mullana, Ambala, Haryana, India and the management who have given me a platform where I am today and a full access to the library for my manuscript.

My thanks to Shri Jitendar P Vij (Chairman and Managing Director), Mr Tarun Duneja (Director-Publishing) and the editorial staff of M/s Jaypee Brothers Medical Publishers (P) Ltd, New Delhi, India, who have done a great job "to put an icing on the cake" by way of their professional expertise to make my work reader-friendly and reach it to your desk.

I gratefully acknowledge my debt to my father-in-law Dr JC Bathla for nurturing the seeds of this endeavor at its infancy. My brother Mr Pankaj Chandna, sister-in-law Mrs Neelu Chandna and nephew Raghav has selflessly and lovingly been there for me. For the continuous blessing and encouragement I wish to express my gratitude to my parents Smt Santosh Chandna and Shri GR Chandna; mother-in-law Smt Pushpa Bathla for blessing me at all stages of life.

I wish to express my deepest thanks to my husband Dr Manish Bathla for great assistance in typing the manuscript and unconditional love and support during the many hours of forced isolation and commitment required to accomplish this feat.

The acknowledgment would not be complete if I do not express my thanks and love to my dear son Milind who unknowingly helped me by his smiles and love at times of difficulty and always motivated me by saying three little words "Buck-up Mummy"!

Contents

Section Two: Classification and Epidemiology

Section Three: Etiology

Section Four: Pathology of Gingival and Periodontal Diseases

Section Five: Diagnosis

Section Six: Treatment

A. Non-surgical Therapy

B. Surgical Therapy

Section Seven: Interdisciplinary Approach

Section Eight: Implantology

Section Nine: Advances

Veenu Madaan Hans, Shaveta Sood, Shalu Bathla

Lasers

Photodynamic Therapy

Tissue Engineering

Gene Therapy

Nanotechnology

Periodontal Vaccine

Minimally Invasive Surgery

Section Ten: Maintenance Phase

Section Eleven: Miscellaneous

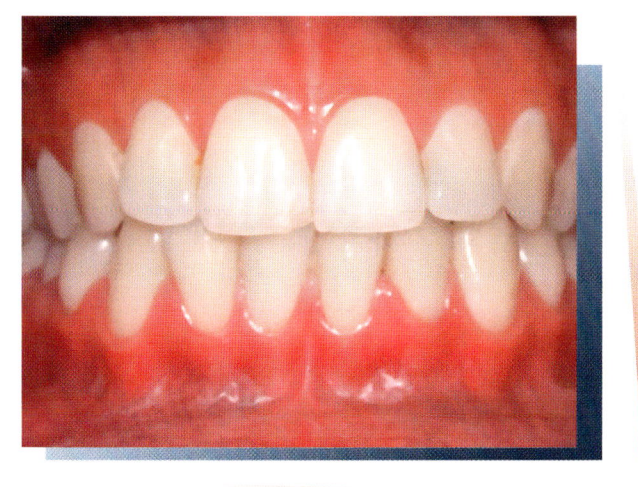

SECTION

ONE

NORMAL
PERIODONTIUM

CHAPTER 1

Gingiva

Shalu Bathla

DEFINITION

Gingiva is the part of oral mucosa that covers the alveolar processes of the jaws and surrounds the necks of the teeth.

MACROSCOPIC FEATURES

Anatomically, the gingiva is classified into three distinct domains: Free/marginal gingiva, attached gingiva and interdental gingiva **(Fig. 1.1).**

1. Free gingiva
2. Interdental gingiva
3. Attached gingiva

1. Marginal gingiva is the terminal edge of the gingiva surrounding the teeth in a collar – like fashion. The marginal gingiva is called free as it is not attached to the underlying periosteum of alveolar bone. The gingival margin is demarcated from attached gingiva by an indentation called as free gingival groove which is positioned at a level corresponding to the level of the cementoenamel junction (CEJ). Free gingival groove is only present in about 30-40% of adults. Functionally, the marginal gingiva forms the soft tissue wall of the V - shaped gingival sulcus. Gingival sulcus is a shallow groove between the tooth and normal gingiva that extends from the free surface of the junctional epithelium coronally to the level of free gingival margin.

2. Interdental gingiva is the part of the gingiva which is present in the interdental space beneath the area of tooth contact. In the presence of diastema the interdental papilla is absent **(Fig. 1.2).**

   Col is a valley like depression which connects the facial and lingual papillae and conforms to the shape of the interproximal contact areas **(Fig. 1.3)**. Col epithelium is identical to junctional epithelium having the same origin (from dental epithelium), non-keratinized and gradually replaced by continuing cell division.

3. Attached gingiva is firm, resilient and tightly bound to the underlying periosteum of alveolar bone and cementum by connective tissue fibers. The attached gingiva is thus, firmly entrenched between two movable structures – the marginal gingiva coronally and the alveolar mucosa apically.

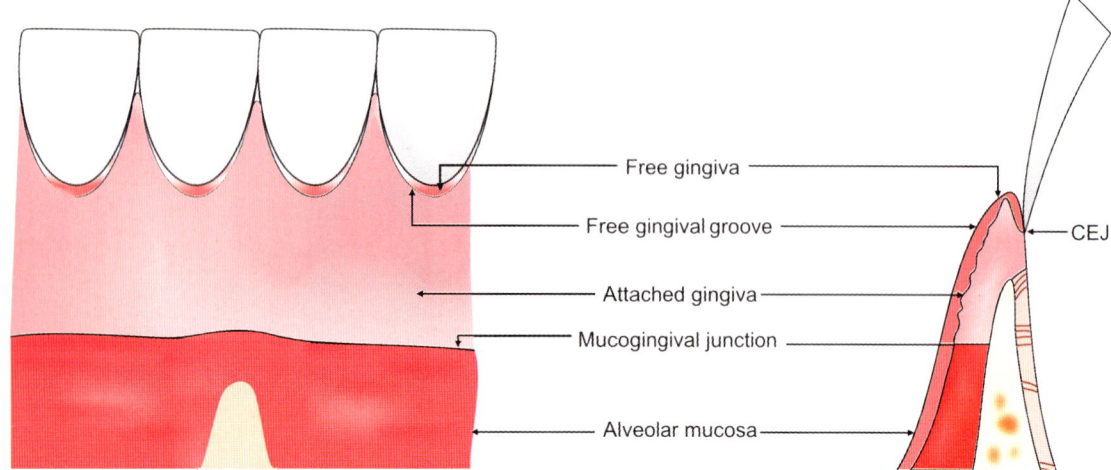

Fig. 1.1: Macroscopic features of gingiva

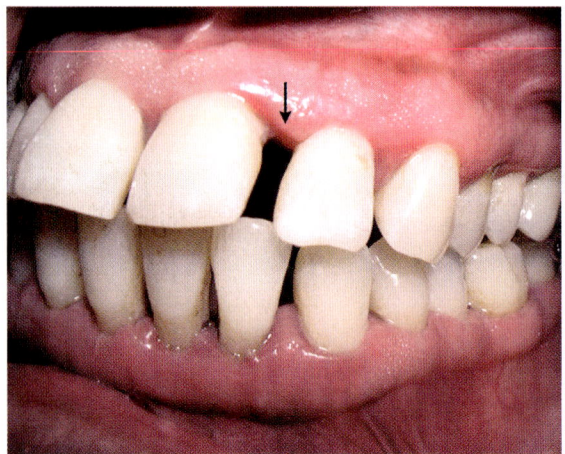

Fig. 1.2: Absence of interdental papilla in the diastema

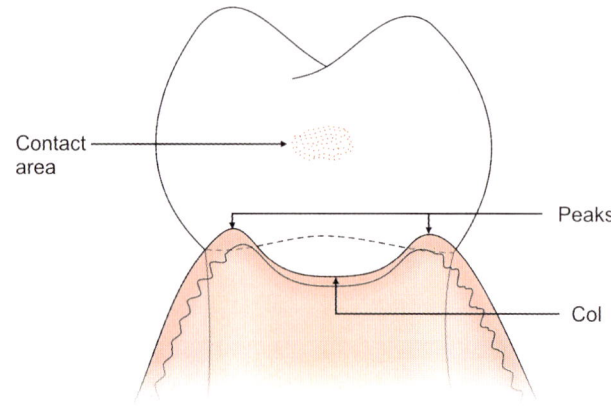

Fig. 1.3: Showing col and peaks

Width of attached gingiva: It is the distance between mucogingival junction and the projection on the external surface of the bottom of gingival sulcus/periodontal pocket. The dimensions of the attached gingiva vary from the anterior to the posterior teeth. Width of attached gingiva on facial aspect of – maxillary incisor region is 3.5 to 4.5 mm, mandibular incisor region is 3.3 to 3.9 mm, maxillary first premolar is 1.9 mm and mandibular first premolar is 1.8 mm approx. Width of attached gingiva increases with age and in supraerupted teeth. This increase in dimension occurs as a result of an increase in the height of the alveolar process which in turn is the result of passive eruption.

Significance of attached gingiva:

a. It gives support to the marginal gingiva.

b. It provides attachment or a solid base for the movable alveolar mucosa for the action of lips, cheeks and tongue.

c. It can withstand frictional and functional stresses of mastication and toothbrushing. When the marginal tissue is alveolar mucosa, it does not resist the functional stresses of toothbrush trauma imposed on it. Frequently, the result is apical shifting of the marginal tissue and additional recession. Attached gingiva has more densely organized connective tissue and is more firmly bound to the underlying periosteum and bone. Consequently, it is more resistant to the functional stresses placed upon it. Alveolar mucosa is thin, delicate tissue, poorly attached to bone and cementum and is not capable of withstanding these same functional stresses.

d. Attached gingiva acts as a barrier for passage of inflammation. A tooth having alveolar mucosa at its margin seems to show clinical signs of inflammation in the presence of microbial flora more readily than does a corresponding tooth that has a sufficient band of attached gingiva. Such marginal tissue appears to be more susceptible to the products of inflammation that may result in pocket formation or apical migration of both attachment apparatus and marginal tissues.

e. It provides resistance to tensional stresses. Attached gingiva serves as a buffer between the mobile free gingival margin and mobile alveolar mucosa. There are skeletal muscle fibers within the alveolar mucosa that exert a force in an apical direction on the attached gingiva. This force is dissipated by bound down keratinized tissue.

Width of attached gingiva can be measured:

a. *Anatomically*: Stretch the lip/cheek to demarcate the mucogingival line while pocket is being probed. Measure the total width of gingiva (gingival margin to mucogingival line) and subtract the sulcus/pocket depth from it to determine width of attached gingiva.

b. *Functionally*:
   • *Tension test*: Stretch the lip or cheek outward and forward to mark mucogingival line. Measure the total width of gingiva (gingival margin to mucogingival line) and subtract the sulcus/pocket depth from it to determine width of attached gingiva.
   • *Roll test*: Push the adjacent mucosa coronally with a dull instrument to mark mucogingival line. Measure the total width of gingiva (gingival margin to mucogingival line) and subtract the sulcus/pocket depth from it to determine width of attached gingiva. A more reliable method of identifying the mucogingival junction would be to take the side of a periodontal probe or similar blunt instrument and jiggle the alveolar mucosa in an apicoronal direction. Since the alveolar mucosa is mobile, it will roll up ahead of the blunt instrument.

c. *Histochemically*: Iodine staining test: Paint the gingiva and oral mucosa with Schiller's or Lugol's solution (iodine and potassium iodide solution). The alveolar mucosa takes on a brown color owing to its glycogen content, while the glycogen free, attached gingiva remains unstained. Measure the total width of the unstained gingiva and subtract the sulcus/pocket depth from it to determine width of attached gingiva.

The other dimension that may play a significant role in the maintenance of the periodontal health is the thickness of the gingiva. Gingival phenotype or biotype has been classified by Eger and Muller into thick and thin or Class I, IIA and IIB. Thick gingival phenotype seems to be more conducive to periodontal health. A thin phenotype predisposes to gingival recession and increased tendency to gingival inflammation **(Fig. 1.4).**

Mucogingival junction is the interface between the apically located alveolar mucosa and the coronally located attached gingiva which remains stationary throughout life. Mucogingival junction is present on the three gingival surfaces namely facial gingiva of the maxilla, facial and lingual gingiva of the mandible. The palatal gingiva of the maxilla is continuous with the tissue of the palate, which is bound down to the palatal bones. Because the palate is devoid of freely movable alveolar mucosa, there is no mucogingival junction.

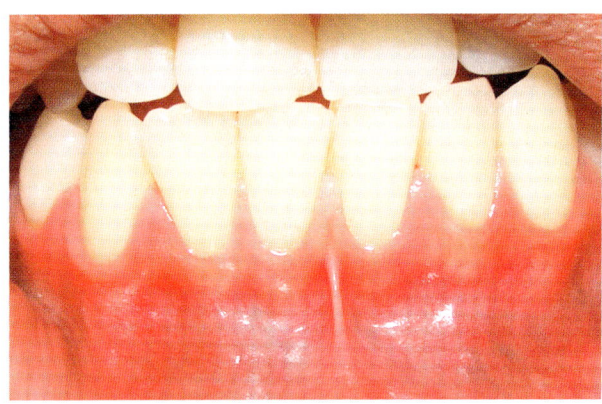

Fig. 1.4: Thin gingival phenotype

TABLE 1.1: Differences between alveolar mucosa and attached gingiva

		Alveolar mucosa	Attached gingiva
1.	Color	Red	Pink
2.	Surface texture	Smooth and shiny	Stippled
3.	Epithelium	• Thinner	• Thicker
		• Rete pegs absent	• Rete pegs present
		• Nonkeratinized	• Parakeratinized
4.	Connective tissue	• More loosely arranged	• Not so loosely arranged
		• More blood vessels	• Moderate blood vessels

MICROSCOPIC FEATURES

Histologically, gingiva is composed of gingival epithelium, epithelium-connective tissue interface and underlying connective tissue.

Gingival Epithelium

The gingival epithelium is comprised of oral epithelium, sulcular epithelium and junctional epithelium (**Fig. 1.5 and Table 1.2**).

i. Oral epithelium/outer epithelium: It covers the crest and outer surface of marginal gingiva and surface of the attached gingiva. It is a keratinized stratified squamous epithelium.

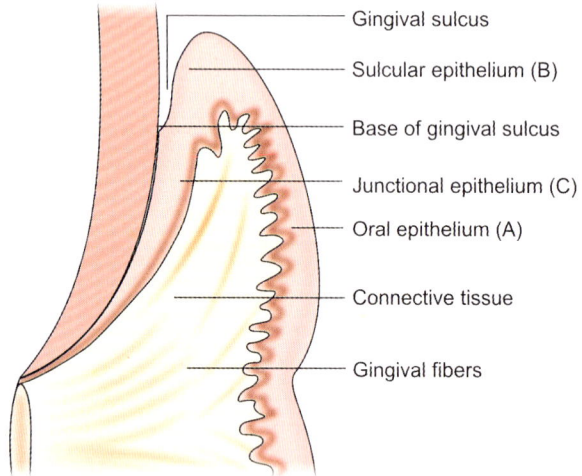

Fig. 1.5: Microscopic features of gingiva: A. Oral epithelium, B. Sulcular epithelium, C. Junctional epithelium

Following are the layers of oral epithelium (**Fig. 1.6**):

*   *Stratum basale*: The cells are either cylindric or cuboid. The basal cells are found immediately adjacent to the connective tissue and are separated from connective tissue by a basement membrane. It is the germinative layer, having the ability to divide. When two daughter cells have been formed by cell division, an adjacent older basal cell is pushed into the spinous cell layer and starts, as a keratinocyte, to traverse the epithelium. It takes approximately 1 month for a keratinocyte to reach the outer epithelial surface, where it is shed from the stratum corneum.
*   *Stratum spinosum*: It is a prickle cell layer in which large polyhedral cells with short cytoplasmic processes are present. The uppermost cells of this layer contain granules called as keratinosomes or Odland bodies, which are modified lysosomes. They contain a large amount of acid phosphatase, an enzyme which is involved in the destruction of organelle membranes.
*   *Stratum granulosum*: Cells of this layer are flattened in a plane parallel to the gingival surface. Keratohyaline granules which are associated with

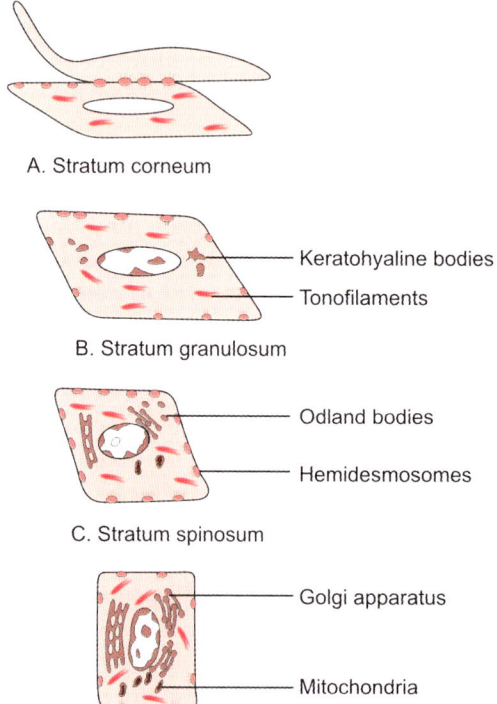

Fig. 1.6: Representative cells of various layers of stratified squamous epithelium

TABLE 1.2: Differences between oral, sulcular and junctional epithelium

	Oral	Sulcular	Junctional
1. Keratinization	Keratinized	Non-keratinized	Non-keratinized
2. Rete pegs	Present	Absent	Absent
3. Strata granuloma and corneum	Present	Lacking	Lacking
4. Merkel cells	Present	Absent	Absent
5. Langerhans cells	Present	Few	Absent
6. Type IV collagen in basal lamina	Present	Absent	Absent
7. Tight junctions	More	Few	Few
8. Acid phosphatase activity	Present	Lacking	Lacking
9. Glycolytic enzyme activity	High	Lower	Lower
10. Intercellular space	Narrower	Narrower	Wider

keratin formation are (1 μm in diameter) round in shape and appear in the cytoplasm of the cell.

- *Stratum corneum*: It consists of closely packed, flattened cells that have lost nuclei and most other organelles as they become keratinized. The cells are densely packed with tonofilaments. Clear, rounded bodies probably representing lipid droplets appear within the cytoplasm of the cell.

ii. Sulcular epithelium: It lines the gingival sulcus. It is a non-keratinized, stratified squamous epithelium which extends from the coronal end of the junctional epithelium to the crest of the gingival margin.

iii. Junctional epithelium (JE): Junctional epithelium consists of collar like band of stratified squamous nonkeratinized epithelium. The normal length of junctional epithelium is 0.25 -1.35 mm.

Development/Origin of Junctional Epithelium

Before the tooth begins its eruptive movements, the crown of the tooth is covered by a double layer of epithelial cells. The inner layer of cells called ameloblasts which have completed their formative function, develops hemi-desmosomes and becomes firmly attached to the enamel surface. The outer layer consists of more flattened cells, the remnants of all the remaining layers of the dental organ. Together these two layers are called as reduced enamel epithelium. Connective tissue present between this reduced enamel epithelium and the overlying oral epithelium breaks down, and degenerates when the tooth eruption begins in the oral cavity. The cells of the outer layer of reduced enamel epithelium and the basal cells of the oral epithelium proliferate and migrate into the degenerative connective tissue and thus eventually fuse to establish a mass of epithelial cells over the erupting tooth. Cell death in the middle of this epithelial plug leads to the formation of an epithelium-lined canal through which the tooth erupts without hemorrhage. From this mass of epithelium, together with the remaining reduced dental epithelium, the epithelial component of dentogingival junction is established. The reduced ameloblasts, which have lost and do not regain the ability to divide, change their morphology and are transformed into squamous epithelial cells that retain their attachment to the enamel surface. The cells of the outer layer of reduced enamel epithelium which retain their ability to divide, become and function as basal cells of a forming junctional epithelium.

It was first named epithelial attachment (Epithelansatz) by Gottlieb, but later it was examined electron microscopically and was renamed as junctional, or attachment epithelium by Stern. This epithelium synthesizes the material that attaches it to the tooth. This material, its morphology, mode and mechanism of function, is what is now called the epithelial attachment. Thus, the cellular structure is referred to as junctional or attachment epithelium and its extracellular tooth attaching substance is referred to as the epithelial attachment.

Junctional epithelium is divided into three zones: the apical, middle and coronal zone. The middle zone is the zone with the maximum adhesiveness, and the coronal zone is the most permeable of the three zones.

Junctional epithelium has three surfaces: Internal surface which faces the tooth surface, external surface which faces the gingival connective tissue and coronal surface of the junctional epithelium forms the base of the sulcus. Junctional epithelium is attached to the tooth surface by means of internal basal lamina and to gingival connective tissue by an external basal lamina. The attachment of junctional epithelium to the tooth is mediated through an ultramicroscopic mechanism defined as the epithelial attachment apparatus. It consists of hemidesosomes at the plasma membrane of the cells directly attached to the tooth (DAT cells) and a basal lamina like extracellular matrix, termed the internal basal lamina, on the tooth surface **(Fig. 1.7)**.

Junctional epithelium is easily penetrated because of the following factors:

i. Along the junctional epithelium, subepithelial vessels are parallel to the surface and are made up mostly of venules rather than capillaries. These venules have a greater disposition towards increased permeability

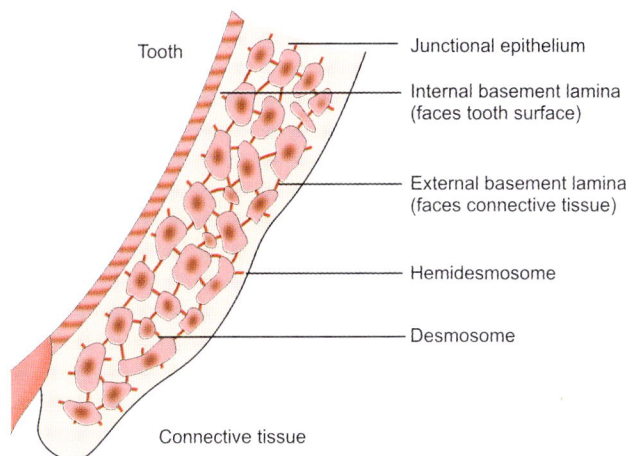

Fig. 1.7: Junctional epithelium

than do capillaries and arterioles and they are more susceptible to hemorrhage and thrombosis.

ii. Few intercellular tight junctions
iii. Minimal cytoplasmic filaments
iv. Higher number of intercellular spaces
v. Lower number of desmosomes.

Functions: Junctional epithelium serves many roles in regulating tissue health:

i. Provides attachment to the tooth.
ii. Acts as barrier attached to the tooth and thus forms an epithelial barrier against the plaque bacteria. External basement membrane laterally forms an effective barrier against invading microbes.
iii. Rapid cell division and funneling of junctional epithelial cells towards the sulcus hinder bacterial colonization and repair of damaged tissue occurs rapidly.
iv. Allow GCF flow—Junctional epithelium allows the access of GCF, inflammatory cells and components of the immunological host defense to the gingival margin. Junctional epithelium allows two - way movement of variety of substances: a.From connective tissue into crevice – Gingival fluid exudates, PMNs, Ig, complement and various cells of immune system; b. From crevice to connective tissue – Foreign material such as carbon particles, trypan blue.
v. Active antimicrobial substances are produced by junctional epithelial cells. These include defensins, lysosomal enzymes, calprotectin and cathelicidin.
vi. Epithelial cells activated by microbial substances secrete chemokines, e.g. IL-1, IL-6, IL-8 and TNF-α that attract and activate professional defense cells such as lymphocytes and PMNs.

Cells present in the gingival epithelium are namely keratinocytes and non- keratinocytes:

1. *Keratinocytes:* These make up 90% of the total gingival cell population. They originate from the ectodermal germ layer. Structurally, keratinocytes are like any other cells having cell organelles like nucleus, cytosol, ribosomes, Golgi apparatus. Keratinocytes have melanosomes, which are the pigment bearing granules present in these cells only and not in the other cells of periodontium. The main function of the gingival epithelium, i.e. protection and barrier against the oral environment is achieved by the proliferation and differentiation of the keratinocytes. Keratinocytes have to move from basal to superficial layers of the epithelium as the process of differentiation occurs in a basocoronal direction culminating in the formation of a keratin barrier. The microfilaments present in the keratinocytes help in cell motility and maintenance of the polarity.

Keratinocyte motility requires the following steps:

- Development of lamellopodia, i.e. extensions on the leading edge of the cell towards the direction of movement.
- Attachment of this portion of the cell to the substratum.
- Movement of the cytosolic material towards the leading edge of the cell.
- Detachment of the rear end.

2. *Non-keratinocytes/Clear cells*: The various non-keratinocytes are Langerhans cells, merkel cells and melanocytes.

Langerhans cells (LCs) are modified monocytes belonging to reticuloendothelial system which reside chiefly in suprabasal layers. They are responsible for communication with immune system by acting as antigen – presenting cells for lymphocytes. These cells containg - specific elongated granules called as Birbecks granules and have marked adenosine triphosphatase activity. Paul Langerhans used gold impregnation technique 100 years ago to visualize LCs. They are the only epidermal cells which express receptors for C3 and Fc portion of IgG. Langerhans cells can move in and out of the epithelium unlike melanocytes.

Merkel cells are located in deeper layers of epithelium. These are not dendritic cells as melanocytes and Langerhans cells. These cells possess keratin tonofilaments and occasional desmosomes which link them to adjacent cells. Merkel cells are sensory in nature and respond to touch.

Melanocytes originate from neural crest cells found in the stratum basale of the gingival oral epithelium. Oral mucosal melanocytes were identified in gingiva by Laidlaw and Cahn in 1932. These cells have long dendritic processes that are found interspersed between the keratinocytes of the epithelium. They lack tonofilaments and desmosomal connection to adjacent keratinocytes. Melanocytes are the cells which are responsible for the barrier to UV damage and synthesize melanin which is responsible for providing color to gingiva. Melanin is synthesized in organelle called premelanosomes/melanosomes in melanocytes cells. Melanosomes are transported along microtubules and actin filaments to the cell periphery. Melanocytes bind to the plasma membrane and transfer the melanosomes to adjacent keratinocytes **(Fig. 1.8)**. The precise mechanism is unknown, but has been described as cytocrine secretion. Sometimes, in the connective tissue

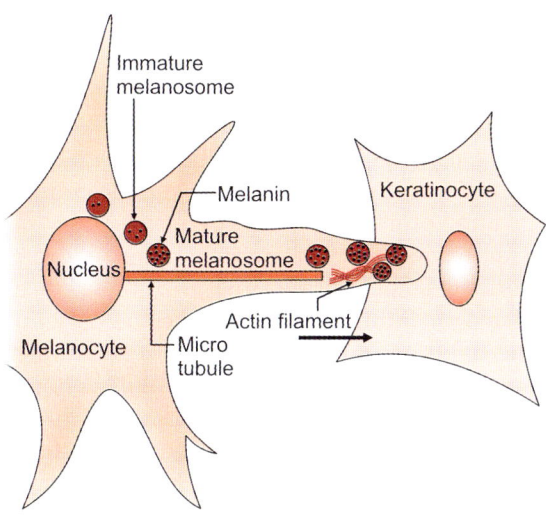

Fig. 1.8: Mechanism of melanosome transport

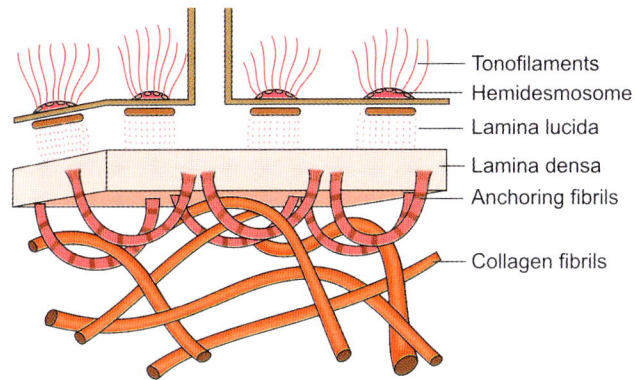

Fig. 1.9: Basal lamina—Junction between epithelium and connective tissue

macrophages take up the melanosomes produced by melanocytes in the epithelium and are called as melanophages/melanophores. Melanocytes may be classified as active or inactive, depending on presence or absence of mature melanosomes. The ratio of melanocytes to keratinocytes producing epithelial cells is approx. 1:36 cells.

Epithelium—Connective Tissue Interface

Ultrastructurally, epithelial – connective tissue interface is composed of 4 elements namely *basal cell plasma membrane* with its specialized attachment devices (hemidesmosomes), *lamina lucida* an electrolucent zone of 25 to 45 nm wide and *lamina densa* an electrodense zone of 40 to 60 nm thickness where type IV collagen is present and last is *reticular layer*. From the lamina densa so called anchoring fibrils project in a fan-shaped fashion into the connective tissue **(Fig. 1.9)**.

The various junctional complexes present in gingiva are:

- Tight/occluding junctions are formed by the fusion of external leaflets of adjacent cell membranes at a series of points.
- Adhesive junctions:
  Cell to cell
  - Zonula adherens
  - Desmosomes: It is the most common type of junction which consists of two adjacent attachment plaques one from each cell that are separated by an interval of approx. 30 nm.

Cell to matrix
  - Focal adhesions
  - Hemidesmosomes
- *Communicating (gap) junctions*: They have intercellular pipes/channels that apparently bridge both the adjacent membranes and intercellular space. The intercellular space in gap junction is approx. 3 nm and is the major pathway for direct intercellular communication.

Gingival Connective Tissue / Lamina Propria

The gingival connective tissue consists of gingival fibers, various cells and ground substance.

Gingival Fibers

Fibers in human gingiva are made up of collagen, reticulin and elastin. Collagen fibers make up more than 50% of the volume of human gingiva. Types I, III, IV, V, VI of collagen are present in gingiva. Type I collagen predominates. The structural formula for type I collagen is $[\alpha1\,(I)\,]_2\,\alpha2$. Type III collagen is fetal collagen which is important in the early phases of wound healing and remains in an unmineralized form. Type III collagen in the gingiva is partly responsible for the maintenance of space in the healing matrix. Type IV collagen is present in the lamina densa layer of the basement membrane of the epithelium. Type VI collagen is distributed with the elastin fibers along the blood vessels. The type VI collagen fibers impart rigidity required to maintain the elastic blood vessel wall from undergoing permanent deformation. Type VII collagen acts as anchoring fibrils that help to reinforce epithelial attachment to the underlying connective tissue.

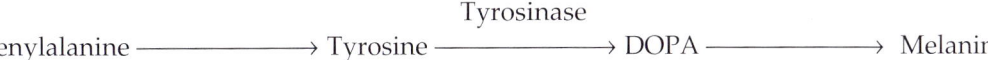

$$\text{Phenylalanine} \xrightarrow{\hspace{2cm}} \text{Tyrosine} \xrightarrow{\text{Tyrosinase}} \text{DOPA} \xrightarrow{\hspace{2cm}} \text{Melanin}$$

PERIODONTICS REVISITED

The functions of these fibers are:
a. To stabilize the attached gingiva to the alveolar process.
b. To stabilize the attached gingiva to the tooth.
c. Helps to maintain the epithelial seal to the tooth.
d. To provide stability to the tooth.
e. To brace marginal/free gingiva firmly against the tooth and adjacent attached gingiva.
f. To provide rigidity to withstand forces of mastication without being deflected away from the tooth surface.

Gingival fibers are arranged into following groups **(Fig. 1.10)**:
i. *Dentogingival group*: These fibers extend from the cementum apical to junctional epithelium and course laterally and coronally into lamina propria of the gingiva. These provide gingival support.

ii. *Alveologingival group*: These fibers arise from the alveolar crest and insert coronally into lamina propria of the gingiva. Attaches attached gingiva to alveolar bone.
iii. *Circular group*: This group of fibers encircle the teeth in a cuff or ring like fashion. Maintain contour and position of free marginal gingiva.
iv. *Transseptal fibers*: These are the group of prominent horizontal fibers located interproximally that extend from cementum of one tooth to the cementum of the neighboring tooth. Maintain relationship of adjacent teeth, protect interproximal bone. The transseptal fibers collectively form an interdental ligament connecting all the teeth of the arch. This ligament, although belonging to the supraalveolar fiber apparatus, appears to be uniquely important in maintaining the integrity of the dental arch. It is

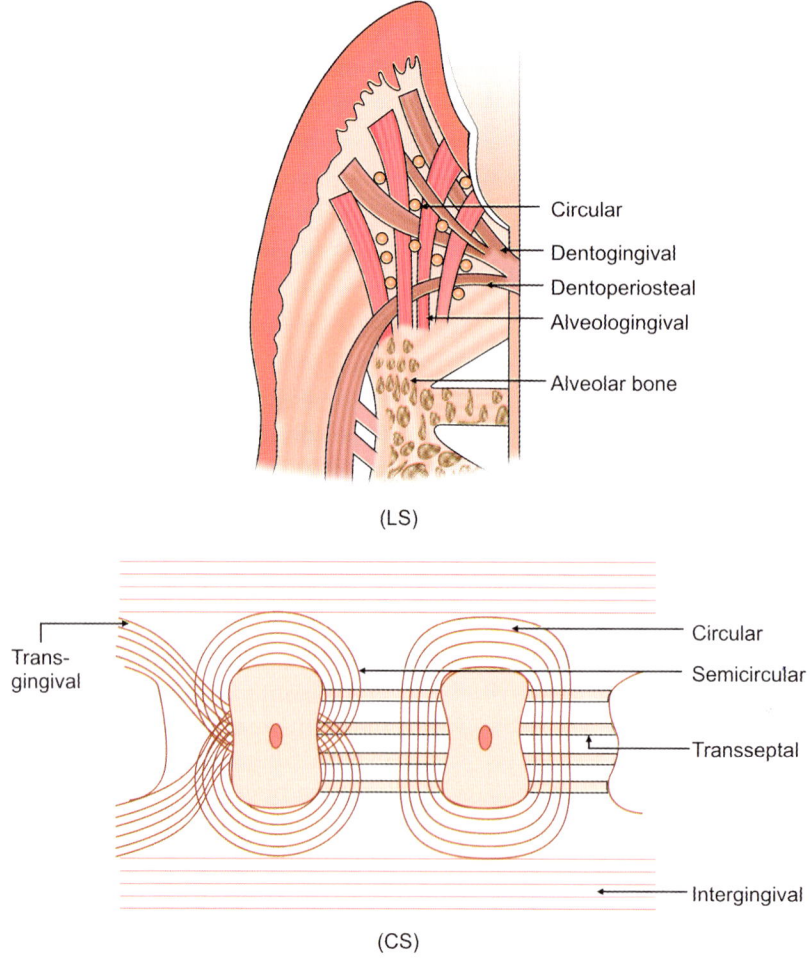

(LS)

Trans-
gingival

Circular
Semicircular
Transseptal
Intergingival

(CS)

Fig. 1.10: Gingival fibers

rapidly reformed after excision. Residual portions of transseptal fibers are seen, even in advanced stages of resting periodontal disease.

v. *Dentoperiosteal group*: On the oral and vestibular surfaces of jaws, dentoperiosteal group of fibers extends from the tooth, passing over the alveolar crest to blend with fibers of the periosteum of the alveolar bone. Anchors tooth to bone, protect periodontal ligament.

vi. *Semicircular group*: Group of fibers which attach at the proximal surface of a tooth, immediately below the cementoenamel junction, go around the facial or lingual marginal gingiva of the tooth and attach on the other proximal surface of the same tooth.

vii. *Transgingival group*: Fibers that attach in the proximal surface of one tooth, transverse the interdental space diagonally, go around the facial or lingual surface of the adjacent tooth, again traverse diagonally the interdental space and attach in the proximal surface of the next tooth. Secure alignment of teeth in the arch.

viii. *Intergingival group*: These fibers run parallel to dentition on vestibular and oral surfaces. They provide contour and support for the attached gingiva.

ix. *Interpapillary group*: They are seen in the interdental gingiva extending in a faciolingual direction. Provide support for interdental gingiva.

Dentogingival, dentoperiosteal and alveologingival fibers group provide the attachment of gingiva to the tooth and to the bony structure. Fibers of circular, semicircular, transgingival, intergingival and transseptal bundles connect teeth to one another.

Cells

- Fibroblasts are derived from the undifferentiated progenitor mesenchymal cells that are present in the follicle. These are elongated or spindle shaped cells having prominent rough endoplasmic reticulum and golgi apparatus. Their cytoplasm is usually rich in mitochondria, vacuoles and vesicles. They play important role in the development, maintenance and repair of the gingival connective tissue. These cells have the ability to not only respond to paracrine as well as autocrine signals but also synthesize and secrete a number of growth factors, cytokines and metabolic products.
- Mast cells are located perivascularly and are identified by their unique cytoplasmic granules which produce heparin and histamine.

- Other cells are eosinophils, macrophages, adipose and inflammatory cells (neutrophils, plasma cells and lymphocytes).

Ground Substance

The cells, fibers, nerves and vessels of the gingiva are embedded in a viscous, gel-like ground substance. The ground substance is composed of proteoglycans and glycoproteins, which facilitates cell movement and diffusion of various biologically active substances. A number of proteoglycans have been identified in the gingival tissues including decorin, biglycan, versican and syndecan. Glycoproteins identified in gingival connective tissue are fibronectin, tenascin, osteonectin and laminin.

BLOOD SUPPLY

Arterial supply: Blood vessels are easily evidenced in tissue sections by means of immunohistochemical reactions. Earlier techniques like histoenzymatic reactions and perfusion with India ink into experimental animals techniques were used. There are three sources of blood supply to gingiva namely *supraperiosteal arterioles, vessels of periodontal ligament and arterioles emerging from the crest of the interdental septa* **(Fig. 1.11)**. Supraperiosteal arterioles mainly supply free gingiva and gingival sulcus. These arterioles are the terminal branches of sublingual artery, mental artery, buccal artery, facial artery, greater palatine artery, infraorbital artery and posterior superior dental artery. Vessels of periodontal ligament mainly supply col area. Arterioles

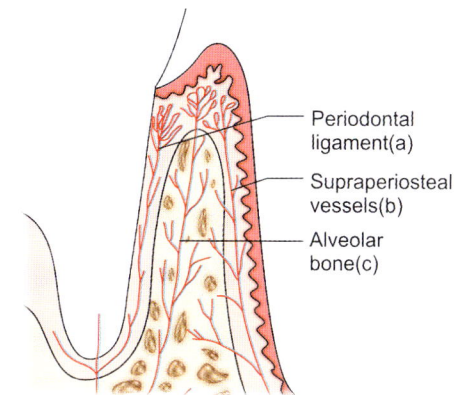

Fig. 1.11: Gingival blood supply derives from: a. Periodontal ligament, b. Supraperiosteal vessels, c. Alveolar bone

Periodontal ligament(a)

Supraperiosteal vessels(b)

Alveolar bone(c)

PERIODONTICS REVISITED

emerging from the crest of the interdental septa mainly supply attached gingiva.

Dentogingival plexus are plexus of blood vessels beneath junctional epithelium. The blood vessels in this plexus have a thickness of approximately 40 μm, which means that these are mainly venules. No capillary loops occur in it, in healthy gingiva. Subepithelial plexus are plexus of blood vessels beneath oral epithelium of free and attached gingiva, yield thin capillary loops of 7 μm to each connective tissue papilla.

The venous and lymphatic vessels follow a course closely paralleling that of arterial supply. Lymphatic drainage starts in the connective tissue papillae and drains into regional lymph nodes. Buccal gingiva of maxilla, buccal and lingual gingiva of mandibular premolar and molar region drains into submandibular lymph nodes. Mandibular incisor region drains into submental lymph nodes whereas third molars region drains into jugulodigastric lymph nodes. Their main function is to return fluids and filterable plasma components to the blood via the thoracic duct.

NERVE SUPPLY

The various regions of gingiva are innervated by end branches of trigeminal nerve. The gingiva on the labial aspect of maxillary incisors, canines, premolars is innervated by the superior labial branches from infraorbital nerve. Buccal gingiva in maxillary molar region is innervated by branches from posterior superior dental nerve. Palatal gingiva is innervated by greater palatal nerve except incisors area which is innervated by sphenopalatine nerve. Lingual gingiva in mandible is innervated by sublingual nerve, a branch of lingual nerve. Gingiva on the labial aspect of mandibular incisiors and canines is innervated by mental nerve. Buccal aspect of molars is innervated by buccal nerve. Innervations of mandibular premolars is by both mental and buccal nerve. In the attached gingiva, most nerves terminate within the lamina propria, and only a few endings occur between epithelial cells. Meissner type tactile corpuscles, Krause type end bulbs and encapsulated spindles are the types of neural terminals.

CLINICAL CRITERIA OF NORMAL GINGIVA

Color

Color of the gingiva is described as coral pink which depends upon vascular supply, thickness of epithelium,

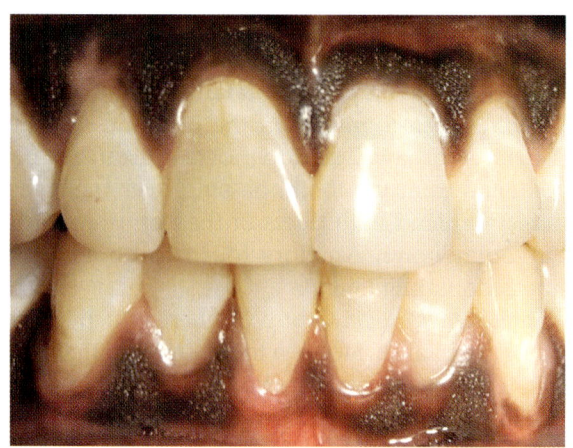
Fig. 1.12: Generalized melanin pigmentation

degree of keratinization of epithelium and presence of pigment containing cells **(Fig. 1.12)**.

A variation in gingival pigmentation is not produced by variation in the number of pigment forming melanocytes but by genetically determined variation in their pigment producing capacity. Thus, variations in gingival pigmentation are related to complexion and race. It is lighter in blond individuals with a fair complexion than in dark complexioned individuals. In the Caucasian individuals pigmentation is minimal, in African or Asian individuals there are brown or blue-black areas of pigmentation while in Mediterranean people occasional patches of pigmentation are found.

Gingival pigmentation was classified according to modification of melanin index:

Category 0: No pigmentation
Category 1: Solitary unit(s) of pigmentation in papillary gingiva without formation of continuous ribbon between solitary units.
Category 2: At least 1 unit of formation of continuous ribbon extending from two neighboring solitary units.

Surface Texture

The surface texture of free gingiva is smooth whereas of attached gingiva is stippled. Pitted surface texture giving orange peel appearance is called as stippling which is more prominent on the labial than on the lingual gingival surfaces. Stippling is normally present on attached gingiva and center of interdental papilla. It is best viewed by drying the gingiva and switching off the chair light. Stippling varies with age, it appears usually in children of about 5 years and increases with age but is absent in old age.

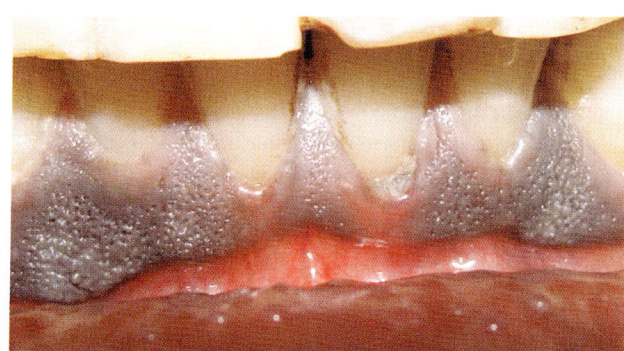

Fig. 1.13: Stippling seen on attached gingiva and center of interdental papilla

Histologically: The bottom of the pits correspond to deep ridges or projections of epithelium into lamina propria of the connective tissue. The protruding parts correspond to thinner epithelium overridges or projections of the connective tissue. The ridge and the peg arrangements between the epithelium and connective tissue provide excellent mechanical stability between the two tissue components as well as large contact interphase for metabolic interchange. In erythematous tissue stippling may disappear, although it may be present in thick fibrotic tissue **(Fig. 1.13),** which is diseased. Stippling is not an absolute sign of health and the absence of it is not necessarily a sign of disease.

Contour

The marginal gingiva follows a scalloped outline normally and straight line along teeth with relatively flat surfaces. Attached gingiva has festooned appearance with intermittent prominence corresponding to contour of roots. When the teeth are placed more labially, then the normal arcuate contour is accentuated and gingiva is located farther apically. When teeth are lingually placed, the gingiva is horizontal and thickened. Thus, contour of gingiva depends upon shape and alignment of the teeth in the arch. It also depends upon the location and size of the area of proximal contacts and dimensions of the embrasures.

Shape

Shape of interdental gingiva depends upon contour of the proximal tooth surface, location and shape of the proximal contact and dimensions of the gingival embrasures. The interdental papilla is pointed and pyramidal in normal contact areas and in anterior regions. But it is flat or saddle shaped in ... and in molar regions.

Size

The size of the gingiva corresponds to the sum total o. the bulk of cellular and intercellular elements and their vascular supply.

Consistency

On palpation with a blunt instrument, attached gingiva should be firm, resilient and tightly bound to the underlying hard tissues. The abundant collagen fibers and the non-collagenous protein combines to give gingiva, the firm consistency.

LANDMARK STUDIES RELATED

Ainamo A, Ainamo J. The width of attached gingiva on supraerupted teeth. Journal of Periodontal Research 1978;13:194–18.

This study comprised 28 first and second maxillary molars which in the lack of antagonists had erupted beyond the occlusal plane. The maxillary mucogingival junction was marked with short pieces of metal wires, orthopantograms were taken and the distance from the mucogingival junction to the floor of the nasal cavity and to the cementoenamel junction were measured to the nearest mm. Eleven measurable occluding contralateral teeth were used as controls. A comparison was also made between the supraerupted teeth and the previously measured normally occluding teeth. The results indicated that even during pronounced supraeruption, the teeth tend to erupt with their investing tissues while the location of the mucogingival junction remains constant. This finding is of special interest as it would make possible to treat the problem of a too narrow zone of attached gingiva by grinding the tooth out of occlusion and allowing it and its gingival margin to erupt. The anatomical width of attached gingiva, i.e. the distance from the mucogingival junction to the cementoenamel junction was found to be 3.7 mm wider in the supraerupted teeth than in the normal occluding control teeth.

Caffesse RG, Nasjleti CE, Castelli WA. The role of sulcular environment in controlling epithelial keratinization. Journal of Periodontology 1979; 50:1-6.

The influence of the sulcular environment on the keratinization of the outer surface gingival epithelium

sted in three young adult rhesus monkeys. A
of 40 mucoperiosteal flaps were raised and
erted so as to bring the outer surface epithelium in
ontact with the tooth and were sutured. The monkeys
were sacrified after giving H$_3$ thymidine one hour
prior. The material was prepared for histologic and
radioautographic evaluation. Results indicated that
the outer surface epithelium changes its morphology
to a nonkeratinized epithelium devoid of deep rete
pegs when in close contact with the tooth, resulting in
the anatomical characteristics normally seen in
sulcular epithelium. It was concluded that the sulcular
environment has the capability of controlling the
keratinizing potential of the outer surface epithelium.
The constant irritation of bacterial plaque and its
product may be responsible for the premature
desquamation of the sulcular epithelium which in turn
might not allow its full differentiation.

POINTS TO PONDER

✓ The junctional epithelium and gingival fibers together
forms a functional unit called as dentogingival unit.
✓ The pH of the gingiva ranges from 6.5 to 8.5.
✓ Junctional epithelium is the only attachment in the
body between soft tissue and a calcified tissue which
is exposed to the external environment.
✓ Gingival fiber groups enable the gingiva to form a
rigid cuff around the tooth that add stability
especially when a significant portion of the
periodontal ligament and alveolar support is lost.
This explains that the increased mobility in
periodontally involved teeth immediately after
surgical procedures is because these procedures
disrupt or remove the gingival fiber groups.

BIBLIOGRAPHY

1. Baktold PM, Walsh LJ, Narayanan AS. Molecular and cell
biology of the gingiva. Periodontol 2000;24: 28-55.
2. Eley BM, Manson JD. The periodontal tissues. In, Periodontics
5th ed Wright 2004; 1-20.
3. Grant DA, Stern IB, Listgarten MA. Gingiva and dentogingival
junction. In, Periodontics. 6th ed CV Mosby Company 1988; 25-55.
4. Itoiz ME, Carranza FA. The Gingiva. In, Newman, Takei, Carranza.
Clinical Periodontology. 9th ed WB Saunders 2003; 16-35.
5. Lindhe J, Karring T, Araujo M. Anatomy of the Periodontium.
In, Lindhe J, Karring T, Lang NP. Clinical Periodontology and
Implant dentistry. 4th ed Blackwell Munksgaard 2003; 3-49.
6. Ramfjord SP, Ash MM. Connective tissue. In, Periodontology
and Periodontics, Modern Theory and Practice. 1st ed AITBS
Publisher and distributor India, 1996; 15-20.
7. Ramfjord SP, Ash MM. Epithelium. In, Periodontology and
Periodontics, Modern Theory and Practice. 1st ed AITBS
Publisher and distributor India, 1996; 5-14.
8. Stern IB. Oral mucous membrane. In, Bhaskar SN. Orban's Oral
histology and Embroylogy. 11th ed Mosby 1991; 260-336.
9. Squier CA, Finkelstein. Oral mucosa. In, Tencate AR. Oral
histology Development, Structure and Function. 5th ed Mosby
1998; 345-87.

MCQs

1. The mucogingival junction is located between the:
   A. Free gingiva and attached gingiva
   B. Free gingiva and tooth
   C. Base of the sulcus and alveolar mucosa
   D. Attached gingiva and alveolar mucosa
2. Stippling is seen in:
   A. Marginal gingiva
   B. Attached gingiva
   C. Interdental gingiva
   D. Attached gingiva and center of interdental
   papilla
3. The area of periodontium more susceptible to tissue
   breakdown is:
   A. Free gingiva
   B. Gingival sulcus
   C. Interdental col
   D. Interdental papilla
4. Dentogingival unit comprises:
   A. Gingival fibers
   B. Gingival fibers and junctional epithelium
   C. Periodontal fibers and ligament
   D. None of the above
5. Gingiva is supplied by:
   A. Supraperiosteal vessels
   B. Vessels of periodontal liagment
   C. Arterioles emerging from alveolar crest
   D. All of the above
6. Which of the following fiber group is not attached to
   alveolar bone:
   A. Transseptal fibers
   B. Oblique fibers
   C. Horizontal fibers
   D. Dentoperiosteal fibers

7. Odland bodies are:
   A. Modified mitochondria
   B. Modified lysosomes
   C. Modified ribosome
   D. Modified centrioles
8. Which of the following cells of the gingival epithelium is not a clear cell?
   A. Keratinocyte
   B. Langerhans cell
   C. Merkel cells
   D. Melanocytes
9. The length of the junctional epithelium ranges from:
   A. 0.25 - 0.75 mm
   B. 0.15 - 0.75 mm
   C. 0.25 - 1.35 mm
   D. 0.5 - 1.0 mm
10. The width of attached gingiva is greatest in:
    A. Maxillary anterior region
    B. Maxillary molar region
    C. Maxillary premolar region
    D. Mandibular premolar region

11. The color of attached gingiva in health, is determined by:
    A. The presence of melanophores
    B. Degree of keratinization of epithelium
    C. Vascular supply
    D. All of the above
12. If a diastema is present, the interdental papilla is:
    A. Larger in size
    B. Smaller in size
    C. Absent in the region
    D. None of the above
13. Which of the following enzymes increase their activity towards surface in gingival oral epithelium?
    A. Succinic dehydrogenase
    B. Nicotinamide adenine dinucleotide
    C. Cytochrome oxidase
    D. Glucose -6-phosphatase

Answers

1. D	2. D	3. C	4. B	5. D
6. A	7. B	8. A	9. C	10. A
11. D	12. C	13. D		

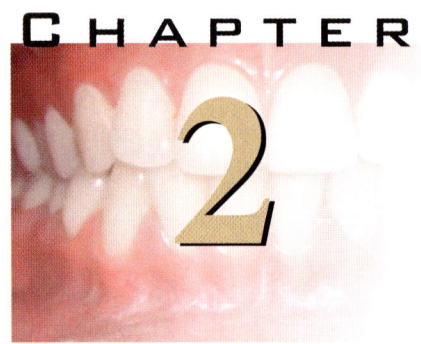

CHAPTER 2

Periodontal Ligament

Shalu Bathla

INTRODUCTION

The attachment apparatus of the tooth includes the periodontal ligament, cementum and alveolar bone. *Periodontal ligament is the soft, specialized connective tissue situated between the cementum covering the root of the tooth and bone forming the socket wall.* Its width ranges from 0.15 to 0.38 mm. Periodontal ligament's shape is like an hourglass apicocoronally, corresponding to the rotation point of the tooth. Periodontal ligament is thinnest at the axis of rotation in the middle and widens coronally and apically. The synonyms of periodontal ligament are periodontal membrane, alveolodental ligament, desmodont, pericementum, dental periosteum and gomphosis.

DEVELOPMENT

As the crown approaches the oral mucosa during tooth eruption, the fibroblasts of dental follicle become active and start producing collagen fibrils. These fibers initially lack orientation, but they soon acquire an orientation oblique to the tooth. The first collagen bundles appear in the region immediately apical to the cementoenamel junction and give rise to the gingivodental fiber groups. As tooth eruption progresses, additional oblique fibers appear and become attached to the newly formed cementum and bone. The transseptal and alveolar crest fibers develop when the tooth merges into the oral cavity. Alveolar bone deposition occurs simultaneously with periodontal ligament organization **(Fig. 2.1)**. During eruption, cemental Sharpey's fibers appear first, followed by Sharpey's fibers emerging from bone. Sharpey's fibers of bone are fewer in number and more widely spaced than those emerging from the cementum. At a later stage, alveolar fibers extend into the middle zone to join the lengthening cemental fibers and attain their classic orientation, thickness and strength when occlusal function is established.

CONSTITUENTS

A. Periodontal ligament fibers
B. Cellular elements
C. Ground substances
   i. Glycosaminoglycans
   ii. Glycoproteins

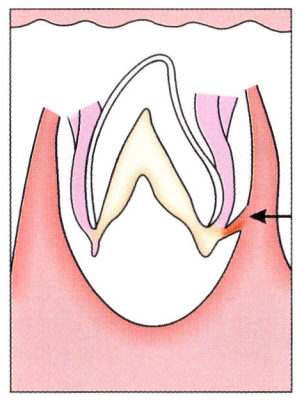
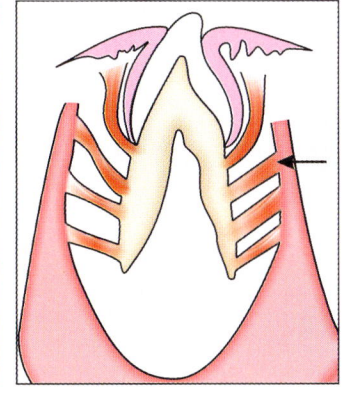

Alveolar crest fibers are
forming

Alveolar crest fibers are
initially oblique

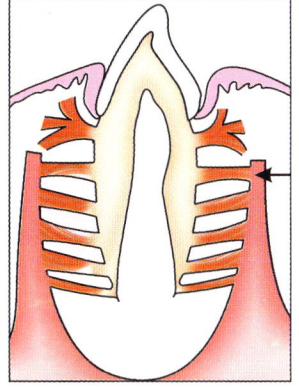
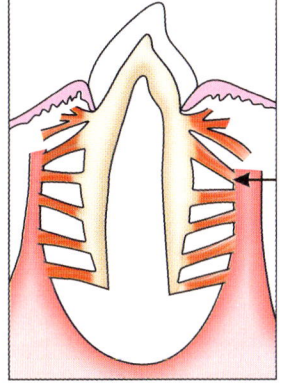

Alveolar crest fibers are
horizontal

Alveolar crest fibers
direction are again oblique
(but in opposite direction)

Fig. 2.1: Development of principal periodontal ligament fibers

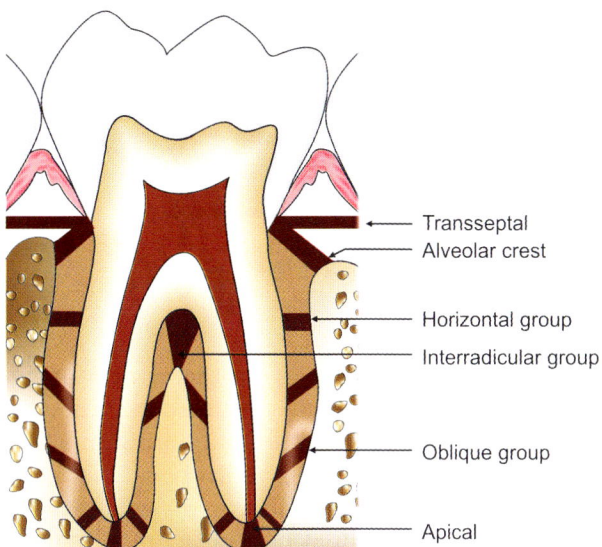

Fig. 2.2: Principal periodontal ligament fiber groups

Periodontal Ligament Fibers

Fibers in human periodontal ligament are made up of collagen and oxytalan. Elastic fibers are present only in the wall of blood vessels. Oxytalan are immature elastic fiber. The orientation of these fibers are different from collagen fibers been in axial direction instead of collagen fibers running from bone to tooth. The one end of these fibers is embedded in cementum or bone and the other end in the wall of blood vessel. Thus, they support the blood vessels of periodontal ligament. These are numerous and dense in cervical region of the ligament.

Collagen: There are at least 19 recognized collagen types encoded by 30 separate genes, dispersed among at least 12 chromosomes. Three polypeptide alpha chains coil around each other to form typical triple helix configuration. It is a protein composed of different amino acids, the most important being glycine, proline, hydroxylysine and hydroxyproline. It always contains hydroxylysine and hydroxyproline. Types I, III,V, VI, XII (FACIT) of collagen are present in periodontal ligament. Collagen is synthesized by fibroblasts, chondroblasts, osteoblasts, odontoblasts and other cells. It is secreted in an inactive form called as procollagen, which is then converted into tropocollagen. In the extracellular space, tropocollagen is polymerized into collagen fibrils which are then aggregated into collagen bundles by the formation of crosslinkages. There is rapid turnover rate of periodontal ligament collagen, with half life of only 10 – 15 days, which is about 5 times faster than gingival collagen.

The principal fibers of periodontal ligament are arranged in six groups **(Fig. 2.2)** and are named according to their location and direction of attachment:

1. *Transseptal group*: Extends interproximally over alveolar bone crest and are embedded in the cementum of adjacent teeth. They are reconstructed even after destruction of the alveolar bone has occurred in the periodontal disease and are responsible for returning teeth to their original state after orthodontic therapy.

2. *Alveolar crest group*: Extends obliquely from the cementum just beneath the junctional epithelium to the alveolar crest. They prevent extrusion and lateral tooth movements.

3. *Horizontal group*: Extends at right angles to the long axis of the tooth from cementum to alveolar bone. This fiber group resists horizontal pressure against the crown of the tooth.

The labels in Fig. 2.2: Transseptal, Alveolar crest, Horizontal group, Interradicular group, Oblique group, Apical

PERIODONTICS REVISITED

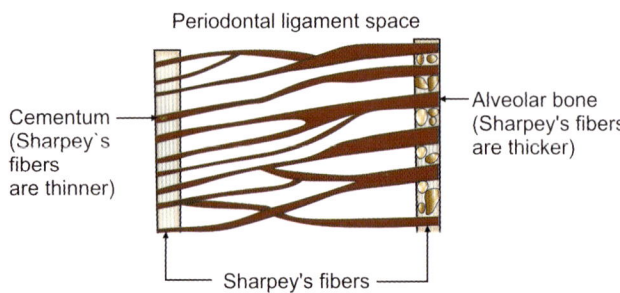

Periodontal ligament space

Cementum
(Sharpey's
fibers
are thinner)

Alveolar bone
(Sharpey's fibers
are thicker)

Sharpey's fibers

Fig. 2.3: Sharpey's fibers

4. *Oblique group*: Extends from the cementum in a coronal direction obliquely to the bone. They bear vertical masticatory stresses and transform vertical stress into tension on the alveolar bone.

5. *Apical group*: The apical fibers radiates in irregular fashion from cementum to bone at apical region of socket. They prevent tooth tipping, resist luxation and protect neurovascular supply to the tooth.

6. *Interradicular group*: These are found only between roots of multirooted teeth running from cementum into bone, forming crest of interradicular septum. They prevent luxation, tooth tipping and torquing.

The ends of the periodontal fibers that are embedded in alveolar bone and cementum are called Sharpey's fibers. On the cementum side these Sharpey's fibers are much thinner in diameter and insert at closer intervals as compared with the alveolar bone side **(Fig. 2.3)**. These differences in the pattern of insertion have clinical importance in the distribution of forces that are generated within the periodontal ligament during occlusion, traumatic forces and tooth movement. These forces are more evenly distributed along the cementum surface and are more concentrated along the more widely spaced insertions on the alveolar bone side. As a result, in response to mechanical forces, there is generally a remodeling of the periodontal housing on the alveolar bone side and not on the cementum side, preventing the possibility of significant cementum and root resorption.

Cellular Elements

1. Connective tissue cells:
   a. Synthetic cells
      • *Fibroblasts*: These are the most predominant connective tissue cells. Fibroblast are a spindle shaped or stellate cells with an oval-shaped nucleus containing one or more nucleoli. They originate from mesenchymal cells. Fibroblasts have the ability to synthesize and secrete a wide range of extracellular molecules like collagen fibers, elastic fibers, proteoglycans, glycoproteins, growth factors and enzymes (collagenase). These cells are capable of both synthesizing and degrading collagen.
      • *Cementoblasts*: These are the cells responsible for secreting the organic matrix of cementum within the periodontal ligament.
      • *Osteoblasts*: These are found on the surface of the alveolar bone. Their gross appearance and ultrastructure is similar to that of osteoblasts found elsewhere in the body.
   b. Resorptive cells
      • *Osteoclasts*: These are bone resorbing cells which are formed by fusion of mononuclear cells arising from bone marrow.
      • *Fibroblasts*: These cells are also responsible for degrading collagen fibers.
      • *Cementoclasts*: These are mononuclear cells resembling osteoclast located in howships lacunae.

2. Epithelial cells: These are remnants of Hertwig's root sheath which are present close to cementum throughout the periodontal ligament and more in apical and cervical areas. When stimulated they proliferate and participate in the formation of periapical cysts and lateral root cysts. It has been proposed that epithelial cell rests of Malassez play an important role in the maintenance of periodontal ligament space. In physiologic conditions, it is therefore thought that these cells, that are devoid of any mineralization propensity, may contribute to maintain a non-mineralized area. These cells are involved in pathogenesis of several disorders including pocket formation. The presence of c – met receptors in the epithelial cell rests of Malassez suggest that these cells can respond to the inflammatory cytokine, Hepatocyte growth factor. This scatter factor is thought to be capable of aiding migration of these cells and hence aid in the pathogenesis of pocket. These cells are also thought to be responsible for cementum repair as they are found in areas of resorption when mechanical injury was created in experimental animals. It has been suggested that cells retain the capacity to differentiate into cementoblasts and lay down matrix. Thus, epithelial cell rests of Malassez are thought to play a role in physiological maintenance of periodontal ligament space; may play a role in pathogenesis of

pocket formation and probably may mediate process involved in regeneration.

3. Immune system cells: Various defense cells present in periodontal ligament are neutrophils, lymphocytes, macrophages, mast cell and eosinophils
4. Cells associated with neurovascular elements
5. Progenitor cells

Ground Substance

It is an amorphous, nonfibrous and noncellular matrix which forms the major constituent of the periodontal ligament. Ground substance helps in the transportation of water, electrolytes, nutrients and metabolites to and from the connective tissue cells, thus is essential for the maintenance of the normal function of connective tissue. It is thought to have a significant effect on the tooth's ability to withstand stress loads.

The main constituents are protein-carbohydrate macromolecules. These complexes are divided into proteoglycans and glycoproteins. Proteoglycans are the large group of extracellular macromolecules that consist of protein core to which are attached glycosaminoglycan chains. The proteoglycans that are involved in the organization and regulation of collagen fibers are decorin and biglycan abundantly present in the periodontal ligament. Decorin, especially is present bound to collagen and is important to regulate fibrillogenesis. Decorin is also bound to Transforming Growth Factor-β (TGF-β) and prevents excessive fibrosis and thus prevents excessive cross-linking of the collagen fibers of the periodontal ligament. Glycoproteins are the macromolecules with carbohydrate core. Glycoproteins have adhesive properties which bind cells to extracellular elements. These glycoproteins are grouped into two fibronectin and tenascin. Fibronectin is a large protein which binds cells to collagen and proteoglycans. It promotes the adhesion of fibroblasts to the extracellular matrix and plays a role in the alignment of collagen fibers.

Cementicles are globular masses of cementum arranged in concentric lamellae that lie free in the periodontal ligament or adhere to the root surface. These cementicles may develop from calcified epithelial rests or from calcified Sharpey's fiber or from calcified thrombosed vessels within periodontal ligament.

FUNCTIONS

Periodontal ligament serves the following functions:
1. Supportive:
   - Attaches the teeth to the bone.
   - It maintains gingival tissues in their proper relationship to the teeth.

- Periodontal ligament protects the blood vessels and nerves from injury by mechanical forces.
- Periodontal ligament transmits occlusal forces to the bone.
- It resists the impact of occlusal forces and thus acts as a shock absorber.

Resistance to the impact of occlusal forces:

There are different theories to explain the mechanism of tooth support:

Tensional theory: According to this theory, the principal fibers of periodontal fibers play the major role in supporting the tooth and transmitting forces to the bone. When the force is applied to the crown, principal fibers unfold and straighten, transmitting the forces to alveolar bone, which leads to elastic deformation of the bony socket and then alveolar bone transmits the load to the basal bone.

Viscoelastic system theory: According to this theory, the displacement of the tooth is largely controlled by fluid movement and fibers play a secondary role. When the forces are transmitted to the tooth, the extracellular fluid passes from the periodontal ligament into marrow spaces of bone through foramina. Periodontal fiber bundles absorb the slack and tighten, after the depletion of tissue fluids. This leads to blood vessel stenosis. Arterial back pressure cause ballooning of the vessels. The tissue fluid replenishes as the blood ultrafiltrates pass into the tissues.

Thixotropic theory: According to this theory, periodontal ligament has the rheologic behavior of a thixotropic gel (i.e. the property of becoming fluid when shaken/stirred and then becoming semisolid again).

Transmission of occlusal forces to the bone:

The arrangement of the principal fibers is similar to a suspension bridge or hammock. When an axial force is applied to a tooth, a tendency towards displacement of the root into the alveolus occurs. The oblique fibers alter their wavy, untensed pattern; assume their full length; and sustain the major part of the axial force. But when the horizontal or tipping force is applied, two phases of tooth movement occur. One is within the confines of the periodontal ligament, and the other produces a displacement of the facial and lingual bony plates. The tooth rotates about an axis that may change as the force is increased.

2. Sensory: Periodontal ligament is capable of transmitting tactile, pressure and pain sensations by trigeminal pathways.

3. Nutritive: It supplies nutrients to cementum, bone and gingiva through blood vessels and lymphatics.
4. Formative: The tissues have the regenerative capacity in providing the cell lineage namely osteoblast, cementoblast and fibroblast. Thus, it helps in the formation and resorption of cementum and bone during physiologic tooth movement and repair of injuries.
5. Homeostasis: With the presence of both formative and resorptive activity the periodontal ligament provides a homeostasis in the tissue environment.

BLOOD SUPPLY

The blood supply is derived from the inferior and superior alveolar arteries to mandible and maxilla respectively. Blood supply reaches the periodontal ligament from 3 sources:
  i. Apical vessels
 ii. Penetrating vessels from the alveolar bone
iii. Anastomosing vessels from the gingiva
    Blood vessels are present in the interstitial spaces of loose connective tissue between the principal fibers and are connected in the net like plexus that runs longit-udinally. These blood vessels are closer to the bone than to cementum. The blood supply increases from the incisors to the molars; is greatest in the gingival third of single rooted teeth, less in the apical third, and least in the middle; is equal in the apical and middle thirds of multirooted teeth; is slightly greater on the mesial and distal surfaces than on the facial and lingual; and is greater on the mesial surfaces of mandibular molars than on the distal. The capillaries of periodontal ligament are fenestrated while in other connective tissues they are continuous. Due to fenestration, they have greater ability of diffusion and filtration which is related to high metabolic requirements of periodontal ligament and its high rate of turnover.
    The venous drainage of the periodontal ligament accompanies the arterial supply. Venules receive the blood through the abundant capillary network; there are also, arteriovenous anastomoses that bypass the capillaries. These are more frequent in apical and interradicular regions.

NERVE SUPPLY

The periodontium receives both autonomic and sensory innervations. Autonomic nerves are sympathetic arising from the superior cervical ganglion and terminating in the smooth muscles of the periodontal arterioles. Activation of the sympathetic fibers induces constriction of the vessels. Sensory nerves that supply the periodontium arise from maxillary and mandibular divisions of trigeminal nerve. They are mixed nerves of large and small diameter. They have four types of sensory endings including nocioceptive free nerve endings receptors, two kinds of mechanoreceptors and spindle like receptors. Unmyelinated sensory fibers terminate as nocioceptive free endings. Coiled endings are present mainly in midregion of periodontal ligament. Ruffini endings are low threshold, slowly adapting mechanoreceptors located primarily in the apical areas. They have dendritic ramifications with expanded terminal buttons. Spindle like receptors are for pressure and vibration which are surrounded by a fibrous capsule and located mainly at the apex. About 75% of the mechanoreceptors within the periodontal ligament have their cell bodies in the terminal ganglion while the remaining 25% have their cell bodies in the mesencephalic nucleus.

MAINTENANCE OF THE PERIODONTAL LIGAMENT SPACE

One of the most remarkable features of periodontal ligament is the maintenance of the space in spite of its constant exposure to mechanical forces or orthodontic tooth movement. Following factors have been thought to contribute to this maintenance of periodontal ligament:
1. Periodontal fibroblasts lack osteoblast differentiating genes coding for protein namely bone sialoprotein which is thought to be an initial nucleator of hydroxyapatite crystal. Therefore, in vitro formation of crystals does not occur within the periodontal ligament space. Osteocalcin expression within the periodontal fibroblasts under physiological conditions is also less or absent.
2. Inhibitors of mineralization: This is the most important mechanism by which periodontal fibroblasts maintain their space.
   a. Msx protein: The greater expression of msx homeobox protein within the periodontal ligament is thought to be a defense mechanism that prevents periodontal mineralization.
   b. S100 protein: Periodontal ligament shows a greater expression of S100, a calcium binding protein. Increased expression of S100 seems to regulate expression of osteoblast differentiation genes

coding for proteins such as osteocalcin and alkaline phosphatase and thus, inhibits mineralization.

c. *Periodontal ligament associated protein 1 (PLAP1)*: It is a potent inhibitor of mineralization as it can bind with BMP and antagonize its action. This binding prevents cytodifferentiation and as a result expression of the osteoblast phenotype is restricted.

3. Epithelial cells of Malassez: The presence of epithelial cells of Malassez in the periodontal ligament space is thought to be deterrent to osteoblast differentiation and is, therefore, an important regulator, especially in the coronal areas of the tooth.

4. Nitric oxide (NO): On application of mechanical stress, increased NO production from the periodontal ligament is thought to result in osteoclast activity and bone resorption thereby maintaining the periodontal space.

Characteristic features of periodontal ligament

Hour glass shape

0.15- 0 .38 mm width

Supportive, nutritive, regenerative and sensory functions

POINTS TO PONDER

✓ Oblique group is the largest group of periodontal ligament fibers.

✓ Intermediate plexus (Sicher 1966): Fibers arising from cementum and bone are joined in mid region of periodontal ligament space giving rise to a zone of distinct appearance in light microscope. It was believed that the intermediate plexus provides a site where rapid remodeling of fibers occurs, allowing adjustment in the ligament to be made to accommodate small movements of tooth. However, evidence derived from electron microscope provide no support for this and was believed to be an artifact.

✓ Fibroblasts are described as architect, builder and caretaker of connective tissue and play dual role in collagen synthesis and degradation.

✓ Gla proteins are important for the regulation of mineralization in the extracellular matrix. These proteins are called so due to the presence of amino acids that are – carboxylated, called the gla residues. The important members of the gla protein family are Bone gla protein (osteocalcin) and Matrix gla protein

(MGP). MGP has been detected in the periodontal ligament and is thought to play a contributory role in the maintenance of the periodontal ligament space.

BIBLIOGRAPHY

1. Bartold PM, Narayanan AS. The Biochemistry and Physiology of the Periodontium. In, Wilson TG, Kornman KS. Fundamentals of Periodontics.Quintessence Publishing Co.1996; 61 – 108.
2. Berkovitz BKB, Schore RC. Cells of the periodontal ligament. In, Berkovitz BKB, Moxham BJ, Newman HN.The Periodontal Ligament in Health and Disease. 2nd ed Mosby – Wolfe 1995; 9–33.
3. Bernard GW, Carranza FA. The tooth supporting structures. In, Newman, Takei, Carranza. Clinical Periodontology. 9th ed WB Saunders 2003; 36-57.
4. Freeman E. Periodontium. In, Tencate AR. Oral histology Development, Structure and Function. 5th ed Mosby 1998; 253-88.
5. Holmstrup P. The macroanatomy of the Periodontium. In, Wilson TG, Kornman KS. Fundamentals of Periodontics. Quintessence Publishing Co.1996; 17 – 26.
6. Holmstrup P. The microanatomy of the Periodontium. In, Wilson TG, Kornman KS. Fundamentals of Periodontics. Quintessence Publishing Co.1996; 27 – 46.
7. Linden RWA, Billar BJ, Scott BJJ. The innervations of the periodontal ligament. In, Berkovitz BKB, Moxham BJ, Newman HN. The Periodontal Ligament in Health and Disease. 2nd ed Mosby – Wolfe 1995; 133 – 59.
8. Lindhe J, Karring T, Araujo M. Anatomy of the Periodontium. In, Lindhe J, Karring T, Lang NP. Clinical Periodontology and Implant dentistry. 4th ed Blackwell Munksgaard 2003; 3-49.
9. Melcher AH, McCulloch CAH. Periodontal ligament. In, Bhaskar SN. Orban's Oral histology and Embroylogy. 11th ed Mosby 1991; 203-38.
10. Moxham BJ, Grant DA. Development of the periodontal ligament. In, Berkovitz BKB, Moxham BJ, Newman HN.The Periodontal Ligament in Health and Disease. 2nd ed Mosby – Wolfe 1995; 161 – 81.
11. Nanci A, Bosshardt DD. Structure of Periodontal tissues in health and disease. Periodontol 2000 2006;40: 11-28.
12. Organization of the matrix. In, Arun KV. Molecular biology of periodontium. 1st ed Jaypee brothers 2010; 35-69.
13. Periodontal ligament. In, Grant DA, Stern IB, Listgarten MA. Periodontics. 6th ed CV Mosby Company 1988; 56-75.

MCQs

1. Periodontal fibers which are consistent and reconstructed even after the destruction of the alveolar bone:
   A. Apical fibers
   B. Alveolar crest fibers
   C. Oblique fibers
   D. Transseptal fibers

2. Predominant connective tissue cells of periodontal ligament are:
   A. Fibroblasts
   B. Epithelial rests of Malassez
   C. Osteoclasts
   D. Osteoblasts

3. Radiograph of a periodontal ligament of a tooth which has lost its antagonist shows:
   A. Widening of the periodontal ligament space
   B. Narrowing of the periodontal ligament space
   C. Increased density
   D. Sclerotic changes

4. Which of the following amino acid is at every third position of collagen molecule?
   A. Alanine
   B. Glycine
   C. Hydroxylysine
   D. Hydroxyproline

5. The periodontal ligament fibers that mainly prevent the extrusion of teeth are:
   A. Alveolar crest fibers
   B. Transseptal fibers
   C. Horizontal fibers
   D. Interradicular fibers

6. The function of fibroblast in periodontal ligament:
   A. Synthesis of collagen
   B. Degradation of collagen
   C. Both A and B
   D. None of the above

7. Which of the following is not correct about periodontal ligament:
   A. It is shaped like hourglass
   B. It is thicker on mesial side of root
   C. It is narrow at axis of rotation
   D. None of the above

8. Largest fiber group in periodontal ligament is:
   A. Transseptal fibers   B. Oblique fibers
   C. Horizontal fibers   D. Apical fibers

9. The thickness of periodontal ligament is maximum in:
   A. Teeth with heavy function
   B. Teeth with light function
   C. Teeth which are functionless
   D. The third molar teeth

10. The vascular supply of periodontal ligament is:
    A. Greatest in the middle third of the single rooted teeth
    B. In the form of net-like plexus that runs closer to cementum than to alveolar bone
    C. Greatest in the middle third of the multirooted teeth
    D. In the form of net-like plexus that runs closer to alveolar bone than to cementum

11. The following group of fibers is absent in an incompletely formed root:
    A. Alveolar crest group
    B. Oblique group
    C. Horizontal group
    D. Apical group

12. Which of the following fibers regulate the blood flow of periodontal ligament?
    A. Mature elastin fibers
    B. Oxytalan fibers
    C. Eluanin fibers
    D. Collagen Type III

Answers

1. D	2. A	3. B	4. B	5. A
6. C	7. B	8. B	9. A	10. D
11. D	12. B			

Cementum

Shalu Bathla

INTRODUCTION

Cementum is calcified avascular mesenchymal tissue that forms the outer covering of the anatomic root. Two pupils of Purkinje in 1835 first demonstrated cementum microscopically. The hardness and calcification of cementum, when it is fully mineralized is less than that of dentin. Cementum is light yellow in color, with dull surface. It does not has the ability to remodel and is resistant to resorption.

DEVELOPMENT

The enamel organ including the epithelial root sheath as it develops is surrounded by a layer of connective tissue known as the dental sac. The zone immediately in contact with the dental organ and continuous with the ectomesenchyme of the dental papilla is called the dental follicle which consists of undifferentiated fibroblasts. The rupture of Hertwig's root sheath allows the mesenchymal cells of the dental follicle to contact the dentin, where they start forming a continuous layer of cementoblasts. Cementum formation begins by deposition of a meshwork of irregularly arranged collagen fibrils sparsely distributed in a ground substance or matrix called precementum or cementoid. This is followed by a phase of matrix maturation, which subsequently mineralizes to form cementum. Cemen-toblasts, which are initially separated from the cementum by uncalcified cementoid, sometimes become enclosed within the matrix and are trapped. Once they are enclosed, they are referred to as cementocytes and will remain viable in a fashion similar to that of osteocytes.

FUNCTIONS

1. Cementum provides attachment to the collagen fibers of periodontal ligament to the root.
2. Cementum functions as a covering for the root surface, a seal for the open dentinal tubules thus, preventing dentinal sensitivity.
3. Cementum aids in maintaining the teeth in functional occlusion.
4. It contributes to the process of repair after damage to the root surface.

COMPOSITION

i. Inorganic: 40 - 50% – Hydroxyapatite
ii. Organic: 50%
   • Collagen Type I (90%), III, V, XII (FACIT), XIV are present in cementum. The sources of collagen fibers are fibroblasts which produce extrinsic Sharpey's fibers and cementoblasts which produce intrinsic fibers of the cementum matrix.

- Non-collagenous: Fibronectin, Bone sialoprotein, Osteopontin, Osteocalcin, Osteonectin and Alkaline phosphatase. Osteocalcin is a mineral regulatory protein related to bone matrix formation and mineralization which is expressed by cementoblasts lining the roots of developing and fully formed teeth.
- Formative cells: Cementoblast
- Degradative cells: Cementoclast/Odontoclast
- Adhesion molecule: Cementum attachment protein (CAP) is present on the outer surface of the cementum. CAP is known to play a role in chemotaxis and differentiation of cementoblasts prior to laying down of the cementoid matrix. In addition, CAP mediates the attachment of the periodontal ligament fibers to the root surface.
- Growth factor: Insulin like growth factor

CLASSIFICATION

Cementum can be classified as:
1. According to location: **(Fig. 3.1)**
   i. Radicular cementum
   ii. Coronal cementum
2. According to cells present:
   i. Acellular cementum is the first cementum to be formed and covers approximately the cervical third or half of the root; it does not contain cells. This cementum is formed before the tooth reaches the occlusal plane.
   ii. Cellular cementum, forms after the tooth has reached the occlusal plane. It contains cementocytes in individual spaces (lacunae) that communicate with each other through a system of anastomosing canaliculi.

3. According to fibers present:
   Schroeder through light and electron microscopy, has enabled cementum to be classified into 5 different subtypes based on the source of collagen fibers:
   i. *Acellular afibrillar cementum (AAC)*: 1 to 15 µm. It consists of only mineralized ground substance, which is a product of cementoblasts. Cells and collagen (extrinsic and intrinsic) fibers are absent. It forms coronal cementum. Loss of the cervical part of the reduced enamel epithelium at the time of tooth eruption may place portions of mature enamel in contact with the connective tissue, which then will deposit over it an acellular afibrillar type of cementum.
   ii. *Acellular extrinsic fiber cementum (AEFC)*: 30 to 230 µm. It consists of only Sharpey's fibers, which is a product of fibroblasts and cementoblasts. This type of cementum lacks cells and is found in cervical third of the root.
   iii. *Cellular mixed stratified cementum (CMSC)*: 100 to 1000 µm. It consists of extrinsic and intrinsic fibers and cells which is a product of fibroblasts and cementoblasts. It is found in apical third of roots and in furcation areas.
   iv. *Cellular intrinsic fiber cementum (CIFC)*: It consists of cells and intrinsic fibers, lacking extrinsic

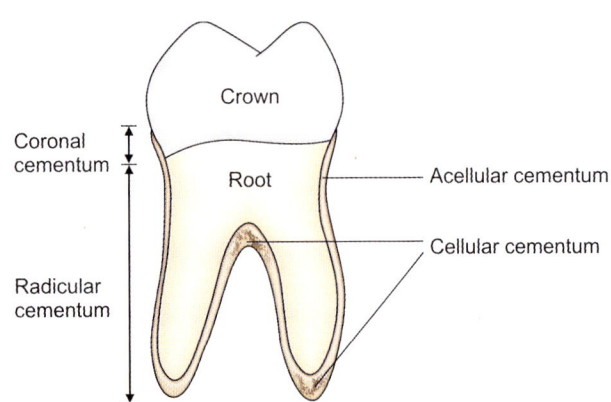

Fig. 3.1: Distribution of cementum on tooth surface

TABLE 3.1: Differences between acellular and cellular cementum		
	Acellular cementum	Cellular cementum
1. Formation	Forms before tooth reaches occlusal plane	Forms after tooth reaches occlusal plane
2. Cells	Does not contain any cells	Contains cementocytes
3. Location	Coronal portion of the root	Apical portion of the root
4. Rate of formation	Slower	Faster
5. Incremental lines	More	Sparse
6. Function	Forms after regenerative periodontal surgical procedure	Contributes to the length of root during growth
7. Calcification	More calcified	Less calcified
8. Sharpey's fibers	More	Less
9. Regularity	Regular	Irregular
10. Thickness	20 - 50 µm near the cervix, 150 - 200 µm near the apex	Thickness of 1 to several mm

collagen fibers, which is a product of cemento-blasts. It fills resorption lacunae.

v. *Intermediate cementum*: It is an ill defined zone near the cementodentinal junction of certain teeth that appears to contain cellular remnants of Hertwig's epithelial root sheath embedded in a calcified ground substance. It is also called as Layer of Hopewell Smith.

Thickness of Cementum

The thickness of cementum varies from 16 to 60 μm (thickness of hair) near cervix to 150 to 200 μm (thickest) near the apex. Cementum is thicker in distal surfaces than mesial surfaces due to functional stimulation during mesial drift/migration. It is a continuous process and rate varies throughout life.

VARIOUS JUNCTIONS OF CEMENTUM

Cementodentinal junction: It is the interface between dentin and cementum. The collagen fibers of cementum and dentin intervene at their interface in a very complex manner. It is not possible to determine which fibrils are cemental in origin and which are of dentinal origin.

Cementoenamel junction (CEJ): The relation between cementum and enamel at the cervical region of teeth is variable **(Fig. 3.2)**.

• In about 60-65%—Cementum overlaps enamel. This occurs when the enamel epithelium degenerates at its cervical termination permitting connective tissue to come in direct contact with the enamel surface.

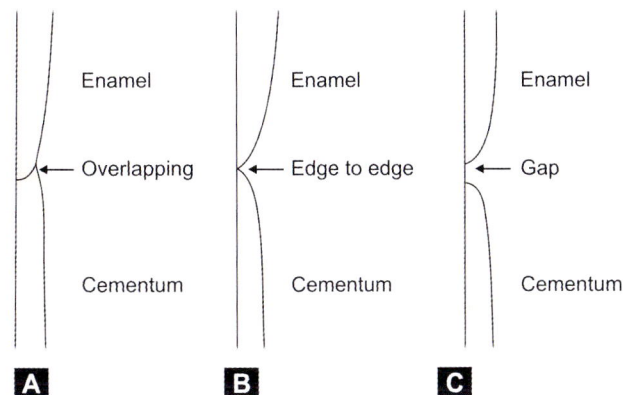

A. Cementum overlaps enamel (60–75%)
B. Edge to edge (30%)
C. Enamel and cementum do not meet (5–10%)

Fig. 3.2: Cementoenamel junction (CEJ)

• In about 30%—Edge to edge butt joint is there.
• In about 10%—Space is present between cementum and enamel and there is no cementoenamel junction, the cervical portion of the root is delayed in its separation from dentin.

Significance of CEJ: It helps in determining the level of attachment and the amount of bone loss.

CLINICAL CONSIDERATIONS

1. *Repair and resorption of cementum*: Cementum on the root surface undergoes resorption and repair alternately according to the change in the environment faced by it. There may be local or systemic causes of cemental resorption. Local causes: Trauma from occlusion, cysts and tumors, periapical pathology, excessive orthodontic forces, embedded teeth, replanted and transplanted teeth, idiopathic, pressure from malaligned erupting teeth and teeth without functional antagonists. Systemic causes: Deficiency of calcium, Vitamins A and D, hypothyroidism and hereditary fibrous osteodystrophy.

2. *Cementum anomalies*:
   • Hypercementosis refers to a prominent thickening of the cementum. It may be localized to one tooth or affect the entire dentition. Hypercementosis occurs as a generalized thickening of the cementum, with nodular enlargement of the apical third of the root. Hypercementosis of the entire dentition may occur in patients with Paget's disease.
   • Cementoblastoma is the only neoplasm of cementum.
   • Cementoma is not a true neoplasm but it is a fibro-osseous lesions.
   • Cementicles are the calcified round or ovoid bodies sometimes seen in the periodontal ligament. These are present singly or in multiple numbers near the cemental surface. There are two types of cementicles – free (lie free in the periodontal ligament) and attached cementicles (attached to the root surface).

Cementum formation is altered in the following diseases:
Paget's disease – hypercementosis
Hypopituitarism – decrease cementum formation
Cleidocranial dysplasia – defective cementum formation
Hypophosphatasia – total absence of cementum formation

3. *Ankylosis*: Fusion of the cementum and alveolar bone with obliteration of the periodontal ligament is termed ankylosis. Ankylosis occurs in teeth with cemental resorption, which suggests that it may represent a form of abnormal repair.

4. *Exposure of cementum to the oral environment*: Cementum becomes exposed to the oral environment in cases of gingival recession and as a consequence of loss of attachment in pocket formation. The cementum is sufficiently permeable to be penetrated in these cases by organic substances, inorganic ions, and bacteria. Bacterial invasion of the cementum occurs commonly in periodontal disease.

POINTS TO PONDER

✓ Acellular extrinsic fiber cementum type of cementum is desired following regenerative periodontal surgical procedure.
✓ Both acellular cementum and cellular cementum are arranged in lamellae separated by incremental lines parallel to the long axis of the root. These lines represent rest periods in cementum formation.

BIBLIOGRAPHY

1. Armitage GC. Cementum. In, Bhaskar SN. Orban's Oral histology and Embroylogy. 11th ed Mosby 1991; 180-202.
2. Bartold PM, Narayanan AS. The Biochemistry and Physiology of the Periodontium. In, Wilson TG, Kornman KS. Fundamentals of Periodontics. Quintessence Publishing Co.1996; 61–108.
3. Bernard GW, Carranza FA. The tooth supporting structures. In, Newman, Takei, Carranza. Clinical Periodontology. 9th ed WB Saunders 2003; 36-57.
4. Cementum. In, Grant DA, Stern IB, Listgarten MA. Periodontics. 6th ed CV Mosby Company 1988; 76-93.
5. Freeman E. Periodontium. In, Tencate AR. Oral histology Development, Structure and Function. 5th ed Mosby 1998; 253-288.
6. Holmstrup P. The macroanatomy of the Periodontium. In, Wilson TG, Kornman KS. Fundamentals of Periodontics. Quintessence Publishing Co.1996; 17 – 26.
7. Holmstrup P. The microanatomy of the Periodontium. In, Wilson TG, Kornman KS. Fundamentals of Periodontics. Quintessence Publishing Co.1996; 27 – 46.
8. Lindhe J, Karring T, Araujo M. Anatomy of the Periodontium. In, Lindhe J, Karring T, Lang NP. Clinical Periodontology and Implant dentistry. 4th ed Blackwell Munksgaard 2003; 3-49.

MCQs

1. Cementum was first demonstrated microscopically by:
   A. Two pupils of Purkinje in 1835
   B. Two pupils of Purkinje in 1935
   C. William Sharpey
   D. None of the above
2. The most common presentation of CEJ is:
   A. Butt-joint
   B. Failing to meet each other
   C. Enamel overlaps cementum
   D. Cementum overlaps enamel
3. Which of the following is more mineralized?
   A. Acellular extrinsic fiber cementum
   B. Cellular mixed stratified cementum
   C. Cellular intrinsic fiber cementum
   D. Intermediate cementum
4. Adhesion molecule present in cementum:
   A. Cementum attachment protein
   B. Vascular adhesion molecule
   C. Insulin growth factor
   D. None of the above
5. Cementum that usually fills resorption lacunae:
   A. Cellular intrinsic fiber cementum
   B. Intermediate cementum
   C. Acellular extrinsic fiber cementum
   D. None of the above
6. The following are true about cementicles:
   A. Calcified round or ovoid bodies
   B. Usually seen in the periodontal ligament near the cemental surface
   C. Both A and B
   D. None of the above
7. Mineral regulatory protein present in cementum:
   A. Osteopontin   B. Bone sialoprotein
   C. Osteocalcin   D. None of the above

Answers

1. A   2. D   3. A   4. A   5. A
6. C   7. C

Alveolar Bone

Shalu Bathla

INTRODUCTION

It is the portion of maxilla and mandible that forms and supports the tooth sockets (alveoli). Alveolar bone is a specialized connective tissue that is mainly characterized by its mineralized organic matrix. Together with the root cementum and periodontal ligament, the alveolar bone constitutes the attachment apparatus of the teeth. The main function is to distribute and reabsorb forces generated by mastication and other tooth contact. In addition, the jaw bones consist of the basal bone, which is the portion of the jaw located apically but unrelated to the teeth **(Fig. 4.1)**.

DEVELOPMENT

The alveolar bone begins to first form by an intramembranous ossification within the ectomesenchyme surrounding the developing tooth. This first bone formed called as woven bone is less organized and is replaced with a more organized lamellar bone. When a deciduous tooth is shed, its alveolar bone is resorbed. The succedaneous permanent tooth moves into place,

developing its own alveolar bone from its own dental follicle. As the tooth root forms and the surrounding

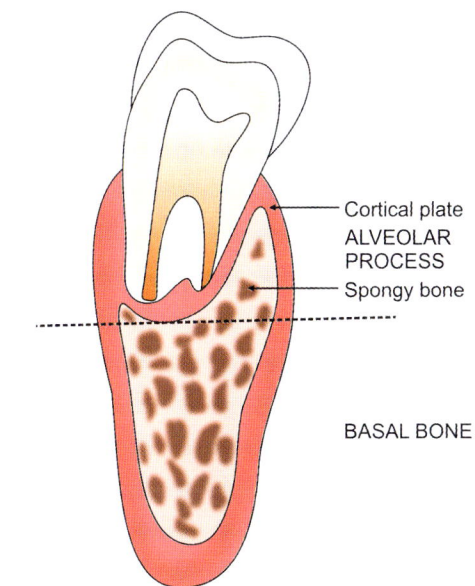

Cortical plate
ALVEOLAR
PROCESS
Spongy bone

BASAL BONE

Fig. 4.1: Dotted line indicates the separation between alveolar bone and basal bone

tissues develop and mature, alveolar bone merges with the separately developing basal bone and the two become one continuous structure. Although alveolar bone and basal bone have different intermediate origins, both are ultimately derived from neural crest ectomesenchyme. Mandibular basal bone begins mineralization at the exit of the mental nerve from the mental foramen, whereas the maxillary basal bone begins at the exit of the infraorbital nerve from the infraorbital foramen.

PARTS

The alveolar process is divisible into separate areas on an anatomic basis **(Fig. 4.2)**, but it functions as a unit, with all parts interrelated in the support of the teeth.

1. *Alveolar bone proper*: Thin lamella of bone that surrounds the root of the tooth and gives attachment to principal fibers of the periodontal ligament is called as alveolar bone proper. The alveolar bone proper forms the inner wall of the socket. It is perforated by many openings that carry branches of the interalveolar blood vessels and nerves into the periodontal ligament and is called as Cribriform plate. The bone in which principal fibers called Sharpey's fibers of periodontal ligament are anchored is known as bundle bone. The bundle bone contains few fibrils in the intercellular substances. This bone is not unique to the jaws, it occurs throughout the skeletal system wherever ligament and muscles are attached. Radiographically, this bundle bone appears as a thin radiopaque line surrounding the roots of teeth and is called as lamina dura. Lamina dura appears more dense than the adjacent supporting bone, but this radiographic density may be due to the mineral orientation around the fiber bundles and the apparent lack of nutrient canals. But there is no difference in mineral content between lamina dura and the supporting bone. The lamina dura is evaluated clinically for periapical or periodontal pathology.

2. *Supporting alveolar bone*: Bone that surrounds the alveolar bone proper and gives support to the socket is called as supporting alveolar bone.

   It consists of 2 parts:
   i. *Cortical plates*: Which consists of compact bone and form the outer and inner plates of the alveolar bone.
   ii. *Spongy bone*: Which fills the area between these plates and alveolar bone proper. It is also called as trabecular bone or cancellous bone.

   Most of the facial and lingual portions of the sockets are formed by compact bone alone; cancellous bone surrounds the lamina dura in apical, apicolingual, and interradicular areas.

INTERDENTAL SEPTUM

The interdental septum consists of cancellous bone bordered by the socket wall cribriform plates (lamina dura or alveolar bone proper) of approximating teeth and the facial and lingual cortical plates. If the interdental space is less than 0.5 mm, i.e. in kissing roots, cancellous bone is lacking **(Fig. 4.3)**. The septum may consist of only the cribriform plate leading to diminished blood supply. If roots are too close together, an irregular "window" can appear in the bone between adjacent roots **(Fig. 4.4)**. Determining root proximity radiographically is important. The mesiodistal angulation of the crest of the interdental septum usually parallels a line drawn between the cementoenamel junctions of the approxi-

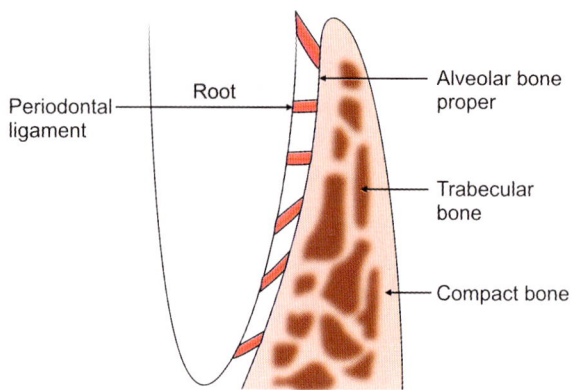

Fig. 4.2: Tooth supporting alveolar process

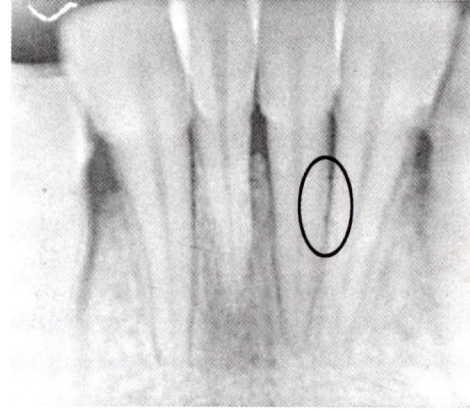

Fig. 4.3: Kissing roots where cancellous bone is lacking

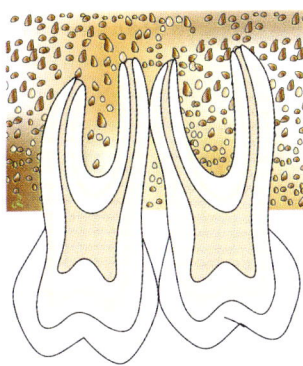

Fig. 4.4: Boneless window between adjoining close roots of molars

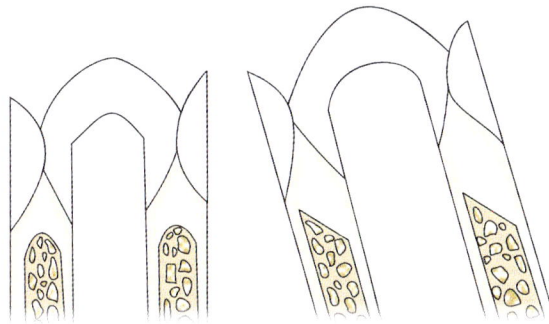

Fig. 4.5: Variations in shape of interdental alveolar crest according to the position of teeth

mating teeth. The distance between the crest of the alveolar bone and the cementoenamel junction in young adults varies between 0.75 and 1.49 mm (average 1.08 mm). The mesiodistal and faciolingual dimensions and shape of the interdental septum are governed by the size and convexity of the crowns of the two approximating teeth, as well as by the position of the teeth in the jaw and their degree of eruption **(Fig. 4.5)**.

COMPOSITION

1. Inorganic: 67% Hydroxyapatite
2. Organic: 33%
   - Collagen – 28% Type I – (Mainly), Types III, V, XII and XIV
   - Non-collagenous protein – 5%. The various non-collagenous proteins are osteonectin, osteopontin, bone sialoprotein, osteocalcin, bone proteoglycan, biglycan, bone proteoglycan II decorin, thrombospondin and bone morphogenetic proteins (BMPs).

Osteonectin functions primarily to link collagen to the mineralized matrix of bone.

Osteopontin is an important glycoprotein of bone and is vital for chemotaxis of bone forming cells. Osteopontin is synthesized by a variety of mesenchymal cells especially fibroblasts, osteoblasts, osteoclasts and the differentiating mesenchymal cells. Osteopontin has been shown to respond to mechanical stimulus and its upregulation is thought to play an important role in the turnover of bone following mechanical stress. Osteopontin through its chemotactic ability is able to bring in osteoblasts and osteoclasts into area in which it is expressed. It has been detected in GCF and its potential as a marker for periodontal disease has been explored.

Bone sialoprotein is more specific to bone forming cells than osteopontin. Bone sialoprotein plays a role in chemotaxis of osteoblasts. However, its primary role is to act as an initial nucleator to hydroxyapatite crystal formation and is thus essential to the mineralization process.

Gla proteins are important for the regulation of mineralization in the extracellular matrix. The important members of the gla protein family are Bone gla protein (osteocalcin) and Matrix gla protein (MGP). These proteins are called so due to the presence of amino acids that are γ - carboxylated, called the gla residues. Bone gla protein regulates crystal growth and limits the size of the hydroxyapatite crystals so that they form a three dimensional integrated mineralized mass.

Chondroitin 4-sulfate is especially found in greater proportion in alveolar bone, it has been used as a marker of periodontal disease activity. This ability to promote mineralization has been utilized in regenerative periodontal therapy.

CELLULAR COMPONENTS

Osteoblast: These are generally cuboidal or slightly elongated cells that line a large percentage of bone surfaces. Osteoblasts are uninucleated cells that synthesize both collagenous and non-collagenous bone proteins and are thought to be derived from multipotent mesenchymal cells. These cells exhibit high level of alkaline phosphatase on the outer surface of their plasma membrane. This enzyme is used as a cytochemical marker to distinguish preosteoblasts from fibroblasts. Functions of osteoblast are bone formation by synthesizing organic matrix of bone, cell to cell communication and maintenance of bone matrix and bone resorption by producing proteases which are involved in matrix degradation and maturation.

Osteoblasts produce type I collagen, non-collagenous proteins (osteocalcin, osteopontin, osteonectin) and various proteoglycans. These also produce cytokines and growth factors like BMPs (BMP-2 and BMP-7), TGF-β, IGF and PDGF.

Osteocyte: As osteoblasts secretes bone matrix, some of them become entrapped in lacunae and are then called osteocytes. The number of osteoblasts that become osteocytes varies depending on their rapidity of bone formation, the more rapid the formation; the more osteocytes are present per unit volume. The osteocyte extends processes called canaliculi that radiate from the lacunae. These canaliculi bring oxygen and nutrients to the osteocytes through blood and remove metabolic waste products. They have decreased quantity of synthetic and secretory organelles and indeed are smaller cells than osteoblasts.

Bone lining cells: These cells cover most, but not all quiescent bone surfaces in the adult skeleton. Together with osteocytes, bone forming cells and their connecting cell processes appear to form an extensive homeostatic network of cells capable of regulating plasma calcium concentration.

Osteoclast: These are multinucleated giant cells of 50 to 100 μm size. These are irregular oval or club shaped having branching processes. They are derived from circulating blood cell monocytes. Osteoclasts are found in baylike depressions in the bone called Howship's lacunae. The part of the cell in contact with bone shows convoluted surface, the ruffled border which is the site of great activity due to ion transport and protein secretion. Ruffled border is surrounded by a clear zone that has no organelles other than microfilaments **(Fig. 4.6)**. Peripheral region of apical membrane is tightly juxtaposed to matrix which is called as sealing zone. Clear zone and sealing zone are responsible for

attachment of osteoclast to bone matrix. Basolateral membrane is the major site for receipt and integration of regulatory signals. The enzymes released by Osteoclast are acid phosphatase, aryl sulfatase, β-glucuronidase, several cysteine proteinases such as cathepsin B and L, tissue plasminogen activator (TPA), MMP- 1 and lysosymes.

Osteoprogenitor cells: They are long, thin stem cell population to generate osteoblast.

Periosteum consists of an inner layer of osteoblasts surrounded by osteoprogenitor cells, which have the potential to differentiate into osteoblasts, and an outer layer rich in blood vessels and nerves and composed of collagen fibers which penetrate the bone, binding the periosteum to the bone. Periostin is a recently identified protein which is termed so because it was initially identified in the periosteum. It is secreted cell adhesion protein that is 90Kda in size. Structurally, it is a disulfide linked protein that favors osteoblast attachment and spreading. Osteoblast adherence is mediated through the presence of $\alpha_v\beta_3$ and $\alpha_v\beta_5$ integrins that are upregulated in the presence of periostin.

Endosteum is composed of a single layer of osteoblasts and a small amount of connective tissue. The inner layer is the osteogenic layer and the outer is the fibrous layer.

FENESTRATION AND DEHISCENCE

The anatomy of the alveolar processes depends upon the alignment and position of the teeth. When the teeth are in extreme buccal or lingual version the alveolar process is extremely thin or missing on that side of the teeth. Fenestrations are the isolated areas in which root is denuded of bone and marginal bone is intact. Dehiscences are the denuded areas that extend through the marginal bone **(Figs 4.7 and 4.8)**. Dehiscence and fenestration are both associated with extreme buccal or

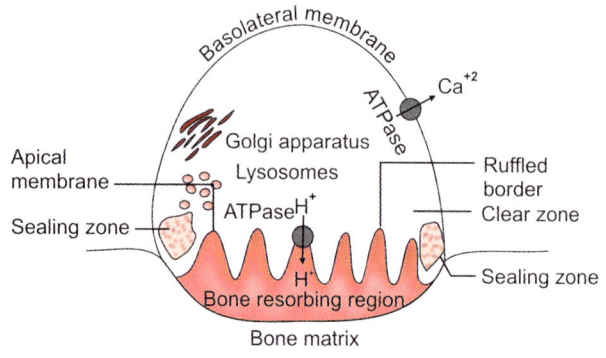

Fig. 4.6: Activated osteoclast

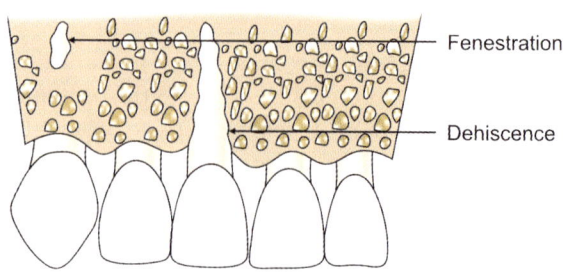

Fig. 4.7: Dehiscence and fenestration

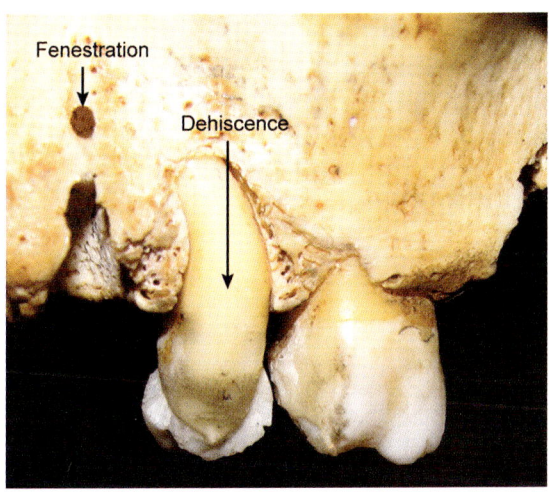

Fig. 4.8: Dehiscence and fenestration

lingual version of teeth. It occurs in 20% of all teeth. The defects are very important clinically because where they occur the root is covered only by the periosteum and overlying gingiva, which may atrophy under irritation and expose the root.

COUPLING

It is interdependency of osteoblasts and osteoclasts in remodeling of the bone **(Fig. 4.9)**.

Osteoblast–osteoclast Coupling

The development of osteoclasts is controlled by the stromal cells through the RANK/ RANKL/ OPG axis. RANK (Receptor activator of nuclear factor kappa) is activated through its ligand RANKL. RANKL is produced from the osteoblasts/stromal cells. Upon RANK/RANKL binding, activation of osteoclasts occurs which subsequently leads to bone resorption. On the other hand, osteoprotegrin (OPG) is also produced by

various mesenchymal cells and acts as a soluble decoy receptor of RANKL. OPG binds to RANKL and prevents downstream activation. As downstream signaling does not occur, there is no activation of transcription factors and therefore no osteoclastogenesis.

BONE MODELING AND REMODELING

Process by which the overall size and shape of bone is established is called as bone modeling. It extends from embryonic bone development to the pre-adult period of human growth, which is continuous and covers a large surface. It represents a change that occurs within the mineralized bone without a concomitant alteration of the architecture of the tissues. Thus, there is change in the initial bone architecture.

Bone remodeling or bone turnover occur in order to allow the replacement of old bone by new bone. It does not stop when adulthood is reached, although its rate slows down, which is cyclical and usually covers a small area. It involves two processes - bone resorption and bone apposition. Thus, modeling and remodeling occur throughout life to allow bone to adapt to the external and internal demands.

As the osteoclasts move through the bone, the leading edge of resorption is termed the cutting cone and is characterized in cross section by a scalloped array of Howship's lacunae, each housing osteoclasts. When portion of an earlier osteon is left unresorbed, it becomes an interstitial lamella. Behind the cutting cone is the migration of mononucleated cells onto the roughened cylinder. As these cells differentiate into osteoblasts, they produce a coating termed the cement or reversal line. It is a thin layer of glycoproteins comprising atleast bone sialoprotein and osteopontin that acts as a cohesive, mineralized layer between the old bone and the new bone to be secreted. On top of the cement line osteoblasts begin

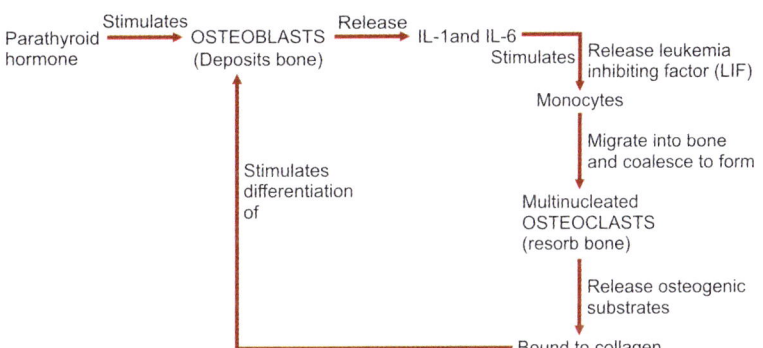

Fig. 4.9: Coupling mechanism

to lay down new bone matrix, mineralizing it from the outer to inner side. The entire area of the osteon where active formation occurs is termed the filling cone. As formation proceeds, some osteoblasts become osteocytes. Once formation is complete, the Haversian canal contains a central blood vessel and a layer of inactive osteoblasts, the lining cells that communicate by means of cell processes with the embedded osteocytes.

The repeated deposition and removal of bone tissue accommodates the growth of a bone without losing function or its relationship to neighboring structures during the remodeling phase.

The various bone resorbing factors are: Systemic factors (parathyroid hormone, parathyroid related peptide, Vitamin D_3 and thyroid hormone); Local factors (prostanoids, lipoxygenase metabolites, IL – 1, TNF – α, TNF – β, IL – 6); Growth factors (EGF, TGF – α, TGF – β, PDGF) and Bacterial factors (lipopolysaccharides, capsular material, peptidoglycans, lipoteichoic acids).

Ten Cate described the sequence of events in the resorptive process as below:

1. Attachment of osteoclasts to the mineralized surface of bone.
2. Creation of a sealed acidic environment through action of the proton pump, which demineralizes bone and exposes the organic matrix
3. Degradation of the exposed organic matrix to its constituents amino acids by the action of released enzymes, such as acid phosphatase and cathepsine
4. Sequestering of mineral ions and amino acids within the osteoclast. Rest is explained in chapter no. 24 Bone Defects.

VASCULAR SUPPLY

The vascular supply to the bone enters the interdental septa through nutrient canals together with veins, nerves and lymphatics. Dental arterioles, which also branch off the alveolar arteries, send tributaries through the periodontal ligament and some small branches enter the marrow spaces of the bone through the perforations in the cribriform plate. Small vessels emanating from the facial and lingual compact bone also enter the marrow and spongy bone.

POINTS TO PONDER

✓ Alveolar bone is the least stable periodontal tissue.
✓ Fenestration is window like circumscribed defect where as dehiscence is cleft like split defect.

✓ Osteoblasts are bone builder where as osteoclast are bone consumers.
✓ Matrix gla protein is a negative regulator of mineralization.

BIBLIOGRAPHY

1. Alveolar process. In, Grant DA, Stern IB, Listgarten MA. Periodontics. 6th ed CV Mosby Company 1988; 94-118.
2. Bartold PM, Narayanan AS. The Biochemistry and Physiology of the Periodontium. In, Wilson TG, Kornman KS. Fundamentals of Periodontics. Quintessence Publishing Co.1996; 61 – 108.
3. Bernard GW, Carranza FA. The tooth supporting structures. In, Newman, Takei, Carranza. Clinical Periodontology. 9th ed WB Saunders 2003; 36-57.
4. Bhaskar SN. Maxilla and Mandilble (Alveolar process). In, Bhaskar SN. Orban's Oral histology and Embroylogy. 11th ed Mosby 1991; 239-59.
5. Embery G, Waddington RJ, Hall RC, Last KS. Connective tissue elements as diagnostic aids in periodontolgy. Periodontol 2000 2000;24:193-214.
6. Freeman E. Periodontium. In, Tencate AR. Oral histology Development, Structure and Function. 5th ed Mosby 1998; 253-88.
7. Holmstrup P. The macroanatomy of the Periodontium. In, Wilson TG, Kornman KS. Fundamentals of Periodontics. Quintessence Publishing Co.1996; 17 – 26.
8. Holmstrup P. The microanatomy of the Periodontium. In, Wilson TG, Kornman KS. Fundamentals of Periodontics. Quintessence Publishing Co.1996; 27 – 46.
9. Lindhe J, Karring T, Araujo M. Anatomy of the Periodontium. In, Lindhe J, Karring T, Lang NP. Clinical Periodontology and Implant dentistry. 4th ed Blackwell Munksgaard 2003; 3-49.

MCQs

1. Coupling phenomenon is:
   A. Association of osteoclast with bone surface for resorption
   B. Association of osteoblast with the matrix for bone mineralization
   C. Interdependency of osteoblasts and osteoclasts in remodeling
   D. Contact between various osteocytes with in haversian system for exchange of nutrients.
2. The inactive osteoblasts are:
   A. Osteocytes
   B. Osteoclasts
   C. Osteoproginator cells
   D. Bone lining cells
3. The enzyme closely associated with new bone formation is:
   A. Acid phosphatase
   B. Alkaline phosphatase

C. Succinic dehydrogenase

D. Both A and B

4. Which of the following is bone gla protein?

A. Osteonectin

B. Bone sialoprotein

C. Osteocalcin

D. Osteopontin

5. Following is true about osteoclast *except*:

A. Mononucleated cells

B. Having branching processes

C. Derived from circulating blood cells monocytes

D. Found in Howship's lacunae.

6. Function of osteoblast:

A. Bone formation by synthesizing organic matrix of bone

B. Cell to cell communication

C. Bone resorption

D. All of the above

7. The term lamina dura refers to the radiographic image of the:

A. Periodontal ligament space

B. Alveolar bone proper

C. Cortical plates

D. Cancellous bone

E. Alveolar crest

8. Following is true about fenestration and dehiscence *expect*:

A. Fenestration is the isolated area in which root is denuded of bone and marginal bone is intact.

B. Dehiscence is the denuded area that extends through the marginal bone.

C. Dehiscence and fenestration are both associated with extreme buccal or lingual version of teeth

D. None of the above

Answers

1. C	2. D	3. B	4. C	5. A
6. D	7. B	8. D		

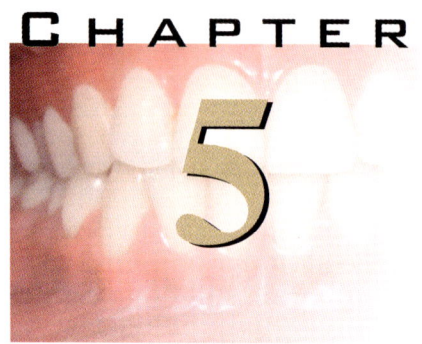

CHAPTER 5

Aging and Periodontium

Shalu Bathla

INTRODUCTION

Aging is slowing of a natural function, a disintegration of the balanced control and organization that characterizes the young adult. General features of aging found in all tissues are tissue desiccation, reduced elasticity, altered cell permeability and diminished reparative capacity. The vasculature, gingiva, periodontal ligament, cementum and alveolar bone all demonstrate the age changes.

VARIOUS AGE CHANGES OF PERIODONTIUM

A. Gingiva: Stippling usually disappears with age. The width of the attached gingiva increases with age (Fig. 5.1)
   a. Gingival epithelium: Aging results in:
      • Thinning and decreased keratinization
      • Rete pegs flatten
      • Migration of junctional epithelium to more apical position
      • Reduced oxygen consumption.
   b. Gingival connective tissue: Aging results in:
      • Increased rate of conversion of soluble to insoluble collagen
      • Increased mechanical strength of collagen
      • Increased denaturing temperature of collagen
      • Decreased rate of synthesis of collagen
      • Greater collagen content.
B. Periodontal ligament:
   • Decreased number of fibroblasts
   • More irregular structures
   • Decrease organic matrix production
   • Decrease epithelial cell rests of Malassez
   • Increased amount of elastic fibers.
C. Cementum:
   • Increase in cemental width
   • Decrease in permeability.
D. Alveolar bone:
   • Bone undergoes osteoporosis with aging
   • Reduction in bone metabolism
   • Decreased vascularity
   • Decreased healing capacity
   • Ability of alveolar bone to withstand occlusal forces decreases after the age of 30.

Dentogingival plaque accumulation has been suggested to increase with age. It has been speculated that a ecological shift occurs in certain periodontal pathogens with age, specifically including an increased role of *Porphyromonas gingivalis* and a decreased role of *Aggregatibacter actinomycetemcomitans*.

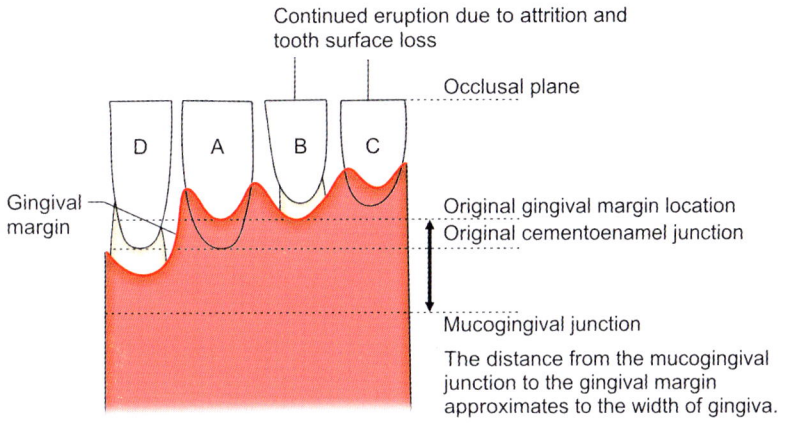

Fig. 5.1: Relationship of the gingival margin with the crown and root surface.
A. Normal relationship of gingival margin 1 to 2 mm above the cementoenamel junction.
B. Clinical recession case where gingival margin remains in same position, as the incisal edge wears off and tooth eruption continues.
C. The gingival margin has moved with the tooth, the entire dentogingival complex has moved coronally increasing the width of attached gingiva.
D. No wear of incisal edge, gingiva has moved apically and clinical recession is evident. The width of attached gingiva is reduced.

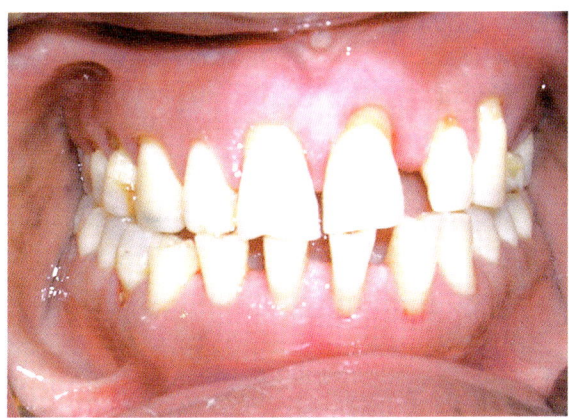

Fig. 5.2: Periodontal changes associated with aging

Tooth - Periodontium Relationships: The most obvious change in the teeth with aging is a loss of tooth substance caused by the attrition. Occlusal wear cause reduction in cusp height and inclination. Wear of teeth also occurs on the proximal surfaces, accompanied by mesial migration of the teeth. Attrition and proximal wear result in a reduced maxillary mandibular overjet in the molar area and an edge-to-edge bite anteriorly **(Fig. 5.2)**.

EFFECTS OF AGING ON THE PROGRESSION OF PERIODONTAL DISEASES

One theory is that many sites of advanced periodontal disease have resulted in tooth loss earlier in life, suggesting that older age is not a risk factor for periodontal disease. Thus, age has been suggested to be not a true risk factor but a background or an associated factor for periodontitis. The relationship between age and periodontal disease is age associated and not a consequence of aging. Advanced age does not decrease plaque control; however, older adults may have difficulty performing adequate oral hygiene because of compromised health, mental status, medications, altered mobility and dexterity. Older adults may change toothbrush habits due to disabilities such as hemiplegia, visual difficulties, dementia, and arthritis. The newer, lightweight, electric-powered toothbrushes may be more beneficial than a manual toothbrush for older adults with physical and sensory limitations.

EFFECTS OF AGING ON THE RESPONSE TO TREATMENT OF THE PERIODONTIUM

Despite the histologic changes in the periodontium with aging, no differences in response to nonsurgical or surgical treatment have been shown for periodontitis patient. Periodontal healing and recurrence of disease are not influenced by age. Factors to consider are medical and mental health status, medications, functional status and lifestyle behaviors that influence periodontal treatment. For older adults, a nonsurgical approach is often the first treatment of choice. Depending on the nature and extent of periodontal disease, surgical therapy may be indicated. Surgical technique should minimize the amount of additional root exposure. Individuals responding best to surgical therapy are those who are able to maintain the surgical result. Thus, age alone is not a contraindication to surgery and implant placement.

Common age changes in all periodontal tissues are

Narrowing of vessel lumen
Thickening of vessel walls
Loss of cellularity
Increasing fibrosis

BIBLIOGRAPHY

1. Eley BM, Manson JD. The Periodontal Tissues. In, Periodontics. 5th ed Wright 2004; 1-20.
2. Fedele DJ, Niessen LC. Periodontal treatment for older adults. In, Newman, Takei, Carranza. Clinical Periodontology. 9th ed WB Saunders 2003; 551-7.
3. Grant DA, Stern IB, Listgarten MA. Periodontal structure in aging humans. In, Periodontics. 6th ed CV Mosby Company 1988; 119-34.
4. Needleman I. Aging and the Periodontium. In, Newman, Takei, Carranza. Clinical Periodontology. 9th ed WB Saunders 2003; 58–63.

MCQs

1. With the increase in age; keratinization of gingiva:
   A. Increases
   B. Decreases
   C. Remains the same
   D. Increases and then decreases
2. With aging, the solubility of the collagen in gingival connective tissue:
   A. Increases
   B. Decreases
   C. Remains constant
   D. First increase then decrease
3. Which of the following fibers increases with age in periodontal ligament?
   A. Type I collagen
   B. Type II collagen
   C. Elastic fibers
   D. Oxytalan fibers
4. Which of the following organism's role is decreased with age:
   A. *P.gingivalis*
   B. *Aggregatibacter actinomycetemcomitans*
   C. *F. nucleatum*
   D. *P. intermedia*
5. The width of the attached gingiva with age:
   A. Increases   B. Decreases
   C. No change   D. None of the above

Answers

1. B   2. B   3. C   4. B   5. A

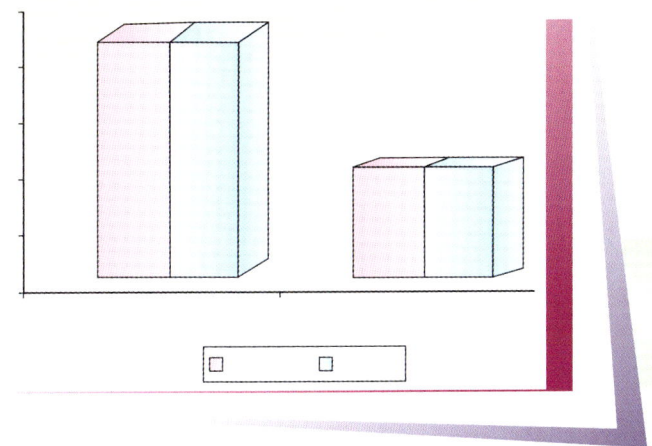

SECTION

TWO

CLASSIFICATION AND EPIDEMIOLOGY

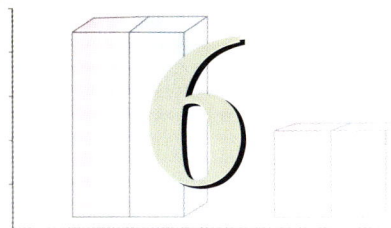

CHAPTER

Classification of Periodontal Diseases

Shalu Bathla

INTRODUCTION

Classification should be a systematic arrangement of groups that possess common attributes. This arrangement should provide insight into the relationship between groups and between members of the same group. Classification of disease is necessary to separate conditions into distinct categories so as to aid clinical and laboratory diagnosis and specific treatments. A system of classifying or grouping the pathologic processes affecting the periodontium serves to identify the etiology and to facilitate communication among clinicians, students and epidemiologists. Over the years a number of classification systems have been developed to organize and name various disease entities or conditions affecting the periodontium.

PURPOSE OF CLASSIFICATION SYSTEM

1. Communicating clinical findings accurately to other dental health care providers and to dental insurance providers.
2. Presenting information to the patient about his or her disease.
3. Formulating individualized treatment plans.
4. Predicting treatment outcomes.

DOMINANT PARADIGM IN THE HISTORICAL DEVELOPMENT OF PERIODONTAL CLASSIFICATION SYSTEM

Development and evolution of classification systems for periodontal disease have been largely influenced by paradigms that reflect the understanding of the nature of periodontal disease during a given historical period. Thoughts that guided the classification of periodontal diseases can be placed into three dominant paradigms primarily:

I. *Clinical characteristics paradigm (1870-1920)*: From the periods 1870 to 1920, very little was known about the etiology and pathogenesis of periodontal disease. Accordingly, the diseases were classified almost entirely on the basis of their clinical characteristics supplemented by unsubstantiated theories about their cause.

II. *Classical pathology paradigm (1920-1970)*: The classification systems of this period were dominated by the classical pathology paradigm which was based on the principles of general pathology and included disease categories labeled as dystrophic, atrophic or degenerative.

In 1928, Gottlieb classified periodontal diseases as:
1. Inflammatory
   - Schmutz pyorrhea (poor oral hygiene)
2. Degenerative or atrophic
   - Diffuse alveolar atrophy
   - Paradental pyorrhea

In 1940, Box classified periodontal diseases as:
1. Gingivitis
   - Acute
   - Chronic
2. Periodontitis
   - Acute
   - Chronic
   - Periodontitis simplex
   - Periodontitis complex

III. *Infection/Host response paradigm (1970-present)*: Classification systems for periodontal disease currently in use are firmly based on and dominated by Infection/Host response paradigm.

In 1977, Schluger, Yuodelis and Page classified periodontal diseases as:
1. Gingivitis
   - Plaque associated gingivitis
   - ANUG
   - Hormonal gingivitis
   - Drug - induced gingivitis
2. Marginal periodontitis
   - Adult type
   - Juvenile type

In 1982, Page and Schroeder classified periodontal diseases as:
   Periodontitis
   - Prepubertal (Generalized/Localized)
   - Juvenile
   - Rapidly progressing periodontitis
   - Adult type periodontitis.

AAP 1989 CLASSIFICATION (WORLD WORKSHOP IN CLINICAL PERIODONTICS)

AAP World workshop in clinical periodontics classified periodontal diseases as:
1. Adult periodontitis
2. Early periodontitis (may be prepubertal, juvenile, rapidly progressive)
3. Periodontitis associated with systemic disease
4. Necrotizing periodontitis
5. Refractory periodontitis

This classification was a refinement of one that had been proposed by Page and Schroeder in 1982. Main features—This classification was based on the infection/host response paradigm depended heavily on the age of the affected patients (Prepubertal and Juvenile periodontitis), rate of progression (Adult and Early periodontitis), host factors (Periodontitis associated with systemic disease) and response to the conventional therapy (Refractory periodontitis).

Drawbacks associated with 1989 AAP classification:
  i. It does not include gingivitis/gingival disease category.
 ii. Periodontitis categories had nonvalidated age dependent criteria.
iii. There was extensive crossover in rates of progression of the different categories of periodontitis. Rapidly progressive periodontitis was a heterogeneous category.
 iv. There was extensive overlap in the clinical characteristics of the different categories of periodontitis.
  v. Refractory periodontitis was a heterogeneous category.
 vi. Prepubertal periodontitis was a heterogeneous category.
vii. Finally, different forms of periodontitis proposed in the classification shared many microbiologic and host response features, which suggested extensive overlap and heterogeneity among the categories.

As a consequence of these drawbacks, the 1989 classification was criticized shortly after it was published and different system was proposed and new classification was developed in 1993, by European workshop on Periodontology as:
1. Adult periodontitis
2. Early onset periodontitis
3. Necrotizing periodontitis.

This classification lacked adequate categorization of broad spectrum of periodontal disease. Moreover, gingival diseases were also not included.

AAP 1999 CLASSIFICATION (INTERNATIONAL WORKSHOP FOR CLASSIFICATION OF PERIODONTAL DISEASES)

CLASSIFICATION OF PERIODONTAL DISEASES AND CONDITIONS

1. Gingival diseases
   - Plaque – induced gingival diseases
   - Non- plaque – induced gingival diseases
2. Chronic periodontitis
   - Localized
   - Generalized
3. Aggressive periodontitis
   - Localized
   - Generalized
4. Periodontitis as a manifestation of systemic diseases
5. Necrotizing periodontal diseases
   - Necrotizing ulcerative gingivitis (NUG)
   - Necrotizing ulcerative periodontitis (NUP)
6. Abscesses of the periodontium
   - Gingival abscess
   - Periodontal abscess
   - Pericoronal abscess
7. Periodontitis associated with endodontic lesions
   - Endodontic – periodontal lesion
   - Periodontal – endodontic lesion
   - Combined lesion
8. Developmental or acquired deformities and conditions
   - Localized tooth – related factors that predispose to plaque– induced gingival diseases or periodontitis
   - Mucogingival deformities and conditions around teeth
   - Mucogingival deformities and conditions on edentulous ridges
   - Occlusal trauma

GINGIVAL DISEASES

Dental plaque - Induced gingival diseases

These diseases may occur on a periodontium with no attachment loss or on one with attachment loss that is stable and not progressing.

I. Gingivitis associated with dental plaque only
   A. Without local contributing factors
   B. With local contributing factors
II. Gingival diseases modified by systemic factors
   A. Associated with endocrine system
      1. Puberty – associated gingivitis
      2. Menstrual cycle – associated gingivitis
      3. Pregnancy associated
         a. Gingivitis
         b. Pyogenic granuloma
      4. Diabetes mellitus – associated gingivitis
   B. Associated with blood dyscrasias
      1. Leukemia – associated gingivitis
      2. Other

III. Gingival diseases modified by medications
   A. Drug – influenced gingival diseases
      1. Drug – influenced gingival enlargements
      2. Drug – influenced gingivitis
         a. Oral contraceptive – associated gingivitis
         b. Other
IV. Gingival diseases modified by malnutrition
   A. Ascorbic acid deficiency gingivitis
   B. Other

Non Plaque induced gingival diseases

I. Gingival diseases of specific bacterial origin
   A. Neisseria gonorrhea
   B. Treponema pallidum
   C. Streptococcal species
   D. Other
II. Gingival diseases of viral origin
   A. Herpes virus infections
      a. Primary herpetic gingivostomatitis
      b. Recurrent oral herpes
      c. Varicella Zoster
   B. Other
III. Gingival diseases of fungal origin
   A. Candida - species infections: Generalized gingival candidiasis
   B. Linear gingival erythema
   C. Histoplasmosis
   D. Other
IV. Gingival diseases of genetic origin
   A. Hereditary gingival fibromatosis
   B. Other
V. Gingival manifestations of systemic conditions
   A. Mucocutaneous lesions
      1. Lichen planus
      2. Pemphigoid
      3. Pemphigus vulgaris
      4. Erythema multiforme
      5. Lupus erythematosus
      6. Drug induced
      7. Other
   B. Allergic reactions
      1. Dental restorative materials
         a. Mercury
         b. Nickel
         c. Acrylic
         d. Other
      2. Reactions attributable to
         a. Toothpastes or dentifrices
         b. Mouthrinses or mouthwashes
         c. Chewing gum additives
         d. Food and additives
      3. Other
VI. Traumatic lesions (factitious, iatrogenic,or accidental)
   A. Chemical injury
   B. Physical injury
   C. Thermal injury
VII. Foreign body reactions
VIII. Not otherwise specified

DEVELOPMENTAL/ACQUIRED DEFORMITIES AND CONDITIONS

Developmental or acquired deformities and conditions

Localized tooth related factors that modify or predispose to plaque induced gingival diseases or periodontitis
1. Tooth anatomic factors
2. Dental restorations or appliances
3. Root fractures
4. Cervical root resorption and cemental tears

Mucogingival deformities and conditions around teeth

1. Gingival or soft tissue recession
   A. Facial or lingual surfaces
   B. Interproximal (papillary)
2. Lack of keratinized gingiva
3. Decreased vestibular depth
4. Aberrant frenum or muscle position
5. Gingival excess
   A. Pseudopocket
   B. Inconsistent gingival margin
   C. Excessive gingival display
   D. Gingival enlargement
   E. Abnormal color

Mucogingival deformities and conditions on edentulous edges

1. Vertical and or horizontal ridge deficiency
2. Lack of gingiva or keratinized tissue
3. Gingival or soft tissue enlargements
4. Aberrant frenum or muscle position
5. Decreased vestibular depth
6. Abnormal color

Occlusal trauma

1. Primary occlusal trauma
2. Secondary occlusal trauma

Main features of AAP 1999 classification system are:

i. Comprehensive section of gingival diseases is included in this classification.
ii. There is replacement of the term adult periodontitis with chronic periodontitis, since epidemiological evidence suggests that chronic periodontitis may also be seen in adolescents.
iii. There is elimination of separate categories of rapidly progressive periodontitis and refractory periodontitis because of the lack of evidence that they represent separate conditions.
iv. There is replacement of the term early onset periodontitis with aggressive periodontitis largely because of the clinical difficulties in determining the age of onset in many of these cases. The author of this new classification also questions the use of the term juvenile periodontitis for the same reasons. They have replaced the term with localized and generalized aggressive periodontitis. The term aggressive was added because bone and tissue destruction occurs rapidly as compared with other periodontitis.
v. A new classification group of periodontitis as a manifestation of systemic disease has been created and this includes those cases of prepubertal periodontitis directly resulting from known systemic diseases.
vi. There are also new group categories of abscesses of the periodontium, periodontic–endodontic lesions and developmental/acquired deformities/conditions.

BIBLIOGRAPHY

1. Armitage GC. Classifying periodontal diseases—a long-standing dilemma. Periodontol 2002; 30:9-23.
2. Armitage GC. Diagnosis and Classification of Periodontal diseases. In, Rose LF, Mealey BL, Genco RJ, Cohen DW. Periodontics, Medicine, Surgery and Implants. Elsevier Mosby 2004; 19-31.
3. Eley BM, Manson JD. Classification of periodontal diseases. In, Periodontics 5th ed Wright 2004;120-22.
4. Grant DA, Stern IB, Listgarten MA. Examination and diagnosis: classification. In, Periodontics. 6th ed CV Mosby Company 1988; 525-72.
5. Genco RJ. Classification and clinical and radiographic features of periodontal disease. In, Genco RJ, Goldman HM, Cohen DW. Contemporary Periodontics. CV Mosby Company 1990; 63-81.
6. Novak MJ. Classification of diseases and conditions affecting the periodontium. In, Newman, Takei, Carranza. Clinical Periodontology 9th ed WB Saunders 2003; 64-73.

MCQs

1. According to the 1999 classification of disease and conditions affecting periodontium the ascorbic acid deficiency gingivitis is included in:
   A. Gingival disease modified by systemic factors
   B. Gingival manifestation of systemic condition
   C. Gingival disease modified by malnutrition
   D. Gingival disease modified by medication.
2. In 1989 AAP classification following condition is not included:
   A. Dental plaque induced gingival diseases
   B. Refractory periodontitis
   C. Necrotizing ulcerative periodontitis
   D. Adult periodontitis
3. In 1999 AAP classification following condition is not included:
   A. Localized aggressive periodontitis
   B. Generalized chronic periodontitis
   C. Refractory periodontitis
   D. Non-plaque induced gingival lesion

Answers

1. C   2. A   3. C

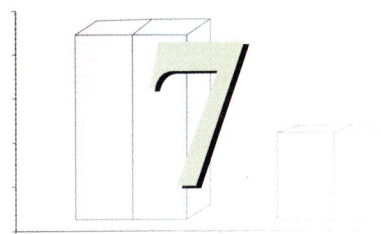

Epidemiology of Gingival and Periodontal Diseases

Shalu Bathla

DEFINITION OF EPIDEMIOLOGY

John M. Last (1988) defined epidemiology as *"the study of the distribution and determinants of health related states or events in specified populations and the application of this study to the control of health problems"*.

AIMS OF EPIDEMIOLOGY

The International Epidemiological Association has listed three main aims of epidemiology, which were put forward by Lowe and Kost Rzewski in 1973 as follows:
1. To describe the size and distribution of the disease problems in human populations.
2. To provide the data essential for the planning, implementation and evaluation of health services for the prevention, control and treatment of diseases.
3. To identify etiological factors in the pathogenesis of disease.

USES OF EPIDEMIOLOGY

Morris has identified seven distinct uses of epidemiology:
1. To study historically, the rise and fall of disease in the population
2. Community diagnosis
3. Planning and evaluation
4. Evaluation of individuals risks and chances
5. Syndrome identification
6. Completing the natural history of disease
7. Searching for causes and risk factors

EPIDEMIOLOGICAL METHODS

Epidemiology as a science is organized into 3 distinct divisions as:
1. *Descriptive Epidemiology*: Descriptive studies are used to observe and document the occurrence, progression and distribution of a disease or condition in population in relation to host, environmental and agent factors. Descriptive studies are usually the first phase of any epidemiological investigation.
2. *Analytical Epidemiology*: Analytical studies are used to investigate hypothesis derived from descriptive epidemiologic studies or other data sources.
3. *Experimental Epidemiology*: Experimental epidemiology is used to test hypothesis further by introducing a preventive or therapeutic agent and comparing the outcome in test subjects with concurrent observations in control groups.

Descriptive and analytical studies are also called as observational studies.

EPIDEMIOLOGIC STUDY DESIGNS

Analytical epidemiology is observational, the most common observational studies are:

a. Cross-sectional studies
b. Cohort studies
c. Case-control studies

Cross-sectional study: It is based on a single examination of a cross-section of population at one point of time. It is also known as prevalence study. Cross-sectional study designs are often used to investigate the association between risk factors and disease prevalence in situations where less is known concerning the form or type of association. This study design is probably the most commonly used. The focus is on prevalence of disease, not the incidence. The temporal relationship between exposure and the disease is often unknown in cross-sectional studies.

Prevalence: It indicates all current cases both old and new existing at a given point in time or over a period of time in a given population. It is of two types:

- *Point prevalence*: It is defined as the number of all current cases of a specific disease at one point of time in relation to a defined population. The "point" in point prevalence can be either a day or few days or even few weeks, depending upon the time taken to examine the sample of the population.
- *Period prevalence*: It is defined as the total number of existing cases of a specific disease during a defined period of time (e.g. annual prevalence) expressed in relation to a defined population.

Prevalence is dependent on two factors, the incidence and duration of the disease.

Prevalence = Incidence × Mean duration

P = I X D

Incidence: It is defined as the number of new cases of a specific disease occurring in a defined population during a specified period of time.

$$\text{Incidence} = \frac{\begin{array}{c}\text{Number of new cases of a specific}\\\text{disease during a given time period}\end{array}}{\text{The population at risk}} \times 1000$$

Case control study: Case control study involves two populations - cases and controls. In case control studies the unit is the individual rather than the group. The focus is on the disease or some other health problem that has already developed. Thus, these are basically comparison studies. Case-control studies are useful for studying risk factors associated with relatively rare diseases. In case control studies it is possible to select a group of cases and an appropriate group of controls (matched or unmatched) and investigate exposure or risk factors thought to be associated with the occurrence of disease **(Fig. 7.1)**. The usual measure of association is the odds ratio. A case-control study can provide important information related to association between exposure level for rare diseases, but is not capable of providing estimates of disease occurrence.

Odds ratio: It is a measure of the strengths of the association between risk factor and outcome. Odds ratio can be derived from case control study. It is the ratio of exposure among the cases to exposure among the controls.

Cohort study: It is usually undertaken to obtain additional evidence to refute or support the existence of an association between the suspected cause and disease. The cohorts are identified prior to the appearance of the disease under investigation and the study proceeds forward from cause to effect **(Fig. 7.1)**. The cohort study design is useful for comparing disease incidence for relatively common diseases among groups having different exposure levels or risk factors. The usual

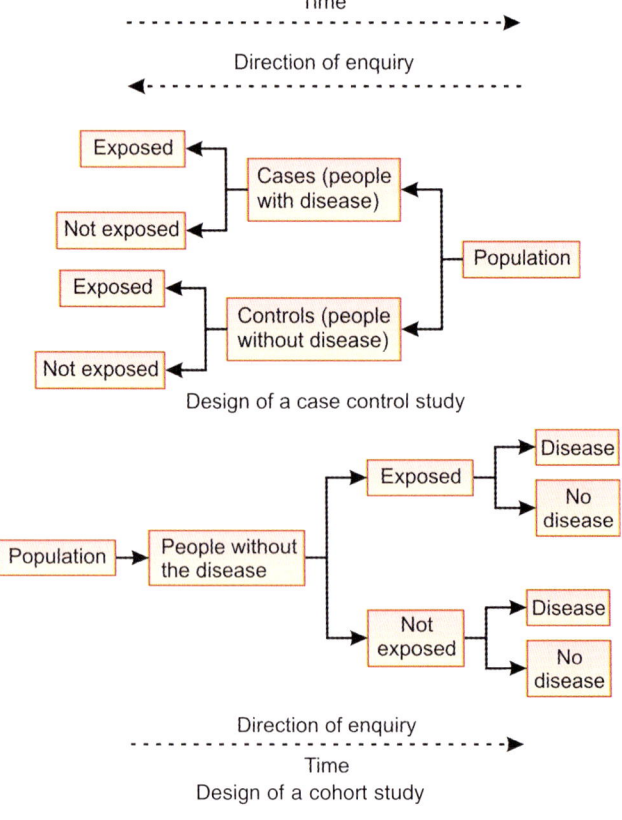

Design of a case control study

Design of a cohort study

Fig. 7.1: Analytical epidemiology

measures of association include the risk ratio, relative risk and attributable risk. This design may be useful for following the natural course or progression of periodontal disease in a group of subjects when little or no control and monitoring are imposed. A cohort design could involve a non-randomized parallel design in which the occurrence or progression of periodontal disease is monitored in subjects with or without a risk factor (high vs. low levels of a microbial infection, smokers vs. non smokers, etc.). A premier cohort study design is the randomized controlled clinical trial in which a high level of control and monitoring is an integral component.

Experimental epidemiology include clinical trials, which may be categorized as
a. Randomized controlled trials
b. Field trials
c. Community trials

In 1986, Lindhe et al stated that there are certain minimal requirements for the design of acceptable clinical trials:

- Testable hypothesis
- An adequate number of subjects
- Test and control groups
- Random assignment of subjects to these groups
- Appropriate and reproducible measurements to assess effects of therapy
- Appropriate statistical methods to test the hypothesis

PERIODONTAL EPIDEMIOLOGY

Periodontal epidemiology literature lacks consistency in methodology of research, which includes various definitions for periodontal disease and health; different approaches to measure periodontal indices of pocket depth and attachment loss; inconsistent study designs and lack of adjustments to known risk factors. These inconsistencies do not allow for effective comparison of epidemiological studies, which is essential to find strong association of risk factors with periodontal disease, which in turn is necessary for the interpretation of risk and causality.

Gingivitis: Epidemiologic studies show that gingivitis is ubiquitous in population of children and adults globally. More than 82% of adolescents in United States have overt gingivitis and signs of gingival bleeding. Similar or higher prevalence of gingivitis has been reported in children and adolescents in other parts of the world. A high prevalence of gingivitis is also found in adults.

Chronic periodontitis: Chronic periodontitis is common worldwide. It may occur in most age groups but is more prevalent among adults. The estimates of chronic periodontitis in various populations vary significantly, in part because populations differ in their demographics and levels of exposure to various etiologic and risk factors of periodontitis. Chronic periodontitis in children and adolescents shows a wide frequency range in various geographic regions and racial/ethnic groups. Low disease frequencies among young Caucasians in Western Europe and North America and relatively high frequencies in Africa and Latin America have been reported.

Aggressive periodontitis: For the most part, epidemiologic studies of aggressive periodontitis have many of inherent weakness of disease definition and study design as studies of chronic periodontitis. Aggressive periodontitis shows a wide range of occurrence frequencies in various geographic regions and demographic groups and the variance seems particularly large between different racial/ ethnic groups. Estimates of disease occurrence by racial/ ethnic groups are 0.1% to 0.2% of Caucasians, 0.4 to 1.0% of Asians and 1.0% to 3.0% of Africans and Africans Americans.

Factors affecting the prevalence and severity of gingivitis and periodontal diseases are:

Age
Oral hygiene
Sex
Race
Occupation
Education
Professional dental care
Geographic location
Social customs and nutrition
Fluoride

Epidemiologic data can form the basis for selection and implementation of strategies to prevent and treat periodontal diseases. Three broad strategies are:
- *Population strategy*: It uses a community wide approach in which health education and other favorable life practices are introduced in the community and unfavorable behaviors are attempted to be changed.
- *Secondary prevention strategy*: It includes detecting and treating individuals with destructive periodontal diseases. Dental health education approaches to improve the oral hygiene of the individual patient, although successful in the short-term, have been shown to be relatively ineffective in making sustained changes in oral hygiene behaviors.
- *Identification of high risk groups for periodontitis*: The early detection of active disease and identification of

subjects and groups who are more likely to develop destructive periodontal diseases in the future are important elements of dental care system planning.

INDICES

According to AL Russell an index has been defined as a *"numerical value describing the relative status of a population on a graduated scale with definite upper and lower limits, which are designed to permit and facilitate comparison with other populations classified by the same criteria and methods"*.

Methods which express clinical observations in numerical values are known as indices. There are many indices for recording and quantifying periodontal and gingival conditions which can be used with reproducible accuracy. Indices may allow a more straight forward approach to gather and interpret data.

Indices may be classified as:
I. According to reversibility of the index:
   • Irreversible index: Index that measures conditions that will not change. e.g an index that measures dental caries.
   • Reversible index: Index that measures conditions that can be changed. For Example, P-M-A index and Gingival index.
II. According to extent of area measured:
   • Full mouth indices: Index that measures the patients entire dentition or periodontium e. g Russel's periodontal index.
   • Simplified Indices: Index that measures only a representative sample of the dental apparatus. e.g. Greene and Vermillion's Oral hygiene Index - simplified (OHI - S).
III. According to entity which they measure:
   • Disease index – The D (decay) portion of the DMF index.
   • Treatment index – The F (filled) portion of the DMF index.
   • Symptom index – The Gingival or sulcular bleeding index.

GINGIVAL INDICES

Papillary Marginal Attached (PMA) Index

It was developed by M Massler and I Schour in 1944. In this index, the number of gingival units affected were counted rather than the severity of the inflammation.

Teeth examined: All of the facial gingival tissues surrounding all the teeth were assessed except third molars. The facial surface of gingiva around a tooth was divided into three component parts:
• Papillary gingiva (P)
• Marginal gingiva (M)
• Attached gingiva (A)

Method: The examination is started from the maxillary left second molar around to the maxillary right second molar and then from the mandibular right second molar to the mandibular left second molar.

For prevalence studies, each PMA unit is scored 0 or 1 for the absence or presence of inflammation respectively. The P, M and A numerical values for all teeth were totaled separately and then added together to calculate the PMA index score per person.

Gingival Index (GI)

It was developed by H Loe and J Silness in 1963. The purpose of this index is to assess the severity of gingivitis based on color, consistency and bleeding on probing.

Teeth examined: The teeth selected as the index teeth are - 16, 11, 24, 36, 31, 44 (FDI system). Gingival index can be determined for selected teeth or for the entire dentition.

Method: Four gingival areas i.e. distal, facial, mesial and lingual are examined systematically for each tooth. Bleeding is assessed by running circumferentially periodontal probe along the soft tissue wall of gingival crevice.

Calculation of index: The score for the four areas of the tooth can be totaled and divided by four to give a tooth score. By adding the tooth scores together and dividing by the number of teeth examined, an individual's gingival index score can be obtained.

Criteria for Gingival index

Score   *Criteria*
0   Normal gingiva
1   Mild inflammation: Slight change in color and slight edema. No bleeding on probing.
2   Moderate inflammation: Redness, edema and glazing. Bleeding on probing.
3   Severe inflammation: Marked redness, edema and ulceration. Tendency towards spontaneous bleeding.

Scoring Criteria

Gingival scores	Condition
0.1 - 1.0	Mild Gingivitis
1.1 - 2.0	Moderate Gingivitis
2.1 - 3.0	Severe Gingivitis

Modified Gingival Index (MGI)

The Modified Gingival Index (MGI), was developed by RR Lobene, J Weatherford, NM Ross, RA Lamm, and C Menaker in 1986.

Following are the modifications in this index:
1. Elimination of gingival probing to assess the presence or absence of bleeding, meaning there is no gentle probing to possibly provoke bleeding on pressure. Thus, the non-invasive index allows repeated evaluations and permits intracalliberation and intercalliberation of examiners.
2. Redefinition of the scoring system for mild and moderate inflammation.

The developers of the MGI decided to eliminate probing, which could disturb plaque and irritate the gingiva.

Modified Gingival Index does not assess the presence of periodontal pockets or attachment loss.

Criteria for MGI

Score	Criteria
0	Absence of inflammation
1	Mild inflammation: Slight change in color, little change in texture of any portion but not the entire marginal or papillary gingival unit.
2	Mild inflammation: Criteria as above but involving the entire marginal or papillary gingival unit.
3	Moderate inflammation: Glazing, redness, edema, and/or hypertrophy of the marginal or papillary gingival unit.
4	Severe inflammation: Marked redness, edema, and/or hypertrophy of the marginal or papillary gingival unit; spontaneous bleeding, congestion, or ulceration.

BLEEDING INDICES

The bleeding indices are based on the objective diagnostic signs of inflammation. These detect early inflammatory changes, which occurs before any changes in gingival color, form and texture. They also detect presence of inflammatory lesions located at the base of periodontal pocket, an area which is inaccessible to visual examination. Bleeding indices can be used to enhance patient's motivation for plaque control because patient can easily understand.

The disadvantages of gingival bleeding index are that – i) Types of probe, angulation depth and force of probing may vary and may bring discrepancy in the results and ii) Bleeding from gingival sulcus may be associated with other forms of periodontal disease, not only gingivitis.

Sulcus Bleeding Index (SBI)

SBI is an index for assessment of gingival bleeding, developed by HR Muhlemann and S Son in 1971. The purpose of this index is to locate areas of gingival sulcus bleeding upon gentle probing and thus, recognizes and record the presence of early inflammatory gingival disease.

Method: The SBI is based on the evaluation of gingival bleeding on probing, gingival contour and gingival color changes. Four gingival units are scored systematically for each tooth; the labial and lingual marginal gingiva (M units) and the mesial and distal papillary gingiva (P units). The probing of the four areas should be carried out under proper illumination. The probe should be held parallel with the long axis of the tooth for M units and directed towards the col area for P units. After the probing is done, wait for 30 seconds before scoring apparently healthy gingival units. The gingiva should be dried gently to observe color changes clearly.

Scoring Criteria: The assessment of gingival bleeding is done on a scale of 0 to 5, according to the following criteria:

Score	Criteria
0	Healthy appearance of P and M, No bleeding upon sulcus probing
1	Apparently healthy P and M showing no color or contour change and no swelling, but bleeding from sulcus on probing.
2	Bleeding on probing and color change caused by inflammation (reddening), No swelling or macroscopic edema.
3	Bleeding on probing, change in color, slight edematous swelling.
4	Bleeding or probing, color change, obvious swelling.
5	Spontaneous bleeding on probing, color change, marked swelling with or without ulceration.

Calculation: Each of the four gingival units (M and P) is scored from 0 to 5 to obtain the SBI of the area. The scores for the four units are totaled and divided by four to obtain the SBI for the tooth. By totaling scores for individual teeth and number of teeth, the SBI is determined.

PERIODONTICS REVISITED

Papillary Bleeding Index (PBI)

The Papillary Bleeding Index (PBI) was developed by H R Muhlemann in 1977. The PBI is based on bleeding following gentle probing of the interdental papilla.

Method: The PBI is performed by sweeping the papillary sulcus on the mesial and distal aspects with a periodontal probe. The mouth is divided into quadrants, with the maxillary right and mandibular left quadrants probed lingually and the maxillary left and mandibular right quadrants probed buccally. The blunt periodontal probe is carefully inserted into the gingival sulcus at the base of the papilla on the mesial aspect, then moved coronally to the papilla tip. This is repeated on the distal aspect of the same papilla. The intensity of any bleeding thus, provoked was recorded on a scale of 0 to 4.

Scoring Criteria

Score	Criteria
0	No bleeding after probing.
1	A single discrete bleeding point appears after probing.
2	Several isolated bleeding points or a single fine line of blood appears.
3	The interdental triangle fills with blood shortly after probing.
4	Profuse bleeding occurs after probing; blood flows immediately into the marginal sulcus.

Calculation: Each papilla is scored according to the criteria. The scores are totaled and divided by the number of papilla examined.

Gingival Bleeding Index (GBI)

The Gingival Bleeding Index (GBI) was developed by HG Carter and GP Barnes in 1974, to record the presence or absence of gingival inflammation as determined by bleeding from interproximal gingival sulci.

Method: All interproximal areas having a mesial and distal sulcus component are considered to be susceptible to gingival inflammation and these areas are recorded as total areas at risk. Each interproximal area has two sulci, which either are scored as one interdental unit or may be scored individually. Certain areas may be excluded from scoring because of accessibility, tooth position, diastema, or other factors, and if exclusions are made, a consistent procedure should be followed for an individual and for a group, if a study is to be made. Third molars are usually excluded and 26 interdental units are scored.

Procedure: Unwaxed dental floss is used. The floss is passed interproximally first on one side of the papilla and then on the other. The floss is then curved around the adjacent tooth and brought below the gingival margin. The floss is moved up and down for one stroke, with care not to lacerate the gingiva. A new length of clean floss is used for each area. Retract for visibility of bleeding from both facial and lingual aspects. A gap of 30 seconds should be allowed for reinspection of an area that does not show blood immediately either in the area or on the floss.

Scoring Criteria: Bleeding indicates the presence of disease. No attempt is made in this index to quantify the severity of bleeding because no bleeding represents healthy tissues.

PLAQUE INDICES

Plaque Component of the Periodontal Disease Index

In this index, six Ramfjord teeth 16, 11, 24, 36, 31, 44 (FDI system) are stained with bismarck brown solution. The criteria is to measure the presence and extent of plaque on a scale of 0 to 3, looking specifically at all interproximal, facial and lingual surfaces of the index teeth.

Scoring Criteria

Score	Criteria
0	No plaque present
1	Plaque present on some but not all interproximal, buccal and lingual surfaces of the tooth
2	Plaque present on all interproximal, buccal and lingual surfaces, but covering less than one half of the surfaces
3	Plaque extending over all interproximal, buccal and lingual surfaces and covering more than one half of these surfaces.

$$\text{Plaque score of an individual} = \frac{\text{Total score}}{\text{No. of teeth examined}}$$

This index is used in longitudinal studies of periodontal diseases and clinical trials of preventive or therapeutic agents.

Plaque index (PI)

This index assesses only the thickness of plaque at the gingival area of the tooth.

Method: The evaluation or scoring is done on the entire dentition or on selected teeth. The surfaces examined are the four gingival areas of the tooth i.e. distofacial, facial, mesiofacial and lingual surfaces. Mouth mirror, light source, dental explorer and air drying of the teeth and gingiva are used in the scoring of this index.

Scoring Criteria

Score   *Criteria*

0   No plaque in the gingival area

1   A film of plaque adhering to the free gingival margin and adjacent area of the tooth. The plaque may be recognized only by running a probe across the tooth surface.

2   Moderate accumulation of soft deposits within the gingival pocket and on the gingival margin and/or adjacent tooth surface that can be seen by the naked eye.

3   Abundance of soft matter within the gingival pocket and/or on the gingival margin and adjacent tooth surface.

$$\text{Score for area} = \frac{\text{Total of the four scores per tooth}}{4}$$

$$\text{Score for person} = \frac{\text{Plaque index scores per tooth}}{\text{No. of teeth examined}}$$

Patient Hygiene Performance Index (PHP)

This index for assessing an individual's oral hygiene performance was introduced by A G Podshadley and J V Haley in 1968. It is simplified index and the assessments are based on six index teeth. It is the first index developed for the sole purpose of assessing an individual performance. It is used as educational and motivational tool for the patient.

Teeth and Surfaces to be examined – Six index teeth

	Tooth	*Surface*
16	Upper right first molar	Buccal
11	Upper right central incisor	Labial
26	Upper left first molar	Buccal
36	Lower left first molar	Lingual
31	Lower left central incisor	Labial
46	Lower right first molar	Lingual

Method: Apply a disclosing agent before scoring. Instruct the patient to swish for 30 seconds and expectorate but not rinse. Examination is made using a mouth mirror. Each tooth surface to be evaluated is divided longitudinally into mesial, middle and distal thirds. The

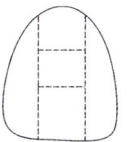

Tooth is divided
into 5 subdivisions

Fig. 7.2: Patient hygiene performance index tooth

middle third is then subdivided horizontally into gingival, middle and occlusal or incisal thirds **(Fig. 7.2)**.

Debris Score for each Subdivision

Each of the five subdivisions is scored for the presence of stained debris as follows:

0 - No debris (or questionable)

1 - Debris definitely present

$$\text{PHP} = \frac{\text{Total debris score}}{\text{No. of teeth scored}}$$

Rating

0 (No debris)	Excellent
0.1 – 1.7	Good
1.8 – 3.4	Fair
3.5 – 5.0	Poor

Turesky Modification of the Quigley-Hein Plaque Index

The Quigley-Hein Plaque index was modified by S Turesky, ND Gilmore and I Glickman in 1970. Plaque is assessed on facial and lingual surfaces of all of the teeth after using basic fuchsin disclosing agent.

Scoring Criteria

Score   *Criteria*

0   No plaque

1   Separate flecks of plaque at the cervical margin of the tooth

2   A thin, continuous band of plaque (upto 1 mm) at the cervical margin of the tooth

3   A band of plaque wider than 1 mm but covering less than 1/3rd of crown of the tooth

4   Plaque covering atleast 1/3rd but less than 2/3rd of the crown of the tooth

5   Plaque covering 2/3rd or more of the crown of the tooth

$$\text{Plaque score per person} = \frac{\text{Total of all plaque score}}{\text{No. of surfaces examined}}$$

CALCULUS INDICES

Calculus Component of the Periodontal Disease Index

Calculus index was described by Ramfjord SP in 1959 as one of the components of periodontal disease index.

Method: The presence and extent of calculus on the facial and lingual surfaces of the six index teeth are evaluated using a mouth mirror and a dental explorer and/or a periodontal probe.

Scoring Criteria

Score	Criteria
0	Absence of calculus
1	Supragingival calculus extending only slightly below the free gingival margin (Not more than 1 mm)
2	Moderate amount of supragingival and subgingival calculus or subgingival calculus alone.
3	An abundance of supragingival and subgingival calculus.

Calculation: The calculus score per tooth are totaled and then divided by the number of teeth examined to yield the calculus score per person.

Calculus Surface Index

The Calculus surface index (CSI) was developed by J Ennever, CP Sturzenberger and AW Radike in 1961. Four mandibular incisiors are examined for the presence or absence of calculus by visual and tactile examination. The Calculus surface index has been shown to have good intra-examiner reproducibility, in a relatively short period of time.

Scoring Criteria

Score	Criteria
0	Indicates the absence of calculus
1	Indicates the presence of calculus

It is used to determine rapidly whether specific agent has any effect on reducing or preventing supragingival or subgingival calculus.

Simplified-Oral Hygiene Index (OHI – S)

Simplified-Oral Hygiene Index was developed in 1964 by John C. Greene and Jack R. Vermillon. It is a composite index which deals both with calculus and oral debris together.

Teeth and Surfaces to be examined – Six index teeth

	Tooth	Surface
16	Upper right first molar	Buccal
11	Upper right central incisor	Labial
26	Upper left first molar	Buccal
36	Lower left first molar	Lingual
31	Lower left central incisor	Labial
46	Lower right first molar	Lingual

Method: The Oral Hygiene Index (OHI – S) has two components, the simplified debris index and the simplified calculus index.

Oral Debris Index (DI-S)

The surface area covered by debris is estimated by running the side of an explorer (Shepherd's Hook) along the tooth surface being examined.

Scoring Criteria

Score	Criteria
0	No debris or stain present
1	Soft debris covering not more than one third of the tooth surface or the presence of extrinsic stain without other debris, regardless of surface area covered.
2	Soft debris covering more than one third but not more than two thirds of the exposed tooth surface.
3	Soft debris covering more than two thirds of the exposed tooth surface.

After the debris scores are recorded, the teeth are then examined for calculus.

Calculus Index (CI-S)

Score	Criteria
0	No calculus present
1	Supragingival calculus covering not more than one third of the exposed tooth surface.
2	Supragingival calculus covering more than one third but not more than two thirds of the exposed tooth surface or the presence of individual flecks of subgingival calculus around the cervical pattern of the tooth or both.
3	Supragingival calculus covering more than two thirds of the exposed tooth surface or a continuous heavy band of subgingival calculus around the cervical portion of the tooth or both.

Calculation of the Index

DI-S and CI-S scores

0.0 - 0.6	Good
0.7 - 1.8	Fair
1.9 - 3.0	Poor

For each individual, the debris and calculus scores are totaled and divided by the number of tooth surfaces examined.

$$\text{Calculation of DI-S score} = \frac{\text{Total score}}{\text{No. of surface examined}}$$

$$\text{Calculation of CI-S score} = \frac{\text{Total score}}{\text{No. of surface examined}}$$

Once the DI-S and CI-S are calculated separately, then they are added together to get the OHI-S score.

OHI-S scores

0.0 - 1.2	Good
1.3 - 3.0	Fair
3.1 - 6.0	Poor

V-M Calculus Assessment

The Volpe-Manhold Probe Method of Calculus assessment was developed by AR Volpe and JH Manhold in 1962 to assess the presence and severity of calculus formation, specifically new deposits of supragingival calculus, following an oral prophylaxis. It is used for longitudinal studies.

Method: A periodontal probe graduated in millimeter divisions is used to measure the deposits in calculus on the lingual surfaces of the six mandibular anterior teeth.

To obtain VMI scores, the three tooth planes, the mesial, distal and gingival, on the lingual surface of the lower six anterior teeth are examined. The periodontal probe is used to measure the linear extent of the supragingival calculus by placing the flat calibrated end of the probe always at the most inferior visible border of the calculus formation.

$$\text{VMI} = \frac{\text{Total VMI score}}{\text{No. of lower anterior teeth examined}}$$

Marginal Line Calculus Index (MLC-I)

The Marginal line calculus index was developed by HR Muhlemann and P Villa in 1967. This index is frequently used in short – term clinical trials (i.e. less than 6 weeks) of anticalculus agents.

This index is used to assess the supragingival calculus along the margins of the gingiva.

It only scores the supragingival calculus formed in the cervical area along the marginal gingiva on the lingual side of the four mandibular incisors. The examination is done using a mouth mirror, after drying the tooth surfaces with air.

PERIODONTAL DISEASE INDICES

Periodontal Index (PI)

It was developed by AL Russell in 1956.

Teeth examined: All the teeth present are examined. This is a composite index because it measures both reversible and irreversible aspects of periodontal disease.

Scoring Criteria

Score	Criteria
0	*Negative*: There is neither overt inflammation in the investing tissues nor loss of function due to destruction of supporting tissues.
1	*Mild gingivitis*: There is an overt area of inflammation in the free gingiva, but this area does not circumscribe the tooth.
2	*Gingivitis*: Inflammation completely circumscribes the tooth, but there is no apparent break in the epithelial attachment.
6	*Gingivitis with pocket formation*: The epithelial attachment has been broken, and there is pocket.

TABLE 7.1: Various Calculus Indices

Name	Year	Authors	Method
Calculus surface index	1961	Ennever, Sturzenberger and Radike	Use air, mirror and explorer to detect calculus
Calculus index simplified (CI-S), part of OHI-S	1964	Greene and Vermillion	With an explorer, detect calculus on tooth surface or around cervical portion of tooth
	1965	Volpe, Manhold and Hazen	Measure with probe in three planes
V-M Calculus assessment Marginal line calculus index (MLC-I)	1967	Muhlemann and Villa	Divide tooth in half (mesial and distal); with air, visualize minute areas of supramarginal calculus next to gingival on lingual four mandibular incisors

PERIODONTICS REVISITED

There is no interference with normal masticatory function, the tooth is firm in its socket, and has not drifted.

8 *Advanced destruction with loss of masticatory function*: The tooth may be loose, may have drifted, may sound dull on percussion with a metallic instrument, or may be depressible in its socket.

Russell chose the scoring values (0, 1, 2, 6, 8) in order to relate the stages of the disease in an epidemiological survey to the clinical conditions observed.

Russell's Rule - The Russell's Rule states that "When in doubt assign the lower score".

0 - 0.2	Clinically normal supportive tissues
0.3 - 0.9	Simple gingivitis
1.0 - 1.9	Beginning destructive periodontal disease
2.0 - 4.9	Established destructive periodontal disease
5.0 - 8.0	Terminal disease

Periodontal Disease Index (PDI)

The PDI is a modification of Russell's Periodontal Index (PI) for epidemiological surveys of periodontal disease. The most important feature of PDI is measurement of the level of the periodontal attachment related to the cementoenamel junction of the teeth.

Components of Periodontal Disease Index: The PDI comprises of three components namely:

1. Plaque Component
2. Calculus Component
3. Gingival and Periodontal Component

Scoring methods: The six-selected index teeth called Ramfjord teeth which include, the maxillary right first molar, maxillary left central incisor, maxillary left first premolar, mandibular left first molar, mandibular right central incisor, and mandibular right first premolar.

Scoring Criteria

Score	*Criteria*
0	Absence of inflammation
1	Mild to moderate inflammatory gingival changes not extending all around the tooth
2	Mild to moderately severe gingivitis extending all around the tooth
3	Severe gingivitis, characterized by marked redness, tendency to bleed and ulceration
4	Gingival crevice in any of the four measured areas (mesial, distal, buccal, lingual), extending apically to CEJ, but not more than 3 mm
5	Gingival crevice in any of the four measured areas extending apically, 3 – 6 mm from CEJ
6	Gingival crevice in any of the four measured areas extending apically more than 6 mm from CEJ

$$PDI = \frac{\text{Total no. of individual tooth scores}}{\text{No. of teeth examined}}$$

Score for individual: The PDI score for a group is obtained by totaling the individual PDI scores and then, dividing by the number of people examined.

Community Periodontal Index of Treatment Needs (CPITNs)

It was developed for the joint working committee of the World Health Organization and Federation Dentaire Internationale (WHO / FDI) by Jukka Ainamo, David Ramies, George Beagrie, Terry Cutress, Jean Martin, and Jennifer Sardo-Infirri in 1982. This index was developed primarily to survey and evaluate periodontal treatment needs rather than determining past and present periodontal status, i.e. the recession of the gingival margin and alveolar bone.

The CPITN records the common treatable conditions, namely

- Periodontal pocket
- Gingival inflammation
- Dental calculus and
- Other plaque retentive factors.

CPITN probe was designed for two purposes, namely measurement of pocket depth and detection of

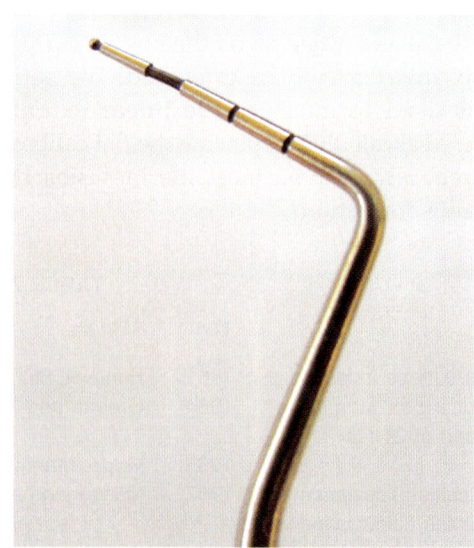

Fig. 7.3: CPITN probe

subgingival calculus. The pocket depth is measured through colour coding with a black mark starting at 3.5 mm and ending at 5.5 mm. The probe has a 'ball tip' of 0.5 mm diameter that allows easy detection of subgingival calculus **(Fig. 7.3)**.

Procedure: The dentition is divided into six parts (sextants), for assessment of periodontal treatment needs. Each sextant is given a score.

Index teeth: For adults, aged 20 years or more, only ten teeth, known as the index teeth are examined. These teeth have been identified as the best estimators of the worst periodontal condition of the mouth. The ten specified index teeth are: 17, 16, 11, 26, 27, 31, 36, 37, 46, 47 (FDI system).

For young people up to 19 years, only six index teeth are examined, because of the high frequency of false pockets. The six index teeth selected are: 16, 11, 26, 31, 36, 46.

Probing procedure: A tooth is probed to determine pocket depth and to detect subgingival calculus and bleeding response. The probing force can be divided into a:

- 'Working component'- to determine pocket depth and
- 'Sensing component'- to detect subgingival calculus.

The working force should not be more than 20 gms. The probe is inserted between the tooth and the gingiva and the sulcus depth or pocket depth is noted against the color code or measuring lines. The ball end of the probe should be kept in contact with the root surface. For sensing subgingival calculus, the lightest possible force which will allow movement of the probe ballpoint along the tooth surface is used. Recommended sites for probing are mesial, midline and distal of facial and lingual/palatal surfaces. Withdrawing the probe between each probing or with the probe tip remaining in the sulcus, the probe may be walked around the tooth.

Extent and Severity Index

The Extent and Severity Index (ESI) of periodontal disease was developed to provide separate estimates of the extent and severity of periodontal disease in individuals and populations. The Periodontal Index and the Periodontal Disease Index yield scores that represent the severity of periodontal disease in individuals or populations, but these scores do not provide information on the extent of disease. Extent and severity index does not assess gingival inflammation instead, it estimates the loss of periodontal attachment at the mesiofacial and facial sites of 14 teeth in one maxillary quadrant and 14 teeth in the contralateral mandibular quadrant using the periodontal probing method developed by Ramfjord for the PDI. A threshold of disease has to be established to calculate the extent score for an individual.

Extent score; for an individual, is the percentage of sites examined that have attachment loss greater than 1 mm. Severity score; for an individual is the average loss

TABLE 7.2: Criteria for the community periodontal index of treatment needs

Periodontal status	Treatment Needs
0 Healthy periodontium	0 = No treatment needed
1 Bleeding observed, directly or by using mouth mirror after sensing	I = Oral hygiene needs improvement
2 Calculus felt during probing, but the entire black area of the probe is visible	II = I+ professional scaling
3 Pocket 4 or 5 mm (gingival margin is situated on black area of probe)	II = I+ professional scaling
4 Pocket> 6 mm (black area of probe not visible)	III = I+II+ complex treatment

TABLE 7.3: Various periodontal disease indices

	Name	Year	Authors	Method
1	Periodontal index (PI)	1956	Russell	Do not use probe; weigh scores and combine gingival and periodontal status.
2	Periodontal disease Index (PDI)	1967	Ramfjord	Select the "Ramfjord" teeth (#3, #9 #12, #19, #25 and #28) and score for gingiva, attachment loss, calculus and plaque.
3	Community periodontal index treatment needs (CPITN)	1982	Ainamo et al	This index is for epidemiological purposes. Use O'leary's sextants with specified index teeth or worst tooth, WHO probe, 0 to 4 codes per sextant; evaluate bleeding, deposits and pocket depth.
4	Extent and severity index	1986	Carlos, Wolfe and Kingman	This index is for epidemiological purposes. Estimates the attachment level from probe depths-14 sites in each of 2 contralateral quadrants.

PERIODONTICS REVISITED

of attachment per site among the disease sites. The ESI is expressed as a bivariate statistic: ESI = (Extent, Severity). For example, an individual's ESI of (20, 3.0) would be interpreted as 20% of sites examined had disease and of the diseased sites the average loss of attachment was 3.0 mm.

The ESI for a population would be the average extent and severity scores for the individuals examined.

POINTS TO PONDER

✓ Case-control studies are also called as retrospective or backward studies.

✓ Cohort studies are also called as prospective or forward studies.

✓ Cross - sectional studies are just like photographs and longitudinal studies are cine films.

✓ Longitudinal studies: Observations are repeated in the same population over a prolonged period of time by means of follow - up examinations.

✓ Periodontal index (PI) by Russell has true biologic gradient.

✓ Disclosing agent used in Plaque component of periodontal disease index (PDI) is Bismarck brown solution and in Turesky – Gilmore – Glickman plaque index, basic fuchsin is used as disclosing agent.

✓ Case–control studies can be more prone to bias than cohort studies.

✓ Clinical trials avoid bias and confounding through the processes of randomization and blinding.

✓ Gindex Index- This periodontal index is a colorimetric test to measure gingival inflammation based on the hemoglobin content of saliva. Abbott and Caffesse in 1978 formed a correlation between the gindex values, gingival index and cervicular fluid flow.

BIBLIOGRAPHY

1. Albandar JM, Brown LJ, Brunelle JA, et al. Gingival state and dental calculus in early onset periodontitis. J Periodontol 1996; 67(10):953-59.
2. Albandar JM. Epidemiology and Risk factors of periodontal diseases. Dent Clin North Am 2005; 49: 517-32.
3. Albandar JM, Rams TE. Global epidemiology of periodontal diseases: an overview. Periodontol 2000 2002; 29: 7–10.
4. Beck JD, Arbes SJ (Jr). Epidemiology of gingival and periodontal diseases. In, Newman, Takei, Carranza. Clinical Periodontology 9th ed WB Saunders 2003; 74-95.
5. Douglass CW. The epidemiology of periodontal diseases. In, Wilson TG, Kornman KS. Fundamentals of Periodontics. Quintessence Publishing Co.1996;9-16.
6. Epidemiology, Etiology and Prevention of Periodontal diseases. In, Soben Peter. Essentials of Preventive and Community Dentistry. Arya (MEDI) Publishing House. 4th ed 2004;110-113.
7. Greene JC. General principles of epidemiology and methods for measuring prevalence and severity of periodontal disease. In, Genco RJ, Goldman HM, Cohen DW. Contemporary Periodontics. CV Mosby Company 1990;97-105.
8. Indices in Dental epidemiology. In, Soben Peter. Essentials of Preventive and Community Dentistry. Arya (MEDI) Publishing House. 4th ed 2004;311-359.
9. Irfan UM, Dawson DV, Bissada NF. Epidemiology of periodontal disease: a review and clinical perspectives. J Int Acad Periodontol 2001; 3: 14-21.
10. Kingman A, Albandar JM. Methodological aspects of epidemiological studies of periodontal diseases. Periodontol 2000 2002; 29:11–30.
11. Lindhe, et al. Design of clinical trials of traditional therapies of periodontitis. J Clin Periodontol 1986; 13: 488.
12. Lobene RR, Weatherford T, Ross NM et al. A modified gingival index for use in clinical trials. Clin Prevent Dent 1986; 8(1):3.
13. Loe H. The gingival index, the plaque index, and the retention index systems. J Periodontol 1967; 38(suppl): 610.
14. Loe H, Morrison E. Epidemiology of periodontal disease. In, Genco RJ, Goldman HM, Cohen DW. Contemporary Periodontics. CV Mosby Company 1990;106 – 116.
15. Park K. Textbook of Preventive and Social Medicine. 17th ed Banarsidass Bhanot Publishers 2002; 44 - 107.
16. Russell AL. A system of classification and scoring for prevalence surveys of periodontal disease. I Dent Res 1954; 35(3):350.

MCQs

1. Which among these serves as highest level of clinical evidence?
   A. Cohort studies
   B. Case control studies
   C. Systematic review of randomized controlled trials
   D. Case reports

2. An epidemiological index with true biological gradient is:
   A. Ramfjord index
   B. Russell's periodontal index
   C. Papillary- Marginal – Attached Index
   D. Modified gingival index

3. The score of 8.0 in Russel's periodontal index (PI) indicates:
   A. Irreversible terminal disease
   B. Established destructive periodontal disease
   C. Beginning of destructive periodontal disease
   D. PI score is always less than 1

4. Which of the following does not assess the presence of periodontal pockets or attachment loss:
   A. Modified Gingival Index (MGI)
   B. Gingival Index (GI)
   C. Both A and B
   D. Papillary Bleeding Index (PBI)

5. Ramfjord teeth are:
   A. Maxillary right first molar (16), Maxillary left central incisor (21), Maxillary left first premolar (24),
   B. Mandibular left first molar (36), mandibular right central incisor (41)
   C. Mandibular right first premolar (44)
   D. All of the above
6. Cementoenamel junction of the teeth is used as fixed landmark for measuring the level of the periodontal attachment loss in:
   A. Papillary bleeding index (PBI)
   B. Periodontal disease index (PDI)
   C. Russell's periodontal index (PI)
   D. None of the above

7. Plaque Index was developed by:
   A. Silness and Loe in 1964
   B. Loe and Silness in 1964
   C. Russell in 1956
   D. None of the above
8. Incidence rate can be measured in:
   A. Case-control study
   B. Cohort study
   C. Cross-sectional study
   D. None of the above

Answers

1. C	2. B	3. A	4. C	5. D
6. B	7. A	8. B		

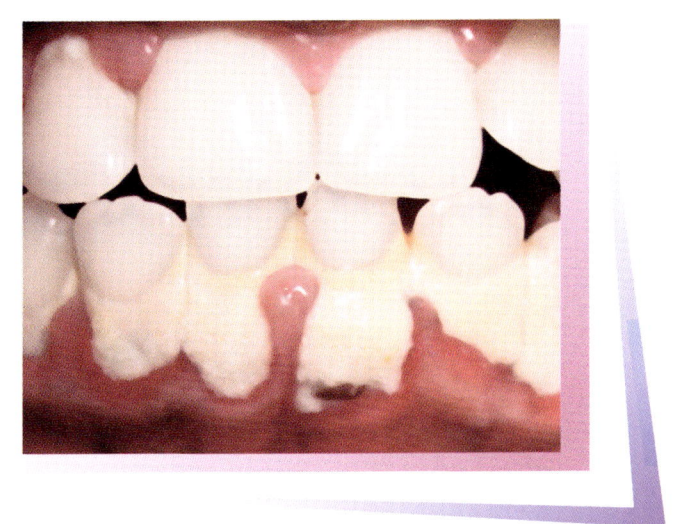

SECTION THREE

ETIOLOGY

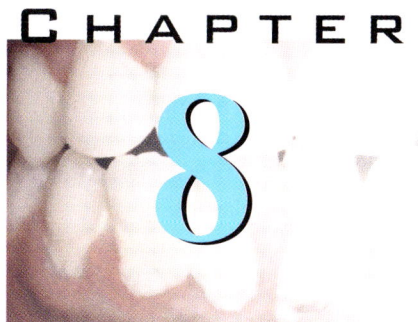

CHAPTER

8

Periodontal Microbiology

Shalu Bathla

INTRODUCTION

Microbial etiology of periodontal diseases is needed to be well understood because of two major reasons: First, knowledge of the etiological agents of periodontal diseases would help in the selection of appropriate treatment. Second, it would provide a useful therapeutic approach to control and prevent periodontal diseases, e.g. manufacturing of vaccines against various pathogens prior to the onset of diseases.

But the microbiology of periodontal diseases is difficult to understand and study due to difficulty in sample collection, cultivation and identification of isolates. Periodontal infections are mixed infections and microbiota is very complex, making hard to distinguish between secondary invaders and true pathogens. Periodontal disease appears to be episodic and thus, there is difficulty in differentiating between active and inactive sites for sampling.

CRITERIA FOR DEFINING PERIODONTAL PATHOGENS

Koch's Postulates

Microorganism can be accepted as the causative agent of an infectious disease only if the following conditions are satisfied **(Fig. 8.1)**.
1. The microorganisms should be constantly associated with the lesions of the disease.
2. It should be possible to isolate the bacterium in pure culture from the lesions.
3. Inoculation of such pure culture into suitable animal model should reproduce the lesions of the disease.
4. It should be possible to reisolate the microbes in pure culture from the lesions produced in the experimental animals.

Limitations of Koch's postulates:
• Inability to culture all the organisms: Large sized spirochetes in periodontitis cannot be grown in pure culture.

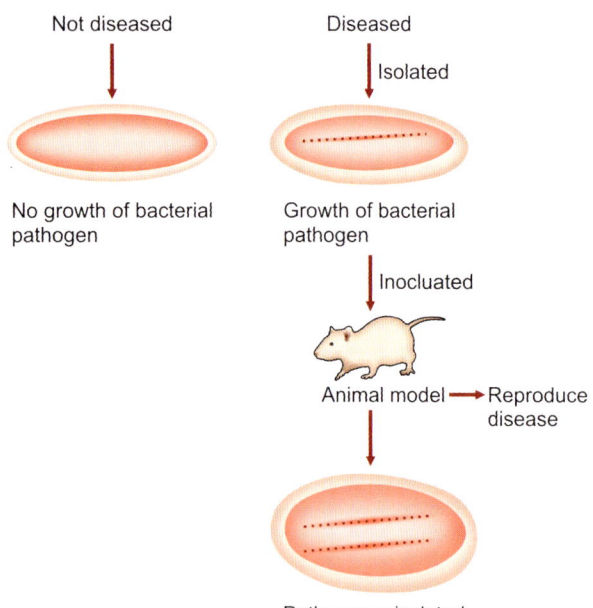

Fig. 8.1: Koch's postulates

- Lack of a good model system: Host range is restricted to humans or to animal species in which the human diseases cannot be reproduced. (*P. gingivalis* does not usually colonize in animals).
- The actual state of periodontal disease progression can be difficult to determine. The same clinical signs and symptoms may be produced by several organisms which may give rise to a variety of clinical disease features.

Thus, the inherent problem with Koch's postulates in showing causality is the primarily concern with the infecting agent and lack of consideration for the environment or the influence of the host in disease development.

Socransky's Criterion

Sigmund Socransky, a researcher at the Forsyth Dental Center in Boston, proposed criteria by which periodontal microorganisms may be judged to be potential pathogens.

1. Association with the lesion: Association is the first requirement for a microbe to cause a periodontal lesion. Pathogen should be associated with disease, as evident by increase in the number of organisms at diseased sites.
2. Elimination of the suspected organism: Organism should be eliminated or decreased in sites that demonstrate clinical resolution of disease with treatment.

3. Host response to organism: Microbe should be able to demonstrate a host response, in the form of an alteration in the host cellular or humoral immune response.
4. Animal studies: Pathogens should be capable of causing disease in experimental animal models.
5. Virulence factors: Potential pathogens should be capable of producing virulence factors which cause destruction of the periodontal tissues.

PERIODONTAL PATHOGENS

The World Workshop in Periodontology (Consensus report 1996) designated *Aggregatibacter actinomycetemcomitans (A.a), P. gingivalis, Tannerella forsythia* as periodontal pathogens.

Aggregatibacter Actinomycetemcomitans

Aggregatibacter actinomycetemcomitans was first isolated by German microbiologist Klinger in 1912 from lesion of cervicofacial actinomycosis. The microorganism was isolated together with *Actinomyces israelli*. Hence, the species name actinomycetemcomitans means together with Actinomyces. Genus name Actinobacillus actino referring to star- shaped internal morphology of the colonies and bacillus referring to cell shape (rod- shaped).

Morphological characteristics: It is a member of the family Pasteurellaecae. It's size is approx $0.4 \pm 0.1 \times 1.0 \pm 0.4$ μm. It is non-motile gram negative coccobacillus, non -sporulating, capnophilic, requires an atmosphere containing 5- 10% CO_2 for good growth. It forms small (0.5 -1.0 mm in diameter), smooth, circular, convex and translucent colonies on solid media with a slightly irregular edge and has an internal morphology described as star shaped.

Biochemical characteristics: *Aggregatibacter actinomycetemcomitans* is non hemolytic, fermentative, oxidase and catalase positive. It does not produce indole.

Ultrastructure: It reveals features typical of gram negative organisms including an outer cytoplasmic membrane, periplasmic space and inner cytoplasmic membrane. A significant feature of *Aggregatibacter actinomycetemcomitans* is its surface ultrastructure which includes fimbriae, vesicles and extracellular amorphous material. Fimbriae are the small filamentous cell surface appendages associated with bacterial colonization of host tissues. It occurs in peritrichous arrays. Vesicles are the structures which are lipopolysaccharide in nature, originate from and are continuous with the outer membrane. The vesicles function as delivery vehicles for *Aggregatibacter actinomycetemcomitans* toxic materials since it exhibit adhesive properties, bone resorption activity, endotoxin and bacteriocin. Certain *Aggregatibacter actinomycetemcomitans* cells have amorphous material on their surface that frequently embeds adjacent cells in a matrix.

Serological characteristics: Zambon et al in 1983 identified 3 serotypes of *Aggregatibacter actinomycetemcomitans* a, b and c. Serotype a and b are commonly found in the human oral cavity, while serotype c comprises only approx 10% of *Aggregatibacter actinomycetemcomitans* human oral isolates. Kaplan et al in 2001 divided *Aggregatibacter actinomycetemcomitans* into 6 serotypes from a to f.

Virulence factors: It elaborates myriad of virulence factors in order to maintain itself in the oral cavity.

- Factors that promote colonization and persistence in the oral cavity are adhesins, bacteriocin, invasins, antibiotic resistance.
- Factors that interfere with host's defenses are leukotoxin, chemotaxis inhibitor, Fc binding protein and immunosuppressive factors. Leukotoxin has the ability to kill human polymorphonuclear leukocytes, monocytes and lymphocytes. LtxA is a 116kDa protein which is a member of a family of pore forming toxin.
- Factors that destroy host tissues are collagenase, cytotoxin, endotoxin, cytolethal distending toxin and epitheliotoxin.
- Factors that inhibit host repair of tissues are fibroblast inhibitory factor and inhibitors of bone formation.

Porphyromonas Gingivalis

In the late 1970s, it was recognized that the black pigmented Bacteroides contained species that were asaccharolytics (*P. gingivalis*), intermediate level of carbohydrate fermenter (*P. intermedia*) or highly saccharolytic (*Prevotella melaninogenica*). *P. gingivalis* is a gram negative, anaerobic, asaccharolytic, non-motile rod shaped bacteria which produces black pigmented colonies. *P. gingivalis* produces virulence factors like collagenase, endotoxin, fatty acids, NH_3, H_2S, indole, hemolysin, fibrinolysin, phospholipase A and bone resportion inducing factor. The ability of *P.gingivalis* to attach to other bacteria, epithelial cells and connective tissue component, fibronectin and fibrinogen are all likely to be important in the virulence of microorganism. The fimbriae not only play a role in the colonization of the microorganism but also activate cytokine production like lipopolysaccharide.

Extracellular cysteine proteinases referred to as gingipains, are considered important virulence factors for *Porphyromonas gingivalis*. Two gingipains referred to as HRgp A and Rgp B are arginine specific proteinase and other one Kgp is a lysine-specific proteinase. The term "gingipain" was originally coined by Travis and colleague. These enzymes activate kallikrein/kinin system, downregulate polymorphonuclear neutrophils, activate blood clotting system, disturb host defense system, stimulate and activate matrix metalloproteinase. *P. gingivalis* causes chemokine paralysis by inhibiting the production of IL- 8 by epithelial cells which is chemotaxin for PMNs. Thus, it inhibits PMN migration.

Tannerella Forsythia (Bacteroides forsythus)

Tannerella forsythia was first isolated at the Forsyth Institute from subjects with progressing advanced periodontitis in the mid 1970s and was described as Fusiform Bacteroides by Tanner et al. It is a gram negative anaerobic, spindle shaped, highly pleomorphic rod. This species is difficult to grow; the growth of organism is enhanced by co-cultivation with *F.nucleatum*. It requires N-acetylmuramic acid for its growth. The various virulence factors produced by *Tannerella forsythia* are endotoxin, fatty acid and methylglyoxal.

Others

Spirochetes are gram negative, anaerobic, helical shaped rods and motile organisms. They penetrate epithelium and connective tissue, degrade collagen and dentin, destroy Ig and complement. Two major problems associated with the areas of investigation are the difficulty in isolating and cultivating spirochetes species and in discriminating and enumerating the different species of oral spirochetes.

Fusobacterium nucleatum is a gram-negative, anaerobic spindle shaped rod.

Prevotella intermedia is a gram-negative, anaerobic short round-ended rod.

Campylobacter rectus is a gram-negative, anaerobic, short, motile vibrio. It forms small convex, corroding or pitting colonies on blood agar plates. It produces leukotoxin and is capable of stimulating fibroblasts.

Others species include Cytomegalovirus, Epstein Barr virus, papilloma and herpes simplex virus that have been proposed to play a role in the etiology of periodontal diseases.

PERIODONTICS REVISITED

Tooth associated plaque microorganisms:
- *Streptococcus mitis*
- *S. sanguis*
- *A. viscosus*
- *A. naeslundii*
- *Eubacterium spp.*

Tissue associated plaque microorganisms:
- *S. oralis*
- *S. intermedius*
- *P. micros*
- *P. gingivalis*
- *P. intermedia*
- *Tannerella forsythia*
- *F. nucleatum*

MICROORGANISMS ASSOCIATED WITH

Periodontal Health

Beneficial species of the host affect the disease progression by preventing the colonization/roliferation of pathogenic microorganisms, e.g. hydrogen peroxide produced by *S.sanguis* is lethal to *Aggregatibacter actinomycetemcomitans*. Sometimes, these species also degrade the virulence factors produced by the pathogens. Following are the beneficial micro-organisms:
- *S. sanguis*
- *S. mitis*
- *Capnocytophaga spp.*
- *Veillonella*
- *Streptococcus*
- *Gemella sp.*
- *Atopobium sp.*

Chronic Gingivitis/Dental Plaque Induced Gingivitis

Gram positive organisms are:
- *S. sanguis*
- *S. mitis*
- *S. intermedius*
- *S. oralis*
- *A. viscosus*
- *A. naeslundii*
- *Peptostreptococcus micros*

Gram negative organisms are:

- *F. nucleatum*
- *P. intermedia*
- *V. parvula*
- *Hemophilus*
- *Capnocytophaga*
- *Campylobacter spp.*

Chronic Periodontitis

- *P. gingivalis*
- *Tannerella forsythia*
- *P. intermedia*
- *C. rectus*
- *Eikenella corrodens*
- *F. nucleatum*
- *Aggregatibacter actinomycetemcomitans (A.a)*
- *P. micros*
- *Treponema*
- *Eubacterium spp.*
- *Herpes virus group*
- *EBV-1*
- *Human CMV*

Localized Aggressive Periodontitis

- *Aggregatibacter actinomycetemcomitans (A.a)*
- *P. gingivalis*
- *E. corrodens*
- *C. rectus*
- *F. nucleatum*
- *B. capillus*
- *Eubacterium brachy*
- *Capnocytophaga spp.*
- *Spirochetes*
- *Herpes viruses including EBV-1*
- *Human CMV*

Necrotizing Periodontal Disease

- *Spirochetes*
- *P. intermedia*

Abscesses of Periodontium

- *F. nucleatum*
- *P. intermedia*
- *P. gingivalis*
- *P. micros*
- *Tannerella forsythia*

LANDMARK STUDIES RELATED

Socransky SS, Haffajee AD, Cugini MA et al. Microbial complexes in subgingival plaque. Journal of Clinical Periodontology 1998; 25: 134-144.

In 185 adult subjects, 13321 subgingival plaque samples were taken from the mesial aspect of each tooth. Using checkerboard DNA-DNA hybridization each

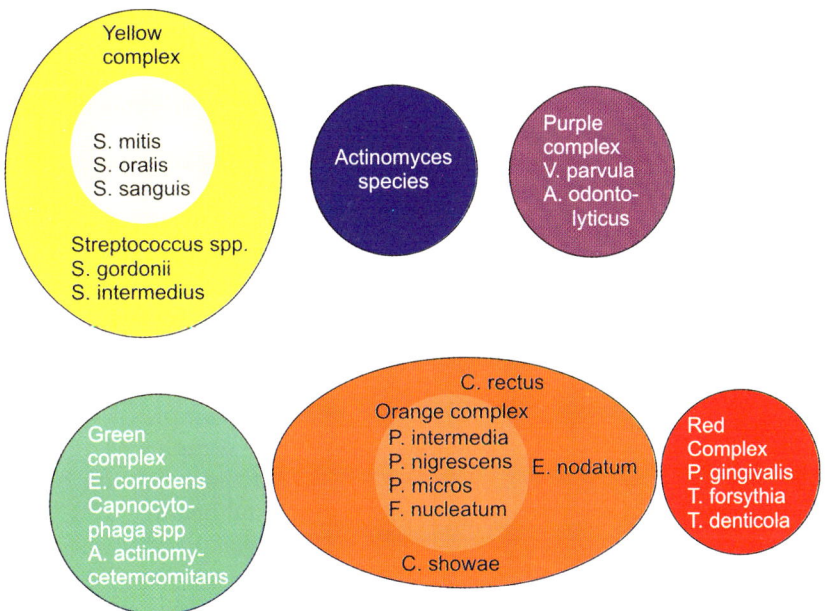

Fig. 8.2: Microbial complexes in subgingival plaque

sample was individually analyzed for the presence of 40 subgingival species. Six bacterial clusters were described in subgingival biofilms **(Fig. 8.2).**

- Yellow complex: *Streptococcus spp., S. sanguis, S. mitis, S. intermedius, S oralis, S. gordonii*
- Purple complex: *Veillonella parvula* and *A. odonto-lyticus*
- Green complex: *Capnocytophaga sp, Aggregatibacter actinomycetemcomitans serotype a* and *Eikenella corrodens*
- Orange complex: *Campylobacter gracilus, F. nucleatum, P. intermedia, P. micros, C. rectus*
- Red complex: *P. gingivalis, Tannerella forsythia, T. denticola*

Significance: Early colonizers include members of yellow, purple and green complexes. Orange complex members are thought to bridge early colonizers. Red complex members are associated with bleeding on probing and more dominant at late stages of plaque development whereas green and orange complexes include species recognized as pathogens in periodontal and non – periodontal infection.

POINTS TO PONDER

✓ Ecosystems/niches present in the oral cavity are: Supragingival hard surfaces – (teeth, implants, restoration, prostheses), periodontal / periimplant pocket, buccal epithelium, palatal epithelium,

epithelium of the floor of the mouth and dorsum of the tongue. Subgingival ecologic niches present in the oral cavity are: tooth / implant surface, gingival exduate fluid medium, surface of epithelial cells and superficial portion of the pocket epithelium.

✓ New names of various periodontal bacteria:

	Previous name	Current name
i.	*Bacteroides gingivalis*	*Porphyromonas gingivalis*
ii.	*Bacteroides intermedius*	*Prevotella intermedia*
iii.	*Bacteroides melaninogenicus*	*Prevotella melaninogenica*
iv.	*Bacteroides forsythus*	*Tannerella forsythia*
v.	*Wolinella recta*	*Campylobacter rectus*
vi.	*Actinobacillus actinomycetemcomitans*	*Aggregatibacter actinomycetemcomitans*

BIBLIOGRAPHY

1. Ellen RP, Galimanas VB. Spirochetes at the forefront of periodontal infections. Periodontol 2000 2005; 38:13-32.
2. Haake SK, Newman MG, Nisengard RJ and Sanz M. Periodontal Microbiology. In, Newman, Takei, Carranza. Clinical Periodontology. 9th ed WB Saunders 2003; 96-112.
3. Historical Introduction. Ananthanarayan, Paniker. Textbook of Microbiology. Orient Longman 6th ed 2002; 1-6.
4. Socransky SS, Haffajee AD. Microbiology of periodontal disease. In, Lindhe J, Karring T, Lang NP. Clinical periodontology and Implant dentistry. 4th ed Blackwell Munksgaard 2003; 106-49.
5. Socransky SS, Haffajee AD. Bacterial etiology of destructive periodontal disease: Current concepts. J Periodontol 1992; 63: 322-31.

PERIODONTICS REVISITED

6. Taylor PM, Meyer DH, Mintz KP, Brissette C. Virulence factors of Actinobacillus actinomycetemcomitans. Periodontol 2000 1999; 20:136-67.
7. Zambon JJ. Actinobacillus actinomycetemcomitans in human periodontal disease. J Clin Periodontol 1985; 12: 1-20.
8. Zambon JJ. Microbiology of periodontal disease. In, Genco RJ, Goldman HM, Cohen DW. Contemporary Periodontics. CV Mosby 1990; 147-60.

MCQs

1. Leukotoxins are produced by which of the following periopathogens:
   A. *P.gingivalis*
   B. *P.intermedia*
   C. *A.actinomycetemcomitans*
   D. *F.nucleatum*
2. Which microorganism is increased in pregnancy:
   A. *Prevotella intermedius*
   B. *Porphyromonas gingivalis*
   C. *Porphyromonas melaninogenicus*
   D. *Eikenella corrodens*
3. Which of the following bacteria have the capacity to invade host tissue cells directly?
   A. *P. gingivalis*
   B. *A. actinomycetemcomitans*
   C. *T. denticola*
   D. All of the above
4. Which of the following is not included in the Green complex?
   A. *Aggregatibacter actinomycetemcomitans* serotype a
   B. *P. gingivalis*
   C. *Eikenella corrodens*
   D. *Capnocytophaga spp.*
5. Which of the following complex is most closely attached to destructive periodontal diseases:
   A. Red complex
   B. Green complex
   C. Orange complex
   D. Purple complex
6. Which of the following bacteria is associated with periodontal health?
   A. *S. sanguis*
   B. *S. mitis*
   C. *Capnocytophaga spp.*
   D. *Veillonella*
   E. All of the above

Answers

1. C   2. A   3. D   4. B   5. A
6. A

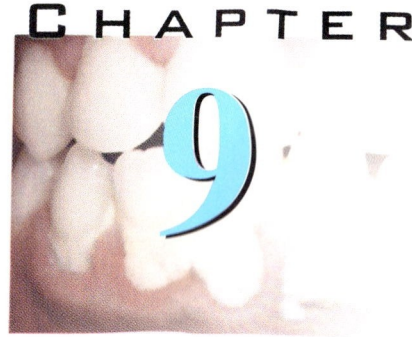

CHAPTER

9

Dental Plaque

Shalu Bathla

BIOFILM

The term biofilm describes relatively undefinable microbial community associated with a tooth surface or any other hard non-shedding material. Biofilms are ubiquitous and are found in oral cavity, the bottom of boats and docks, inside pipes, rocks in streams, catheters, hip and voice prosthesis and contact lenses.

The bacteria in biofilm cluster together to form sessile, mushroom shaped microcolonies. Each microcolony is an independent community with its own customized living environment. In biofilms, microcolonies of bacterial cells are distributed in glycocalyx matrix. Water channels are present between the microcolonies which permit passage of nutrients and bacterial products throughout the biofilm. The main method of transferring information in a biofilm is Quorum sensing which involves the regulation of expression of specific genes through the accumulation of signaling compounds that mediate intercellular communication. The other methods of transferring information in biofilm are conjugation, transformation, plasmid transfer and transpoon transfer. The functions of biofilm are to facilitate processing and uptake of nutrients, protection and cross feeding one species and providing nutrients for another species (Fig. 9.1).

Biofilm bacteria exhibit stronger resistance (1000 to 1500 times) to biocides and antimicrobial agents than do their planktonic counterpart. Following hypothesis may help to explain the increased resistance to antimicrobials. First, the exopolysaccharide of the biofilm matrix may inhibit the diffusion of antimicrobial agents. Second, the physiological differences among biofilm bacteria leave only a part of biofilm bacteria susceptible to growth-dependent antibiotics. Third, the genetic changes occurring in transition from planktonic to biofilm bacteria make the biofilm bacteria insensitive to various biocides and antimicrobial agents. Fourth, slower rate of growth of organisms due the nutrient limitation may also contribute to the resistance to antimicrobial agents by biofilm bacteria. Finally, extracellular enzymes such as β–lactamase, formaldehyde dehydrogenase become concentrated in extracellular matrix, thus inactivating some antibiotics.

DEFINITION OF PLAQUE

According to WHO in 1978, it is defined as *specific but highly variable structural entity resulting from colonization and growing microorganisms on surfaces of teeth and consisting of numerous microbial species and strains embedded in an extracellular matrix.*

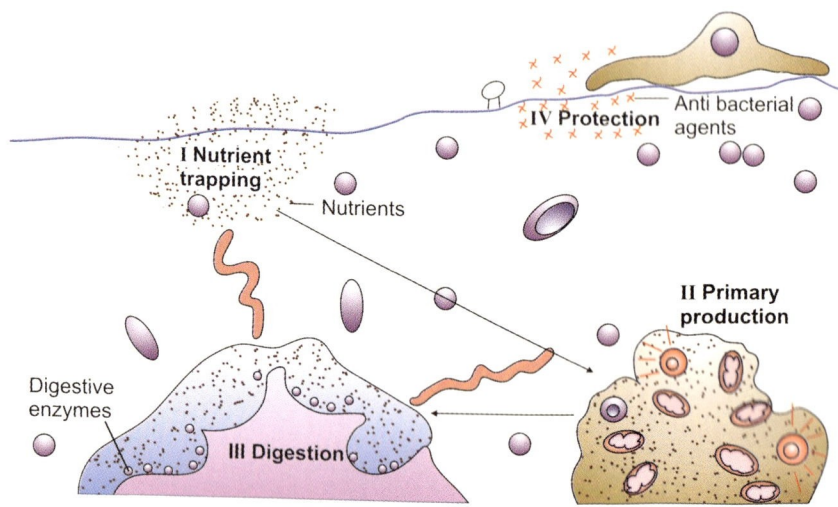

Fig. 9.1: Characteristic features of plaque biofilm
I. Nutrients are trapped
II. Production of their own nutrients
III. Nutrients are digested
IV. Protection from antibacterial agents

It can also be defined as the soft deposits that form the biofilm adhering to the tooth surface or other hard surfaces in the oral cavity, including removable and fixed restorations.

CLASSIFICATION

Dental plaque is broadly classified as supragingival, subgingival or peri-implant plaque based on its position on the tooth and implant surface. Supragingival plaque is found at or above the gingival margin. Subgingival plaque is found below the gingival margin, between the tooth and the gingival sulcular tissue **(Table 9.1)**.

A. Supragingival plaque
B. Subgingival plaque
   a. Tooth associated
   b. Tissue associated
C. Peri-implant plaque

CLINICAL ASSESSMENT

Plaque can be assessed by the following methods:
1. *Direct vision*: Plaque becomes detectable with naked eyes after an uninterrupted formation of 1-2 days.
2. *Use of explorer/probe*: Plaque can be detected by scraping the tooth surface with an explorer/probe.
3. *Using disclosing agents*: Plaque can be easily detected by using disclosing solution or tablet. Disclosing solution contains a dye or other coloring substance, which imparts it's color to calculus, plaque and films on the surface of teeth, tongue and gingiva **(Figs 9.2 and 9.3)**. The various disclosing agents are

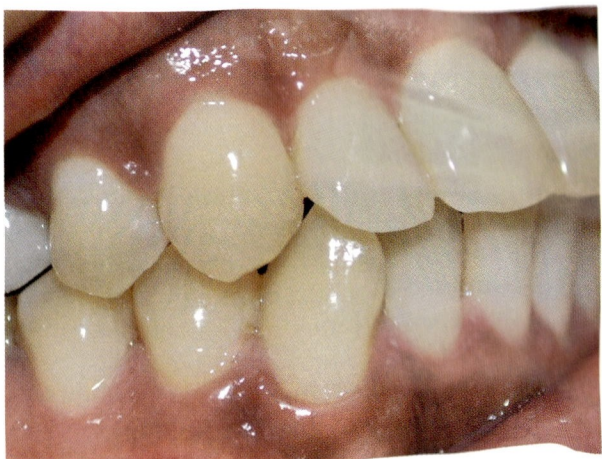

Fig. 9.2: Plaque not visible through naked eye

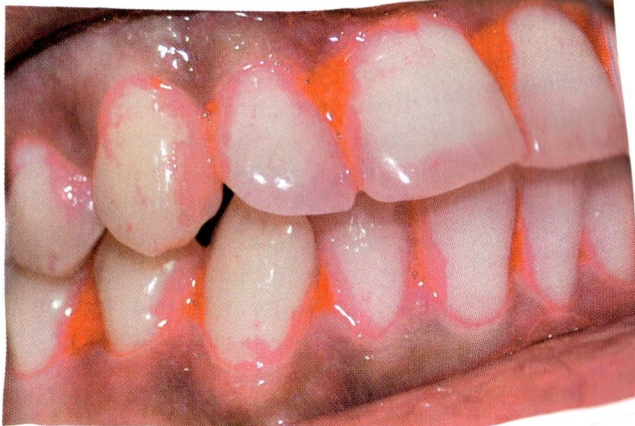

Fig. 9.3: Plaque visible through the use of disclosing

TABLE 9.1: Differences between supragingival and subgingival plaque

		Supragingival plaque	Subgingival plaque
1.	Location	Coronal to the margin of free gingiva	Apical to the margin of free gingiva
2.	Origin	Salivary glycoprotein and salivary microorganisms	Downgrowth of bacteria from supragingival plaque
3.	Distribution	Areas left uncleaned, cervical third and promixal surfaces	Attached plaque covers calculus and unattached plaque extends to the periodontal attachment
4.	Retention	Rough surface of teeth or restoration, malpositioned teeth and carious lesion	Overhanging margins of filling and periodontal pockets
5.	Structure	Adherent, densely packed microbial layer over pellicle on tooth surface	Tooth surface attached plaque, unattached plaque, epithelium attached plaque
6.	Microorganisms	Early plaque: Gram-positive cocci Older plaque: 3-4 days: Increased no. of filaments and fusiforms 4-9 days: More complex flora with rods, filamentous forms 7-14 days: Vibrios, Spirochetes	Anaerobic population Diseased pocket: Primarily Gram-negative, motile, Spirochetes, rods
7.	Source of nutrients for bacterial proliferation	Saliva and ingested food	GCF, exudate and leukocytes
8.	Significance	Causes gingivitis, supragingival calculus and dental caries	Causes gingivitis, periodontal infection and subgingival calculus

Skinner iodine solution, iodine disclosing solution, Basic fuchsin, Bismarck Brown, Erythrosin (FDC Red No. 3), Two tone dye (FDC red no. 3 and FDC green no.3).

4. *Clinical records*: There are various indices for recording and scoring plaque which are explained in chapter no. 7: Epidemiology of gingival and periodontal diseases.

COMPOSITION

Dental plaque is mainly composed of microorganisms. Approximately 2×10^8 bacteria are present in 1 mg of dental plaque. The material present between the bacteria in the dental plaque is called as intermicrobial matrix which is approximately 25% of the plaque volume. Plaque microbes, saliva, gingival exudates are the sources which contribute to the intermicrobial matrix.

1. *Microorganisms*: There are approx. 500 distinct bacterial and non-bacterial (Mycoplasma, yeasts, protozoa and viruses) species.
2. *Host cells*: Epithelial cells, macrophages and leukocytes are the cells present in intermicrobial matrix.
3. *Organic compounds*: These are polysaccharides, proteins, glycoproteins and lipid materials. Glycoproteins from saliva are an important component of the pellicle that initially coats a clean tooth surface. Polysaccharides produced by bacteria, of which dextran is the predominant form, contribute to the organic portion of the matrix. Albumin, probably originating from crevicular fluid, has been identified as a component of the plaque matrix. The lipid material consists of debris from the membranes of disrupted bacterial and host cells and possibly food debris.

4. *Inorganic compounds:* These are calcium, phosphorus, fluoride, sodium and potassium. The primary source of inorganic constituents of supragingival plaque is saliva; as the mineral content increases, the plaque mass becomes calcified to form calculus. The inorganic component of subgingival plaque is derived from crevicular fluid.

FORMATION

The plaque formation is divided into three phases **(Fig. 9.4)**:

I. *Pellicle formation*: Hydrophobic macromolecules begin to adsorb on the tooth surface to form a conditioning film called as acquired pellicle. The pellicle is composed of a variety of salivary glycoproteins (mucins) that are derived from saliva, crevicular fluid, bacterial and host tissue cells. The pellicle alters the charge and free energy of the tooth surface, which in turn increases the efficiency of bacterial adhesion.

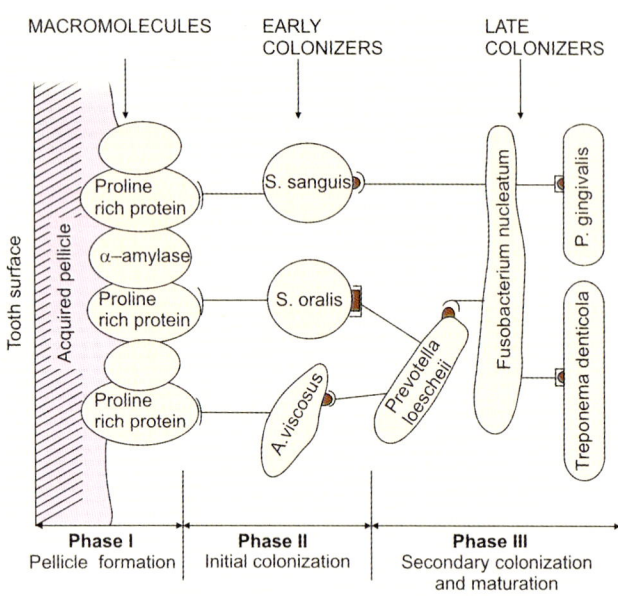

Fig. 9.4: Phases of plaque formation

II. *Initial colonization of microorganisms:* Initial colonizers are gram-positive facultative microbes (*Actinomyces viscosus* and *Streptococcus sanguis*). These bacteria adhere variably to the pellicle coated tooth surfaces. Some possess specific attachment structures such as extracellular polymeric substances and fimbriae, which enable them to attach rapidly upon contact. There is interaction of receptors of the dental pellicle and adhesins of the bacterial surface. *A. viscosus* has fimbriae on which protein adhesins are there which bind specifically to proline rich proteins found in the dental pellicle.

III. *Secondary colonization and maturation of microbes:* *P. intermedia, P. gingivalis, F. nucleatum* are secondary colonizers which do not initially colonize clean or pellicle coated tooth surfaces. In this phase, there is coaggregation, which is the ability of different species and genera of plaque microbes to adhere to one another. Bridging refers to the observation that two non-coaggregating straizns may participate together in a multi generic aggregate if they recognize a common partner by distinct mechanism. *Fusobacterium nucleatum* is believed to be important in bridging between primary and secondary colonizers during plaque maturation. Examples of interaction of secondary colonizers with early colonizers are *Fusobacterium nucleatum* with *Streptococcus sanguis;* *Prevotella loescheii* with *Actinomyces viscosus;*

Capnocytophaga ochraceus with *A. viscosus.* The examples of interaction among secondary colonizers are *F. nucleatum* with *P.gingivalis; F. nucleatum* with *Treponema denticola.*

MICROSCOPIC STRUCTURE

Corn cob structure (Leptothrix racemosa) are common at the surface of the supragingival deposits. The term Corn cob was coined by Jones in 1971 because of their resemblance to an ear of corn. In 1987, Vicentini first described that these structures have inner core of rod-shaped bacterial cells (*F. nucleatum*) and over the surface of which is attached the coccal cells (Streptococci or *P. gingivalis*). Tooth associated plaque is loosely organized containing mainly gram-negative rods and cocci as well as large numbers of filaments, flagellated rods and spirochetes. Tooth associated plaque microorganisms are *Streptococcus mitis, S. sanguis, A. naeslundi* and *Eubacterium* **(Fig. 9.5)**.

With increasing thickness of plaque diffusion into and out becomes more and more difficult. An oxygen gradient develops as a result of rapid utilization by the superficial bacterial layers and poor diffusion of oxygen through the biofilm matrix. Completely anaerobic conditions eventually emerge in the deeper layers of the deposits. Thus, there is transition from gram-positive to gram-negative microorganisms which is paralleled by a physiologic transition in the developing plaque. In the subgingival plaque, test tube brush or bristle brush

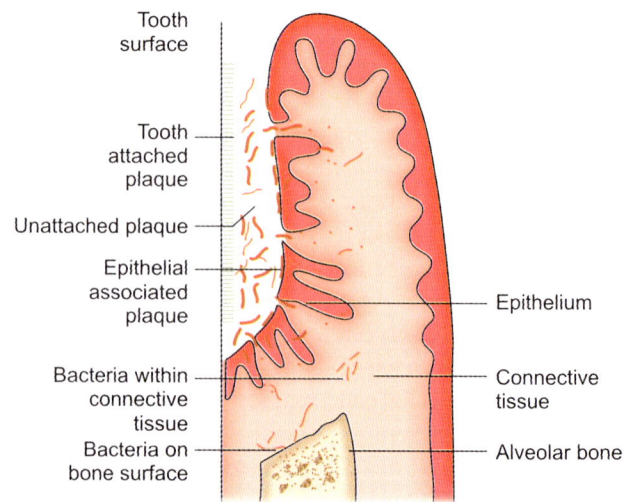

Fig. 9.5: Association of plaque and bacteria with tooth surface and periodontal tissues

structures are common. These are composed of filamentous bacteria to which gram- negative rods adhere. Tissue associated plaque microorganisms are *S. oralis, S. intermedius, P. micros, P. gingivalis, P. intermedia, Tannerella forsythia* and *F. nucleatum* **(Fig. 9.5)**.

METABOLIC INTERACTIONS IN DENTAL PLAQUE

Metabolic interactions among different bacterial species found in plaque are **(Fig. 9.6):**

1. Synergistic/Agonistic interactions:
   - *Streptococcus* and *Actinomyces* produce lactate and formate as metabolic byproducts which are used in the metabolism of *Veillonella* and *Campylobacter* respectively.
   - *Veillonella* produces menadione which is used by *P. gingivalis* and *P. intermedia*.
   - *Campylobacter* produces protoheme which is used by *P. gingivalis*.
   - *P. gingivalis* produces isobutyrate which is utilized by *Treponema*.
   - *Treponema* and *Capnocytophaga* produce succinate which is used by *P. gingivalis*.
2. Antagonistic interactions:
   - *S. sanguis* produces H_2O_2 which kills Aggregatibacter actinomycetemcomitans.
   - *Aggregatibacter actinomycetemcomitans* produces bacteriocin which kills *S. sanguis*.

Metabolic interactions between the host and microorganisms are found in plaque. Host acts as important source of nutrients. The breakdown of host hemoglobin provide hemin iron which is important in the metabolism of *P. gingivalis*. Ammonia released by the degradation of host protein by bacterial enzymes is being used by bacteria as nitrogen source.

VARIOUS PLAQUE HYPOTHESIS

1. *Non-specific plaque hypothesis*: This hypothesis was described by Walter Loesche in 1976. According to this hypothesis, periodontal disease results from the elaboration of noxious products by the entire plaque flora. The shortcomings of this hypothesis were that i) Some individuals with constant amount of plaque and calculus never developed destructive periodontitis and ii) Some sites were not affected whereas advanced disease was found in adjacent sites.

2. *Specific plaque hypothesis*: According to this hypothesis only certain plaque is pathogenic and its pathogenicity depends on the presence of or increase in specific microorganisms, as in the case of well known exogenous bacterial infections of man such as TB, syphilis. The shortcoming was that there were occasions when either disease was diagnosed in the absence of the putative pathogens or when pathogens were present with no evidence of disease.

3. *Modern version of specific theory*: It was described by Socransky in 1979 and according to this theory 6-12 bacterial species may be responsible for the majority of cases of destructive periodontitis and additional species may be responsible for small number of other cases.

4. *Unified theory*: Described by Theilade in 1986. It is the modern version of non-specific and specific plaque hypothesis. According to this theory, all bacterial plaque may contribute to the pathogenic potential of the subgingival flora to a greater or lesser extent. This is due to its ability to colonize and evade host defenses and provoke inflammation and tissue damage.

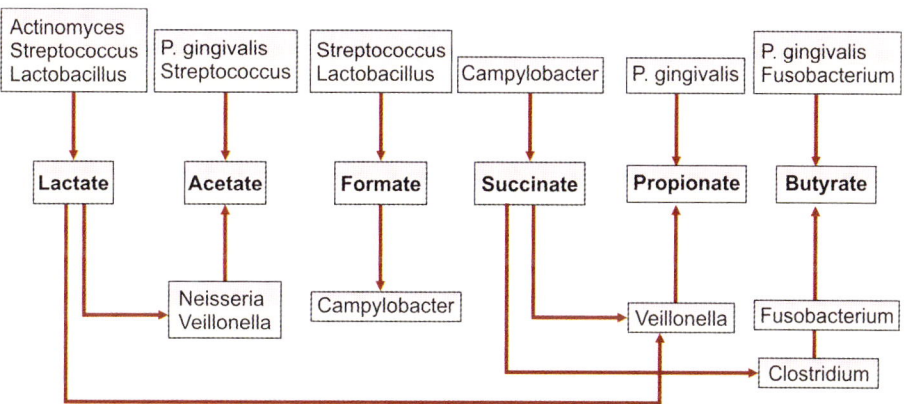

Fig. 9.6: Metabolic interactions among bacterial species in plaque biofilm

PERIODONTICS REVISITED

5. *Ecological plaque hypothesis*: According to this, any change in the nutrient status of a pocket i.e. physical and chemical change to the habitat are considered the primary cause for overgrowth of pathogens.

PLAQUE ACCUMULATION AND RETENTION

Marginal plaque is of prime importance in the development of gingivitis whereas supragingival plaque and tooth associated plaque are critical in calculus formation and root caries. Tissue associated subgingival plaque is important in the soft tissue destruction that characterize different forms of periodontitis. The pathogenic potential of tissue associated subgingival plaque is due to microorganism invasion into connective tissues and release of endotoxins and inflammatory substances.

Plaque accumulates more rapidly on rough surfaces of teeth, restoration and calculus. Plaque accumulation around crowded teeth is much greater than the teeth in good alignment especially in mandibular anterior teeth. Teeth which are not in use during mastication also show more plaque accumulation. Patients who are not motivated and cooperative show more plaque deposition. Plaque also deposits more in areas which are difficult to clean such as under overhanging crown margins and carious lesions.

The various plaque retentive areas are:
1. Natural areas/factors:
   - *Supragingival*: Supragingival calculus, cavitated carious lesions and exposed cementum.
   - *Subgingival*: Subgingival calculus, cavitated carious lesions, furcation involvement, root grooves, rough unplaned cementum, deep, narrow pockets and enamel projections.
2. Iatrogenic factors: Overhanging restoration margins, orthodontic bands, overcontoured and inadequate crown margins and portions of removable prosthesis those impinge on gingiva.

CONTROL AND REMOVAL OF PLAQUE

Dental plaque cannot be easily washed away by vigorous rinsing or water sprays. It also resists disruption by antimicrobial agents that cannot easily penetrate the protective polysaccharide matrix barrier characteristic of biofilms. Therefore, dental plaque is removed by scaling and root planing. It can also be removed by individual mechanical intervention (toothbrushing, flossing) and chemical intervention (antiplaque agents). More is explained in chapter no. 37. Mechanical plaque control and chapter no. 38 Chemotherapeutic agents.

OTHER TOOTH DEPOSITS

Plaque is differentiated from other deposits that may be found on the tooth surface such as pellicle, materia alba, food debris, stains and calculus **(Table 9.2)**.

Pellicle is an organic film derived mainly from the saliva and deposited on the tooth surface. Pellicle contains few or no bacteria in its early stages; however, a few hours after its deposition, oral bacteria deposit on the pellicle changing its composition.

Materia alba is a concentration of microorganisms, desquamated epithelial cells, leukocytes, and a mixture of salivary proteins and lipids, with few or no food particles. It is a yellow or grayish-white, soft deposit which is easily displaced with a water spray.

Pigmented deposits on the tooth surface are called dental stains. Stains are primarily an aesthetic problem and do not cause inflammation of the gingiva. The use of tobacco products, coffee, tea, certain mouthrinses, and pigments in foods can contribute to stain formation **(Fig. 9.7)**.

Calculus is a hard deposit that forms by mineralization of dental plaque and is generally covered by a layer of unmineralized plaque. More is explained in chapter no.10 Dental Calculus and Other Contributing Factors.

POINTS TO PONDER

✓ Corn cob and test tube brush structures are the examples of coaggregation in dental plaque.
✓ *Fusobacterium nucleatum* bridges between primary and secondary colonizers during plaque maturation.

TABLE 9.2: Differences between plaque, materia alba and food debris

	Plaque	Materia alba	Food debris
Structure	Definite, regular	Amorphous	No structure
Effect of rinsing	Do not dislodge	Dislodged by forceful rinsing	Dislodged readily
Adherence	Close	Loose	None

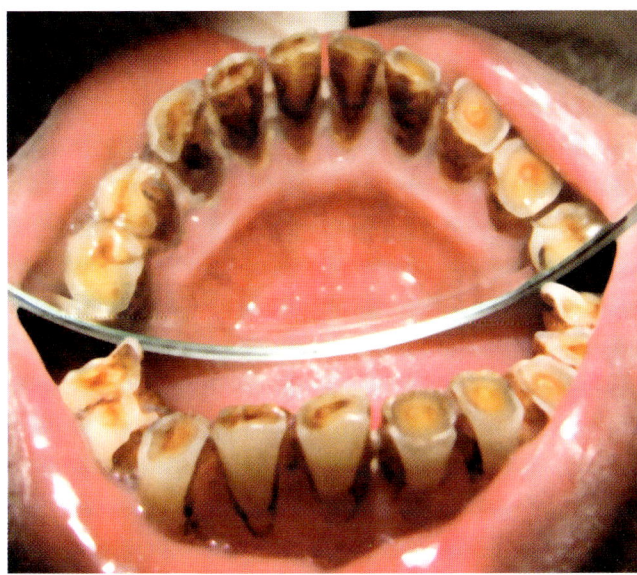

Fig. 9.7: Tobacco stains

BIBLIOGRAPHY

1. Busscher HJ, Evans LV. Oral biofilms and plaque control. Harwood academic publishers.
2. Eley BM, Manson JD. The Aetiology of periodontal diseases. In, Periodontics 5th ed Wright 2004; 39-54.
3. Genco RJ. Microbial dental plaque. In, Genco RJ, Goldman HM, Cohen DW. Contemporary Periodontics. CV Mosby Company 1990; 126-34.
4. Grant DA, Stern IB, Listgarten MA. Microbiology (plaque) In, Periodontics 6th ed CV Mosby Company 1988; 147-97.
5. Haake SK, Newman MG, Nisengard RJ, Sanz M. Periodontal Microbiology. In, Newman, Takei, Carranza. Clinical Periodontology 9th ed WB Saunders 2003; 96-112.
6. Lang NP, Mombelli A, Attstrom R. Dental plaque and Calculus. In, Lindhe J, Karring T, Lang NP. Clinical Periodontology and Implant dentistry 4th ed Blackwell Munksgaard 2003; 81-105.
7. Wilkins EM. Bacterial plaque and other soft deposits. In, clinical practice of the dental hygientist 8th ed Lippincott 1999; 264-76.

MCQs

1. The first bacteria to be deposited on the tooth in bacterial plaque formation are:
   A. Gram-negative rods
   B. Gram-positive rods
   C. Gram-positive cocci
   D. Gram-negative cocci
2. Non-specific plaque hypothesis was put forward by:
   A. Genco
   B. Listgarten
   C. Loesche
   D. None of the above
3. Radius of action of toxins in the bacterial plaque is:
   A. Less than 2.5 mm
   B. Greater than 3.5 mm
   C. Less than 1.5 mm
   D. 1.5-2.5 mm
4. 1 mg of plaque contains approximately:
   A. 2×10^8 bacteria
   B. 2×10^9 bacteria
   C. 2×10^{10} bacteria
   D. 2×10^{11} bacteria
5. Corn cob formation in dental plaque is an example of:
   A. Adhesion
   B. Symbiosis
   C. Attachment
   D. Coaggregation
6. Materia alba differs from dental plaque in:
   A. Absence of microorganisms
   B. Presence of desquamated epithelial cells
   C. Lack of internal structure
   D. Duration of adherence to tooth

Answers

1. C   2. C   3. D   4. A   5. D
6. C

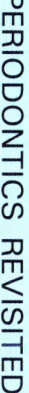

CHAPTER

10

Dental Calculus and Other Contributing Factors

Shalu Bathla

HISTORICAL PERSPECTIVE

Albucasis (936–1013 AD), an Arabian physician and surgeon, defined the relationship between calculus and dental disease and explained the need for the thorough removal of deposits. Albucasis described the way to remove calculus from teeth. Paracelsus (1493-1541) developed an interesting theory called as doctrine of calculus. He understood that pathologic calcification occurred in a variety of organs, and he considered these disease conditions to result from a metabolic disturbance whereby the body takes nourishment from food and discards the refuse as "tartarus", a material that cannot be broken. This tartar consisting of gravel and gluelike components was considered to came from barley, peas, milk, meat and fish, and drinks such as wine, beer, and fruit juice. The amount of tartar formed depended on the region of the body. Paracelsus recognized the extensive formation of tartar on the teeth and related this to toothache. Until the 1960s, the prevalent thinking in dentistry was that dental calculus was the cause of periodontal diseases; that by its roughness it was irritating and that bacteria then had a secondary influence. However, a series of classic studies on experimental gingivitis published from 1965 to 1968 clearly demonstrated the causative relation between dental plaque and gingivitis. Current thinking is that dental plaque is the precursor of calculus, which is mineralized plaque. Calculus is invariably covered with plaque on its surface.

DEFINITION

Dental Calculus is an adherent, calcified or calcifying mass that forms on the surfaces of teeth and dental appliances.

TYPE/CLASSIFICATION

It is classified according to its relation to the gingival margin as supragingival and subgingival calculus **(Table 10.1)**.

The various forms of submarginal and subgingival calculus are shown in **(Fig. 10.1)**.

- *Spicules*: Small isolated pieces of calculus. These are frequently located at line angles and interdental areas.
- *Ledge*: A larger deposit that forms on a section of the tooth and is approximately parallel to the cementoenamel junction (CEJ).
- *Ring form*: A ledge like deposit that encircles the tooth, forming a ring of calculus. In addition to calculus, roughness on the tooth surface may be caused by rough restorations, carious lesion, or necrotic cementum.

TABLE 10.1: Differences between supragingival calculus and subgingival calculus

		Supragingival calculus	*Subgingival calculus*
1.	Color	White or whitish yellow	Dark brown/genuine black
2.	Shape	Amorphous bulky, shape of calculus is determined by anatomy of teeth, contour of gingival margin and pressure of tongue, lips or cheeks	Flattened to conform with pressure from the pocket wall. May be crusty, shiny, thin, finger and fern like.
3.	Consistency	Moderately hard	Flint like, brittle
4.	Attachment	Easily detached from tooth	Firmly attached to the tooth surface
5.	Location	Coronal to the gingival margin **(Fig. 10.2)**	Below the crest of the marginal gingiva **(Fig. 10.3)**.
6.	Visibility	Visible in the oral cavity	Not visible on routine clinical examination
7.	Composition	More brushite and octacalcium phosphate. Less Magnesium whitlockite. Salivary proteins are present. Sodium content is lesser.	Less brushite and octacalcium phosphate. More Magnesium whitlockite. Salivary proteins are absent. Sodium content increases with the depth of pocket.
8.	Source	Derived from salivary secretions	Formed from gingival exudate
9.	Distribution	Symmetrical arrangement on teeth, more on facial surface of maxillary molars and lingual surface of mandibular anterior teeth due to openings of salivary glands ducts **(Fig. 10.4)**.	Related to pocket depth, heaviest on proximal surfaces.

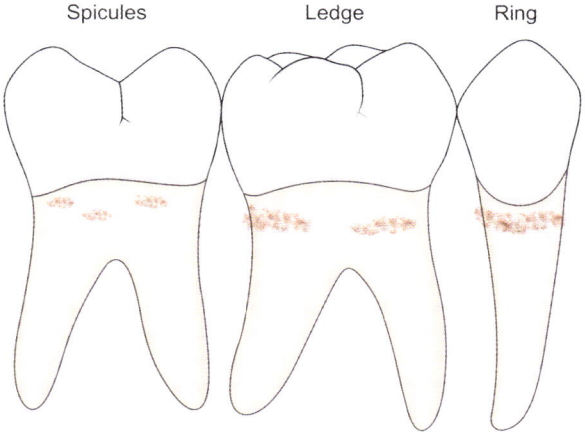

Spicules   Ledge   Ring

Fig. 10.1: Forms of subgingival calculus

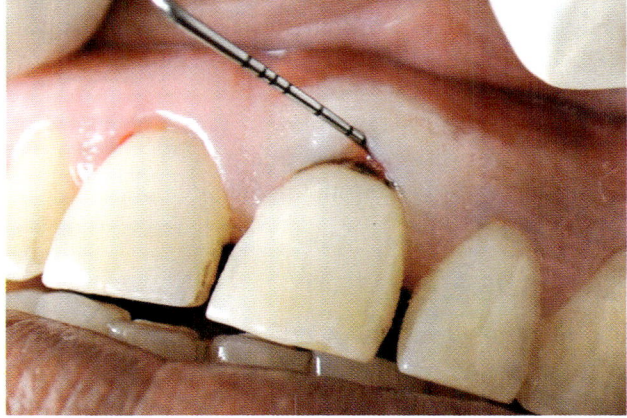

Fig 10.3: Subgingival calculus

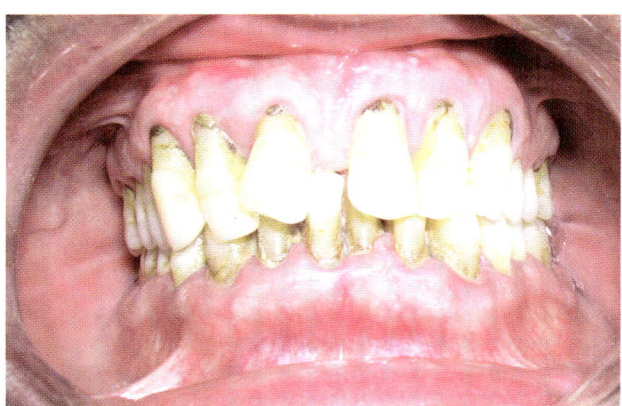

Fig. 10.2: Supragingival calculus

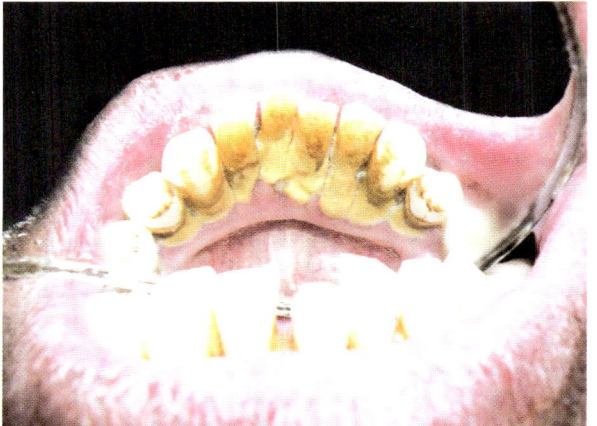

Fig. 10.4: Calculus at lingual surfaces of mandibular anterior teeth

PERIODONTICS REVISITED

COMPOSITION OF CALCULUS

1. *Inorganic content*
   a. Elements: Calcium (39%), phosphorus (19%), carbon dioxide (1.9%), magnesium (0.8%) and traces of sodium, zinc, strontium, bromine, copper, manganese, tungsten, gold, aluminium, silicon, iron, fluorine.
   b. Compounds: Calcium phosphate (75.9%), calcium carbonate (3.1%) and traces of magnesium phosphate and other metals.
   c. Crystals: Hydroxyapatite (58%), magnesium whitlockite (21%), octacalcium phosphate (12%) and brushite (9%) are the four main forms of crystals present.
2. *Organic content*: 1.9 to 9.1% of carbohydrates (galactose, glucose, rhamnose, mannose, glucuronic acid, galactosamine, arabinose, galacturonic acid, glucosamine); 5.9 to 8.2% of proteins; 0.2% of lipids (Neutral fats, fatty acids, cholesterol, phospholipids, cholesterol esters); Protein polysaccharide complexes; Desquamated epithelial cells; Leukocytes and microorganisms.
3. *Bacterial content*: At periphery – Gram-negative rods and cocci predominate. Filamentous organisms, Diphtheroids, Bacterionema and Veillonella species are also present.

CALCULUS FORMATION

Mineralization consists of crystal formation, namely hydroxyapatite, octacalcium phosphate, magnesium whitlockite, and brushite each with a characteristic developmental pattern. The crystal forms in the intercellular matrix, on the surface of bacteria and finally within the bacteria. The mineralization process is considered the same for both supragingival and subgingival calculus. The initiation of calcification and the rate of calculus accumulation vary from person-to-person, for different teeth and at different times in the same person. On the basis of these differences, persons may be classified as heavy, moderate, or slight calculus formers or as noncalculus formers. Heavy calculus formers have higher salivary levels of calcium and phosphorus than do light calculus formers. Light calculus formers have higher levels of parotid pyrophosphate. Pyrophosphate is an inhibitor of calcification.

Theories Related to Mineralization of Calculus

1. *Booster/precipitation theory*: Loss of carbon dioxide and formation of ammonia leads to increase in the pH which leads to the precipitation of calcium phosphate salts.
2. *Epitactic/Nucleation concept*: The carbohydrate – protein complexes may initiate calcification by removing calcium from the saliva and binding with it to form nuclei that induce deposition of minerals. Seeding agents induce small foci of calcification that enlarges and unites together to form calcified mass.
3. *Inhibition theory*: Calcification occurring only at specific site is because of the existence of an inhibiting mechanism at noncalcifying sites. Where calcification occurs, the inhibitor is apparently altered or removed. Inhibiting substance is thought to be pyrophosphate and among the controlling mechanism is the enzyme alkaline pyrophosphatase, which can hydrolyze the pyrophosphate to phosphate. The pyrophosphate inhibits calcification by preventing the initial nucleus from growing, possibly by "poisoning" the growth centers of the crystal.
4. *Transformation theory*: Amorphous noncrystalline deposits and brushite can be transformed to octacalcium phosphate and then to hydroxyapatite.

CLINICAL ASSESSMENT

The clinical assessment can be done by:
1. *Visual examination by use of compressed air*: Small amount of supragingival calculus that have not been stained are frequently invisible when they are wet with saliva. Subgingival calculus deposits can sometimes be detected visually by blowing air down the gingival crevice. Dark edge of calculus may be seen at or just beneath the gingival margin. An explorer may be used when visual examination is not definite.
2. *Probing*: A fine subgingival explorer or probe is needed that can be adapted close to the root surface all the way to the bottom of a pocket. Each subgingival area must be examined carefully to the bottom of the pocket, completely around each teeth. While probing for sulcus/pocket a rough subgingival tooth surface can be felt when calculus is present. Although there are other causes of roughness, subgingival calculus is the most common.
3. *Radiographs*: The deposits may also be visible on radiographs although this is not always reliable.

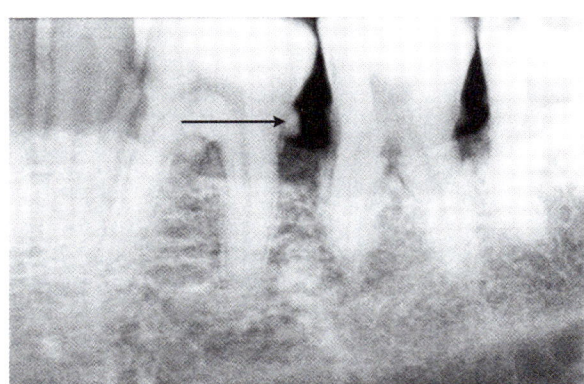

Fig. 10.5: Subgingival calculus seen in radiograph

Radiographs may be useful in diagnosis of subgingival calculus **(Fig. 10.5)**. The location of calculus does not indicate the bottom of the periodontal pocket because the most apical plaque is not sufficiently calcified to be visible on radiographs.

4. *Clinical records*: The various indices for recording and scoring calculus are explained in chapter no. 7 Epidemiology of Gingival and Periodontal diseases.

MODES OF ATTACHMENT OF CALCULUS TO THE TOOTH SURFACE AND IMPLANT

Helmut A. Zander in 1952 described four types of calculus attachment **(Figs 10.6A to D)**:

1. Attachment by means of an organic pellicle.
2. Mechanical locking into surface irregularities such as resorption lacunae and caries. This type of attachment make the removal of calculus difficult as calculus embedded beneath the cementum surface penetrates into the dentin.

3. Penetration of calculus bacteria into cementum.
4. Close adaptation of calculus undersurface depressions to the gently sloping mounds of the unaltered cementum surface.

Shroff later theorized that the type of calculus attachment probably depends on the length of time the calculus has been on the tooth. The attachment of calculus to pure titanium implant is less intimate than to root surface.

ROLE OF CALCULUS IN PERIODONTAL DISEASE

Calculus may be harmful both physically and chemically to adjacent gingiva. Calculus is permeable and thus, may absorb and adsorb toxic products. Calculus is rough and porous which facilitates the retention of dental plaque. Calculus is always covered with unmineralized plaque which provides further retention and promotes new plaque accumulation and thus, causes periodontal destruction in the following manner:

- Calculus brings bacterial overlay closer to the supporting tissues
- Interfere with local self-cleansing mechanism
- Provide nidus for continuous plaque accumulation.
- Make plaque removal more difficult.

LOCAL CONTRIBUTING FACTORS

1. Anatomic factors
   a. *Proximal contact relation*: The integrity and location of the proximal contacts along with the contour of the marginal ridges and developmental grooves typically prevent interproximal food impaction. *Food impaction is the forceful wedging of*

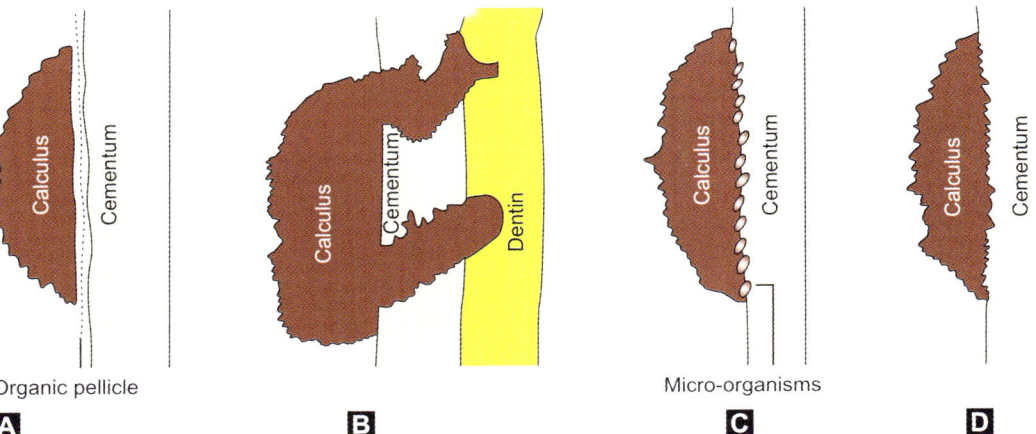

Figs 10.6A to D: Modes of attachment of calculus

PERIODONTICS REVISITED

food into the periodontium by occlusal forces. Hirschfeld in 1930 classified vertical food impaction relative to etiologic factors:

Class I – Occlusal wear

Class II – Loss of proximal support

Class III – Extrusion of a tooth beyond the occlusal plane

Class IV – Congenital morphologic abnormalities

Class V – Improperly constructed restorations

Sequelae of food impaction:

- Feeling of pressure and the urge to dig the material from between the teeth.
- Vague pain which radiates deep in the jaws.
- Gingival inflammation with bleeding and a foul taste in the involved area.
- Gingival recession.
- Periodontal abscess formation.
- Varying degree of inflammatory involvement of the periodontal ligament with an associated elevation of the tooth in its socket, prematurity in functional contact and sensitivity to percussion.
- Destruction of alveolar bone.
- Caries of the tooth.

Plunger cusps are the cusps that tend to forcibly wedge food into interproximal embrasures of opposing teeth. Distolingual cusps of maxillary molars are the most common plunger cusp. Plunger cusp effect may occur with wear or it may be the result of a shift in tooth positions following the failure to replace missing tooth.

b. *Cervical enamel projection (CEP) and enamel pearls*: They appear as narrow wedge-shaped extensions of enamel pointing from the cementoenamel junction (CEJ) toward the furcation area. The clinical significance of CEPs is that they are plaque retentive and can predispose to furcation involvement.

c. *Intermediate bifurcation ridge*: The intermediate bifurcation ridge is a convex excrescence of cementum that runs longitudinally between the mesial and distal roots of a mandibular molar. It may be located at the midpoint between the buccal and lingual surfaces of the area of root division or it may be located in a more lateral position. These ridges are found more frequently on first molars. These irregular contours make plaque and calculus removal more difficult and inadequate plaque and calculus removal can lead to failure of furcation treatment, especially regenerative therapy.

d. *Palatogingival groove*: The palatogingival groove frequently termed the palatoradicular groove,

often begins at the cingulum and extends apically for a variable distance **(Fig. 10.7A)**. Deep pocketing of maxillary incisors, especially isolated, should prompt an examination for this plaque – retentive root anomaly **(Fig. 10.7B)**. If the palatogingival groove is associated with bone loss and attachment loss, the clinician may attempt to remove the groove through odontoplasty or to reduce its depth to minimize plaque retention **(Fig 10.7C)**.

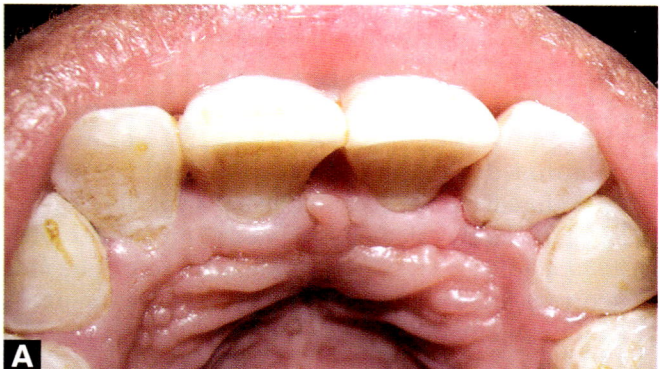

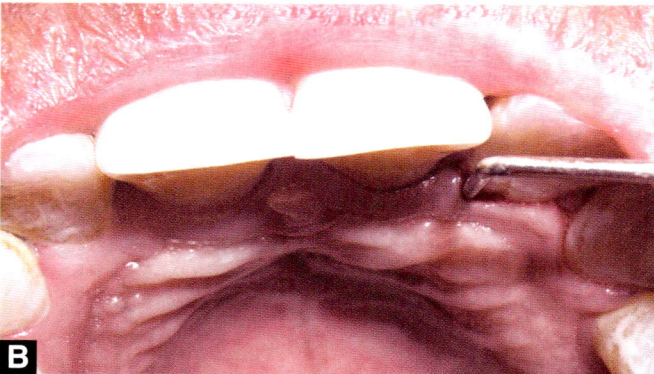

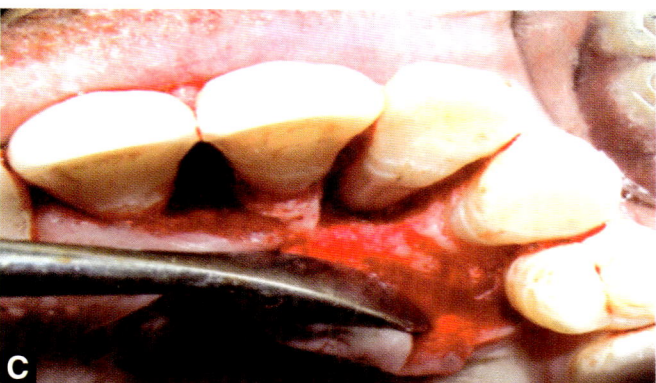

Figs 10.7A to C: (A) Palatogingival groove at the cingulum of lateral incisor, (B) Pocket associated with palatogingival groove, (C) Bone loss associated with palatogingival groove

e. *Root proximity*: Close approximation of tooth roots, with an accompanying thin interproximal septum leads to an increased risk for periodontal destruction.

2. Iatrogenic factors: Inadequate dental procedures that contribute to the deterioration of the periodontal tissues are referred to as *iatrogenic factors.*

a. *Restorative dentistry*: The improper use of rubber dam clamps, matrix bands and burs can lacerate the gingiva resulting in varying degree of mechanical trauma and inflammation. Restorations can do more harm than good to the patient's oral health if performed improperly **(Fig. 10.8)**. Overhanging margins of restorations and crowns accumulate additional plaque by limiting the patient's access.

b. *Prosthesis*: Gross iatrogenic irritants such as poorly designed clasps, prosthesis saddles and pontics exert a direct traumatic influence upon periodontal tissues **(Fig. 10.9)**.

c. *Orthodontic procedures*: Orthodontic therapy may affect the periodontium by favoring plaque retention, by directly injuring the gingiva as a result of overextended bands, chemical irritation by exposed cement **(Fig. 10.10)** and by creating excessive, unfavorable forces, or both.

d. *Extraction of impacted third molar*: The extraction of impacted third molars often results in the creation of vertical bone defects distal to the second molars. Careless use of elevators or forceps during extraction results in crushing of alveolar bone.

3. Malocclusion as contributing factors: Crowded or malaligned teeth can be more difficult to clean than properly aligned teeth. In deepbite, maxillary incisors impinge on the mandibular labial gingiva or mandibular incisors on the palatal gingiva, causing gingival and periodontal inflammation **(Fig. 10.11)**. Failure to replace missing posterior teeth have adverse consequences on the periodontal support for the remaining teeth. When the mandibular first molar is extracted, the initial change is a mesial drifting and tilting of the mandibular second and third molars with extrusion of the maxillary first molar. As the mandibular second molar tips mesially, its distal cusps extrude and act as plungers. The distal cusps of the mandibular second molar wedge between the maxillary first and second molars and open the contact by deflecting the maxillary second molar distally. Subsequently, food impaction may occur and accompanied by gingival inflammation with eventual

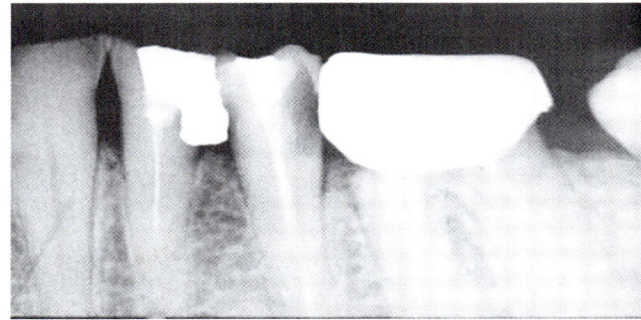

Fig. 10.8: Interproximal bone boss associated with overhanging restoration predisposing to plaque retention

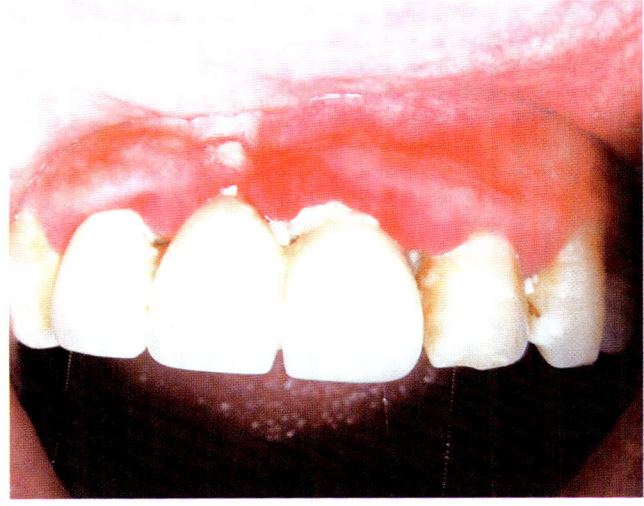

Fig. 10.9: Inflammatory gingival changes around fixed partial prosthesis

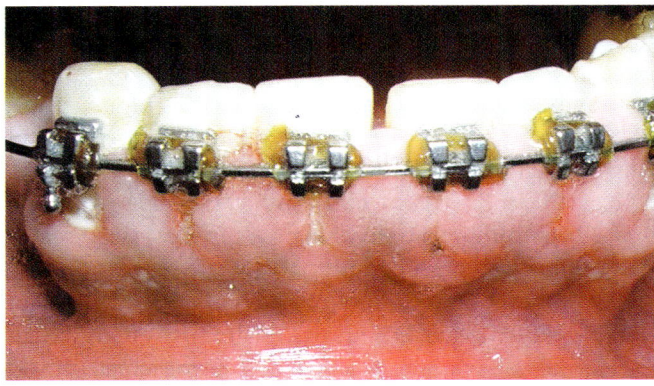

Fig. 10.10: Gingival hyperplasia in lower anteriors due to chemical irritation by exposed cement

loss of the interproximal bone between the maxillary first and second molars.

PERIODONTICS REVISITED

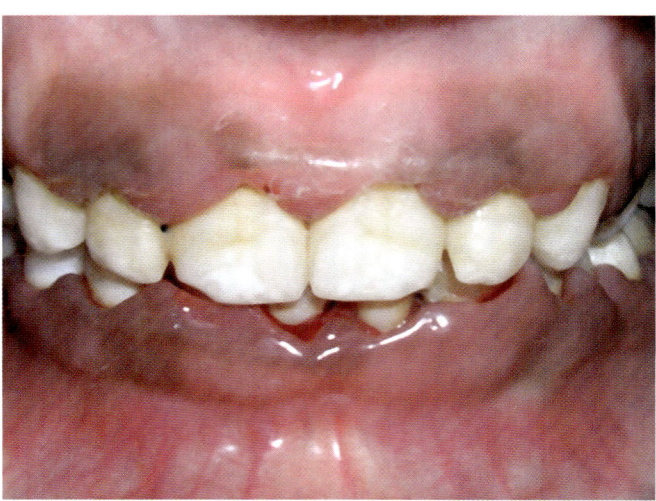

Fig. 10.11: Deep bite causing gingival and periodontal inflammation

4. Habits as contributing factors
    a. *Toothbrush and floss trauma*: The toothbrush may cause damage to dental soft and hard tissues. A new toothbrush, and especially a hard toothbrush, can abrade epithelium and leave painful ulcerations on the gingiva. Thin marginal gingiva that is abraded away can lead to gingival recession and exposure of the root surface. The tooth surface, usually the root surface, can be abraded away by improper toothbrushing technique, especially with a hard toothbrush. The abrasives in toothpaste may contribute significantly to this process. The defect usually manifests as V-shaped notches at the level of the CEJ **(Fig. 10.12)**.

    Flossing can also cause damage to dental hard and soft tissues. Flossing clefts may be produced when floss is forcefully snapped through the contact point so that it cuts into the gingiva. Also, an aggressive up and down cleaning motion can produce a similar injury.
    b. *Mouth breathing and tongue thrusting*: Mouth breathing can dehydrate the gingival tissues and increase susceptibility to inflammation. These patients may or may not have increased levels of dental plaque. In some cases, gingival enlargement may also occur. Excellent plaque control and professional cleaning should be recommended, although these measures may not completely resolve the gingival inflammation. Tongue thrusting is often associated with an anterior open bite. During swallowing the tongue is thrust forward against the teeth instead of being placed against the palate. When the amount of pressure against the teeth is great, it can lead to tooth mobility and cause increased spacing of the anterior teeth. This problem is difficult to treat but must be recognized in the diagnostic phase as a potentially destructive contributing factor.
    c. *Tobacco use*: Smoking is one of the most significant risk factors currently available to predict the development and progression of periodontitis **(Fig. 10.13)**. Rest is explained in chapter no 16. Smoking and Periodontium.

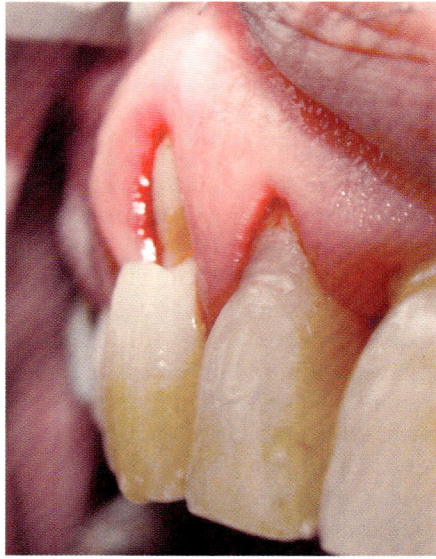

Fig. 10.12 : Toothbrushing abrasion

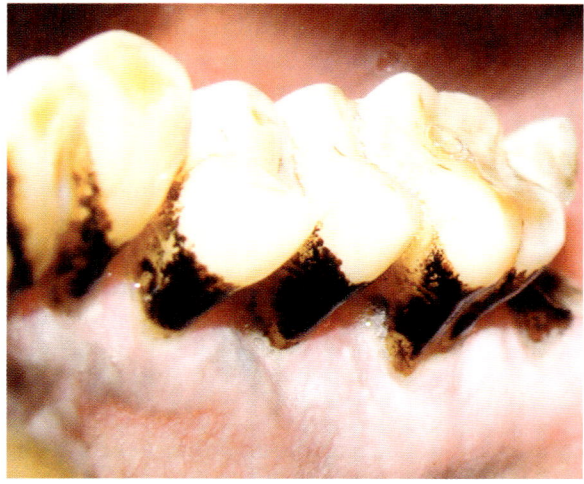

Fig. 10.13: Tobacco stains

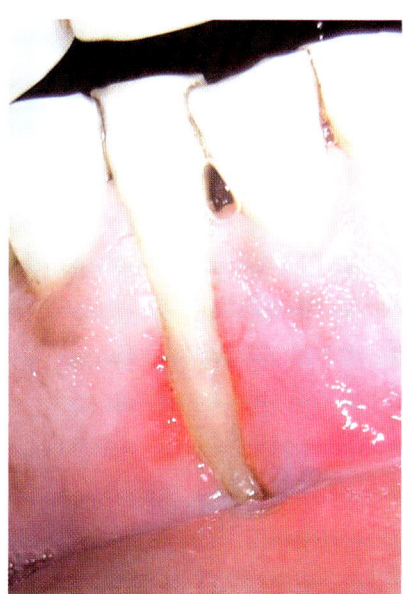

Fig. 10.14: Localized gingival recession due to pricking the gingiva with a fingernail (*Courtesy:* Dr Ajay Mahajan)

d. *Factitious injuries*: Self-inflicted or factitial injuries can be difficult to diagnose because their presentation is often unusual. These injuries are produced in a variety of ways including pricking the gingiva with a fingernail **(Fig. 10.14)**, with knives and by using toothpicks or other oral hygiene devices.

LANDMARK STUDIES RELATED

Lang NP, Hotz P, Graf H, Geering AH, Saxer VP, Sturzenberger OP, Mechel AH. Effects of supervised chlorhexidine mouthrinses in children. Journal of Periodontal Research 1982; 17: 101-11.

The study was done on 158 children (aged 10–12 years). They were divided into four groups, Group A was assigned to daily mouthrinses 6 times per week using a 0.2% solution of chlorhexidine gluconate, Group B used the same solution only twice per week, and Group C was assigned to daily rinsing using a 0.1% solution of chlorhexidine gluconate. Group D served as control and rinsed daily with a placebo solution. All the rinsings were supervised and timed for 30 seconds. No attempt was made to influence the oral hygiene habits of the children. Prior to the initial prophylaxis and after 6 months of supervised rinsing, plaque was scored using the Plaque Index (PlI), and gingivitis was assessed using the gingival index (GI). Calculus was scored according to the calculus surface index (CSI), and stain was also graded. At the end of the study it was found that plaque was significantly reduced whereas, calculus was increased significantly in all the groups when compared with the controls. Thus, it was concluded that there was statistically significant increase in calculus levels in children rinsing with a 0.2% chlorhexidine gluconate solution. It was postulated that dead bacteria had accumulated on the tooth surfaces, acting as sites for calculus deposition.

Gaare D, Rolla G, Aryadi FJ, Vander Ouderaa F. Improvement of gingival health by tooth brushing in individuals with large amounts of calculus. Journal of Clinical Periodontology 1990; 17: 38-41.

This study was conducted on Indonesian soldiers of 20 - 25 years of age having large amount of calculus. In one half of the subjects (Group A) careful professional prophylaxis was performed, while in the other half (Group B), tooth brushing was the sole oral hygiene aid. Gingival health in both groups improved after 2 months: from 63 to 36% bleeding points in group A, and from 61 to 36% in group B. There was thus no obvious benefit from the professional prophylaxis received by group A. The improvement of gingival health through tooth brushing, in spite of the presence of calculus, supports the contention that plaque, rather than calculus, as a non-inflammatory scale, provides the pathogenic potential.

POINTS TO PONDER

✓ Reversal phenomenon is the decline from maximal calculus accumulation. It is due to vulnerability of bulky calculus to mechanical wear from food, cheeks, lips and tongue.
✓ Calculus can also occur readily in germ free animals.
✓ Calculocementum is the calculus embedded deeply in the cementum and which appears morphologically similar to cementum.
✓ Calculus is the most prominent plaque retentive factor and is a secondary etiologic factor for periodontitis.

BIBLIOGRAPHY

1. Grant DA, Stern IB, Listgarten MA. Calculus. In, Periodontics. 6th ed CV Mosby Company 1988; 198-215.
2. Hinrichs JE. The role of calculus and other predisposing factors. In, Newman, Takei, Carranza. Clinical Periodontology 9th ed WB Saunders 2003; 182-203.
3. Lang NP, Mombelli A, Attstrom R. Dental Plaque and Calculus. In, Lindhe J, Karring T, Lang NP. Clinical Periodontology and Implant dentistry. 4th ed Blackwell Munksgaard 2003; 81-105.

PERIODONTICS REVISITED

4. Mandel ID. Dental calculus. In, Genco RJ, Goldman HM, Cohen DW. Contemporary Periodontics. C.V Mosby 1999; 135-46.
5. Wilkins EM. Dental calculus. In, Clinical practice of the dental hygientist. 8th ed Lippincott 1999; 277-84.

MCQs

1. Mineralized plaque is:
   A. Materia alba
   B. Calculus
   C. Food debris
   D. Dental stains
2. Calculus
   A. *Per se* is the irritating cause to gingiva
   B. It is always covered with a non-mineralized layer of plaque
   C. It is formed as all plaque undergoes mineralization
   D. Formation cannot be maintained in germ-free animals
3. The most efficient means of identifying supragingival calculus is by:
   A. Visual observation and compressed air
   B. Tactile detection and periodontal probe
   C. Use of disclosing solution
   D. Transillumination
4. Dental calculus contains:
   A. Vital microorganisms
   B. Non-vital microorganisms
   C. Both of the above
   D. None of the above
5. The most common crystalline forms present in supragingival calculus are:
   A. Hydroxyapatite and magnesium whitlockite
   B. Hydroxyapatite and octacalcium phosphate
   C. Hydroxyapatite and brushite
   D. Magnesium whitlockite and octacalcium phosphate
6. Which of the following crystals is more commonly found in the calculus of mandibular anterior areas?
   A. Hydroxyapatite
   B. Magnesium whitlockite
   C. Octacalcium phosphate
   D. Brushite
7. Calculocementum is:
   A. Calculus similar in composition to cementum
   B. Cementum similar in composition to calculus
   C. Cementum appearing morphologically similar to calculus
   D. Calculus appearing morphologically similar to cementum

Answers

1. B	2. B	3. A	4. B	5. B
6. D	7. D			

Answers

1. B   2. B   3. A   4. B   5. B
6. D   7. D

CHAPTER 11

Immunity and Inflammation

Shalu Bathla

INTRODUCTION

The immune system is a network designed for the homeostasis of large molecules (oligomers) and cells based on specific recognition processes. Recognition of the structural features of an oligomer by receptors on immune cells is an important component of the specificity of the immune system.

Immunity refers to the resistance exhibited by the host towards injury caused by microorganisms and their products.

Inflammation refers to tissue injury or irritation, initiated by the entry of pathogens or of other irritants.

Immune responses are categorized as either non-specific innate or specific adaptive. Nonspecific innate immune responses do not adapt with repeated exposure to the same pathogen. An example of innate immunity is phagocytic cells (i.e. monocytes, macrophages, and neutrophils), which possess a number of inherently antimicrobial peptides and proteins that kill many different, rather than one specific, pathogen. In contrast, the specific adaptive immune responses will increase after exposure to a pathogen and usually maintain higher levels for years. Lymphocytes (e.g. T-cells and B-cells) are important in the fundamental form of specific adaptive immunity referred to as the specific immune response.

NONSPECIFIC IMMUNITY

Nonspecific immunity represents the quite potent first line of defense. The cellular components of nonspecific immune system consist of phagocytic cells namely neutrophils, monocytes, natural killer cells, complement system, mast cells and additional inflammatory mediators.

Macrophages

These are modified monocytes, which exit from bone marrow after 2 days and increase in size to about 22 μm and thus, are called as macrophages. Macrophages are important because they secrete Interleukin – 1, IL – 6, IL – 8, IL – 10, Tumor necrosis factor – γ, Interferon α and γ and Insulin – like growth factor. They also produce prostaglandins, cyclic adenosine monophosphate (cAMP) and collagenase in response to stimulation by bacterial endotoxin, immune complexes, or lymphokines **(Fig. 11.1)**.

Mast Cells

These cells are among the most effective cells in alerting the endothelium of a local problem. They possess receptors for the Fc portion of IgE and IgG (FcϵR, FcγR) and complement components (C3a and

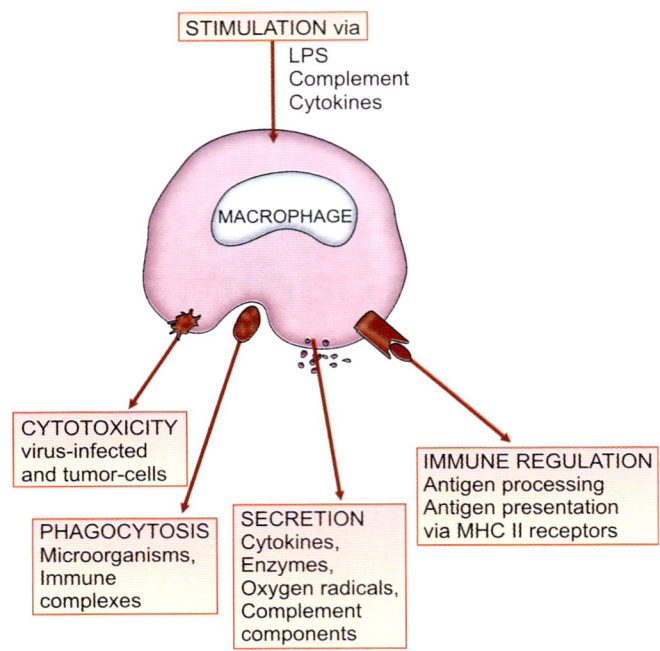

Fig. 11.1: Functions of macrophage

C5a). They contains cytoplasmic granules called as lysosomes, which store – Histamine, heparin, slow reacting substances of anaphylaxis (SRS – A), tumor necrosis factor-α, leukotriene C4, neutrophilic chemotactic factor and eosinophil chemotactic factor.

Neutrophils

Neutrophil are the initial leukocytes recruited into the gingiva. They exit the circulation and migrate into the junctional epithelium and GCF, where they provide the first cellular host defense mechanism to contact and control periodontal bacteria. They act as double edged sword. Neutrophils which differentiate almost completely within bone marrow in 14 days and retain its small size of 10 µm when they exit from bone marrow is called as microphages.

Neutrophils are believed to play an important role in controlling the periodontal microbiota. They are the first leukocytes to arrive at the site of inflammation and are always the dominant cell type within the junctional epithelium and the gingival crevice. For neutrophils to effectively control bacterial infections, their functions-including transendothelial migration, chemotaxis, transepithelial migration, opsonization, phagocytosis and intraphagolysosomal killing must be intact **(Fig. 11.2)**. Disorders of neutrophils are associated with invasive periodontal infection and aggressive periodontitis. For example, severe periodontal destruction involving both the primary dentition and permanent dentition is evident in individuals with disorders affecting neutrophil chemotaxis and phagocytosis. Also, otherwise healthy individuals with severe periodontal problems may have subtle defects in neutrophil function.

A. *Generation of acute phase signals*: Transendothelial migration: It is the selective interaction between leukocytes and endothelium that results in the leukocyte pushing its way between endothelial cells to exit the blood and enter the tissues.

Sequential phases of transendothelial migration of neutrophils are: **(Fig. 11.3)**

1. Rolling: Leukocytes L-selectin interact with addressins on the lumenal surface of endothelial cells, pauses to inspect the endothelium.

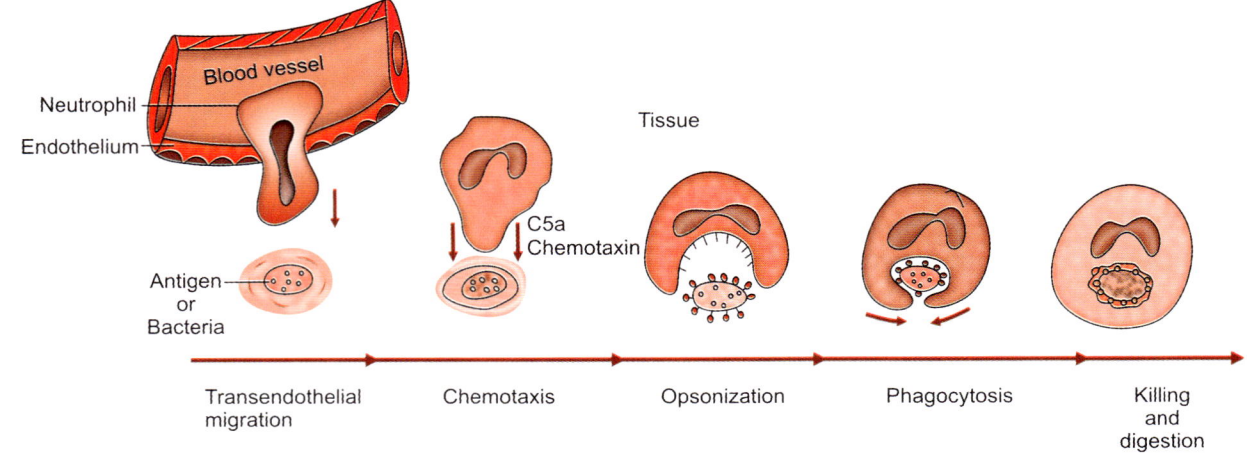

Fig. 11.2: Functions of neutrophil

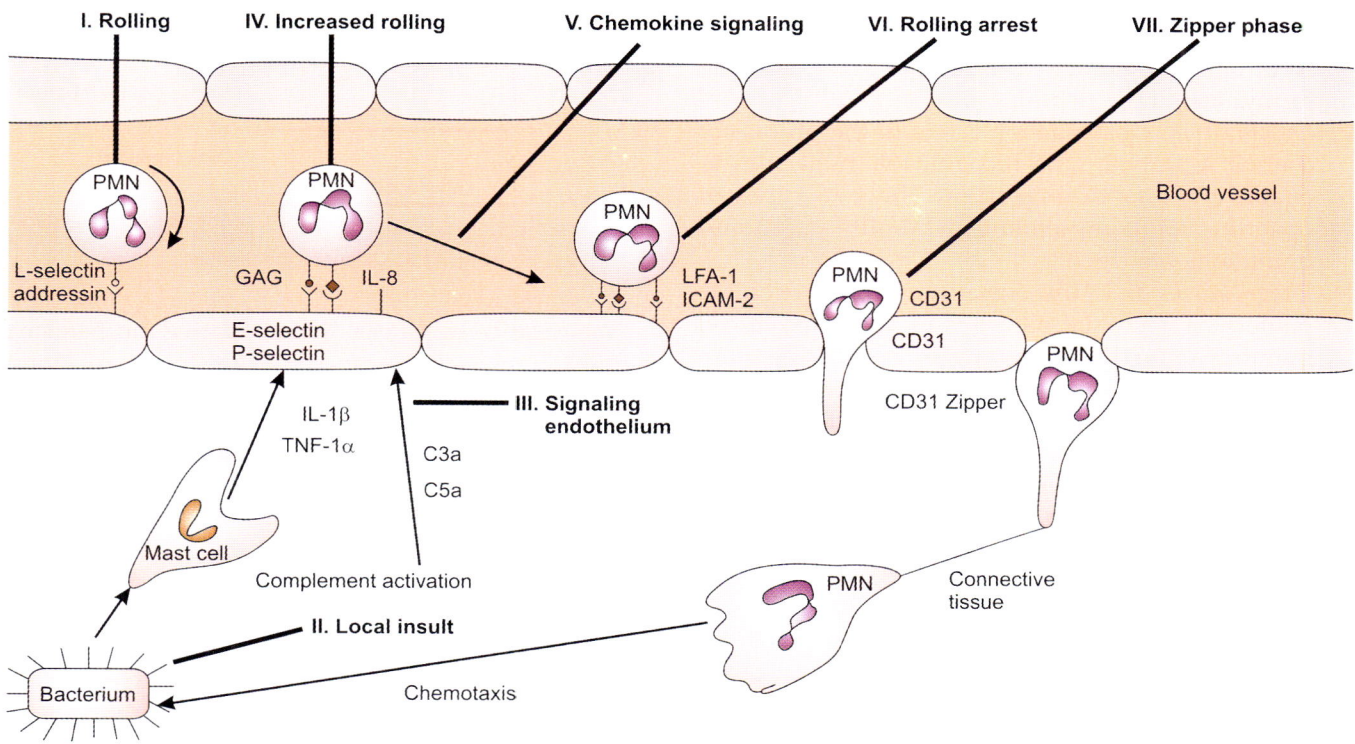

Fig. 11.3: Transendothelial migration

2. An insult to local tissue: Local insult triggers the release of inflammatory mediators IL-1β, TNF-α from mast cell.
3. Signaling the endothelium: TNF-α, C5a, LPS can stimulate endothelial cells to express P- selectin and E- selectin on their lumenal surface.
4. Increased rolling: P-selectin and E-Selectin on the endothelial cells interact with GAG (Carbohydrate molecules) of leukocytes. This increases the number of leukocytes attached to the lumenal surface of endothelium.
5. Signal for rolling arrest: The release of chemokine IL-8 by stimulated endothelium causes the leukocyte to shed L-selectin.
6. Strong adhesions: LFA-1 binds to ICAM-2 which results in arresting of rolling.
7. Zipper phase: CD31 are adhesion molecules present on endothelial cells and leukocytes. The binding of CD31 on endothelium with CD31 of leukocytes, guides leukocytes to the boundaries between endothelial cells.

About 1 to 2% of all neutrophils migrate across the junctional epithelium on a daily basis. This transepithelial migration requires a chemotaxin gradient. The junctional epithelium expresses the chemotactic cytokine (chemokine) IL-8 and intercellular cell adhesion molecule 1 (ICAM-1). A gradient of the membrane bound ICAM-1 and the soluble IL-8 molecules is formed, with increased expression toward the outer surface of the tissue. This distribution is ideal for the migration of neutrophils into the gingival sulcus. Neutrophils may use their adhesins LFA-1, Mac-1, or both to bind ICAM-1 on the epithelial cell in the process of epithelial transmigration.

B. *Chemotaxis*: Once the leukocyte enters the connective tissue, it must be able to locate and migrate to the site of insult, which is accomplished by chemotaxis. It is the directed movement of a cell along a chemical gradient. This is a receptor mediated event that is initiated by chemotactic factors forming a concentration gradient that directs the approach of phagocytic cells.

The chemoattractants are exogenous chemoattractants (bacterial products) and endogenous chemoattractant (C5a and IL-8). The chemotaxins for neutrophils are Tumor necrosis factor (TNF – α), IL-8, Platelet activating factor, Leukotriene B4, C5a, Neutrophilic chemotactic factor, IL-1, IFN-α and N-formyl-methionyl peptides.

C. *Opsonization*: Opsonization refers to the process of coating a particle with recognizable molecules to enable phagocytic ingestion. The two types of opsonins are complement metabolite (C3b) and Immunoglobin (IgG).

D. *Phagocytosis*: It is the engulfment of particulate matters or microbial parasites by the external cell membrane of the phagocyte, resulting in an intracellular, membrane – delimited structure termed phagosome. Bacteria within the phagosome and phagolysosome may be killed by oxidative or nonoxidative mechanisms.

E. *Killing and Digestion:* There are two killing mechanisms one is oxidative mechanism and other is nonoxidative mechanism.

Each neutrophil – posseses 2 types of granules **(Fig. 11.4)**

A. Specific granules are lysozyme, lactoferrin and B_{12} binding protein (Cobalophilin).

B. Azurophilic granules are α defensins (HNP-1, HNP-2, HNP-3, HNP-4), Serprocidin, Elastase, Proteinase 3, Azurocidin, Cathepsin G and lysozyme.

Oxidative mechanism: There is formation of superoxide anion with the help of NADPH oxidase enzyme of neutrophil and this superoxide which is capable of diffusing across the membrane. Hydrogen peroxide is reduced to hydroxyl radical which is capable of causing DNA damage. Myeloperoxidase catalyzes hydrogen peroxide and chloride to hypochlorous acid (HOCl) **(Fig. 11.5)**. This HOCl molecule has antimicrobial properties.

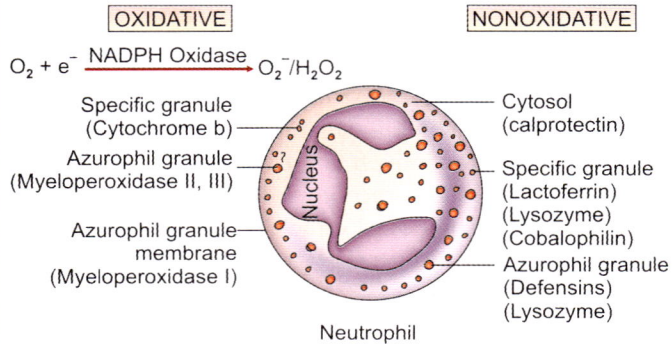

Fig. 11.4: Antimicrobial system of neutrophils

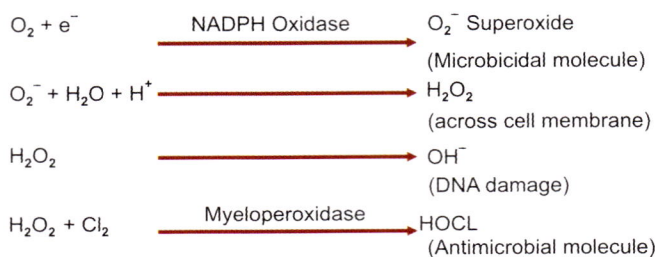

Fig. 11.5: Oxidative mechanism

Nonoxidative mechanism: Nonoxidative mechanisms of killing involve phagosome-lysosome fusion, resulting in secretion of bactericidal substances such as lysozyme, cathepsin G, and α-defensins into the phagolysosome containing the ingested bacterium.

Functions of neutrophil:

Generation of acute phase signals: Involves activation of serum complement components.
Chemotaxis: Directed migration to site of infection
Phagocytosis of microbial invaders
Antimicrobial system: Killing of bacteria

COMPLEMENT SYSTEM

It refers to a series of factors occurring in normal serum that are activated characteristically by antigen – antibody interaction. Complement system is a complex of different protein fractions (C1 to C9) which mediate a number of biologically significant consequences.

The complement cascade can be triggered off by two parallel but independent mechanisms called as classical/direct and alterative or properdin pathway. The reaction sequence in the activation of the complement system has a cascading type pathway. After one component of the complement system is bound with the Fc portion of the antibody in the antibody – antigen complex, the other components of the complement system react in an ordered sequence.

The classical pathway is activated by a reaction of antigen with IgG or IgM antibodies and by aggregated immunoglobulins. The sequence is C1, C4, C2, C3, C5, C6, C7, C8 and C9. C3 is cleaved by the complex C42 into C3b, which binds to the cell membrane, and C3a, which has biologic activity **(Fig. 11.6)**.

An alternative pathway for complement activation also exists. Aggregated antibodies of the IgG, IgA, and IgE classes, endotoxin, fungi, yeast cell walls, viruses, parasites and other substances can initiate the complement sequence by direct activation of the third

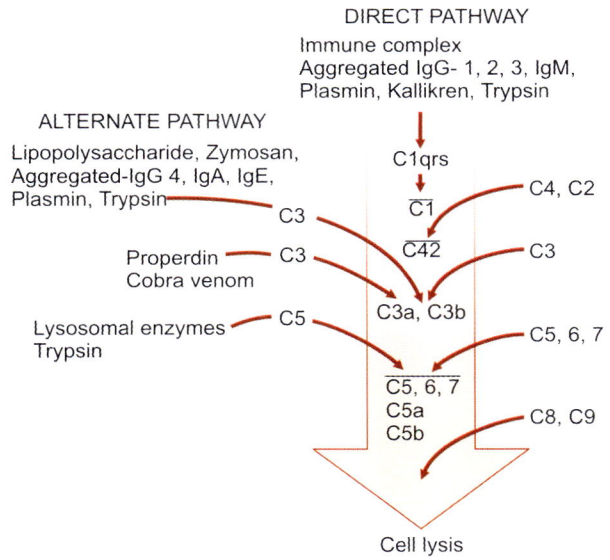

DIRECT PATHWAY
Immune complex
Aggregated IgG- 1, 2, 3, IgM,
Plasmin, Kallikren, Trypsin

ALTERNATE PATHWAY
Lipopolysaccharide, Zymosan,
Aggregated-IgG 4, IgA, IgE,
Plasmin, Trypsin

Properdin
Cobra venom

Lysosomal enzymes
Trypsin

Cell lysis

Fig. 11.6: Complement cascade showing direct and alternate pathways

component of complement (C3) without triggering the beginning of the cascade starting with C1. The alternative pathway begins with the cleavage of C3 after the conversion of C3 proactivator. The sequence after C3 activation is identical to that of the classical pathway: C5, C6, C7, C8, and C9.

Bacterial antigens such as endotoxins and polysaccharides such as dextran are also activators of the alternative pathway. Dental plaque and pure cultures of bacteria can also activate complement by the alternative pathway in the absence of antibody. On activation of complement by endotoxin, biologically active fragmentation products are released.

Complement mediates immunological membrane damage and amplifies the inflammatory responses.

The biologic effects of complement system are:

- Chemotaxis   - C3a, C5a and C5b67
- Kinin production   - C2a
- Opsonization   - C3b
- Cell lysis   - C6, C7, C8 and C9
- Activation of B lymphocytes - C3b
- Enhancement of blood clotting - C6
- Increased vascular permeability - C3a, C5a
- Promotion of clot lysis   - C3, C4

CYTOKINES

The term "cytokine" is derived from the Greek words kytos meaning cell, and kinesis, meaning movement. Cytokines are low molecular weight polypeptides of (5–70 kDa). They function as soluble mediators produced by cells, to regulate or modify the activity of other cells.

IL- 1 is found in two active forms, IL-lα and IL-1β encoded by separate genes. Both are potent proinflammatory molecules and are the main constituents of what was once called "osteoclast activating factor". IL-1 is produced primarily by activated macrophages or lymphocytes but also may be released by other cells, including mast cells, fibroblasts, keratinocytes and endothelial cells. Bacterial lipopolysaccharide is a potent activator of macrophage IL-1 production, whereas TNF-α and IL-1 itself also can activate macrophage IL-1 production. IL-1 is a potent stimulant of osteoclast proliferation, differentiation and activation.

Tumor necrosis factor-α is a multipotential cytokine, produced mainly by macrophages, with a wide variety of biological effects similar to interleukin-1. IL-1 and TNF-α are found in significant concentrations in GCF from periodontally diseased sites, and reductions in IL-1 concentration are associated with successful treatment.

Interleukin-6 is produced by macrophages, fibroblasts, lymphocytes and endothelial cells. Production is induced by interleukin-1 and lipopolysaccharide and suppressed by estrogen and progesterone. Interleukin- 6 causes fusion of monocytes to form multinuclear cells that resorb bone.

Interleukin-10 plays a major role in suppressing immune and inflammatory responses. It is produced by T cells, including human Th0, Th1 and Th2 cells, B cells,

Actions of various cytokines	
Actions	Cytokines
Pro-inflammatory	IL-1, IL-6, IL-8, TNF-α, IFN-γ
Anti-inflammatory	IL-4, IL-10, IL-13, TGF-β
Scarring	IL-6, TGF-β
Anti-Scarring	IL-10
Angiogenic	IL-8, Angiogenins, VEGF
Anti-angiogenic	IL-10

Inflammatory actions of various chemical mediators

Actions	Mediators
Vasoconstriction	Thromboxane A_2, Leukotrienes C_4, D_4, E_4
Vasodilatation	PGI_2, PGE_1, PGE_2, PGD_2, Bradykinin
Increased permeability	Leukotrienes, Histamine, SRS – A, Bradykinin
Chemotaxis	Leukotriene B4, HETE, Lipoxin,
Leukocyte adhesion	Bradykinin
Collagenase activity	$\alpha2$ – macroglobin

monocytes and macrophages after activation. Interleukin-10 inhibits the antigen-presenting capacity of macrophages by downregulating class II major histocompatibility complex expression.

SPECIFIC ACQUIRED IMMUNITY

The component of second line of defense are:
- T lymphocytes
- B lymphocytes
- Plasma cells
- Immunoglobulins

Lymphocytes: Three main types of lymphocytes are distinguished on the basis of their receptors for antigens and they are- T lymphocytes, B lymphocytes and Natural killer cells.

T lymphocytes are derived from the thymus and play a role in cell-mediated immunity. T lymphocytes recognize diverse antigens using a low affinity transmembrane complex called as T cell antigen receptor (TCR). These are of three types: T helper cells (T_H cell), Cytotoxic T cells (T_C cell) and Memory cells.

B lymphocytes which are derived from liver, spleen and bone marrow, are the precursor for plasma cells, and play a role in humoral immunity. B lymphocytes recognize diverse antigens using a high affinity transmembrane complex called as B cell antigen receptor (BCR). Upon contact with antigens and activation via T_H cells, B lymphocytes differentiate into antibody – producing plasma cells.

Natural killer cells recognize and kill certain tumor and virus infected cells. The natural killer cells possesss several classes of antigen receptors including killer inhibitory receptors and killer activating receptors.

Plasma cells are the terminal cells in the progression from B cells. Plasma cells occur in germinal centers and in tissues, where they produce immunoglobulins and antibodies, the effector cells for systemic and local immunity, respectively.

Immunoglobulins: Human immunoglobulins are divided into five classes on the basis of structural differences. The five classes are IgG, IgM, IgA, IgE and IgD. Immunoglobulin molecules are composed of either two κ or two λ light (small) chains and one of five types of heavy (large) polypeptide chains. The class is determined by the type of heavy chain. The basic immunologic structure appears to be Y shaped. The tail of Y contains the ends of two heavy chains and is referred to as Fc fragment. It is in this region where complement binding takes place. The remaining area of the Y shaped

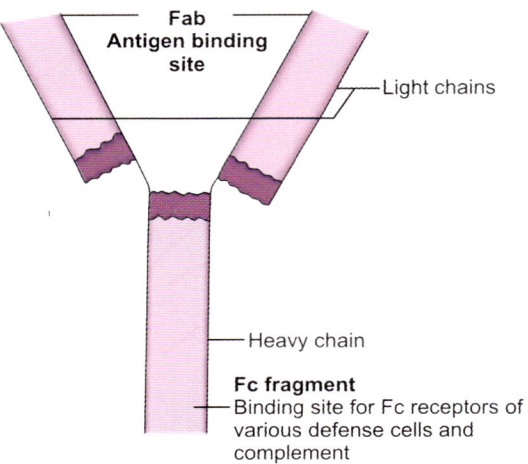

Fig. 11.7: Immunoglobulin Molecule - Y shaped glycoprotein with heavy and light chains

molecule is composed of the light chains and the remainder of the heavy chains. This is the Fab or antigen binding site **(Fig. 11.7)**.

Properties of secretory IgA antibodies make them unique and influence their function on mucosal surfaces. Secretory IgA is more resistant to digestion by proteolytic enzymes than are other immunoglobulins. It has been suggested that the secretory component of a polypeptide chain attached to the Fc portion of secretory IgA stabilizes this portion of the molecule, facilitating its transport across the glandular epithelium. It is also possible that the J chain, the fourth type of polypeptide chain associated with secretory IgA may function in making secretory IgA more resistant to proteolysis.

Functions of immunoglobulins are:

Opsonization of microorganisms
Complement activation
Antigen binding: Antigen antibody complex
Toxin neutralization
Neutralization of viruses
Hypersensitivity reactions (Type I- III)

INTERACTION BETWEEN NONSPECIFIC AND SPECIFIC IMMUNITY

Interaction between nonspecific and specific immunity is well explained in **Figure 11.8**.

IMMUNE MECHANISMS

Immune mechanisms are usually protective responses by the host to the presence of foreign substances such as

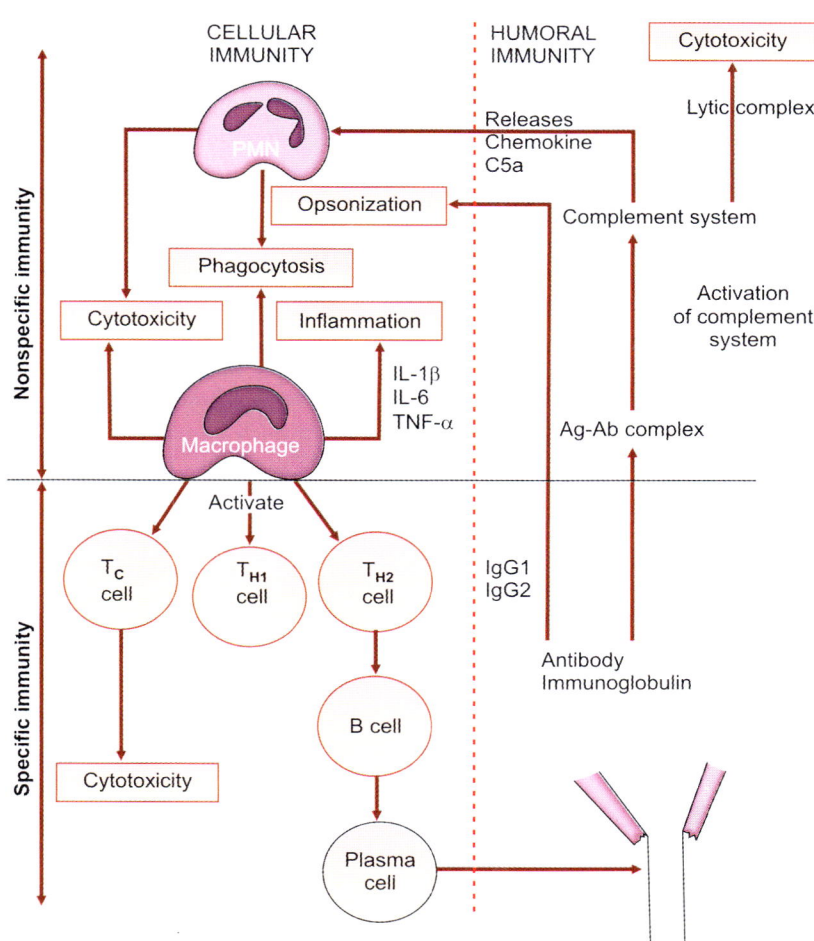

Fig. 11.8: Interaction between nonspecific and specific immunity

bacteria and viruses. They may at the same time cause local tissue destruction by triggering several types of overreaction or hypersensitivity. Tissue damage (immunopathologic changes) may occur in a sensitized host with subsequent exposure to the sensitizing antigen.

Four types of hypersensitivity reactions have been described: I, II, III, and IV. Types I, II and III reactions are humoral and are termed immediate reactions because they occur in minutes to hours. Type IV reactions are cellular or cell mediated and are termed delayed reactions because they occur within days.

Anaphylactic (Type I): IgE plays a direct role in its pathogenesis through its ability to sensitize the skin. This sensitizing capability is referred to as reaginic and the IgE antibody as reagin. IgG antibody combine with antigen in the circulation before it can bind to IgE in mast cells or basophils and prevents sensitization. These IgG antibodies are referred to as blocking antibodies.

IgE antibodies involved in anaphylactic reaction attach strongly at the Fc portion of the antibody to receptors found on mast cells and basophilic leukocytes primarily in connective tissues such as gingiva. This antibody – antigen reaction causes the release of pharmacologically active substances from the sensitized cells. These substances cause the response and have the potential to induce tissue damage in periodontal disease.

Cytotoxic Reactions (Type II): These reactions involve a combination of IgG (or rarely IgM) antibodies with the antigenic determinants on the surface of cells leading to cytotoxic/ cytolytic effects.

Immune Complex (Arthus) Reactions (Type III): When high levels of antigen to which the host has been sensitized are present and persist without being eliminated, antigen – antibody (IgG and IgM) complexes precipitate in and around small blood vessels and with subsequent complement activation, cause tissue damage at the site of local reaction. Inflammation, hemorrhage and necrosis may occur. Tissue damage appears to be due to the release of lysosomal enzymes from PMNs, mast cell activation, platelet agglutination, microthrombi formation and neutrophil chemotaxis. This reaction is referred to as an immune complex, or Arthus reaction and is usually mediated by IgM or IgG antibodies. These antibodies have the ability to fix complement, which is partially responsible for the chemotactic attraction of the PMNs crucial to the Arthus reaction.

Cell – Mediated Immunity or Delayed Hypersensitivity (Type IV): The phenomenon of delayed hypersensitivity belongs to the class of immune responses known as cell – mediated immunity. These reactions are referred to as type IV reactions. Cellular immunity does not involve circulating antibodies but is based on the interaction of antigens with the surface of T lymphocytes releasing lymphokines that cause biological effects on leukocytes, macrophages and tissue cell. There are actually two populations of lymphocytes. Lymphocytes that can develop into plasma cells that produce antibodies are designated as B cells. T and B lymphocytes have been shown to produce biologically active lymphokines.

POINTS TO PONDER

✓ Pan-receptor defect: It is the defect in which all chemotaxin receptors are decreased. It is seen in localized aggressive periodontitis which is characterized by a decrease in chemotactic responses to a variety of chemotactic factors, including C5a, FMLP (formyl peptide) and leukotriene B4.

✓ CD, i.e, cluster of differentiation system are the group of receptors which enable the cell to interact with each other molecules/cells.

BIBLIOGRAPHY

1. Ebersole JL. Immune responses in periodontal diseases. In, Wilson TG, Kornman KS. Fundamentals of Periodontics. Quintessence Publishing Co.1996; 109-58.
2. Eley BM, Manson JD. Host parasite interaction. In, Periodontics 5th ed Wright 2004; 29-38.
3. Genco RJ. Pathogenesis and host responses in periodontal diseases. In, Genco RJ, Goldman HM and Cohen DW. Contemporary Periodontics. CV Mosby Company 1990; 184-93.
4. Grant DA, Stern IB, Listgarten MA. Host response - Inflammation. In, Periodontics. 6th ed CV Mosby Company 1988; 252-65.
5. Grant DA, Stern IB, Listgarten MA. Immunology of periodontal diseases. In, Periodontics. 6th ed CV Mosby Company 1988; 266-92.
6. Haake SK, Nisengard RJ, Newman MG, Miyasaki KT. Microbial interactions with the host in periodontal diseases. In, Newman, Takei, Carranza. Clinical Periodontology 9th ed WB Saunders 2003; 132-52.
7. Kinane DF, Berglundh T, Lindhe J. Host parasite interactions in periodontal disease. In, Lindhe J, Karring T, Lang NP. Clinical Periodontology and Implant dentistry. 4th ed Blackwell Munksgaard 2003; 150-78.
8. Lamster IB. Inflammatory responses in periodontal diseases. In, Wilson TG, Kornman KS. Fundamentals of Periodontics. Quintessence Publishing Co.1996;159-68.
9. Miyasaki KT, Nisengard RJ, Haake SK. Immunity and inflammation, basic concepts. In, Newman, Takei, Carranza. Clinical Periodontology 9th ed WB Saunders 2003;113-31.
10. Nisengard RC, Michael GN, Sanz M. Host Response: Basic Concepts. In, Carranza, Newman. Clinical Periodontology. 8th ed WB Saunders 1996;111-120.

MCQs

1. Macrophages are:
   A. Modified monocytes
   B. Modified neutrophils
   C. Modified lysosomes
   D. None of the above

2. Microphages are:
   A. Neutrophils   B. Basophils
   C. Eosinophils   D. Monocytes

3. Following are the chemotaxins for neutrophil *except*:
   A. Platelet activating factor
   B. IL-1
   C. IL-6
   D. IL-8

4. Coating of microbes with host proteins facilitating phagocytosis:
   A. Chemotaxis   B. Opsonization
   C. Neutralization   D. None of the above

5. Integrin β_2 subunit (CD18) lacks in:
   A. Leukocyte adhesion deficiency II
   B. Leukocyte adhesion deficiency I
   C. Papillon-Lefevre syndrome
   D. Agranulocytosis

6. Osteoclast activating factor is:
   A. IL-1   B. IL-4
   C. IL-8   D. None of the above

7. Pan-receptor defect of neutrophil is found in:
   A. Refractory periodontitis
   B. NUG
   C. Adult periodontitis
   D. Localized juvenile periodontitis

8. Which of these immune cells forms antibodies:
   A. Macrophages   B. PMNs
   C. B lymphocytes   D. T lymphocytes

Answers

1. A	2. A	3. C	4. B	5. B
6. A	7. D	8. C		

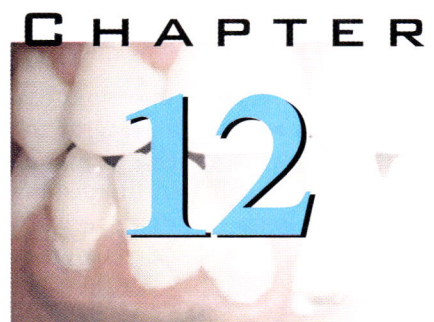

CHAPTER 12

Pathogenesis of Periodontal Diseases and Host Response

Shalu Bathla

INTRODUCTION

The interaction of the microorganisms with the host determines the course and extent of the periodontal diseases. Microorganisms may exert pathogenic effects directly by causing tissue destruction itself or indirectly by stimulating and modulating the host response. The host response is mediated by the microbial interaction and inherent characteristics of the host, including genetic factors that vary among individuals. The host response functions in a protective capacity, preventing the local infection from progressing to a systemic, life-threatening infection. Thus, pathogenesis of periodontal destruction involves a complex interplay between bacterial pathogens and the host tissues.

MICROBIOLOGY AND IMMUNOLOGY IN GINGIVAL HEALTH

The gingival crevice harbors bacteria in both health and disease. In a clinically healthy periodontium, the microbial flora is largely composed of gram-positive facultative microorganisms, predominately species such as *Actinomyces* and *Streptococcus* spp. Gram-negative species and spirochetal forms also may be found, but they are considerably less prevalent and occur in much smaller numbers. Serum antibodies to microorganisms are usually in low titers, suggesting the minimal systemic antigenic stimulation by plaque during gingival health. The gingival tissues typically demonstrate some evidence of inflammation. Tissues are usually infiltrated with chronic inflammatory cells, generally lymphocytes. Neutrophils are common within the junctional epithelium and in the gingival crevice. The infiltration of inflammatory cells is thought to be a response to bacterial plaque. Host defense mechanisms in a healthy individual are effective in managing the bacterial challenge. Physical mechanisms of host defense include the integrity of the epithelial cell layer, as well as the shedding of epithelial cells and the flow of crevicular fluid that may function to clear bacteria and their products from the subgingival environment. It is likely that the complement, neutrophils and antibody production contributes in controlling the sulcular microbiota.

STAGES IN THE PATHOGENESIS OF PERIODONTAL DISEASE

Following are the stages related to the pathogenesis of periodontal diseases:
1. Adhesion and colonization
2. Host tissue invasion
3. Bacterial evasion of host defense mechanisms
4. Host tissue destruction
5. Tissue healing

Adhesion and Colonization

The periodontal environment consists of two fluid systems, i.e. saliva and GCF, both of which are capable of flushing out the bacteria. Bacterial adhesion to a given substrate greatly enhances their ability to stay in the gingival sulcus and multiply. The presence of adhesion in perio-pathogens is a twofold affair in that bacteria can bind to host surfaces and also to other microorganisms. Thus, the surfaces available for attachment of microorganisms include the tooth, tissues, and pre-existing plaque mass.

- *Attachment of microorganisms to tooth surface*: Bacteria that initially colonize the periodontal environment most likely attach to the pellicle or saliva coated tooth surface. A relevant example is the adherence of *Actinomyces viscosus* through fimbriae on the bacterial surface to proline-rich proteins found on saliva coated tooth surfaces.
- *Attachment of microorganisms to tissues*: The adherence of bacteria to host tissues is likely to play a role in colonization and may be a critical step in the process of bacterial invasion. *P. gingivalis* attach through fimbriae to galactosyl residues of epithelial cells. *T. denticola* attach through surface protein to galactosyl or mannose residues of fibroblasts. *A. viscosus* and *A. naeslundii* attach through fimbriae to galactosyl residues of polymorphonuclear leukocytes.
- *Attachment of microorganisms to pre-existing plaque mass*: Bacterial attachment to pre-existing plaque is studied by examining the adherence between different bacterial strains (coaggregation). One of the best characterized interactions is the adherence of *A. viscosus* through surface fimbriae to a polysaccharide receptor of *Streptococcus sanguis*.

Host Tissue Invasion

The properties of a microorganism that enable it to cause disease are referred to as virulence factors. Thus, virulence properties can be broadly categorized into two groups: a) Factors that enable bacterial species to colonize and invade host tissues and b) Factors that enable bacterial species to directly or indirectly cause host tissue damage.

The bacteria or their products penetrate the connective tissue to a variable extent, even to the surface of the alveolar bone. Capability of microorganism to invade tissue has been proposed as a key factor in distinguishing pathogenic from nonpathogenic gram-negative species or strains. Tissue invasion makes it impossible to dislodge these bacteria by mechanical action.

The two means of tissue invasion are:
- Bacteria may enter host tissues through ulcerations in the epithelium of the gingival sulcus or pocket and have been observed in intercellular spaces of the gingival tissues.
- Another means of tissue invasion may involve the direct penetration of bacteria into host epithelial or connective tissue cells. *Aggregatibacter actinomycetemcomitans, P. gingivalis, F. nucleatum* and *Treponema denticola* have the ability to directly invade host tissue cells.

Examples of bacterial host tissue invasion in periodontal diseases are:
- Invasion of deep gingival connective tissue by viable *Aggregatibacter actinomycetemcomitans* in localized aggressive periodontitis.
- Bacteria, particularly spirochetes invade the tissue in NUG.

Thus, the antigens such as collagenase and toxins enter gingival tissues where they trigger host responses and cause direct tissue destruction.

Bacterial Evasion of Host Defense Mechanisms

Bacterial evasion helps the organisms to evade the host responses that attempt to eliminate them. Periodontal bacteria neutralize or evade host defenses via numerous other mechanisms. The periodontium as a whole is endowed with both innate and acquired immune mechanisms to provide defense capabilities against the invading microorganisms. Innate immunity is conferred by the epithelial barrier and the cells of the innate mechanisms, i.e. dendritic cells, neutrophils, monocytes and macrophages. Acquired immunity is provided by B and T lymphocytes.

Following are the examples of host defense mechanisms evaded by bacterial species and bacterial properties:
- *Specific antibodies*: Immunoglobulins facilitate phagocytosis of bacteria by opsonization or block

adherence by binding to the bacterial cell surface and restricting access to bacterial adhesins. The production of immunoglobulin-degrading proteases by specific microorganisms may counteract these host defenses.

- *Polymorphonuclear leukocytes*: Bacteria produce substances that suppress the activity of or kill polymorphonuclear leukocytes normally involved in host defenses. An example of this, is the production of two toxins (leukotoxin and cytolethal distending toxin) by *Aggregatibacter actinomycetemcomitans*, affecting leukocytes.
- *Lymphocytes*: *B. forsythus* and *F. nucleatum* have been shown to induce apoptosis, a form of cellular suicide, in lymphocytes.
- *Interleukin-8*: Interleukin-8 (IL-8) is a proinflammatory chemokine that provides a signal for the recruitment of neutrophils (PMNs) to a local site. *P. gingivalis* is able to inhibit the production of IL-8 by epithelial cells which provide the microorganism with an advantage in evading PMN mediated killing.

Host Tissue Destruction

A central feature of periodontitis is the remodeling of connective tissues that leads to a net loss of local soft tissues, bone and the periodontal attachment apparatus. The fundamental event in the transition from gingivitis to periodontitis is the loss of the soft tissue attachment to the tooth and the subsequent loss of alveolar bone.

The tissue destructive mechanisms can be classified as direct or indirect:

a. Direct mechanism
b. Indirect mechanism

Direct Mechanism

It results from the action of bacterial components that damage tissue directly. The bacterial metabolic by-products such as ammonia, volatile sulfur compounds, fatty acids, peptides and indole inhibit the growth or alter the metabolism of host tissue cells. Periodontal microorganisms also produce variety of enzymes which are capable of degrading essentially all host tissues and intercellular matrix molecules. *P. gingivalis* produces Collagenase, Trypsin-like enzyme, Keratinase, Neuraminidase and Fibronectin-degrading enzymes **(Fig. 12.1)**. Virulence factors of *Aggregatibacter actinomyce-temcomitans* are – Collagenase, Cytotoxin, Leukotoxin, Bacteriocin, Endotoxin, Fc binding protein, Invasins, Immunosuppresive factors, Adhesins, Chemotaxis inhibitor **(Fig. 12.2)**.

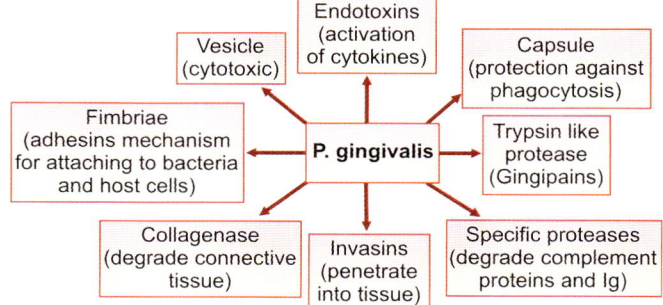

Fig. 12.1: Virulence factors of *P. gingivalis*

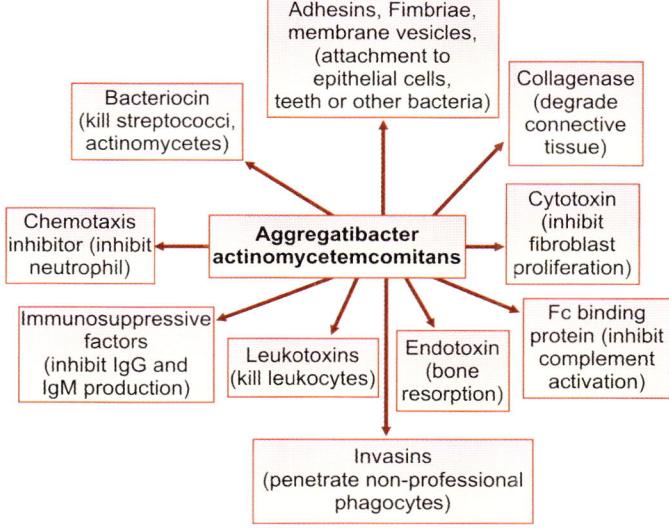

Fig. 12.2: Virulence factors of *Aggregatibacter actino-mycetemcomitans*

Indirect Mechanism

It is through the destructive host responses triggered by the infecting microorganisms. Well characterized interactions involve the release of interleukin-1 (IL-1), tumor necrosis factor (TNF), and prostaglandins from monocytes, macrophages and PMNs exposed to bacterial endotoxin (lipopolysaccharide). These host-derived mediators have the potential to stimulate bone resorption and activate or inhibit other host immune cells. Mediators produced as a part of the host response that contribute to tissue destruction include proteinases, prostaglandins and cytokines.

Proteinases

Proteinases or proteases cleave proteins by hydrolyzing peptide bonds and may be classified into two major classes, endopeptidases and exopeptidases, depending

PERIODONTICS REVISITED

on the location of activity of the enzyme on its substrate. Endopeptidases cleave bonds in their substrate within the polypeptide chain, whereas the exopeptidases cleave their substrate near the end of the polypeptide chain.

Matrix Metalloproteinases (MMPs)

These are considered to be primary proteinases involved in periodontal tissue destruction by degradation of extracellular matrix molecules. Matrix metalloproteinases (MMPs) are a family of homologous Zn^{+2} endopeptidases that collectively cleave most if, not all of the constituents of the extracellular matrix. There are about 28 MMPs:

Protease	MMP Number	Matrix substrate
Collagenase – 1	MMP – 1	Collagen
Collagenase – 2	MMP – 8	Collagen
Collagenase – 3	MMP – 13	Collagen
Collagenase – 4	MMP – 18	Collagen
Gelatinase – A	MMP – 2	Gelatin, Elastin
Gelatinase – B	MMP – 9	Gelatin, Elastin
Stromelysin – 1	MMP – 3	Laminin, Fibronectin, Non – triple helical region of Collagen types II and III
Stromelysin – 2	MMP – 10	
Stromelysin – 3	MMP – 11	Fibronectin
Matrilysin	MMP – 7 (Smallest)	Aggrecan, Laminin
Enamelysin	MMP – 20	Amelogenin

Structure of MMPs (Fig. 12.3)

Catalytic domain harbors the active site Zn^{+2} binding sequence. Catalytic domain is preceded by a propeptide that endows the enzyme with catalytic latency at the time of secretion and is followed by a protein rich hinge region that marks the transition to the largest domain. A plexin–like COOH terminal sequence is there which plays a role in determining substrate specificity. The two gelatinase, in addition, contain a gelatin binding insert (fibronectin type II like inserts) in the catalytic domain. Plexin – like

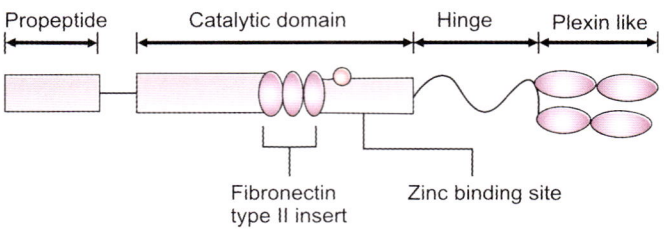

Fig. 12.3: Structure of MMPs

domain is absent from the smallest MMP, Matrilysin (mol. wt. 28,000).

Activations: MMPs are secreted in latent or inactive form. Enzyme activity in the tissues is partly controlled by activation of the latent enzyme and the level of enzyme inhibitors present. Proteases capable of activation MMPs include bacterial enzymes such as the chymotrypsin-like protease produced by *T. denticola*, as well as host cell enzymes such as neutrophil Cathepsin G.

The other activators are:
- Organomercurials, metal ions, thiol reagents and oxidants
- Plasmins, trypsin, tryptase, kallikrein.

Inhibitions: MMPs are inactivated by a-macroglobulins that are found in serum and gingival crevicular fluid.

The other inhibitors are:
- Tissue inhibitors of metalloproteinases – locally produced tissue inhibitors
- IGF, TNF - α, IL – 1, TGF - β, glucocorticoids, retinoic acid.

Prostaglandins

Prostaglandins are arachidonic acid metabolites generated by cyclooxygenases (COX-1, COX-2). Arachidonic acid is a 20-carbon polyunsaturated fatty acid found in the plasma membrane of most cells. The primary cells responsible for PGE_2 production in the periodontium are macrophages and fibroblasts. PGE_2 is increased in periodontal sites demonstrating inflammation and attachment loss. Induction of MMPs and osteoclastic bone resorption is induced by PGE_2. PGE_2 appears to be partly responsible for the bone loss associated with periodontitis.

Cytokines

These are explained in chapter no. 11 Immunity and Inflammation.

Tissue Healing

In the healing stage, resolution of inflammation and healing of the periodontal tissues occur. Periods of remission are characterized by reduction of inflammation, restoration of gingival tissues and often gingival fibrosis. Changes in the alveolar bony contours, with remodeling occur during remission suggesting that healing has occurred. The chronic immune system plays an important role in healing processes which consist of regeneration and repair.

Regeneration involves the replacement of tissues with new, identical tissues that function like the original tissues.

Repair involves replacement of one tissue with another tissue, such as fibrous connective tissue, which may not function like the tissue replaced. After traumatic or surgical injury, healing is initiated as part of the immediate and acute inflammatory responses. The periodontal "healing" cycle during the pathogenesis of periodontal disease is primarily postinflammatory; and cellular elements other than platelets provide important signals in this process. Periodontal repair occurs in overlapping phases of inflammation shutdown, angiogenesis and fibrogenesis.

In the postinflammatory healing process, the shutdown of inflammatory processes and initiation of postinflammatory healing is orchestrated by leukocytes. Some of the important anti-inflammatory signals generated by leukocytes include IL-1 receptor antagonist (IL-Ira) and transforming growth factor (TGF-β). In inflamed periodontal tissues, macrophages are a source of IL-1ra, whereas neutrophils, macrophages, and mast cells and lymphocytes produce TGF-β.

Cytokines such as IL-1β and TNF-β helps to induce angiogenesis and fibrogenesis in both inflammation and healing. PDGF activates fibroblasts and osteoblasts, resulting in the induction of protein synthesis. TGF-β is a multifunctional peptide that stimulates osteoblasts and fibroblasts and inhibits osteoclasts, epithelial cells, and most immune cells.

The immune system can induce regenerative bone healing by preventing osteoclast formation and activation and by activating osteoblasts.

IMMUNOLOGIC ASPECTS OF THE MICROBIAL INTERACTION WITH THE HOST

Periodontal disease is dependent on bacteria, as discussed earlier and bacteria may directly interact with the host tissues in mediating tissue destruction. In addition, many tissue changes associated with periodontal diseases appear to be well-orchestrated responses, suggesting the influence of host regulation. Among the orchestrated responses are the antimicrobial activities by acute inflammatory cells (neutrophils) and the adaptive activities brought about by monocytes/macrophages and lymphocytes. Adaptive responses include the epithelial alterations, angiogenesis, episodic remodeling of the underlying hard and soft connective tissues, and antigen-specific immune responses. Remodeling of the connective tissues appears to be episodic and occurs in cycles of destruction and reconstruction. Excessive destruction or inadequate reconstruction can result in periodontal disease.

Periodontal disease represents a well-regulated response to bacterial infection directed by the inflammatory cells of the host immune system in the following manner:

1. Innate factors such as complement, resident leukocytes, and mast cells play an important role in signaling endothelium, thus initiating inflammation. Complement activation in response to bacterial infection results in generation of the complement-derived anaphylatoxins C3a and C5a. Anaphylatoxins are substances that stimulate vascular changes indirectly by causing degranulation of the resident leukocytes and mast cells. Degranulated mast cells increases within the gingival connective tissue as gingival inflammation increases. Mast cells constitutively transcribe TNF-α, TGF-β, IL-4 and IL-6; when stimulated, they induce transcription of proinflammatory cytokines such as IL-1, IL-6, IFN-α, and others. The stimulation of endothelial cells by C5a, IL-1β, TNF-α, and bacterial lipopolysaccharides result in the expression of selectins on the lumenal surface of the endothelial cells and release of chemokines from the endothelial cells. These processes are central in transendothelial migration of leukocytes, which result in the movement of leukocytes into the local tissues.

2. Acute inflammatory cells (i.e. neutrophils) protect local tissues by controlling the periodontal microbiota within the gingival crevice and junctional epithelium. Neutrophils function to contain the microbial challenge through phagocytosis and killing and may contribute to local tissue changes by the release of tissue degrading enzymes.

3. Chronic inflammatory cells, macrophages, and lymphocytes protect the entire host from within the subjacent connective tissues and do all that is necessary to prevent a local infection from becoming systemic and life threatening. These cells orchestrate connective tissue changes associated with both periodontal infection and periodontal repair and healing. They also function to assist the neutrophils in controlling bacterial infection by forming specific opsonic antibodies. The host response in the connective tissues may result in local destruction of the tissue,

PERIODONTICS REVISITED

which is evident as periodontal disease. In recent years, the potential systemic impact of periodontal disease has been increasingly recognized. However, the end result of the periodontal host response is largely successful for the host in preventing progressive spread of the infection despite local tissue destruction.

CONCEPTS OF PATHOGENESIS OF PERIODONTAL DISEASE

I. *Early concept*: In the mid 1960, concept of pathogenesis was that microorganisms cause periodontal disease. The model in **Figure 12.4** implicated bacterial plaque deposits as the primary, direct factor in the development of periodontitis.

II. *1980s model*: The 1980 model emphasized a central role of host immunoinflammatory response in the clinical development and progression of periodontal disease **(Fig. 12.5)**. Specific bacteria initiated the disease process by activating host responses, which were protective and destructive. The actual destruction of connective tissue and bone resulted primarily from activated tissue mechansims such as MMPs, IL-1 and prostaglandins.

III. *1997 model*: The primary conceptual change was that the role of a number of environmental and acquired risk factors, as modifiers of the immune inflammatory response and in resulting connective tissue and bone metabolism was acknowledged. The 1997 model was non-linear and model implied that there was a range of host responses and a range of clinical expressions of disease that were primarily determined by genetic and environmental factors that modified the host response **(Fig. 12.6)**.

POINTS TO PONDER

✓ Systemic diseases associated with neutrophil disorders and periodontal diseases are diabetes mellitus, Papillon-Lefevre syndrome, Down syndrome, Chediak-Higashi syndrome, drug induced agranulocytosis, cyclic neutropenia and leukocyte adhesion deficiency.

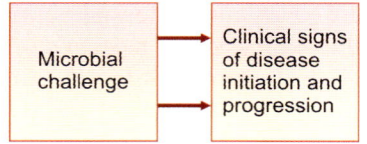

Fig. 12.4: Early Concept - Early linear model depicting the principal etiologic role of bacteria

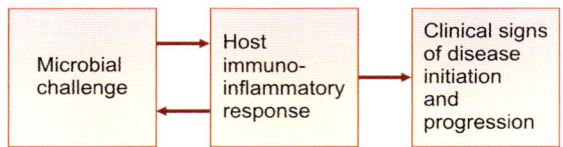

Fig 12.5: 1980's model emphasizing a central role of host immuno-inflammatory response

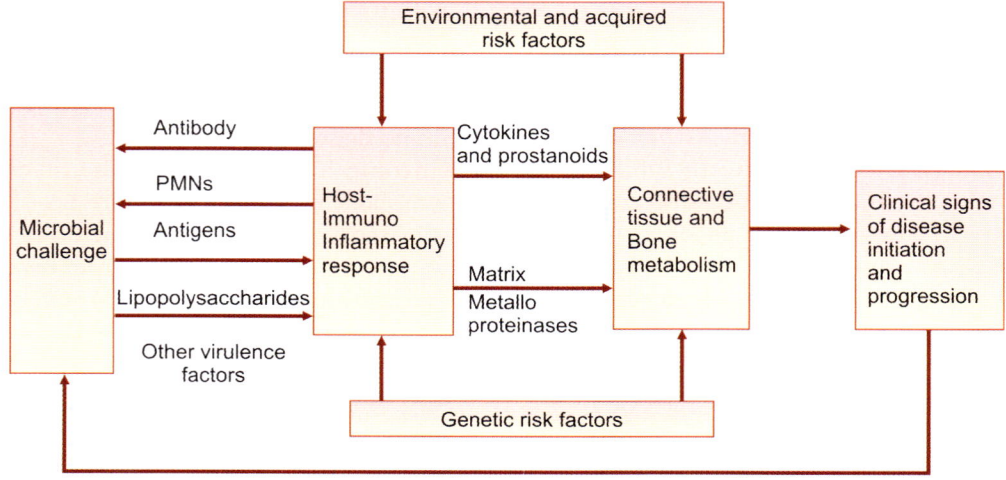

Fig. 12.6: 1997 model demonstrating various factors contributing to the pathogenesis of periodontal disease

✓ Periodontal diseases with neutrophil disorders are NUG, localized aggressive periodontitis and refractory periodontitis.

✓ Chemokine paralysis: *P. gingivalis* impedes transepithelial migration of neutrophils and prevents epithelial cells from secreting IL-8 in response to bacterial challenge. This property may contribute to the virulence of *P. gingivalis* by interfering with the host immune response.

BIBLIOGRAPHY

1. Ebersole JL. Immune responses in periodontal diseases. In, Wilson TG, Kornman KS. Fundamentals of Periodontics. Quintessence Publishing Co.1996;109-58.
2. Eley BM, Manson JD. Host parasite interaction In, Periodontics. 5th ed Wright 2004;29-38.
3. Genco RJ. Pathogenesis and host responses in periodontal diseases. In, Genco RJ, Goldman HM, Cohen DW. Contemporary Periodontics. CV Mosby Company 1990;184-93.
4. Grant DA, Stern IB, Listgarten MA. Host response-Inflammation. In, Periodontics. 6th ed CV Mosby Company 1988;252-65.
5. Grant DA, Stern IB, Listgarten MA. Immunology of periodontal diseases. In, Periodontics. 6th ed CV Mosby Company 1988;266-92.
6. Haake SK, Nisengard RJ, Newman MG, Miyasaki KT. Microbial interactions with the host in periodontal diseases. In, Newman, Takei, Carranza. Clinical Periodontology 9th ed WB Saunders 2003;132-52.
7. Informational paper. The Pathogenesis of Periodontal diseases. J Periodontol 1999;70: 457-70.
8. Kinane DF, Berglundh T, Lindhe J. Host parasite interactions in periodontal disease. In, Lindhe J, Karring T, Lang NP. Clinical Periodontology and Implant dentistry. 4th ed Blackwell Munksgaard 2003;150-78.
9. Kornman KS. Mapping the Pathogenesis of periodontitis: A New Look. J Periodontol 2008;79:1560-68.
10. Lamster IB. Inflammatory responses in periodontal diseases. In, Wilson TG, Kornman KS. Fundamentals of Periodontics. Quintessence Publishing Co.1996; 159-68.
11. Miyasaki KT, Nisengard RJ, Haake SK. Immunity and inflammation, basic concepts. In, Newman, Takei, Carranza. Clinical Periodontology 9th ed WB Saunders 2003;113-31.

MCQs

1. Microorganisms having the ability to directly invade host tissue cells:
    A. *Aggregatibacter actinomycetemcomitans*
    B. *P. gingivalis*
    C. *F. nucleatum*
    D. *Treponema denticola*
    E. All of the above

2. *P. gingivalis* has the ability to inhibit the production of:
    A. IL-1 by epithelial cells
    B. IL-8 by epithelial cells
    C. IL-6 by epithelial cells
    D. None of the above

3. The smallest Matrix metalloproteinases (MMPs) is:
    A. Matrilysin (MMP – 7)
    B. Gelatinase – B (MMP – 9)
    C. Enamelysin (MMP – 20)
    D. Stromelysin – 1 (MMP – 3)

4. The sequence of stages related to the pathogenesis of periodontal diseases are:
    1. Adhesion and colonization
    2. Host tissue invasion
    3. Bacterial evasion of host defense mechanisms
    4. Host tissue destruction
    5. Tissue healing
    A. 1, 2, 3, 4, 5
    B. 1, 3, 2, 4, 5
    C. 1, 4, 3, 5, 2
    D. 3, 1, 2, 4, 5

Answers

1. E   2. B   3. A   4. A

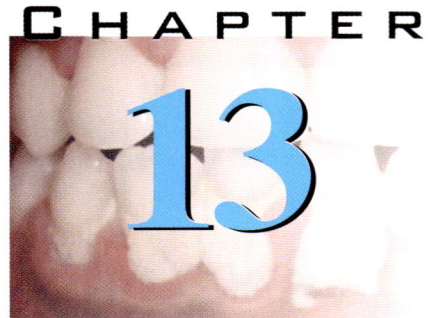

CHAPTER 13

Genetic Basis of Periodontal Diseases

Veenu Madaan Hans, Mayank Hans

INTRODUCTION

Periodontal disease is initiated by plaque which induces an inflammatory response. This inflammation in certain susceptible individuals progress to chronic destructive inflammatory condition termed periodontitis. While microbial and environmental factors are believed to initiate and modulate periodontal disease progression, there is supporting evidence that genes play a role in predisposition and progression of periodontal diseases. Understanding of genetic basis of periodontal disease may have diagnostic and therapeutic value.

GENETIC VARIANCE

Genes can exist in different forms or status. Genetics refers to different forms of gene as allelic variants or alleles. Allelic variants of gene differ in their nucleotide sequence. When specific allele occurs in at least 1% of population, it is said to be genetic polymorphism. When nucleotide changes are very rare and not present in many individuals, it is often called mutation. In contrast to mutation, genetic polymorphism is considered normal variation. When a nucleotide change in codon does not alter the amino acids it is said to be silent. Many single nucleotide polymorphisms that occur in genes do not appear to change the protein products of gene, but many do have an effect on gene product.

GENETIC BASIS OF DISEASE

Genetic variance and environmental exposure are key determinants to phenotypic differences between individuals. Most human diseases have a genetic component to their etiology. However, the extent of this genetic contribution to disease can vary greatly for different diseases.

Genetic diseases can be divided into two main groups: simple Mendelian and complex genetic diseases. Distinction between these groups is based on pattern of transmission.

$$\boxed{\text{Phenotype}} = \boxed{\text{Environment}} + \boxed{\text{Genotype}} + \boxed{\text{Genotype} \times \text{Environment}}$$

Simple Mendelian Diseases

Diseases that follow predictable and generally simple patterns of transmission are called Mendelian conditions. They follow Mendelian mode of inheritance; autosomal dominant, autosomal recessive or X-linked. Prevalence of these conditions are rare (0.1%). Example includes amelogenesis imperfecta, Crouzon syndrome, etc.

Complex Genetic Diseases

These diseases are much more prevalent, usually occurring with a frequency greater than 1% of the population. Complex diseases do not typically follow a simple pattern of familial distribution or transmission. The presence of one disease associated allele is not sufficient to cause disease. There is no one-to-one correlation of presence of a specific genetic allele and occurrence of disease. The alleles reported to be associated with a disease are also found in unaffected individuals and some individuals with disease who do not have the allele. Thus, presence of disease associated allele is not diagnostic for a disease.

METHODS OF GENETIC ANALYSIS

1. *Familial aggregation*: Familial aggregation of a trait can suggest a genetic etiology. However, families also share many aspects of common environment, including diet and nutrition, exposures to pollutants and behavior such as smoking. Certain infectious agents also cluster in the families. Thus, familial aggregation may result from shared genes, environmental exposures and similar socioeconomic influences. To determine the evidence for genetic factors in familial aggregation of a trait, more formal genetic studies are required. Many clinical reports suggest familial aggregation of aggressive periodon-titis.
2. *Twin study*: Through the phenomena of twins, in particular monozygotic twins (MZ) arising from one fertilized egg, nature has provided a wonderful tool for examination of genetic influences in disease and to assess how much this is influenced by environment. Difference in disease experience between monozygotic twins must be due to environmental factors and between dizygotic twins they could arise from both environmental and genetic differences.
3. *Segregation analysis*: Genes are passed from parents to children in a predictable manner and genes segregate in families as predicted by Mendel's law. To study the pattern of trait transmission in families, a method called segregation analysis can be used. By sequentially comparing models with each other, segregation analysis identifies the model that best accounts for observed transmission of trait in given population. It is usually applied to determine if the transmission appears to fit a Mendelian or other mode of genetic transmission. When genetic models of transmission are compared genetic characteristics including mode of transmission, penetrance, frequency of disease and non-disease alleles are included in different models and evaluated. Segregation analysis does not necessarily provide the true model. If important assumptions of model tested are incorrect, this will limit the results. Limitation of segregation analysis must be realized since, it has resulted in inaccurate conclusions for transmission of at least one form of early onset periodontitis. This approach is more appropriately applied to datasets from many families to determine best fitting model. It does not aim to find a specific gene responsible for trait.
4. *Linkage analysis*: It is a technique to localize the gene for a trait to a specific chromosomal location. These studies are based on the fact that genes located in proximity tend to be passed together from generation to generation as a unit. Such genes are said to be linked and violate Mendel's Law of independent assortment. Genetics can apply quantitative analysis to detect the lack of independent assortment of genetic loci and it can be used to map genes to specific chromosome locations. A specific trait is followed as it segregates through family of interest and determined if trait appears to segregate with known genetic polymorphism that has been localized to specific chromosomal location. In this way, it can be determined if a trait appears to segregate in manner consistent with linkage to known genetic marker. Linkage can therefore, prove genetic basis of disease.
5. *Association studies*: Two types of association analysis are commonly used in genetic studies; population based and family based. Population based approach utilizes a standard case control design, in which marker allele frequency is compared between cases and controls. Currently considerable attention is being directed towards the clinical use of disease associated genetic polymorphism for genetic testing. When a positive association is found, several interpretations are possible:
   • Associated allele itself is a disease predisposing allele.

PERIODONTICS REVISITED

- Associated allele is in linkage disequilibrium with actual disease predisposing locus.
- Association is due to population stratification.
- Association is a sampling or statistical artifact.

REQUIREMENTS FOR PROVING A DISEASE AND POLYMORPHISM ASSOCIATION

1. Polymorphism must influence gene product.
2. Biases in study population should be recognized and controlled.
3. Confounders such as smoking should be controlled.
4. Affected gene product should be a part of the disease etiopathology.

GENETIC POLYMORPHISM STUDIES IN PERIODONTITIS

1. *Syndromic form of periodontitis*: Severe periodontitis presents as a part of the clinical monogenetic syndromes as well as gene mutation and biochemical defects are known for many of these conditions. Common point in these conditions is that they are inherited as simple Mendelian traits and are usually due to alteration in single gene locus.
   a. Neutrophil functional disorder
      - *Leukocyte adhesion deficiency (LAD) syndrome*: Generalized form of aggressive periodontitis is an oral manifestation of LAD. It exists in two forms LAD I and LAD II; both of which are autosomal recessive traits.
      - *Chediak higashi syndrome*: In this syndrome the functional capacity of the neutrophils; that is the chemotactic and bactericidal functions are abnormal. This is transmitted as an autosomal recessive trait.
   b. Deficiency in neutrophil number
      - *Infantile genetic agranulocytosis*: It is a rare autosomal recessive disease where neutrophil number is very low. This disease has been associated with aggressive periodontitis.
      - *Cohen syndrome*: This disease is characterized by mental retardation, obesity, dysmorphia and neutropenia. This autosomal recessive disorder shows more frequent and extensive alveolar bone loss.
   c. Genetic defects of structural components
      - *Papillon-Lefevre syndrome (PLS)*: It gives a clinical presentation of various degrees of periodontitis severity as well as great variation in level of abnormal keratosis. Both the primary dentition and secondary dentition are affected. PLS is caused by mutation in the Cathepsin C gene, located on chromosome 11. Cathepsin C is a cysteine protease and functions in protein degradation and activation of proenzymes in immune and inflammatory cells, thus causing severe periodontal bone loss in affected patients.
      - *Haim munk syndrome*: It is a slightly different clinical variant of PLS. Both of these are allelic variants of Cathepsin C gene mutations. This syndrome is also associated with aggressive periodontitis.
      - *Weary-Kindler syndrome*: Aggressive periodontitis has also been reported in this syndrome, where abnormalities in basement membrane occur.

2. *Interleukin-1 (IL-1) and Tumor necrosis factor-α (TNF-α) gene polymorphism*: The genes encoding for interleukin -1 and TNF-α appear to be good candidates for genetic studies for the following reasons:
   - IL-1α, IL-1β and TNF-α are potent immunological mediators with proinflammatory properties.
   - IL-1β and TNF-α have capacity to stimulate bone resorption and they can regulate fibroblast cell proliferation of both gingival and periodontal ligament origin.
   - Various studies suggest that polymorphism in genes of IL-1 cluster and TNF-α could predispose subjects to elevated levels of IL-1 and TNF-α protein levels.
   - Inherent inter-individual differences have been observed for IL-1 and TNF-α production by blood leukocytes isolated from individuals with or without periodontitis.
   Interleukin 1 gene polymorphism: The genes encoding for proteins IL-1α, IL-1β and IL1-RA are located in close proximity in IL-1 gene cluster on chromosome 2. Kornman et al in 1997 first reported polymorphism for IL-1 gene in relation to periodontitis. He evaluated gingival crevicular fluid samples at baseline and three weeks of treatment analyzed by ELISA for IL-1α. At baseline IL-1β in GCF was 2.5 times higher for patients carrying an R-allele at IL-1α -889 and IL-1β + 3954 (Interleukin composite genotype) than those not having composite genotype. After treatment, IL-1β levels in GCF were still 2.2

times higher for IL-1 composite genotype patients. Although other authors have found conflicting results with no significant correlation established between genotype and cytokine production.

For the global population, polymorphisms in the IL-1 gene cluster cannot be regarded as (putative) risk factors for periodontitis or severity of periodontal destruction. For Caucasian patients with chronic periodontitis the role of the IL-1 composite genotype seems to hold some promise; however, to date no clear evidence has emerged and there are currently too many conflicting and negative results.

TNF-α gene polymorphism: TNF-α gene is located on chromosome 6 within the major histocompatibility complex (MHC) gene cluster. Single nucleotide polymorphism (SNP) in gene encoding TNF-α has been studied in promoter regions -1031, -863, -367, -308, -238 and coding region +489. Among Japanese, SNPs at -1031 and -863 were found to be associated with chronic periodontitis. In another study, no association of TNF-α gene polymorphism was found with aggressive periodontitis. At present, very limited data support the association between any reported TNF-α gene variation and periodontitis.

3. *Fc gamma receptor (FcγR) gene polymorphism*: Leukocytes of both myeloid and lymphoid lineage express receptors (FcγR) for constant (Fc) region of IgG molecules. FcγR is likely to play a role in pathogenesis of periodontitis as a bridge between cellular and humoral branches of immune system. Microorganisms can be opsonized by antibodies and are phagocytosed via FcγR on neutrophils. When FcγR mediated leukocyte functions are compromised or exaggerated due to genetic polymorphism in FcγR genes, it is conceivable that susceptibility to and/or severity of periodontitis is affected. FcγR genes are found on chromosome 1 and encode three main receptor classes:

FcγR I (CD 64) - Ia, Ib
FcγR II (CD 32) - IIa, IIb, IIc
FcγR III (CD 16) - IIIa, IIIb

Among these, genetic polymorphism has been identified for FcγRIIa, IIb, IIIa and IIIb. Although many studies have been carried out to associate periodontitis with these polymorphism in many races but the results vary. A recent meta-analysis of these studies associated FcγRIIIb NA1/NA2 polymorphism with chronic as well as aggressive periodontitis. Also, there was a weak evidence for association between FcγRIIa H131R polymorphism and aggressive periodontitis in Asians. In the same meta-analysis, no association between FcγRIIIa F158V and periodontal disease was found.

4. *CD14 gene polymorphism*: R allele in promoter region of CD14 at position-260 (-159) enhances transcriptional activity of gene. Individuals homozygous for R allele have increased levels of soluble CD14 (sCD14) as well as increased density of CD14 in monocytes. Increased serum levels of sCD14 have been associated with periodontitis. Studies in Caucasians subjects on CD14-260 polymorphism, no association was found. In another study, polymorphism at -1359 (N/N genotypes) was found to be associated with severe periodontitis.

5. *TLR2 and TLR4 gene polymorphism*: Toll like receptor 2 exhibits polymorphism at position 677 with transition from arginine to threonine and at position 753 with transition from arginine to glycine. These polymorphisms abrogate the ability of TLR2 to mediate to a response to bacterial cell wall components. A similar polymorphism of TLR 4 at positions 299 and 399 with transition from asparagine to glycine and threonine to isoleucine respectively, affect extracellular domain of TLR 4 protein, leading to an attenuated efficacy of lipopolysaccharide signaling and a reduced capacity to elicit inflammation. Few studies have been done on association of polymorphism of these receptors with periodontitis, but despite the importance of these receptors, the relation with periodontitis has not been established.

6. *IL-10 gene polymorphism*: Gene encoding for interleukin -10 is located on chromosome 1. IL-10 is produced by monocytes and macrophages. It is an anti-inflammatory cytokine and plays a role in downregulation of proinflammatory cytokines such as IL-1 and TNF-α. While few studies found no association between IL-10 polymorphism and chronic as well as aggressive periodontitis, a later study, associated IL-10 1087 polymorphism with susceptibility to periodontitis.

PROBLEMS ASSOCIATED WITH GENETIC STUDIES

1. Exposures such as smoking or systemic disease modifiers have large influences on expression of phenotype, thus interfere with results.
2. There are methodological problems also associated with these studies, for example deciding the study design.
3. Bias against publishing negative results has tremendous impact on literature available on subject.

PERIODONTICS REVISITED

4. Many studies fail to report sensitivity and specificity of their tests and do they describe associated environmental aspects, thus results cannot be universally applied.
5. Number of cases and control may be insufficient to make pronouncement on association between polymorphism and disease.
6. Differences in precise account of racial and ethnic background of both cases and control will render influence of genes questionable.
7. It is not always sure whether the controls are truly not susceptible or they are not exposed to environmental factors required for phenotypic expression.
8. Allele may not always be active and may need environment or other gene to be active. This is the phenomenon of penetrance.

CLINICAL IMPLICATIONS OF GENETIC STUDIES

1. Genetic tests may be developed and prove useful for identifying patients who are most likely to develop disease or suffer from recurrent disease.
2. Genetic risk in an individual, if known can help clinician in environment based prevention and treatment to patient susceptible to periodontal disease.
3. The outcome of the treatment will become more predictable and the maintenance schedule can be varied according to the genetic risk factor of the patient.

It should be remembered that periodontitis has a complex etiology and all the risk factors contribute in the expression of disease. Thus identification of genetic risk factors does not mitigate the importance of recognizing other risk factors and controlling them.

POINTS TO PONDER

✓ PST® genetic susceptibility test is the first and only genetic test that analyze two interleukin-1 (IL-1) genes for variations that identify an individual's predisposition for overexpression of inflammation and risk for periodontal disease. This test employs user-friendly sample collection packets. Samples are collected using a soft brush inside the cheek which is then sent to the laboratory for testing. This sample is assessed for interleukin-1 composite genotype, the presence of which makes the test positive.

BIBLIOGRAPHY

1. Berglundh T, Donati M, Hahn-Zoric M, Hanson LA, Padyukov L. Association of the 1087 IL-10 gene polymorphism with severe chronic periodontitis in Swedish Caucasians. J Clin Periodontol 2003;30:249-54.
2. Kinane DF, Hart TC. Genes and gene polymorphisms Associated With Periodontal Disease. Crit Rev Oral Biol Med 2003;14(6):430-49.
3. Kobayashi T, Westerdaal NA, Miyazaki A, Van derPol WL, Suzuki T, Yoshie H, Van de Winkel JG, Hara, K. Relevance of immunoglobulin G Fc receptor polymorphism to recurrence of adult periodontitis in Japanese patients. Infection and Immunity 1997; 65:3556–60.
4. Kobayashi T, Yamamoto K, Sugita N, Van der Pol WL, Yasuda K, Kaneko S, Van de Winkel JG, Yoshie H. The Fc gamma receptor genotype as a severity factor for chronic periodontitis in Japanese patients. J Periodontol 2001;72:1324-31.
5. Kornman KS, Crane A, Wang HY, di Giovine FS, Newman MG, Pirk FW, Wilson TG Jr, Higginbottom FL, Duff GW. The interleukin-1 genotype as a severity factor in adult periodontal disease. J Clin Periodontol 1997;24:72-7.
6. Loos BG, John RP, Laine ML. Identification of genetic risk factors for periodontitis and possible mechanisms of action. J Clin Periodontol 2005;32 (Suppl 6):159-79.
7. Loos BG, Leppers-Van de Straat FG, Van de Winkel JG, Van der Velden U. Fc gamma receptor polymorphisms in relation to periodontitis. J Clin Periodontol 2003; 30: 595-602.
8. Loos GB, Van der Velden U. Genetics in Relation to Periodontitis In, Lindhe J, Karring T, Lang NP. Clinical Periodontology and Implant dentistry. 4th ed Blackwell Munksgaard 2003;387-403.
9. Michalowicz BS, Pihlstrom. Genetic factors associated with periodontal disease. In, Newman, Takei, Carranza. Clinical Periodontology 9th ed WB Saunders 2003;168-81.

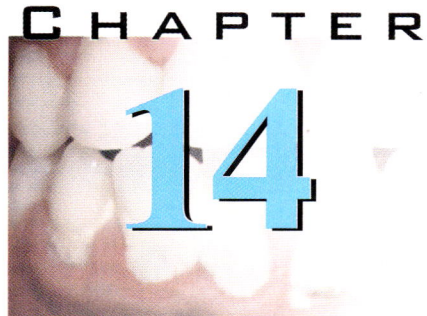

CHAPTER 14

Effect of Systemic Factors Over the Periodontium

Shalu Bathla

INTRODUCTION

The periodontium in health and disease can be affected by an intricate combination of systemic factors such as debilitated systemic diseases, stress, medications or malnutrition. These systemic factors may modify the neuroendocrine- immunologic mechanisms that compose host defenses and thus, are called as systemic modifiers.

HORMONAL FACTORS

Hormonal disturbances may affect the periodontal tissues directly by modifying the tissue response to plaque in gingival and periodontal disease; also by producing anatomic changes in the oral cavity that may favor plaque accumulation.

Diabetes Mellitus

Diabetes Mellitus is a complex metabolic disease characterized by chronic hyperglycemia. Periodontal disease in diabetics follows no consistent or distinct pattern. Very severe gingival inflammation, deep periodontal pockets, rapid bone loss and frequent periodontal abscesses often occur in diabetic patients with poor oral hygiene **(Fig. 14.1)**. Diabetes does not cause gingivitis or periodontal pockets, but there are indications, that it alters the response of the periodontal tissues to local factors, hastening bone loss and

Periodontal findings in diabetes mellitus
Tendency towards enlarged gingiva,
Sessile or pedunculated gingival polyps
Frequent periodontal abscesses.

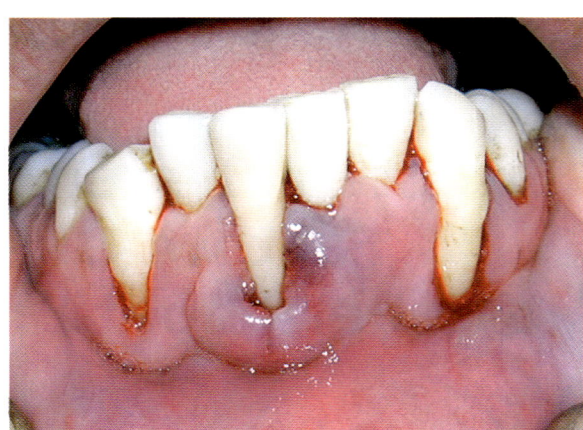

Fig. 14.1: Diabetic patient—Gingival inflammation, periodontal pockets, attachment loss and periodontal abscesses

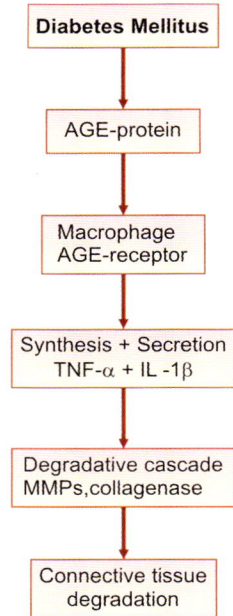

Fig. 14.2: AGE mediated tissue destruction in Diabetes Mellitus. TNF-α—Tumor necrosis factor α; AGE—Advanced glycation end products; IL-1β—Interleukin- 1β

retarding postsurgical healing of the periodontal tissues.

1. *Effects on microbiota*: In uncontrolled diabetic patients, there is increased percentage of spirochetes, motile rods and decreased levels of cocci in periodontal lesions. Patients with type I diabetes with periodontitis have been reported to have a subgingival flora composed mainly of *Capnocytophaga*, anaerobic vibrios, Actinomyces species, *Porphyromonas gingivalis*, *Prevotella intermedia* and *Aggregatibacter actinomycetemcomitans*. Glucose mediated advanced glycation end (AGE) product accumulation affects the migration and phagocytic activity of mononuclear and polymor-phonuclear phagocyte cells resulting in the establishment of more pathogenic subgingival flora.

2. *Effects on the host response*:
   a. Polymorphonuclear leukocytes (PMNs): The increased susceptibility of diabetics to infection has been hypothesized as being due to polymorphonuclear leukocyte deficiencies resulting in impaired chemotaxis, defective phagocytosis and impaired adherence. Advanced glycation end-products also enhance the nicotinamide adenine dinucleotide phosphate (NADPH) oxidases (which are active in the phagosome during phagocytosis) and the respiratory burst of neutrophils. Neutrophils are particularly important in periodontal pathogenesis on the account of extracellular release of their lysosomal contents, which contributes significantly to local tissue damage. Arachidonic acid is a mediator of the AGE-augmented neutrophil respiratory burst, through which neutrophil NADPH is up-regulated, increasing the local production of reactive oxygen species.

   b. Cytokines, monocytes and macrophages: There is hyperglycemia mediated formation of non-enzymatic advanced glycation end products (AGEs) in diabetic patient. AGEs are chemically irreversible, glucose-derived compounds that form slowly and continuously as a function of blood glucose concentration. Macrophages have high affinity receptors for AGE - modified proteins. Binding of the AGE modified protein to the macrophage receptor (RAGE) initiates a cycle of cytokine upregulation, with synthesis of IL - 1 and TNF-α. The synthesis and secretion of these cytokines are increased triggering degradative cascade, resulting in connective tissue degradation **(Fig. 14.2)**.

   c. Altered collagen metabolism: Increased collagenase activity and decreased collagen synthesis is found in diabetic patient. AGE forms cross-linking collagen, making it less soluble and less likely to be normally repaired or replaced. As a result, collagen in the tissues of poorly controlled diabetics is aged and more susceptible to breakdown. Cellular migration through cross-linked collagen is impeded and perhaps more importantly, tissue integrity is impaired as a result of damaged collagen remaining in the tissues for longer periods.

   d. Altered bone metabolism: Diabetes-induced changes in bone metabolism-
- Inhibition of collagen matrix formation
- Alterations in protein synthesis
- Increased time for mineralization of osteoid
- Reduced bone turnover
- Decreased number of osteoblasts
- Reduction in osteocalcin production

Adrenal Insufficiency/Corticosteroid Hormones

The systemic administration of cortisone in experimental animals results in osteoporosis of alveolar bone, capillary dilation with hemorrhage in the periodontal ligament and gingival connective tissue, degeneration and reduction in the number of collagen fibers of the periodontal ligament. The clinical finding of primary adrenal failure is hyperpigmentation of gingiva which may appear as irregular spots that vary in color, ranging from pale brown to black.

    People with primary adrenal insufficiency have no adrenal reserve and thus, have absolutely no means of increasing circulating cortisol levels for stressful situations other than by increasing exogenous steroid dosages. Before treating patients with a history of recent or current steroid use, physician consultation is indicated to determine whether the patient's dental needs and proposed treatment requires supplemental steroids.

Pituitary Gland

In adults, hyperpituitarism results in acromegaly that is characterized by a disproportionate overgrowth of the facial bone and over developed sinuses. The face is large and the lips are greatly enlarged. A marked over growth of the alveolar process causes an increase in the size of the dental arch and consequently affects the spacing of the teeth. This may affect the periodontium by causing food impaction. Hypercementosis is another feature associated with hyperpituitarism.

    Hypopituitarism results in decreased skeletal growth and leads to crowding and malposition of teeth. The periodontal tissues of experimental animals with artificially induced hypopituitarism show increased gingival inflammation, resorption of cementum in the molar furcation areas, reduced apposition of cementum,

decreased osteogenesis in interdental areas, reduced vascularity of the periodontal ligament and cystic degeneration of the ligament and calcification of many of the epithelial rests.

Thyroid Gland

The thyroid gland secretes three hormones: (i) Thyroxine; (ii) Triiodothyronine; and (iii) Calcitonin. Of these three the bulk is made up of thyroxine. In the peripheral tissues, thyroxine is converted into its more active form, triiodothyronine. In animals with thiouracil-induced hypothyroidism, apposition of alveolar bone is retarded and the size of the haversian system is reduced but there is no evidence of periodontal disease. Myxedema develops hyperparakeratosis of gingival epithelium, edema and disorganization of the collagen bundles in the connective tissues, hydropic degeneration and fragmentation of the fibers of periodontal ligament and osteoporosis of the alveolar bone.

Parathyroid Glands

Hyperparathyroidism produces generalized demineralization of the skeleton, increased osteoclasis with proliferation of the connective tissue in the enlarged marrow spaces and formation of bone cysts and giant cell tumors. The disease is called osteitis fibrosa cystica or 'Von Recklinghausen's bone disease'. There is alveolar osteoporosis with loosely meshed trabeculae and widened periodontal ligament space. Loss of the lamina dura and giant cell tumors in the jaws are late signs of hyperparathyroid bone disease, which in itself is uncommon.

Sex Hormones

Explained in chapter no 29. Sex hormones and Periodontium.

HEMATOLOGICAL DISORDERS

All blood cells play a key role in the maintenance of a healthy periodontium. Disorders of the blood or blood-forming organs can have a profound effect on the periodontium. Polymorphonuclear leukocytes, lymphocytes, macrophages and plasma cells are involved in peripheral immune and inflammatory reactions. These leukocytes are critical to the tissues responses and antigenic challenges from the subgingival plaque microbiota. Other nondefense related cells such as the red blood cells have crucial role in maintaining gas exchange and nutrient supply to the periodontium. Platelets are needed for efficient hemostasis of well perfused tissue which, when inflamed, is commonly hyperemic and hemorrhagic. Thus, the pivotal role of blood cells helps in the maintenance of a healthy periodontium. Systemic hematological disorders can have a profound effect on the periodontium. Hematological disorders can be broadly grouped into hemostatic disorders, red blood cell disorders and white blood cell disorders. The white blood cell or leukocyte disorders constitute the major proportion of hematological disorders affecting the periodontium. However, hemostatic and red blood cell disorders may also have a detrimental effect on the integrity of periodontium.

Leukemia

Leukemia is caused by proliferating white blood cell-forming tissues resulting in a marked increase in circulating immature or abnormal white blood cells. These cells infiltrate into tissues and cause enlargement of the spleen, liver and lymph nodes. All leukocyte types may be involved i.e. granulocytes (myeloid), monocytes and lymphocytes. In addition, the disease may be acute or chronic. In acute leukemias, the cell type is commonly a stem cell precursor or blast cell and patients are usually under 20 or over 55 years of age. Chronic leukemias occur mainly in people over 40 years of age and the typical cell type is well differentiated. In all leukemias, the normal marrow function is impaired and thus anemia, infections and thrombocytopenia are common.

1. *Leukemic gingival enlargement*: Leukemic gingival enlargement consists of a basic infiltration of the gingival corium by leukemic cells that creates gingival pockets where bacterial plaque accumulates,

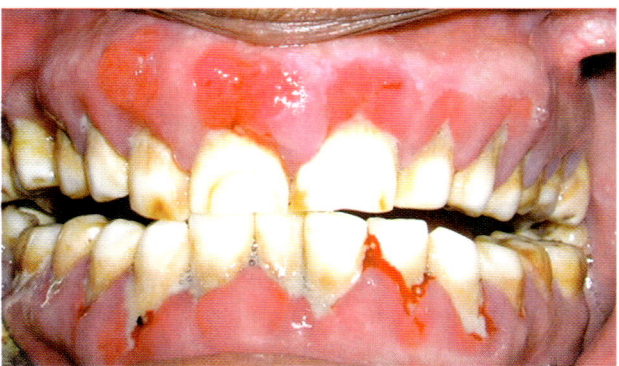

Fig. 14.3: Gingival changes associated with leukemia: The gingiva is inflamed, enlarged and edematous which bleeds spontaneously

initiating a secondary inflammatory lesion that also contributes to the enlargement of the gingiva. The gingiva appears initially bluish red and cyanotic, with rounding of the gingival margin **(Fig. 14.3)**. A marked improvement is brought about by systemic management of the disease and the institution of an effective oral hygiene program.

2. *Gingival bleeding*: It is a common sign in both acute and chronic leukemia. This probably relates to the associated thrombocytopenia and the fact that gingival epithelium may be thin and atrophic.

3. *Oral Ulceration and Infection*: The granulocytopenia resulting from the replacement of bone marrow cells by leukemic cells reduces the tissue resistance to opportunistic microorganisms and leads to ulcerations and infections. Markedly altered and degenerated tissue is extremely susceptible to bacterial infection causing acute gingival necrosis and pseudomembrane formation.

A classification for the etiology of gingival lesions in leukemic patients has been proposed by Barrett (1984). This classification consists of four categories and distinguishes between lesions resulting directly from the disease, treatment and lesions caused by secondary effects i.e. bone marrow and lymphoid tissue depression.

- Category 1 is concerned with lesions caused by direct leukemic infiltration and includes gingival enlargement.
- Category 2 deals with direct drug toxicity caused by chemotherapeutic agents. These drugs cause several distinct gingival changes including erosion and ulceration. The immunosuppressive drug cyclosporine, used to prevent graft rejection after transplantation, can contribute to gingival hyperplasia.
- Category 3 comprises the detrimental effects of graft-versus-host reactions. In this disease, the transplanted lymphocytes react against host antigens. Mucosal lesions include lichenoid striae, epithelial detachment, erosions and ulceration and in themselves can be useful markers of graft-versus-host activity.
- Category 4 involves secondary effects from the depression of marrow/lymphoid tissue and includes hemorrhage, neutropenic ulceration and an increased susceptibility to microbial infections.

Treatment plan for leukemic patient includes chemotherapy, radiation therapy and bone marrow transplantation, each of which has the potential to produce a wide range of oral complications. Mucositis, xerostomia and secondary infection with a variety of bacterial, viral, and fungal agents may occur. Candidiasis is almost universally seen in hospitalized leukemic patients undergoing chemotherapy. Absorbable gelatin sponge with topical thrombin or placement of microfibrillar collagen is used to stop gingival bleeding. Oral rinses of antifibrinolytic agents may also help in controlling bleeding.

Red Blood Cell Disorders

Erythrocyte disorders do not profoundly affect the periodontium.

Acatalasia is a rare, inherited disorder caused by the lack of catalase in cells, especially red and white blood cells. The cells use the enzyme catalase to convert reactive hydrogen peroxide to oxygen and water. The neutralization of H_2O_2 protects these cells from harmful oxidizing agents which could denature hemoglobin and produce local hypoxia and necrosis of the gingiva.

Aplastic anemia is a form of normocytic-normochromic anemia that results from a lack of bone marrow production of erythrocytes and other blood cells. The disorder may be genetic or acquired. The acquired form usually follows exposure to certain drugs, toxic chemicals, or ionizing radiation. Because all bone marrow-derived cells are affected, including the defensive leukocytes and platelets, hemorrhage and infection are the major threats to patients with aplastic anemia. Oral manifestations include petechiae, gingival swelling and bleeding (often spontaneous), gingival overgrowth, and herpetic infections. Rapid bone loss has been reported, and periodontal infections have led to severe, life-threatening systemic infections.

Thrombocytopenia

Thrombocytopenic purpura may be idiopathic or it may occur secondary to some known etiologic factor responsible for a reduction in the number of circulating platelets. Such etiologic factors include aplasia of marrow, destruction of marrow by irradiation or by drugs such as benzene, arsenical agents.

Two forms of Idiopathic thrombocytopenic purpura (ITP) are recognized: acute and chronic. Acute ITP is a self-limited disease that generally remits permanently without sequelae. The onset is usually sudden, with thrombocytopenia manifested by bruising, bleeding, and petechiae a few days to several weeks after an otherwise uneventful viral illness. Conversely, chronic ITP is usually a disease of adults and can be sudden or insidious

in onset. The oral manifestations of thrombocytopenia may be the first clinical sign of the disease. There is spontaneous gingival hemorrhage and prolonged bleeding after trauma and toothbrushing. Good oral hygiene and complete removal of plaque and calculus helps to minimize gingival inflammation and reduce gingival bleeding associated with thrombocytopenia. Periodontal therapy should be limited unless platelet counts exceed a minimum of 50,000/ mm^3 and surgery should be avoided until platelet counts are greater than 80,000/ mm^3. Any drug like aspirin associated with the onset of thrombocytopenic episodes should be avoided.

Coagulation Disorders

The hemostatic disorders do not predispose to periodontal disease but do present management problems during periodontal therapy. Hemorrhaging after scaling in these patients is predictable. Supplementing hemostatic mechanisms by alterations in anticoagulant therapy, platelet transfusions or clotting factor supplements should be considered, particularly prior to surgery.

IMMUNODEFICIENCY DISORDERS

Leukocyte Disorders

Neutropenia: The term neutropenia covers a heterogeneous group of diseases characterized by a decrease or an absence of circulating PMNs. Various types and descriptions of neutropenia exist, including agranulocytosis, familial neutropenia and chronic idiopathic neutropenia. Cyclic neutropenia is a rare condition characterized by cyclic depletion of PMN numbers, typically in three week cycles, although this can be between two and five weeks. Periodontal manifestations include inflamed gingiva, gingival ulceration, periodontal attachment and bone loss. In the severe form, which is often drug-induced, there is ulceration and necrosis of the marginal gingiva. This is associated with bleeding and occasional involvement of the attached gingiva. Histologically, the ulcerated areas exhibit little or no PMN infiltration. The gingiva may be edematous, hyperemic and hyperplastic with areas of partial desquamation. These features are often accompanied by deep periodontal pockets and extensive generalized bone loss involving the permanent dentition.

Agranulocytosis: Agranulocytosis, by strict definition, means depletion of all granulocytes (neutrophils, eosinophils, monocytes and basophils) in the blood. The term is generally used to describe an extremely severe neutropenia, which is often due to adverse drug reactions. It is characterized by a reduction in the number of circulating granulocytes and results in severe infections including ulcerative necrotizing lesions of the oral mucosa, skin, gastrointestinal and genitourinary tracts. Drug idiosyncrasy is the most common cause of agranulocytosis. Striking feature is the absence of a notable inflammatory reaction due to lack of granulocytes. Clinical features of agranulocytosis are gingival hemorrhage, necrosis, increased salivation and fetid odor. The microscopic changes seen in the periodontium are hemorrhage into the periodontal ligament with destruction of the principal fibers and small fragments of necrotic bone. Osteoporosis of the cancellous bone with osteoclastic resorption is there. There may be formation of new bony trabeculae.

Papillon-Lefevre syndrome: Papillon and Lefevre in 1924 discovered this syndrome. It is a rare autosomal recessive disorder characterized by mutation in Cathepsin C gene located on chromosome 11 (11q14 – q21). Cathepsin C is a protease, normally found in high levels in epithelium and immune cells such as neutrophils, which acts to degrade proteins and activate proenzymes in immune cells. Patients with Papillon – Lefevre syndrome have little or no cathepsin C activity. There are alterations in cementum. Collagenolytic activity in periodontal ligament and osteoblastic activity of alveolar bone leads to rapid generalized destruction of alveolar bone affecting both the deciduous and permanent dentition. Systemic administration of retinoids, when combined with meticulous plaque control, debridement, topical antimicrobials along with systemic antibiotic therapy may give the best chance for preventing the progression of periodontitis.

Chediak-Higashi syndrome: It is an autosomal recessive mode of inheritance disease localized to chromosome 1q43. The hallmark of this syndrome is that there is fusion of azurophil and specific granules into giant granules called Megabodies in neutrophils. The average lifespan for children with the Chediak - Higashi syndrome is only 6 years, although some patients may live into early childhood. Oral findings include ulcerations of tongue and buccal mucosa, severe gingivitis and periodontitis. Bone loss is usually generalized and severe. Patients do not respond to periodontal therapy, leading to premature loss of both deciduous and permanent dentitions. It is characterized by decreased chemotaxis, degranulation and microbial activity. A mutation in the LYST (Lysosomal trafficking regulator) gene - the only gene known to cause this syndrome may be responsible for this phenomenon. Bone marrow transplantation appears to be the most effective treatment for correcting these neutrophil abnormalities.

Leukocyte adhesion deficiency: It is an inherited disorder that follows an autosomal recessive pattern. Leukocyte adhesion deficiency is caused by a deficiency in cell surface integrins that prevents the neutrophils from adhering to the vessel wall at the site of an infection. Neutrophils are unable to migrate into the affected tissues and remain within the vasculature.

Leukocyte adhesion deficiency Type I: There is deficiency of integrin β2 subunit (CD18) resulting in impairement in leukocyte function. This defect is usually associated with aggressive periodontitis.

Leukocyte adhesion deficiency Type II: Neutrophils fail to express the ligand (CD15) for P and E selectins, resulting in impaired transendothelial migration in response to inflammation.

Lazy leukocyte syndrome: It is a rare disorder which is characterized by quantitative and qualitative neutrophil defects. Deficiency in neutrophil chemotaxis combined with systemic neutropenia results in recurrent infections. There is rapidly progressive bone loss and tooth loss at an early age.

Glycogen storage diseases: These are caused by abnormalities of enzymes that control glycogen synthesis and degradation. Patients with glycogen storage disease type 1b often have qualitative and quantitative neutrophil defects, leading to an increased susceptibility to infection. Gingivitis and periodontitis are common in patients with glycogen storage disease type 1b.

Antibody Deficiency Disorders

Agammaglobulinemia: There is deficiency of B cells whereas T-cell function remains normal. It can be congenital (X-linked or Bruton's agammaglobulinemia) or acquired. The disease is characterized by recurrent infections, including destructive periodontitis in children.

Acquired immunodeficiency syndrome: It is caused by the human immunodeficiency virus (HIV) and is characterized by destruction of lymphocytes, rendering the patient susceptible to opportunistic infections. Periodontal findings in HIV infected individuals are mainly: linear gingival erythema; necrotizing ulcerative gingivitis (NUG); severe localized periodontitis; and severe destructive necrotizing stomatitis affecting gingiva and bone (similar to noma or cancrum oris). More is explained in chapter no. 27 AIDS and Periodontium.

INFLUENCE OF NUTRITION

Periodontal health relies on a delicate balance between the host, environmental and bacterial factors. The primary etiology of periodontal disesase is bacterial plaque , but a susceptible host is also necessary for disease initation. Nutrition is one of the modifiable factors that impact the host's immune response and integrity of the hard and soft tissues of the oral cavity. The diet which contains different constituents of food (proteins, fats, carbohydrates, vitamins and minerals) in such quantities and proportions that the need for energy is adequately met for maintaining health is called *balanced diet*. Nutritional disorders are not only the result of inadequate dietary intake, but also may be due to disturbances in absorption and utilization and self-imposed dietary restrictions. The components of host - defence that may be adversely affected by inadequate nutrition include:

1. Inflammatory and immune response.
2. Functional capacity of salivary glands and composition of saliva
3. Gingival crevicular fluid production
4. Responsiveness of the repair process, and
5. Integrity of oral mucosa.

The relation between nutritional factors and maintenance of periodontal health, or the role of nutritional factors in the pathogenesis of periodontal disease, is controversial because most of the scientific evidence is derived from laboratory or animal studies.

Nutritional Deficiencies

There are nutritional deficiencies that produce changes in the oral cavity. These changes include alterations of the lips, oral mucosa and periodontal tissues. These changes are considered to be periodontal or oral manifestations of nutritional diseases. There are no nutritional deficiencies that by themselves can cause gingivitis or periodontal pockets.

Vitamins

Vitamins have been defined as organic components in natural foods which are required in minute amounts for normal growth, maintenance and reproduction. They are also called as "miracle workers". They are classified as water soluble (B and C), which are not stored in the body and fat soluble (A, D, E and K), which are stored in the body.

Vitamin A: The deficiency of vitamin A leads to hyperplasia and hyperkeratinization of the gingival epithelium with proliferation of the junctional epithelium and retardation of gingival wound healing. There is little information regarding the effects of vitamin A deficiency on the oral structures in humans. Several epidemiological studies have failed to demonstrate any relation between this vitamin and periodontal disease.

Vitamin B complex deficiency: Oral changes common to B-complex deficiencies are gingivitis, glossitis, glossodynia, angular cheilitis and inflammation of the entire oral mucosa. The gingivitis in vitamin B deficiencies is non-specific, as it is caused by bacterial plaque rather than by the deficiency. The following oral disturbances have been attributed to thiamine deficiency: Hypersensitivity of the oral mucosa, minute vesicles on the buccal mucosa under the tongue, or on the palate and erosion of the oral mucosa. Changes observed in riboflavin deficient animals include severe lesions of the gingiva, periodontal tissues and oral mucosa (including noma). Oral manifestations of vitamin B complex and niacin deficiency in experimental animals include black tongue and gingival inflammation with destruction of the gingiva, periodontal ligament and alveolar bone. Necrosis of the gingiva and other oral tissues and leukopenia are terminal features of niacin deficiency in experimental animals. Folic acid – deficient animals also demonstrate necrosis of the gingiva, periodontal ligament and alveolar bone without inflammation.

Vitamin C (Ascorbic Acid) Deficiency

Vitamin C plays an important role in the formation of amino acids hydroxyproline and hydroxylysine, which are almost unique to collagen, the major protein of periodontium. Its deficiency causes scurvy, which is characterized by hemorrhagic diathesis and retardation of wound healing. There is defective formation and maintenance of collagen and increased capillary permeability. Following are the possible etiologic relationships between vitamin C and periodontal diseases:

• Low levels of vitamin C influence the metabolism of collagen within the peridontium, thereby, affecting the ability of the tissue to regenerate and repair itself.
• Its deficiency interferes with bone formation leading to loss of alveolar bone.

PERIODONTICS REVISITED

- Its deficiency increases the permeability of the oral mucosa to endotoxins and tritiated inulin and of normal human crevicular – epithelium to tritiated dextran. Optimal levels of this vitamin, therefore would maintain the epithelium's barrier function to the various bacterial products.
- Increasing levels of vitamin C enhance both the chemotactic and the migratory action of leukocytes without influencing their phagocytic activity.
- An optimal level of vitamin C is apparently required to maintain the integrity of the periodontal microvasculature.
- Deficiency of vitamin C interferes with the ecologic equilibrium of bacteria in plaque and thus increases its pathogenicity.

Vitamin D deficiency: In vitamin D deficiency, there is generalized bone resorption in jaws, fibro-osteoid hemorrhage in the marrow spaces and destruction of the periodontal ligament. The effect of such deficiency or imbalance on periodontal tissues results in osteoporosis of alveolar bone. Osteoid forms at a normal rate but remains uncalcified. Radiographically, there is generalized partial to complete disappearance of the lamina dura and reduced density of the supporting bone, loss of trabeculae, increased radiolucency of the trabecular interstices and increased prominence of the remaining trabeculae. Microscopic and radiographic changes in the periodontium are almost identical with those seen in experimentally induced hyperparathyroidism.

Vitamin E deficiency: No relationship has been demonstrated between deficiencies in vitamin E and oral disease but in experimental rats systemic vitamin E appears to accelerate gingival wound healing .

Protein deficiency: Protein deprivation causes the following changes in the periodontium of experimental animals: Degeneration of the connective tissue of the gingiva and periodontal ligament, osteoporosis of alveolar bone, retardation in the deposition of cementum and delayed wound healing. Protein deficiency will retard growth, alter physiologic functions and significantly reduce host defenses and wound healing. Protein deprivation adversely affects immunoglobulin A in saliva, PMN phagocytosis and complement activation and both cell mediated and humoral immune responses. Severe protein deficiency (Kwashiorkor) or general starvation (Marasmus) has long been associated with glossitis, increase gingival inflammation and alveolar bone loss.

Antioxidants

In periodontal diseases, proteases released from inflammatory cells, especially polymorphonuclear leukocytes, contain free radicals, which may damage adjacent periodontal tissues. Ongoing research is underway to determine whether or not antioxidant nutritional supplements namely beta carotene, retinol, ascorbic acid, alpha-carotene and selenium, are of benefit in reducing the tissue destruction occurring in plaque induced periodontal diseases. The use of antioxidants in the treatment of oral leukoplakia and perhaps oral cancer shows promising results.

STRESS AND PSYCHOSOMATIC DISORDERS

The systemic reactions that affect the body generally or produce an interrelated nonspecific tissue change resulting from continued exposure to stress have been termed the general adaptation syndrome (GAS) by Selye in 1946. Selye considered GAS to be the basis of the pathogenesis of various diseases. The three stages of this syndrome are-a) Initial response (alarm reaction); b) adaptation to stress (resistant stage); c) Final stage, marked by inability to maintain adaptation to stress (exhaustion stage).

Stress is known to alter immune responsiveness and increase the susceptibility to periodontal infection. The most commonly studied periodontal disease in relation to stress is necrotizing ulcerative gingivitis (Rest is explained in chapter no. 57 Periodontics-Psychiatry).

OTHER SYSTEMIC CONDITIONS

Metal Intoxication

Systemic absorption of certain heavy metal such as, mercury, lead, arsenic and bismuth can produce pigmentation or discoloration of gingival surfaces. These metals may come from environmental exposure or from certain medications.

Bismuth pigmentation: It usually appears as a narrow, bluish-black discoloration of the gingival margin in areas of pre-existent gingival inflammation. Such pigmentation results from the precipitation of particles of bismuth sulphide associated with vascular changes in gingival inflammation.

Lead pigmentation: Lead is slowly absorbed, and toxic symptoms are not particularly definitive when they do occur. The pigmentation of the gingiva is linear (burtonian line), steel gray, and associated with local irritation.

Mercury pigmentation: Gingival pigmentation in linear form results from the deposition of mercuric sulfide. The chemical also acts as an irritant, which accentuates the pre-existent inflammation and commonly leads to notable ulceration of the gingiva and adjacent mucosa and destruction of the underlying bone.

Arsenic and chromium: It may cause necrosis of the alveolar bone with loosening and exfoliation of the teeth. Inflammation and ulceration of the gingiva are usually associated with destruction of the underlying tissues.

PERIODONTAL MANIFESTATIONS OF SYSTEMIC DRUG THERAPY

There are varieties of medications to control one or more chronic conditions. Many of these medications produce changes in the oral cavity because of toxic overdoses, side effects, allergic reactions, or as a consequence of the primary action of the drug.

The effect of systemic drug therapy on the periodontium can be categorized as follows:
- An adverse effect on the periodontal tissues;
- Affording some degree of protection against periodontal breakdown;
- Causing an increased risk of periodontal breakdown.

Adverse effects of systemic medications on the periodontal tissues:

1. *Drug induced xerostomia*: It may result in increased plaque and calculus formation. Drugs with xerostomic potential include diuretics, antihypertensives, antipsychotics and antidepressants.
2. *Leukoplakia*: Drugs of abuse such as cannabis and cocaine can induce gingival leukoplakia and erythema.
3. *Agranulocytosis*: Drug induced agranulocytosis may result in severe gingival necrosis resembling generalized necrotizing ulcerative gingivitis. Drugs implicated in causing agranulocytosis include the phenothiazines, sulphur derivatives, indomethacin and some antibiotics.
4. *Gingival enlargement*: Therapeutic intake of sex hormones such as estrogen, progesterone has been reported to be associated with gingival enlargement. Drug-induced gingival overgrowth remains the most widespread unwanted effect of systemic medication on the periodontal tissues. Three groups of drugs most frequently implicated are – anticonvulsants, immunosuppressants and antihypertensives.

Anticonvulsant drugs associated with gingival enlargement are— Phenytoin, Phenobarbital, Carbamazepine, Sodium Valproate, Primidone and Felbamate. Antihypertensive drugs associated with gingival enlargement are: Nifedipine, Amlodipine, Nimodipine, Nicardine, Nitrendipine, Diltiazem, Felodipine and Bepridil.

Calcium channel blockers group of drugs are antianginal and antihypertensive medications. They are considered to influence gingival fibroblasts to overproduce collagen matrix and ground substance when stimulated by gingival inflammation following plaque build-up. They clearly have major effects in terms of gingival overgrowth and, although it could be argued that an unfavorable gingival form and false pocketing may be plaque retentive and thus, might be local modifiers of periodontitis.

Phenytoin is an anticonvulsant drug commonly used for prevention of seizures. Gingival overgrowth occurs in about half of all individuals who take phenytoin on a chronic regimen. Teenagers and young adults to about 30 years of age are affected more frequently than middle aged or elderly persons. The anterior labial surfaces of the maxillary and mandibular gingiva are most commonly and severely affected **(Fig. 14.4)**. The earliest clinical signs of gingival changes may occur 2-3 weeks after phenytoin therapy is started. Gingival overgrowth often becomes clinically apparent during the first 6-9 months of therapy. Interdental papillae overgrow and extrude, forming firm, mobile, triangular tissue

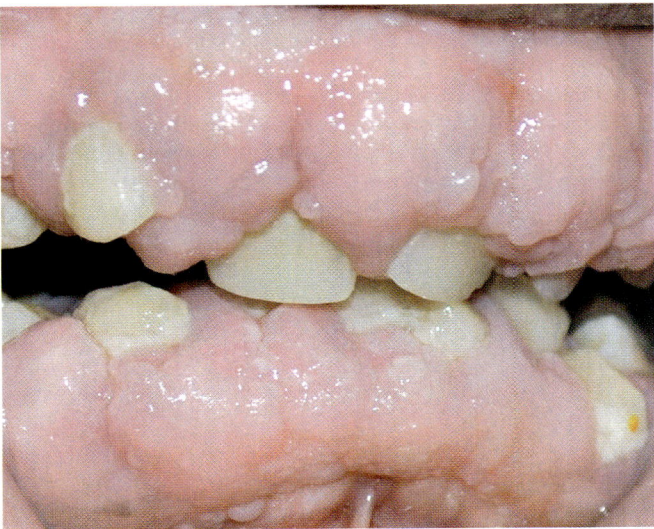

Fig. 14.4: Phenytoin induced gingival enlargement

masses which may fuse mesially and distally and form a continuous curtain of overgrown marginal gingiva.

Cyclosporine is an immunosuppressant drug widely prescribed to control rejection of solid organ transplantation and autoimmune diseases. It exerts effect by selective suppression of specific subpopulations of T lymphocytes, interfering with production of lymphokines and interleukins 1 and 2. The gingival lesions associated with cyclosporine are often clinically and histologically indistinguishable from those elicited by phenytoin. The clinical course is also similar, in that the lesions generally originate in the interdental area and then all segments of the dental arch may be affected.

5. *Halitosis*: Some of the psychiatric medications can cause halitosis namely lorazepam, carbamazepine, amitriptyline, fluoxetine and haloperidol.

6. *Abnormal pigmentation*: A number of drugs may induce unusual pigmentation in the oral cavity. Implicated drugs include minocycline, zidovudine, phenothiazines, bismuth, gold salts and anticancer drugs. Minocycline may produce a gray blue black pigmentation of alveolar mucosa and attached gingiva.

BIBLIOGRAPHY

1. Grant DA, Stern IB, Listgarten MA. Diet and nutrition. In, Periodontics. 6th ed CV Mosby Company 1988;293-306.
2. Grossi SG, Genco RJ. Periodontal disease and diabetes mellitus: A two –way Relationship. Ann Periodontol 1998;3:51-61.
3. Klokkevold PR, Mealey BL, Carranza FA. Influence of Systemic disease and disorders on the periodontium. In, Newman, Takei, Carranza. Clinical Periodontology. 9th ed WB Saunders 2003;204-28.
4. Lundgren T, Grossner CG, Tentman S, Ullbro C. Systemic retinoid medication and periodontal health in patients with Papillon - Lefevre syndrome. J Clin Periodontol 1996;23:176-79.
5. Mealey BL, Rees TD, Rose LF, Grossi SG. Systemic factors Impacting the Periodontium. In, Rose LF, Mealey BL, Genco RJ, Cohen DW. Periodontics. Elsevier Mosby 2004;790-845.
6. Palmer R, Soory M. Modifying factors: Diabetes, Puberty, Pregnancy and the Menopause and Tobacco Smoking. In, Lindhe J, Karring T, Lang NP. Clinical Periodontology and Implant dentistry. 4th ed Blackwell Munksgaard 2003;179-97.
7. Rose LF. Diseases of other organ or tissue systems with periodontal manifestations. In, Genco RJ, Goldman HM, Cohen DW. Contemporary Periodontics. CV Mosby Company 1990; 251-68.
8. Wilson TG, Kornman KS. Systemic modifiers. In, Fundamentals of Periodontics. Quintessence Publishing Co.1996;293-306.

MCQs

1. Drug induced gingival enlargement can be due to:
   A. Nifedipine
   B. Cyclosporine
   C. Phenytoin
   D. All of the above

2. Scurvy is due to the deficiency of:
   A. Vitamin A
   B. Vitamin B
   C. Vitamin C
   D. Vitamin D

3. Advanced glycation endproducts (AGEs) are formed in:
   A. Protein deficiency
   B. Diabetes mellitus
   C. Leukemia
   D. None of the above

4. Following are the findings seen in leukemia:
   A. Gingival enlargement
   B. Gingival bleeding
   C. Oral ulceration and infection
   D. All of the above

Answers

1. D   2. C   3. B   4. D

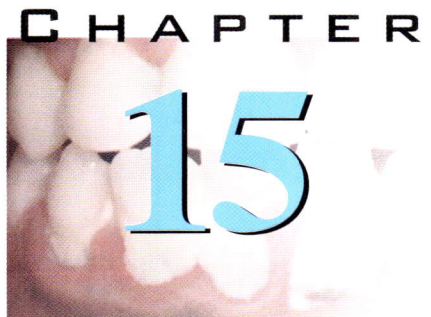

CHAPTER 15

Effect of Periodontal Diseases on Systemic Health

Sanjay Kalra, Shalu Bathla

INTRODUCTION

Periodontal disease is an infectious disease affected by various risk factors and systemic disorders. Since, the early 1990s emerging new evidences are showing the converse side of the relationship between systemic health and periodontal health. Thus, implicating periodontal infection as a risk factor for several systemic conditions such as coronary heart disease, preterm low birth weight infants, diabetes and pulmonary diseases.

RE-EMERGENCE OF FOCAL INFECTION THEORY

In 1900s WD Miller, a microbiologist in Philadelphia and William Hunter, a London physician gave the concept that oral bacteria and infection were the likely cause of most of a person's systemic illnesses. Hunter believed that teeth were liable to septic infection primarily due to their structure and their relationship to alveolar bone. He stated that the degree of systemic effect produced by oral sepsis depends on the virulence of the oral infection and the degree of resistance of the individual. Hunter believed that the connection between oral sepsis and resulting systemic conditions could be shown by removal of the causative sepsis via tooth extraction and observation of the improvement in systemic health. For the next 40 years physicians and dentists would embrace the idea that infections, especially those originating in the mouth, caused most of man's suffering and illness leading to wholesale extraction of teeth. This era, came to be known as the era of focal infection. The focal infection theory fell into disrepute in the 1940s and 1950s when widespread extraction, often of the entire dentition failed to reduce or eliminate the systemic conditions to which the supposedly infected dentition had been linked. The focal infection theory as proposed and defended in the early part of the 20th century, was based on almost no evidence. Today's era of evidence based medicine and dentistry provides an excellent environment to examine the possible relationship between oral infections and systemic disorders.

THE SUBGINGIVAL ENVIRONMENT AS A RESERVOIR OF BACTERIA

The subgingival microbiota in patients with periodontitis provides a significant and persistent gram-negative bacterial challenge to the host. These organisms and their products such as lipopolysaccharides (LPS), have ready access to the periodontal tissues and to the circulation via the sulcular epithelium, which is frequently ulcerated and discontinuous. Even with treatment, complete eradication of these organisms is difficult and their re-emergence is often rapid. The total surface area of pocket epithelium in contact with subgingival bacteria and their products in a patient with generalized moderate periodontitis has been estimated to be approximately the size of the palm of an adult hand, with even larger areas of exposure in cases of more advanced periodontal destruction. Bacteremias are common after mechanical periodontal therapy and also occur frequently during normal daily function and oral hygiene procedures. Thus, the potential for distant seeding of oral infections is ever present. In this manner, periodontal biofilm infection contributes not only to local inflammation resulting in destruction of tooth supporting structures, but also to systemic inflammation as well.

EFFECT OF PERIODONTAL DISEASES ON CARDIOVASCULAR SYSTEM

Atherosclerosis

Atherosclerosis is a focal thickening of the arterial intima, the innermost layer lining the vessel lumen and the media, the thick layer under the intima consisting of smooth muscle, collagen, and elastic fibers.

Following are the proposed mechanisms **(Fig. 15.1)** by which infections may contribute to atherosclerosis:

1. *Direct effects of infectious agents in atheroma formation*: Oral organisms may be involved in coronary thrombogenesis. Aggregation of platelets is induced by the platelet aggregation-associated protein (PAAP) expressed on some strains of *Streptococcus sanguis* and *Porphyromonas gingivalis*. Platelet aggregation plays a major role in thrombogenesis and most cases of acute myocardial infarction are precipitated by thromboembolism.

2. *Indirect or host mediated effects triggered by infection*: One possible mechanism that has gathered considerable support is that periodontitis induces an inflammatory response that is manifested, in part, by the production

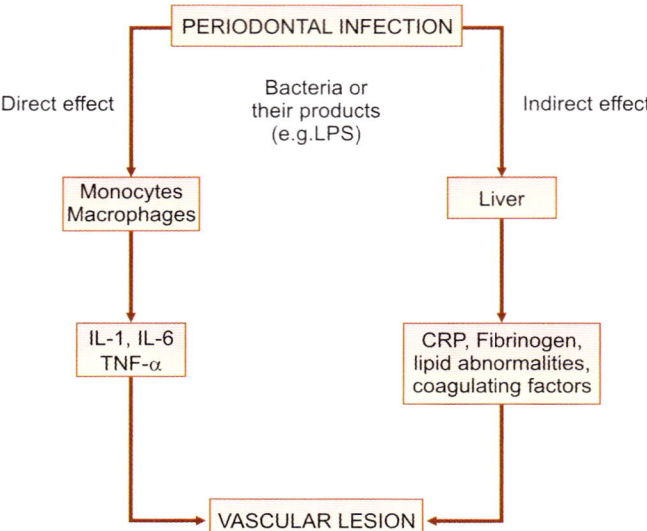

Fig. 15.1: Systemic spread of periodontal infection

of acute – phase proteins, such as C- reactive protein and fibrinogen, by the liver. C-reactive protein and fibrinogen are independent risk factors for coronary artery disease, hence if they are induced, in part at least by periodontal infection, this may helps to explain the link between periodontal disease and heart disease.

Another indirect effect of periodontal infection that may explain the association between periodontal disease and heart disease is that periodontal organisms contain proteins which cross react with the heart. In fact, the heat shock protein-60, which is produced by *Bacteroides forsythus* and *P. gingivalis* has about 60% homology with the mammalian heat–shock protein. It is known that antibodies to the heat–shock protein are found in patients with periodontal disease. These antibodies are cross–reactive with the heat–shock protein that is exposed in an injured epithelium or atheramatous plaque. This could lead to autoimmune phenomena and contribute to atheroma formation.

3. *Common genetic predisposition for periodontal disease and atherosclerosis*: There may be common genetic mechanisms which provide the link between periodontal disease and cardiovascular disease. Beck and colleagues have provided a model proposing that there is a genetically determined hyperinflammatory macrophage phenotype in periodontal disease, which contributes to the susceptibility for atherosclerosis.

4. *Common risk factors for both periodontal disease and atherosclerosis such as lifestyle*: DeStefano and colleagues found that periodontal disease and poor oral hygiene are stronger risk indicators of total mortality and of coronary heart disease. They suggest that oral hygiene may be an indicator or a surrogate for lifestyle affecting personal hygiene and health care and might explain the relationship between periodontal disease and heart disease.

5. Early in the formation of atherosclerotic plaques, circulating monocytes adhere to the vascular endothelium. This adherence is mediated through several adhesion molecules on the endothelial cell surface, including intercellular adhesion molecule-1 (ICAM- 1), endothelial leukocyte adhesion molecule-1 (ELAM-1), and vascular cell adhesion molecule-1 (VCAM-1). These adhesion molecules are up-regulated by a number of factors including bacterial LPS, prostaglandins and proinflammatory cytokines. After binding to the endothelial cell lining, monocytes penetrate the endothelium and migrate under the arterial intima. The monocytes ingest circulating low-density lipoprotein (LDL) in its oxidized state and become engorged and form foam cells characteristic of atheromatous plaques **(Fig. 15.2)**. Once within the arterial media, monocytes may also transform to macrophages. A host of proinflammatory cytokines such as interleukin-1 (IL-1), tumor necrosis factor-alpha (TNF-α), and prostaglandin E_2 (PGE$_2$) are then produced, which propagate the atheromatous lesion. Mitogenic factors such as fibroblast growth factor and platelet-derived growth factor stimulate smooth muscle and collagen proliferation within the media, thickening the arterial wall.

EFFECT OF PERIODONTAL DISEASES ON ENDOCRINE SYSTEM

Diabetes Mellitus

Diabetes mellitus is a clinically and genetically heterogeneous group of metabolic disorders manifested by abnormally high levels of glucose in the blood. The hyperglycemia is due to the deficiency of insulin secretion caused by pancreatic β-cell dysfunction or of resistance to the action of insulin in liver and muscle, or a combination of these.

Periodontitis has been determined to be a potential risk factor for poor glycemic control in patients with diabetes. Periodontal infection increase tissue resistance to insulin, preventing glucose from entering target cells, causing elevated blood glucose levels and requiring increased pancreatic insulin production to maintain normal glucose level. In Diabetes where there is significant insulin resistance, further tissue resistance to insulin induced by periodontal infection exacerbate poor glycemic control. In the hyperglycemic state, numerous proteins and matrix molecules undergo a non-enzymatic glycosylation, resulting in advanced glycation end product (AGEs). Macrophages have high affinity receptors for a common structural elements an AGE - modified proteins. Binding of the AGE modified protein to the macrophage receptor (RAGE) initiates a cycle of cytokine upregulation, with synthesis mostly of IL - 1 and TNF-α. The synthesis and secretion of cytokines are increased which trigger degradative cascade, resulting in connective tissue degradation as explained in **Figure 15.3**. The interaction of AGEs with RAGE perturbs the specific cellular functions. In homeostasis, RAGE is present at low levels in a number of cell types, including endothelial cells, smooth muscle cells, neurons and monocytes. However, in perturbed states, such as diabetes, renal failure, Alzheimer's disease and inflammation, the expression of RAGE on critical target cells is strikingly enhanced.

EFFECT OF PERIODONTAL DISEASES ON REPRODUCTIVE SYSTEM

Pregnancy Outcome

Preterm birth (PTB) infants are those infants who are born before the thirty-seventh weeks of gestation. Low birth weight (LBW) infants are those born at term but weighing

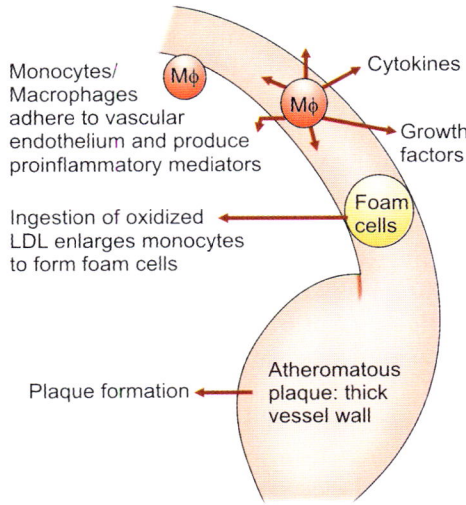

Monocytes/ Macrophages adhere to vascular endothelium and produce proinflammatory mediators

Mϕ

Mϕ

Cytokines

Growth factors

Foam cells

Ingestion of oxidized LDL enlarges monocytes to form foam cells

Plaque formation

Atheromatous plaque: thick vessel wall

Fig. 15.2: Pathogenesis of atherosclerosis

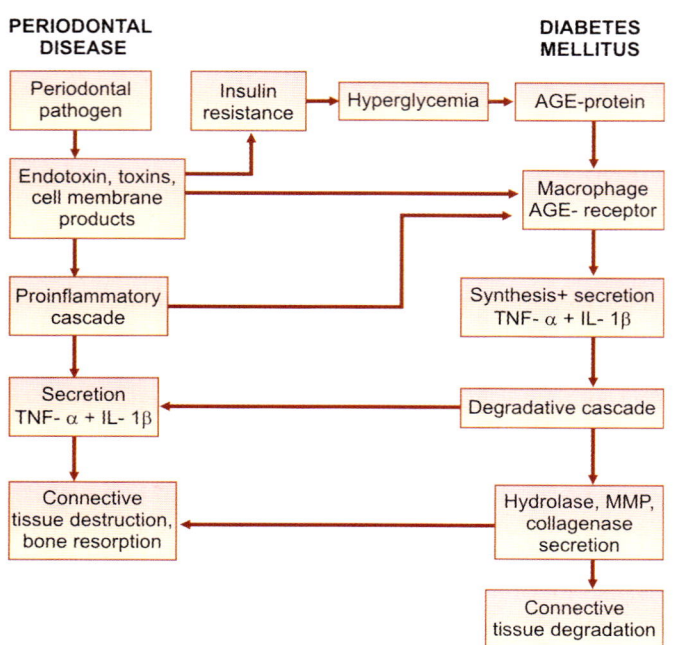

Fig. 15.3: Two way relationship between periodontal disease and diabetes mellitus

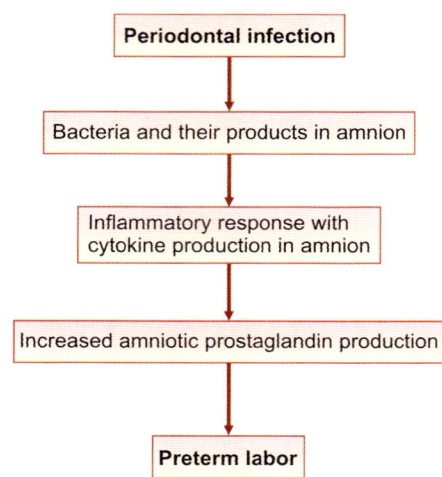

Fig. 15.4: Effect of periodontal infection on pregnancy outcome

less than 2500 gms. In recent years, subclinical and chronic infections such as periodontal disease have been proposed to play a role in premature birth and they significantly increase the risk for both LBW and PTB.

The proposed hypothesis for chronic infection and premature birth is that, the microorganisms or their products such as LPS, enter the uterine cavity either through the ascending route in genitourinary tract infections or through the circulation in nongenital infections. Once the microorganisms or their products have gained access to the uterine cavity, they can stimulate an inflammatory cytokine cascade, with increased production of proinflammatory mediators such as IL-1α and TNF-α. These eventually lead to elevated prostaglandin synthesis, which causes uterine muscle contraction, cervical dilation and premature rupture of membranes **(Fig. 15.4)**.

EFFECT OF PERIODONTAL DISEASES ON RESPIRATORY SYSTEM

Chronic Obstructive Pulmonary Disease

Chronic obstructive pulmonary disease (COPD) is a disease state characterized by airflow obstruction due to chronic bronchitis or emphysema. Bronchial mucous glands enlarge, and an inflammatory process occurs in which neutrophils and mononuclear inflammatory cells accumulate within the lung tissue. COPD shares similar pathogenic mechanisms with periodontal disease. In both diseases, a host inflammatory response is mounted in response to chronic challenge; by bacteria in periodontal disease and by factors such as cigarette smoke in COPD. Several mechanisms have been proposed to explain how oral bacteria can participate in the pathogenesis of respiratory infections:

1. Oral pathogens (such as *P. gingivalis, A. actinomyce-temcomitans*) may be aspirated into the lung to cause infection.
2. Periodontal disease – associated enzymes in saliva may modify mucosal surfaces to promote adhesion and colonization by respiratory pathogens.
3. Cytokines originating from periodontal tissues may alter respiratory epithelium to promote infection by respiratory pathogen. In untreated periodontal disease, oral pathogens continuously stimulate the cells of the periodontium (epithelial cells, endothelial cells, fibroblasts, macrophages, white cells) to release a wide variety of cytokines and other biologically active molecules. Cytokines produced by epithelial and connective tissue cells in response to these bacteria are interleukin IL - 1α, IL - 1β, IL - 6, IL - 8, and TNF - α. Oral bacteria can also stimulate the peripheral mononuclear cells to release cytokines (IL-1α and TNF - α). Thus, resulting neutrophil influx leads to release of oxidative and hydrolytic enzymes that cause tissue destruction directly. Recruitment of monocytes and macrophages leads to further release of proinflammatory mediators.

LANDMARK STUDIES RELATED

Offenbacher S, Katz V, Fertik G, Collins J, Boyd D, Maynor G, McKaig R, Beck J. Periodontal infection as a possible risk factor for preterm low birth weight. Journal of Periodontology 1996;67:1103-13.

A case-control study of 124 pregnant or postpartum mothers was performed. Preterm low birth weight (PLBW) cases were defined as a mother with a birth of less than 2,500 g and one or more of the following: gestational age <37 weeks, preterm labor (PTL), or premature rupture of membranes (PROMs). Controls were mothers with normal birth weight infants (NBW). Each subject received a periodontal examination to determine clinical attachment level. PLBW cases and primiparous PLBW cases had significantly worse periodontal disease than the respective NBW controls. It was demonstrated that periodontal disease is a statistically significant risk factor for PLBW with adjusted odds ratio of 7.9 and 7.5 for all PLBW cases and primiparous PLBW cases, respectively. These data indicate that periodontal diseases represent a previously unrecognized and clinically significant risk factor for preterm low birth weight as a consequence of either PTL or preterm PROM.

BIBLIOGRAPHY

1. Corgel JO. Periodontal Medicine and the female patient. In, Rose LF, Genco RJ, Mealey BL, Cohen DW. Periodontal Medicine; 151-166.
2. Genco RJ, Offenbacher S, Beck J. Cardiovascular Diseases and Oral infections. In, Rose LF, Genco RJ, Mealey BL, Cohen DW. Periodontal Medicine; B.C. Decker Inc. 2000;63-82.
3. Grossi SG, Mealey BL, Rose LF. Effect of periodontal diseases on systemic health. In, Rose LF, Mealey BL, Genco RJ, Cohen DW. Periodontics, Medicine, Surgery and Implants. Elsevier Mosby 2004;846-59.
4. Grossi SG, Genco RJ. Periodontal Disease and Diabetes Mellitus: A Two-way Relationship. Ann Periodontol 1998;3:51-61.
5. Mealey BL. Diabetes mellitus. In, Rose LF, Genco RJ, Mealey BL, Cohen DW. Periodontal Medicine; B.C. Decker Inc. 2000;121-150.
6. Mealey BL, Klokkevold PR. Periodontal Medicine. In, Newman, Takei, Carranza. Clinical Periodontology 9th ed WB Saunders 2003;229-44.
7. Nishimura F, et al. Periodontal Disease as a complication of Diabetes Mellitus. Ann Periodontol 1998;3:20-9.
8. Scannapieco FA. Relationships between periodontal and respiratory diseases. In, Rose LF, Genco RJ, Mealey BL, Cohen DW. Periodontal Medicine B.C. Decker Inc. 2000;83-98.
9. Williams RC, David PD. Periodontitis as a risk for systemic disease. In, Lindhe J, Karring T, Lang NP. Clinical Periodontology and Implant dentistry. 4th ed Blackwell Munksgaard 2003;366-86.

PERIODONTICS REVISITED

Smoking and Periodontium

Shalu Bathla

INTRODUCTION

Tobacco smoking, mostly in the form of cigarette smoking, is recognized as the most important environmental risk factor for periodontal diseases. Smokeless tobacco use has been associated with oral leukoplakia and carcinoma. However, there do not appear to be any generalized effects on periodontal disease progression, other than localized attachment loss and recession at the site of tobacco product placement. Pindborg (1947) was one of the first investigators to study the relationship between smoking and periodontal disease. Smoking is associated with a wide spectrum of disease including hypertension, atherosclerosis, cancer, chronic lung disease, ischemic heart disease, hypercoagulability, coronary artery disease, stroke, esophageal reflux, peripheral vascular disease, peptic ulcer disease, spontaneous abortion, prematurity, low birth weight and delayed wound healing. Tobacco smoking affects the oral environment and ecology, the vasculature, the inflammatory response, the immune response and homeostasis and healing potential of the periodontal tissues. Thus, considered as a risk factor for periodontal diseases.

CLASSIFICATION OF SMOKERS

A. According to Centers for Disease Control (CDC) and Prevention, the smokers are classified as:
   i. *Current smokers*: Those that had smoked ≥ 100 cigarettes over their lifetime and smoked at the time of interview.
   ii. *Former smokers*: Those that had smoked ≥ 100 cigarettes over their lifetime but were not currently smoking.
   iii. *Non-smokers*: Those that had not smoked ≥ 100 cigarettes in their lifetime.
B. According to number of cigarettes smoked/day, smokers can be classified as:
   i. Heavy smokers-smoked ≥ 20 cigarettes/day.
   ii. Light smokers-smoked ≤ 19 cigarettes/day.

CONSTITUENTS OF TOBACCO SMOKE

Cigarette smoking is a very complex mixture of substance with over 4000 known constituents.
A. *Particulate phase include Nicotine and Cotinine*: The patient's exposure to tobacco smoke can be measured

in a number of ways including interviewing the subject using simple questionnaire and biochemical analysis. Cotinine is a metabolite of nicotine and cotinine measurements are more reliable in determining a subject's exposure to tobacco smoke because the half-life is 14-20 hours compared with the shorter half-life of nicotine which is 2-3 hours. Nicotine produces a wide variety of effects, i.e. inhibits apoptosis in certain cell lines (e.g. fibroblasts, osteoclasts), exaggerates immune system activities, etc. Tar (compound of many chemicals), Benzene and Benzo(a)pyrene are the other particulate constituents.

B. *Gas phase include*: Carbon monoxide (decreases the oxygen capacity of Haemoglobin), Ammonia, Dimethyl-nitrosamine, Formaldehyde, Hydrogen cyanide (inhibits enzyme system necessary for oxidative metabolism) and Acrolein.

EFFECTS OF SMOKING ON THE PREVALENCE AND SEVERITY OF PERIODONTAL DISEASE

Gingivitis: Following are the impact of smoking on gingival disease **(Fig. 16.1)**.

- *Gingival inflammation*: Smoking causes decrease in gingival inflammation.
- *Ginigival blood flow*: Smokers have less bleeding on probing due to vasoconstrictive action of nicotine on gingival tissues.
- *Oxygen tension*: Smokers do have lower oxygen saturation.

The suppressive effect on the gingival vasculature can be observed through less gingival redness, lower bleeding on probing and fewer vessels visible clinically and histologically.

Periodontitis: Following are the impact of smoking on periodontal disease **(Fig. 16.2)**.

- Prevalence and severity of periodontal destruction increases with smoking.

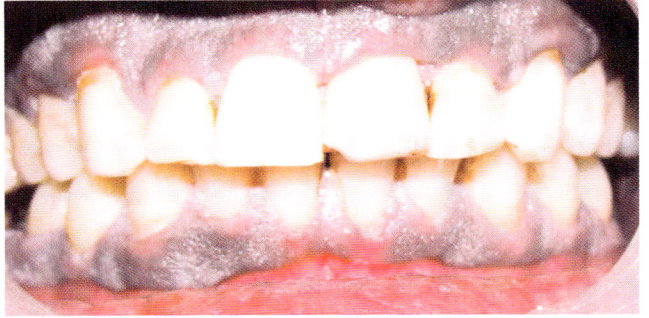

Fig. 16.1: Effects of smoking on gingiva—Decreased gingival inflammation and increased gingival pigmentation

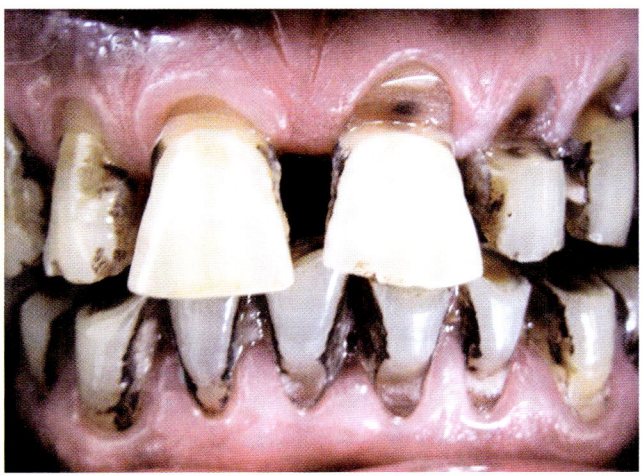

Fig. 16.2: Effect of smoking on periodontium—More attachment loss and bone loss

- *Pocket*: There are deeper probing depth and larger number of deep pocket in smokers.
- *Attachment and bone loss*: More attachment loss and bone loss are seen in smokers.
- In smokers there is increased rate of periodontal destruction and tooth loss.

EFFECTS OF SMOKING ON THE ETIOLOGY AND PATHOGENESIS OF PERIODONTAL DISEASE

Role of smoking in the pathogenesis of periodontal disease: Tobacco smoke contains powerful reducing agents such as carbon monoxide that produce a marked immediate reduction of redox potential at mucosal surfaces. The powerful physicochemical reducing activity of carbon monoxide is more likely a direct mechanism to promote growth of anaerobes at superficial sites. A second mechanism through which smoking might influence progression of periodontal disease, is an indirect microbiological effect through enhancing growth of bacteria that provide growth factors for anaerobes at shallow sites. A third mechanism through which the molecular byproducts of smoking influence progression of periodontitis by damaging the cells that normally protect the periodontal environment. Damage to leukocytes can interfere with clearance of bacteria from the periodontal environment. In the oral cavity, polymorphs are adversely affected by smoking. In common with diabetes, smoking produces advanced glycation endproducts (AGEs). AGE has recently been implicated in diabetes – associated periodontitis. AGE has damaging effects on vasculature, and AGE interferes

PERIODONTICS REVISITED

with cells such as polymorphs, proteins and lactoferrin involved in control of bacteria in tissues and at mucosal surfaces.

Microbiology: There is an alteration in the microbial challenge in smokers which is due to a qualitative rather than quantitative alteration in the plaque. Smoking has no effect on the rate of plaque accumulation but there is increase in colonization of shallow periodontal pockets by periodontal pathogen. Smokers had higher level of *Bacteroides forsythus* and were 2.3 times more likely to habor this microorganism than nonsmokers.

Physiology: Decreased GCF flow, blood flow and bleeding on probing is seen in smokers. The clinical signs of inflammation are less pronounced in smokers when compared with nonsmokers. Subgingival temperatures are lower in smokers than nonsmokers. Time needed to recover from local anesthesia is more in smoker as compared to non-smokers because recovery from the vasoconstriction caused by local anesthetic administration takes longer in smokers.

Immunology: Smoking exerts a major effect on the protective elements of the immune response, resulting in an increase in the extent and severity of periodontal destruction. In smokers, there is downregulation of the immune response to bacterial challenge **(Fig. 16.3)**.

Effects of smoking on the immune system:

There is altered neutrophil, chemotaxis and phagocytosis in smokers.
There is increased TNF-α, PGE$_2$ in smoker's GCF.
There is increased production of neutrophil, collagenase and elastase in smoker's GCF.
Nicotine suppresses osteoblast proliferation.
Nicotine adversely affect fibroblast functions.

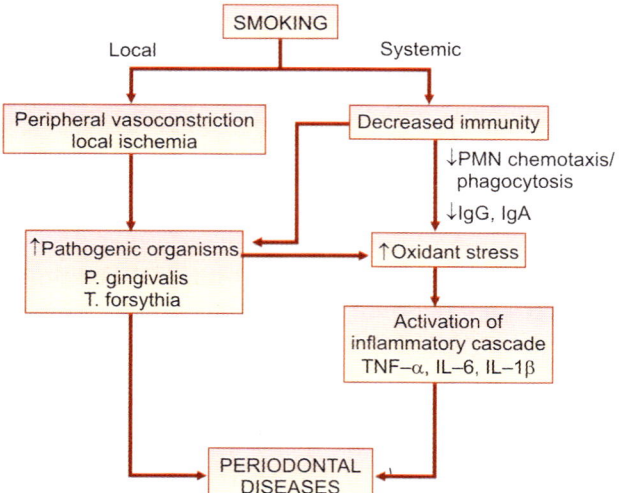

Fig. 16.3: Relationship between smoking and periodontal diseases

I. Effect of smoking on neutrophil function:
    a. Neutrophils transmigration across the periodontal microvasculature is impeded in tobacco smokers.
    b. *Neutrophils receptors*: Neutrophils express functional receptors for several components and metabolites of tobacco smoke, such as nicotine, cotinine (primarily the α3 β4 subtype of nicotinic receptors). The number of nicotinic receptors expressed by human neutrophils are increased in smokers and decline on cessation. Neutrophils also express several receptors for endogenous factors such as IL-8, ICAM-1 and TNF- α, whose natural agonists have been reported to be dysregulated in tobacco smokers.
    c. *Neutrophil derived degradative proteases*: Tobacco smoking increases the production of collagen - degrading enzymes, elastase, MMP-1 and MMP-8 and decreases the levels of major endogenous MMP inhibitors (tissue inhibitors of MMP-1, alpha-1-antitrypsin and alpha-2-macroglobulin).
    d. *Neutrophil respiratory burst*: The respiratory burst represent the oxygen-dependent processes by which neutrophils kill phagocytosed bacterial cells through the generation of multiple reactive oxygen and reactive nitrogen species. The cigarette smoke constitutents inhibit the respiratory burst of neutrophils. The gas-phase cigarette smoke may lead to a suppression of neutrophil NADPH oxidase.
    e. *Neutrophil migration and chemotaxis*: Smoking alter neutrophil chemotaxis and phagocytosis. The actin cytoskeleton is critical in facilitating neutrophil motility that is required for extravasation across the periodontal microvasculature and subsequent migration of neutrophils towards inflammatory stimuli and tobacco smoke exposure impair f-actin kinetics.

II. *Effect of smoking on T and B cell function*: In peripheral blood, there is decrease in proliferative response to polyclonal B cell activators (B cell mitogens) in smokers. Tobacco glycoprotein (a polyphenolic protein in tobacco) is potent B cell mitogens and stimulates production of immunoglobulin classes (IgM, IgG and IgA).

III. *Effect of smoking on osteoblasts*: Smoking suppress cellular proliferation and alkaline phosphatase activity in osteoblasts, thereby decrease the synthesis of bone matrix protein by interfering with oxygen levels in osteoblasts. Osteoclast cell remain longer and are able to continue resorption long after their normal lifecycle would have permitted.

IV. *Effect of smoking on fibroblasts*: Nicotine significantly inhibits proliferation of gingival fibroblast at high concentration. Thus, showing reduction in the production of type I collagen and fibronectin. Nicotine also inhibit periodontal fibroblast growth and attachment.

EFFECT OF SMOKING ON THE RESPONSE OF PERIODONTAL THERAPY

Phase I or non-surgical therapy:
- There is decreased clinical response to scaling and root planing.
- Pocket depth reduction is less in smokers.
- There is less gain in clinical attachment level.

Phase II or surgical phase therapy:
- There is less pocket depth reduction after surgery in smokers.
- After GTR procedure, there are greater chances of membrane exposure in smokers.
- There is less gain in clinical attachment level and bone fill.

Effect of Smoking on Implant surgery:

Smoking addiction is directly related to implant failure. Use of tobacco directly compromise the osseointegration of root-form dental implants. The combination of smoking and plaque-induced inflammation significantly influences bone loss around the implants.

Phase IV or Maintenance therapy:
- There is increase in pocket depth during maintenance phase in smokers.
- Gain in clinical attachment level is lesser in smoker as compared to nonsmokers.

SMOKING CESSATION

Basic Steps of Smoking Cessation Program

Basic steps known as 4 A's for smoking cessation was first proposed by Marc Manley and Thomas Glynn of National Cancer Institute.
- Ask- Identify the tobacco use status of every patient
- Advice- Increase the tobacco user's interest in quitting
- Assist- Help those who are ready with their problem solving skills and with pharmacotherapy
- Arrange- Arrange follow-up support throughout the quitting process.

Periodontal Effects of Smoking Cessation

Smoking cessation is beneficial to periodontal health and periodontal treatment outcomes. Periodontal disease progression slows down in patients who quit smoking. Smoking cessation may even restore the normal periodontal and microbial healing responses. The healing response of ex-smokers can even become similar to that of nonsmokers. Smoking is known to influence the composition of subgingival microflora in patients with periodontitis. Therefore, a combination of antibiotic therapy and participation in a smoking cessation program may be the most effective treatment of smoking induced periodontal diseases.

LANDMARK STUDIES RELATED

Haffajee AD, Socransky SS. Relationship of cigarette smoking to attachment level profiles. Journal of Clinical Periodontology 2001;28;283-95.

In this study 289 chronic periodontitis subjects ranging in age from 20 to 86 years with at least 20 teeth and at least 4 sites with pocket depth and or attachment level >4 mm were recruited. Subjects were subset according to smoking history into never, past and current smokers. Measures of plaque accumulation, overt gingivitis, bleeding on probing, suppuration, probing pocket depth and probing attachment level were taken at 6 sites per tooth. It was found that current smokers had significantly more attachment loss, deeper pockets and fewer sites exhibiting bleeding on probing than past or never smokers.

Haffajee AD, Socransky SS. Relationship of cigarette smoking to the subgingival microbiota. Journal of Clinical Periodontology 2001;28:377-88.

A total of 272 adult subjects ranging in age from 20 - 86 years with at least 20 teeth who were never, past or current smokers were recruited for study. Counts, proportions and prevalence of 29 subgingival species determined using checkerboard DNA-DNA hybridization and compared among the subjects. Subgingival plaque samples were taken from the mesial surface of all teeth in each subject and assayed individually. Members of orange and red complexes including: *E. nodatum, F. nucleatum, P. intermedia, P. micros, P. nigrescens, B. forsythus, P. gingivalis* and *T. denticola* were significantly more prevalent in current smokers than in the other two groups.

PERIODONTICS REVISITED

POINTS TO PONDER

✓ *Relationship of smoking and vitamin C*: Cigarette smoking is known to contain numerous oxidants causing tissue damage. OH⁻ radical can mediate tissue damage and accumulation of hydroperoxide, which can disrupt membrane functions. Vitamin C is known as scavenger of OH⁻ radicals, hypochlorous acid, strong oxidative agent. These radicals can activate both neutrophil derived and GCF collagenase and this oxidative activation can be prevented by Vitamin C, which is a potent antioxidant.

BIBLIOGRAPHY

1. Bain CA, May PK. The association between the failure of dental implants and cigarette smoking. Int J Oral Maxillofacial Implants 1993;8:609-15.
2. Eggert FM, McLeod MH, Flowerdew G. Effects of smoking and treatment status on periodontal bacteria: evidence that smoking influences control of periodontal bacteria at the mucosal surface of the gingival crevice. J Periodontol 2001;72:1210-20.
3. Grossi SG, Zambon J, Machtie EE, et al. Effects of smoking and smoking cessation on healing after mechanical periodontal therapy. JADA 1997; 128: 599 - 607.
4. Henemyre CL, Scales DK, Hokett SD, Cuenin MF, Peacock ME, Parker MH, Brewer PD, Chuang AH. Nicotine Stimulates Osteoclast Resorption in a Porcine Marrow Cell Model. J Periodontol 2003;74:1440-46.
5. Lindhe J, Karring T, Lang NP. Modifying factors: Diabetes, Puberty, Pregnancy and the Menopause and Tobacco smoking. In, Clinical Periodontology and Implant dentistry. 4th ed Blackwell Munksgaard 2003;179-97.
6. Novak MJ, Novak KF. Smoking and periodontal disease. In, Newman, Takei, Carranza. Clinical Periodontology 9th ed WB Saunders 2003;245-53.
7. Palmer RM, Wilson RF, Hasan AS, Scott DA. Mechanism of action of environmental factors- tobacco smoking. J Clin Periodontol 2005;32:180-95.
8. Winkel EG, Van Winkelhoff AJ, Timmerman MF, et al. Amoxicillin plus metronidazole in the treatment of adult periodontitis patients. A double-blind placebo controlled study. J Clin Periodontol 2001;28:296-305.
9. Zambon JJ, Grossi SG, Machtei EE et al. Cigarette smoking increases the risk for subgingival infection with periodontal pathogens. J Periodontol 1996;67:1050.

MCQs

1. Smoking affects periodontal inflammation in following ways:
   A. Clinical signs of inflammation are less pronounced
   B. Increases the GCF flow, bleeding on probing are less pronounced
   C. Clinical signs of inflammation are more pronounced
   D. Both A and B
2. Smoking has adverse effect on the following:
   A. B cells   B. T cells
   C. Neutrophils   D. All of the above
3. Those that had not smoked ≥ 100 cigarettes in their lifetime are:
   A. Nonsmoker
   B. Former smoker
   C. Current smoker
   D. All of the above

Answers

1. D   2. D   3. A

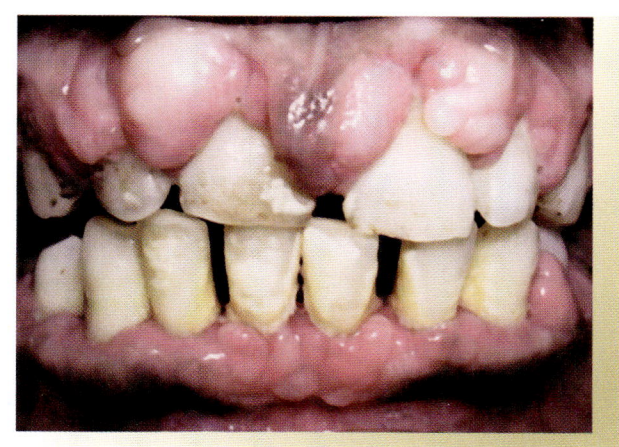

PATHOLOGY
OF
GINGIVAL
AND
PERIODONTAL
DISEASES

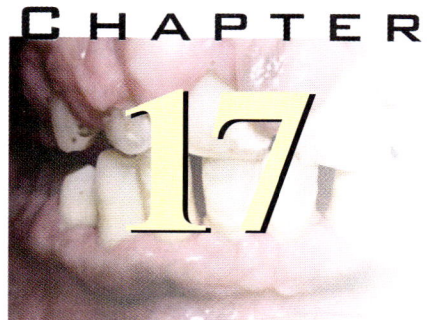

CHAPTER
17

Defense Mechanisms of Gingiva

Shalu Bathla

INTRODUCTION

The gingival tissue is constantly subjected to mechanical and bacterial aggressions. The saliva, the epithelial surface and the initial stages of the inflammatory response provide resistance to these actions. In this chapter defensive role of junctional epithelium, PMNs, saliva and gingival crevicular fluid (GCF) are discussed.

JUNCTIONAL EPITHELIUM

It is commonly accepted that the junctional epithelium exhibits several unique structural and functional features that contribute to prevent pathogenic bacterial flora from colonizing the subgingival tooth surface. First, junctional epithelium is firmly attached to the tooth and thus forms an epithelial barrier against the plaque bacteria. Second, it allows the access of GCF, inflammatory cells and components of the immunological host defense to the gingival margin. Third, junctional epithelial cells exhibit rapid turnover, which contributes to the host-parasite equilibrium and rapid repair of damaged tissue. Junctional epithelium consists of active populations of

cells and antimicrobial functions, which together form the first line of defense against microbial invasion into the underlying tissue **(Fig. 17.1)**.

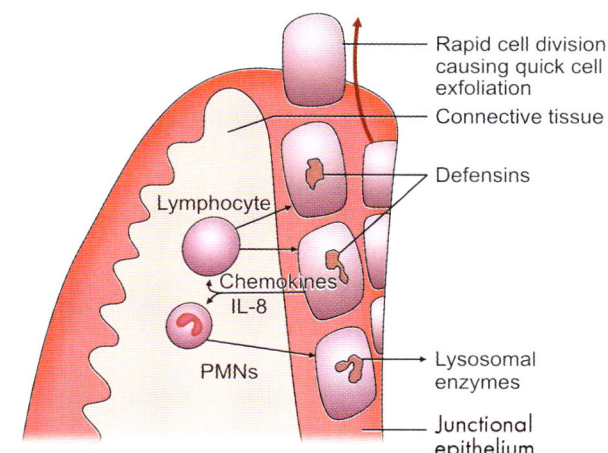

Junctional epithelial cells release chemokines IL-8 that attract and activate neutrophils and lymphocytes. Defensins and lysosomal enzymes and the active antimicrobial substances are also produced by junctional epithelial cells

Fig. 17.1: Antimicrobial mechanisms of junctional epithelium

POLYMORPHONUCLEAR LEUKOCYTES

Polymorphonuclear leukocytes form the most important line of defense against bacterial plaque at the gingival margin. When the polymorphonuclear leukocytes reach the bacteria, they release the contents of their granules and adhere to bacteria and phagocytose them. The polymorphonuclear leukocytes form a protective wall against plaque. Therefore, polymorphonuclear leukocytes are a major contributor in the host–parasite equilibrium but have a limited capacity to reclaim any tooth surface once lost to the plaque bacteria. On the other hand, activated polymorphonuclear leukocytes can cause tissue damage as a result of a variety of enzymes, oxygen metabolites, and other components that are released from their granules during the battle against microbes. (Rest is explained in chapter no. 11 Immunity and Inflammation).

SALIVA

Saliva exerts a major influence on plaque initiation, maturation and metabolism. Salivary flow and composition also influence calculus formation, periodontal disease and caries. In humans, an increase in inflammatory gingival diseases, dental caries, and rapid tooth destruction associated with cervical or cemental caries is partially a consequence of decreased salivary gland secretion (xerostomia). The normal and xerostomic values of stimulated saliva is approx. 1-2 ml/min and less than 0.5 ml/min respectively. Xerostomia may result from a variety of factors, among them are sialolithiasis, sarcoidosis, Sjögren's syndrome, Mikulicz's disease, irradiation and surgical removal of the salivary glands. Salivary secretions are protective in nature because they maintain the oral tissues in a physiologic state. Saliva exerts a major influence on plaque by mechanically cleansing the exposed oral surfaces, by buffering acids produced by bacteria, and by controlling bacterial activity.

Composition of Saliva

1. Electrolytes include potassium, sodium, chloride, bicarbonate, calcium, magnesium and phosphorus
2. Organic:
   A. Protein includes:
      - Acinar cell families: Mucin, proline rich proteins and glycoproteins, histatins, statherin, cystatins, amylase, peroxidases and carbonic anhydrases
      - Ductal and stromal products include lactoferrin, lysozyme, secretory IgA, kallikrein and fibronectin.
   B. Lipids
   C. Carbohydrates
   D. Sulfates.

Role of Saliva

In Oral Health

1. Saliva provides physical protection via mucin and glycoprotein.
2. It helps in lubrication via glycoprotein and mucin.
3. Antibacterial action of saliva is because of the presence of IgA, salivary amylase, lactoferrin, salivary peroxidase, proline rich protein and lysozyme.

   Secretory IgA (sIgA) present in saliva provides the first line of defense via immunologic means in the oral cavity. sIgA binds to microbes which inhibit their adherence to hard and soft tissue surfaces and thus, hindering microbial invasion into deeper host tissues. It plays important role in viral neutralization, attenuation of viral growth and replication on oral surfaces. It also neutralizes and disposes toxins and food antigens.

   Lactoferrin acts against *Actinobacillus* and *Streptococcus*.

   Salivary lacto-thiocyanate peroxidase enzyme catalyses the oxidation of thiocyanate ion (SCN) by H_2O_2, generating highly reactive, oxidized form of thiocyanate ($OSCN^-$), causing direct toxicity to *Streptococcus*. It neutralizes deleterious effects of H_2O_2 produced by a number of oral microorganisms. Lysozyme causes lysis of cell wall of *Aggregatibacter actinomycetemcomitans* and *Veilonella*.
4. Saliva aids in tooth integrity via histatin, statherin and cystatin.
5. Cleansing action of saliva is due to its physical flow.
6. Buffering action of saliva is due to presence of urea and arginine rich protein. *Carbonic anhydrase* causes the reversible hydration of carbon dioxide leading to the formation of bicarbonate, which contributes to the buffering capacity.
7. Saliva provides data for diagnostic testing.
8. Saliva hasten the blood coagulation and protects wound from bacterial invasion due to presence of some coagulating factors.
9. Saliva helps in swallowing and formation of food bolus.
10. Saliva also helps in speech.

In Oral Diseases

1. Saliva helps in the formation of pellicle and thus, plaque deposition.
2. It also aids in plaque mineralization to form calculus.
3. Saliva affects dental caries by cleansing mechanically and by direct antibacterial activity.

Defense mechanisms of oral cavity are due to:

Saliva
Sulcular fluid
Intact epithelial barrier- Junctional epithelium
Presence of normal beneficial flora
Local antibody production
Migrating PMNs and other leukocytes.

GINGIVAL CREVICULAR FLUID (GCF)

GCF is an exudate of varying composition found in the sulcus/periodontal pocket between the tooth and marginal gingiva. GCF is a complex mixture of serum, inflammatory cells, connective tissue, epithelium, and microbial flora inhabiting the gingival margin or the sulcus/pocket. In the healthy sulcus, the amount of GCF is very small. GCF provides a unique window for analysis of periodontal condition.

Methods of Collection of GCF

Many collection methods have been tried some of them are:

I. Absorbing filter paper strips **(Fig. 17.2)**.
   1. *Intracrevicular:* The strip is being inserted into gingival crevice. The intracrevicular method is the most frequently used method which can be further subdivided depending upon whether the strip is inserted just at the entrance of the crevice or is inserted to the base of the pocket until resistance is encountered.
   2. *Extracrevicular*: The strips are overlaid on the gingival crevice region in an attempt to minimize trauma.
      The advantages associated with this method of collection of GCF are:
      a. Quick, easy to use
      b. Can be applied to individual sites.
      c. Least traumatic when correctly used.
II. *Preweighed twisted threads:* Preweighed twisted threads were used by Weinstein et al. The threads are placed in the gingival crevice around the tooth

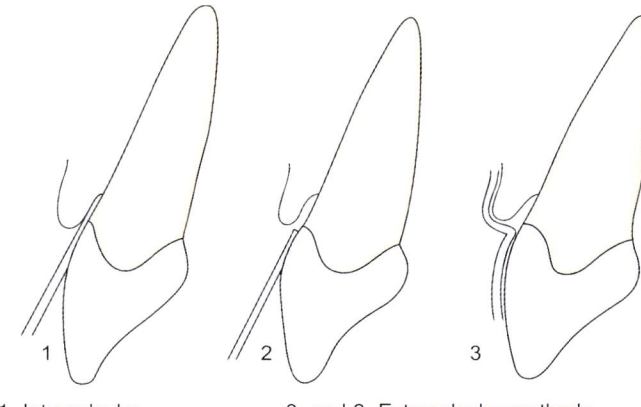

1. Intrasulcular   2. and 3. Extrasulcular methods

Fig. 17.2: Collection of GCF through filter strip in gingival sulcus

and the amount of fluid collected is estimated by weighing the sample thread.

III. *Micropipettes or capillary tubing:* Following the isolation and drying of a site, capillary tubes of known internal diameter are inserted at the entrance of the gingival crevice. GCF from the crevice migrates into the tube by capillary action and because the internal diameter is known the volume of the fluid collected can be accurately determined by measuring the distance, the GCF has migrated. Advantage of this technique is that it provides an undiluted sample of native GCF whose volume can be accurately assessed. The limitations of this technique are that it is difficult to hold capillary tube at the entrance of gingival crevice for such lengthy periods and it is also difficult to remove the complete sample from the tubing.

IV. *Gingival washing methods:* Gingival sulcus is perfused with an isotonic solution such as Hank's balanced salt solution of fixed volume. Two methods are used: one is the simplest method involving the instillation and re-aspiration of 10 µl of Hank's balanced salt solution at the interdental papilla. It is repeated 12 times to allow thorough mixing of transport solution and GCF, second method is more complicated which involves the construction of a customized acrylic stent that isolates the gingival tissue from the rest of the mouth. The tissues are irrigated for 15 minutes with a saline solution, using a peristaltic pump and the diluted GCF is removed.

Limitations of this method are:

- Production of customized acrylic stents is complicated and technically demanding.

PERIODONTICS REVISITED

- It is been useful only in maxillary arch, due to the difficulties of producing a technically satisfactory appliance for the mandibular arch.
- GCF from individual sites cannot be analyzed.
- All the fluid may not be recovered during the aspiration and re-aspiration procedures.
- Precise dilution factor cannot be determined.

V. Other strips like plastic strips or platinum loops are placed along the long axis of the tooth or inserted into the sulcus and pressure is applied to collect the crevicular fluid.

Measurement of GCF

Amount of GCF collected is measured by the following ways:

i. *By direct viewing and staining:* Stain the strip with ninhydrin to produce purple color in the area, where GCF has accumulated and then measure. The disadvantage of this method is that it is not easily applied at the chairside.

ii. *By weighing:* Strip is weighed before and after collecting the GCF sample.

iii. *By electronic device periotron:* Sample strip paper (Periopaper), is inserted between the two jaws of periotron. The wetness of the paper strip affects the flow of an electronic current and gives a digital readout on the screen. The technique is rapid and has no discernible effect upon the GCF sample. Three models of Periotron have been produced (the 600, 6000 and now the 8000) to measure the volume of fluid collected on filter paper strips.

Translation of Periotron values to clinical conditions and Gingival Index with which they are associated:

The amount of GCF is extremely less, i.e. 0.5 to 2.4 µl/day. The mean GCF volume in proximal spaces of anterior and molar teeth are 0.24 to 0.43 µl and 0.43 to 1.56 µl respectively.

Following are the problems associated with GCF collection and data interpretation:

Periotron reading	Level of gingival inflammation	Gingival Index
0–20	Healthy	0
21–40	Mild	1
41–80	Moderate	2
81–200	Severe	3

- *Contamination:* Usually sample is contaminated with blood, saliva or plaque. Frank blood contamination is usually dealt with by discarding the sample and removing the data from analysis.
- *Small sample size:* The amount of GCF collected is extremely small.
- *Sampling time:* Prolonged sampling at the site resulted in protein concentrations approaching those of serum.
- *Volume determination:* Evaporation is a significant problem in accurate volume determination of GCF samples.
- *Recovery of strips:* It depends on type of paper, binding of GCF protein to the filter paper and concentration of the original protein sample.

Composition of GCF

1. *Cellular elements:* Epithelial cells, leukocytes and bacteria
2. *Electrolytes:* Sodium, potassium and calcium
3. *Organic compounds:* Carbohydrates, proteins (immunoglobulins and complement components) and lipids.
4. *Metabolic and bacterial products:* Lactic acid, hydroxyproline, prostaglandins, urea, endotoxins, cytotoxic substances and antibacterial factors.
5. *Enzymes and enzyme inhibitors:* Acid phosphatase, alkaline phosphatase, pyrophosphatase, β–glucuronidase, lysozymes, hyaluronidase, proteolytic enzymes (Mammalian proteinases, bacterial proteinases, serum proteinases inhibitors), lactic dehydrogenase, etc.

Functions of GCF

1. It washes the sulcus, carries out shed epithelial cells, leukocytes and microbes.
2. It contains many antimicrobial agents.
3. It carries neutrophils and macrophages for phagocytosing bacteria.
4. It transports immunoglobins and other immune factors to destroy microorganisms.
5. The monitoring of GCF and quality of its contents is used diagnostically to assess the severity of gingival inflammation, effectiveness of oral hygiene, response of tissues to periodontal therapy and effectiveness of chemotherapeutic agents.

Clinical Significance

1. *Inflammation:* During inflammation the GCF flow increases and its composition starts to resemble that of an inflammatory exudate. The increased GCF flow contributes to host defense by flushing bacterial colonies and their metabolites away from the sulcus and restricting their penetration into the tissue. Thus, the amount of GCF is greater when inflammation is present and is proportional to the severity of inflammation.

2. *Mechanical stimulation:* GCF production is increased by toothbrushing and gingival massage.

3. *Sex hormones:* Estrogen and progesterone increases the flow by increasing the permeability of gingival blood vessels. Pregnancy, ovulation, and hormonal contraceptives all increase gingival fluid production.

4. *Periodontal therapy:* GCF production is increased during the healing period after periodontal surgery.

5. *Smoking:* Smoking produces an immediate transient increase in GCF flow.

6. *Circadian periodicity:* There is increase in the GCF production from 6 am to 10 pm and decreases afterward.

7. The majority of new diagnostic tests for periodontal disease utilize gingival crevice fluid (GCF). The major attraction of GCF, as a diagnostic marker is the site-specific nature of the sample. This allows laboratory investigations of GCF constituents to be linked to clinical assessments at the site of sample collection.

LANDMARK STUDIES RELATED

Brill N, Krasse B. The passage of tissue fluid into clinically healthy gingival pocket. Acta Odontol Scand 1958;16:233-45.

The fluorescein dye was injected intravenously into animal's hind legs and discovered that it could penetrate into the epithelial lining of the gingival sulcus. Fluorescein could also be collected on the strips of filter paper introduced into the sulcus in over 90% of the animals as quickly as one and a half minutes after administration. These findings suggested that the epithelium lining of the gingival sulcus was permeable to small molecular weight compounds and that the passage of tissue fluid into the sulcus acts as a possible defense mechanism that may play an important role in the homeostasis of the crevicular environment.

POINTS TO PONDER

✓ Organulocytes are the living PMNs in saliva.

✓ Factors VIII, IX, X, Plasma thromboplastin antecedent (PTA) and Hageman factor are the coagulation factors present in saliva.

✓ The drugs that cause xerostomia are anticholinergics, antipsychotics, antiparkinsonian, antidepressants, antihistaminics and antihypertensives.

✓ 1:3 ratio is the normal ratio of B lymphocytes to T lymphocytes in GCF.

✓ Various drugs excreted through GCF are Tetracyclines, Metronidazole, Clindamycin, Tinidazole and Erythromycin.

BIBLIOGRAPHY

1. Bulkacz J, Carranza FA. Defence mechanisms of gingiva. In, Newman, Takei, Carranza. Clinical Periodontology 9th ed WB Saunders 2003;254-62.
2. Delima AJ, VanDyke TE. Origin and function of the cellular compoments in gingival crevice fluid. Periodontol 2000 2003;31:55-76.
3. Griffiths GS. Formation, collection and significance of gingival crevice fluid. Periodontol 2000 2003;31:32-42.
4. Grant DA, Stern IB, Listgarten MA. Saliva. In, Periodontics. 6th ed CV Mosby Company 1988;76-93.
5. Scannapieco FA, Levine MJ. Saliva and dental pellicles. In, Genco RJ, Goldman HM, Cohen DW. Contemporary Periodontics CV Mosby Company 1990;117-25.
6. Pollanen MT, Salonen JI, Vitto VJ. Structure and function of the tooth–epithelial interface in health and disease. Periodontol 2000 2003;31:12-31.
7. The periodontal tissues. In, Eley BM, Manson JD. Periodontics 5th ed Wright 2004;1-20.
8. Uitto VJ. Gingival crevice fluid – an introduction. Periodontol 2000 2003;31:9-11

MCQs

1. Electronic instrument used to measure GCF is:
   A. PeriCheck
   B. Periotemp
   C. Perioscan
   D. Periotron

2. Drug which reaches maximum concentration in gingival fluid is:
   A. Tetracycline   B. Penicillin
   C. Erythromycin   D. Sulphonamide

3. The sources of collagenase in GCF can be:
   A. Fibroblast   B. PMN leukocyte
   C. Bacteria   D. All of the above

PERIODONTICS REVISITED

4. Which of the following does not increase the flow of crevicular fluid:
   A. Gingival inflammation
   B. Smoking
   C. Trauma from occlusion
   D. Toothbrushing
5. The gingival fluid can be collected by:
   A. Absorbing paper strips
   B. Microcapillary pipettes
   C. Gingival washings
   D. Any of the above

6. The predominant immunoglobulin in gingival fluid is:
   A. IgA
   B. IgG
   C. IgM
   D. IgE

Answers

1. D   2. A   3. D   4. C   5. D
6. B

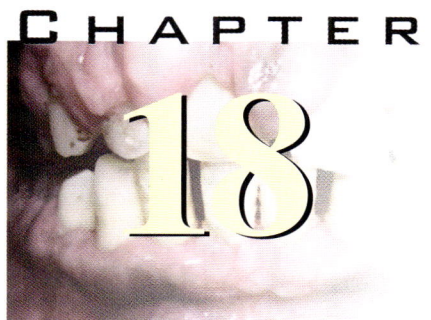

CHAPTER 18

Gingival Inflammation

SK Salaria, Shalu Bathla

INTRODUCTION

Inflammation of gingiva is called gingivitis. Most forms of periodontal diseases are plaque-associated disorders which start as an overt inflammation of the gingiva. In susceptible individuals, if inflammation is left untreated it may spread to involve deeper portions of the periodontium. This chapter will describe extent, duration, distribution, stages, clinical manifestations and sequelae of gingival diseases induced by bacterial plaque.

CLASSIFICATION

I. According to duration:
    1. *Acute gingivitis:* It is sudden in onset and of short duration which is painful.
    2. *Chronic gingivitis:* It is slow in onset and of long duration, and is painless, unless complicated by acute or subacute exacerbations. It is the most common type of gingivitis.
II. According to distribution:
    1. *Localized gingivitis:* Gingivitis confined to the gingiva of a single tooth or group of teeth **(Fig. 18.1)**.
    2. *Generalized gingivitis:* Involves the entire mouth.

3. *Marginal gingivitis:* Involves the gingival margin and may include a portion of the contiguous attached gingiva **(Fig. 18.2)**.

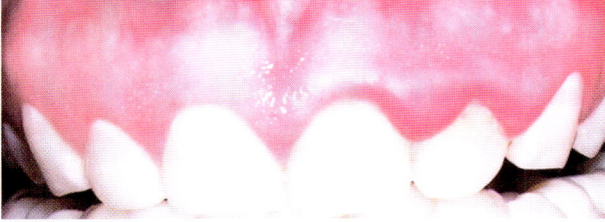

Fig. 18.1: Localized gingivitis in left maxillary anterior region

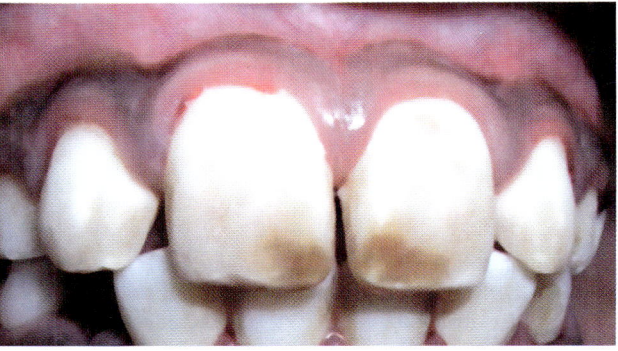

Fig. 18.2: Marginal gingivitis

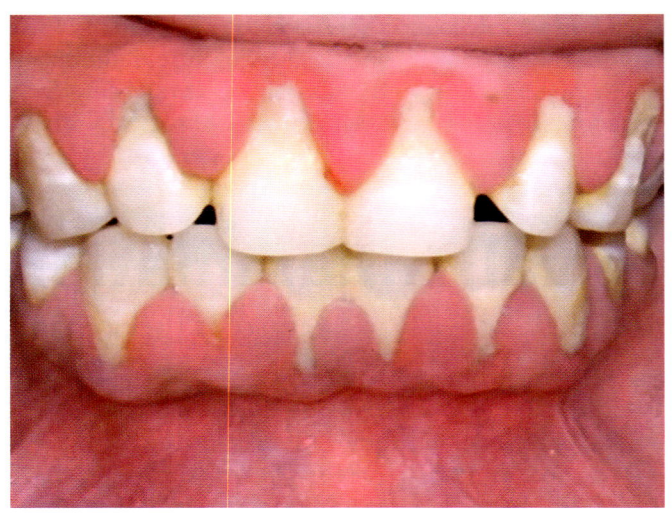

Fig. 18.3: Papillary gingivitis

4. *Papillary gingivitis:* Involves the interdental papillae and often extends into the adjacent portion of the gingival margin **(Fig. 18.3)**.
5. *Diffuse gingivitis:* Affects the gingival margin, the attached gingiva and the interdental papillae.

STAGES OF GINGIVITIS

Page and Schroeder developed a system to categorize the clinical and histopathological stages of periodontal diseases and defined four histopathological stages of periodontal inflammatory changes: The initial, early and established gingival lesions and an advanced periodontal lesion **(Fig. 18.4)**. It is important to note that the evidence available at that time largely consisted of animal and human adolescent biopsies. Their description, based on these material, is now considered to be not fully applicable to the normal adult situation.

Kinane and Lindhe recently classified healthy gingiva into two types:
• Super healthy or 'pristine' state, which histologically has little or no inflammatory infiltrate.
• 'Clinically healthy' gingiva, which looks similar clinically, but histologically, has features of an inflammatory infiltrate.

In everyday, clinical situations one would normally see the healthy gingiva type and only in exceptional circumstances, such as in a clinical trial with supervised daily cleaning and professional assistance, one would

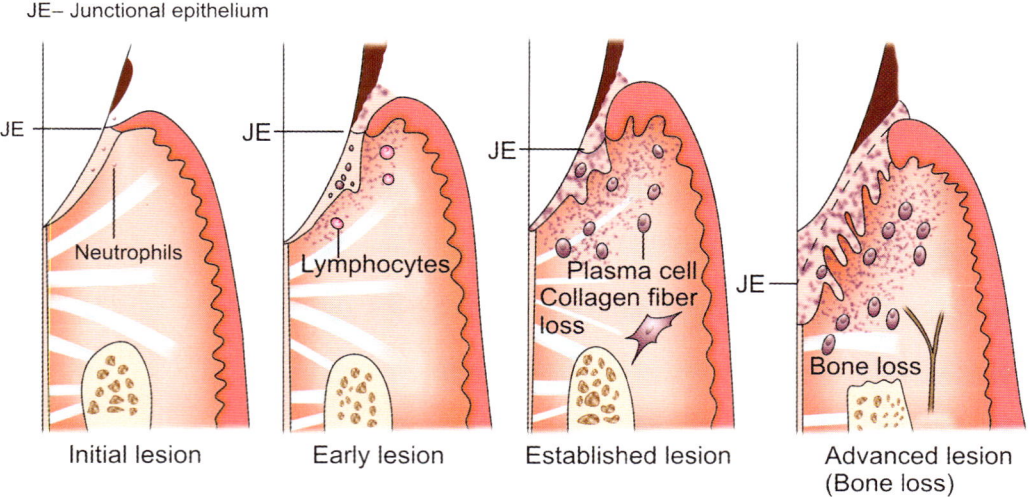

Fig. 18.4: Stages of gingivitis

Stage	Time	Immune cells	Clinical findings
I Initial lesion	2-4 days	PMNs	Increase in gingival flow
II Early lesion	4-7 days	Lymphocytes	Erythema, bleeding on probing
III Established	14-21 days	Plasma cells	Change in color, size, texture

see pristine gingiva. The initial and early lesion descriptions were thought to reflect the histopathology of clinically early stages of gingivitis, while the established lesion reflected the histopathology of more chronic gingivitis. The description of the histopathology of the advanced lesion was considered to reflect the progression of gingivitis to periodontitis.

Stage I: The Initial Lesion

Initial changes in the development of gingivitis occur after 2 to 4 days of plaque accumulation. The first manifestations of gingival inflammation are vascular changes which include dilation of arterioles, capillaries and venules of the dentogingival plexus and increased blood flow. There is increase in the permeability of the microvascular bed resulting in exudation of fluids and proteins into the tissues. As the lesion enlarges, and gingival crevicular fluid flow increases, noxious substances from microbes will be diluted both in the tissue and the crevice. The quantities of leukocytes, mainly polymorphonuclear neutrophils (PMNs) are increased in the connective tissue, the junctional epithelium and the gingival sulcus. The recruitment of leukocytes (predominantly PMNs) from the tissues to the crevice is due to the chemoattractant actions of the host systems (interleukin-8, C5a) and products derived from the biofilm (lipopolysaccharide). Thus, the increase in the migration of leukocytes and their accumulation within the gingival sulcus is correlated with an increase in the flow of gingival fluid into the sulcus. There is little or no proliferation of junctional epithelium laterally (rete pegs). Collagen depletion within the infiltrated area is noted along with an increase in vascular structures. Exudative and transudative fluid and plasma proteins arrive in the gingival crevice region.

Stage II: The Early Lesion

Initial lesion may be transitory and may be quickly repaired after the removal of plaque. But after 4 to 7 days of plaque accumulation, the clinical signs of erythema appear. There is proliferation of capillaries and increased formation of capillary loops between rete pegs or ridges and thus, bleeding on probing is evident. Lymphocytes (mainly T lymphocytes) and PMNs are predominant at this stage and very few plasma cells are noted within the lesion. 70% of the collagen is destroyed around the cellular infiltrate. The main fiber groups affected appear to be the circular and dentogingival fiber assemblies. The junctional epithelium develops widened intracellular spaces that are infiltrated mainly by neutrophils and small numbers of mononuclear cells, especially monocytes.

Stage III: The Established Lesion

The gingiva gives bluish hue due to engorged and congested blood vessels. Venous return is impaired, and the blood flow becomes sluggish. Extravasation of red blood cells (RBCs) into the connective tissue and breakdown of hemoglobin into its component pigments can also deepen the color of the chronically inflamed gingiva. There is increased fluid exudation and leukocyte migration into the tissues and the gingival crevice. The established lesion as defined by Page and Schroeder is dominated by plasma cells. Collagen loss continues in both lateral and apical directions as the inflammatory cell infiltrate expands, resulting in collagen depleted spaces extending deeper into the tissues which are then available for leukocytic infiltration. The dentogingival epithelium continues to proliferate and the rete pegs extend deeper into the connective tissue in an attempt to maintain epithelial integrity and a barrier to microbial entry. The junctional epithelium is no longer closely attached to the tooth surface. There is no evidence of alveolar bone loss at this stage, or of apical migration of junctional epithelium. Within 2 to 4 weeks after the beginning of plaque accumulation, the gingivitis become established. Migrating leukocytes are found in the junctional epithelium, within widened intercellular spaces.

Stage IV: Advanced Lesion

This is the final stage called as the advanced lesion. The inflammatory cell infiltrate extends laterally and further apically into the connective tissue. The advanced lesion has all the characteristics of the established lesion but differs importantly in that alveolar bone loss occurs, fiber damage is extensive and the junctional epithelium migrates apically from the cementoenamel junction (CEJ). It is generally accepted that plasma cells are the dominant cell type in the advanced lesion.

CLINICAL FEATURES OF GINGIVITIS

Gingival Bleeding

Gingival bleeding is one of the earliest symptoms of gingival inflammation. Gingival bleeding varies in severity, duration, and the ease with which it is provoked. Gingival bleeding is mainly due to the dilation and engorgement of capillaries. Permeability of the sulcular epithelium is increased by degradation of

PERIODONTICS REVISITED

intercellular cementing substances and widening of intercellular spaces. As the inflammation becomes chronic, ulceration of sulcular epithelium takes place. Because the capillaries are engorged and closer to the surface and epithelium being ulcerated and less protective, stimuli that are ordinally innocuous causes rupture of capillaries and gingival bleeding.

Etiological factors responsible for gingival bleeding are:

A. Local factors:
   a. *Acute bleeding*: Aggressive toothbrushing, sharp pieces of hard food, gingival burns from hot food or chemicals and necrotizing ulcerative gingivitis.
   b. *Chronic bleeding*: Chronic gingival inflammation.
B. Systemic factors:
   a. *Vascular abnormality*: Vitamin C deficiency and allergy such as Henoch Schönlein purpura
   b. *Vitamin K deficiency*.
   c. *Platelet disorder*: Idiopathic thrombocytopenic purpura.
   d. *Deficient platelet thromboplastic factors*: Uremia, multiple myeloma and postrubella purpura.
   e. *Coagulation defects*: Hemophilia, Christmas disease.
   f. *Malignancy*: Leukemia.
   g. *Drugs*: Salicylates and anticoagulants (dicoumarol, heparin).

Significance of gingival bleeding: Bleeding on probing is easily detectable clinically and therefore, is of value for the early diagnosis and prevention of more advanced gingivitis. It is a more objective sign and therefore requires less subjective estimation by the examiner. It appears earlier than other visual signs of inflammation. Thus, several gingival indices have been developed based on this earliest sign. Gingival bleeding on probing helps to determine whether the lesion is an active or inactive.

Changes in Gingival Color

The normal gingival color is coral pink which is produced mainly by the vascular supply and modified by overlying keratinized layer. The gingiva become red when there is an increase in vascularization and reduction of keratinization. Color changes vary with the intensity of the inflammation. Initially, there is an increasingly red erythema.

Factors responsible for change in gingival color are:

A. Color changes associated with local factors:
   a. Acute gingivitis:
      • NUG- marginal bright red erythema. In severe acute inflammation, the red color gradually

becomes a dull, whitish gray **(Fig. 18.5)**. The gray discoloration produced by tissue necrosis is demarcated from the adjacent gingiva by a thin, sharply defined erythematous zone.
      • Herpetic gingivostomatitis: Diffuse
      • Chemical irritations: Patch like/diffuse
   b. *Chronic gingivitis*: Chronic inflammation intensifies the red or bluish red color because of vascular proliferation and reduction of keratinization due to epithelial compression by the inflamed tissue.
   c. *Metallic pigmentation*: Gingival pigmentation from systemically absorbed metals results from perivascular precipitation of metallic sulfides in the subepithelial connective tissue. Gingival pigmentation is not a result of systemic toxicity. It occurs only in areas of inflammation, where the increased permeability of irritated blood vessels permits seepage of the metal into the surrounding tissue.
      • Bismuth pigmentation – Black line
      • Arsenic pigmentation – Black
      • Mercury pigmentation – Black line
      • Lead pigmentation – Bluish red, deep blue or gray (Burtonian line)
      • Silver pigmentation – Voilet marginal line
B. Color changes associated with systemic factors:
   a. Endogenous factors:
      • Addison's disease – Increased Melanin pigmentation
      • Peutz-Jeghers syndrome – Increased Melanin pigmentation
      • Albright's syndrome – Increased Melanin pigmentation

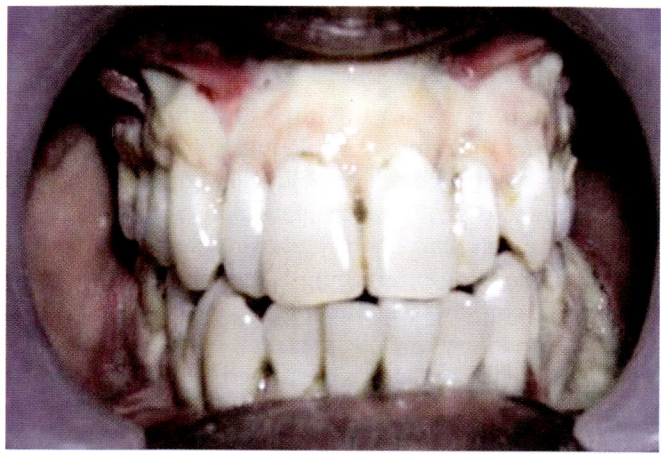

Fig. 18.5: NUG (*Courtesy:* Dr Ambika)

- Jaundice – Yellowish color due to depostion of bilirubin
- Hemochromatosis – Bluish gray due to depostion of Iron
- Diabetes
- Pregnancy
- Blood dyscrasias
- Hyperthyroidism
- Drugs—Chloroquine (slate gray), Minocycline (brown), Chlorpromazine, Zidovudine, Ketoconazole, Methyldopa and Busulphan.
  b. Exogenous factors:
- Tobacco/smoking—Grayish color due to increased melanin pigmentation
- Amalgam – Localized bluish black areas **(Fig. 18.6)**
- Coloring agents in food, lozenges and betel.

Changes in Gingival Contour

Normally the contour of marginal gingiva is scalloped and knife-edged. Interdental papilla is pointed and pyramidal in anterior region whereas in posterior region it is tent - shaped, filling the area.

The various diseased conditions related to gingival contour are:

a. *Acute and chronic gingivitis*: Marginal gingiva may be rounded or rolled.
b. *Gingival enlargement*: Papilla may be bulbous.
c. *Stillman's clefts*: These are apostrophe – shaped identations which extend from and into gingival margin along the root surface, most frequently on

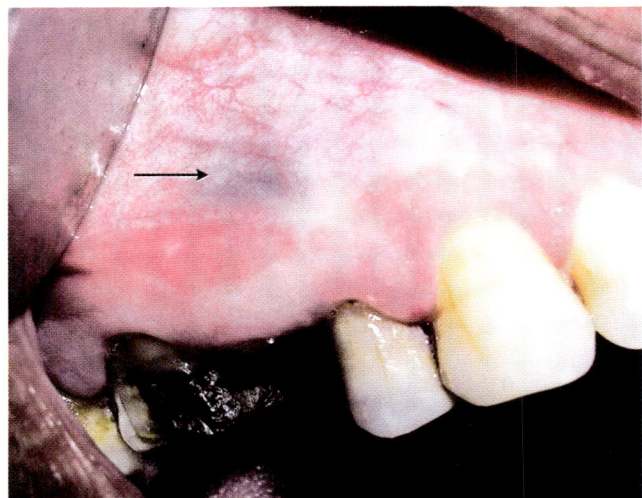

Fig. 18.6: Amalgam tattoo (*Courtesy:* Dr Ambika)

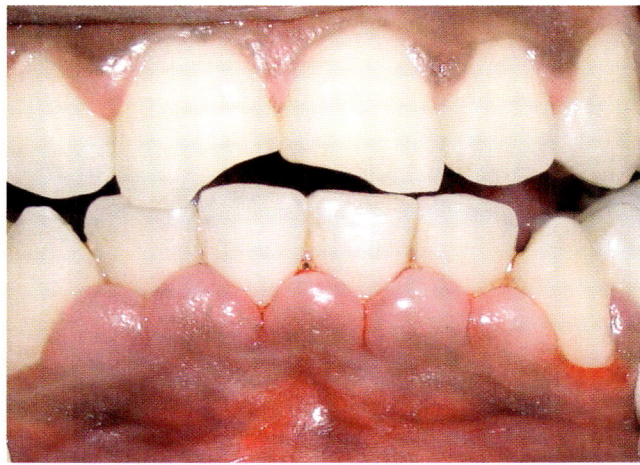

Fig. 18.7: Gingival clefts

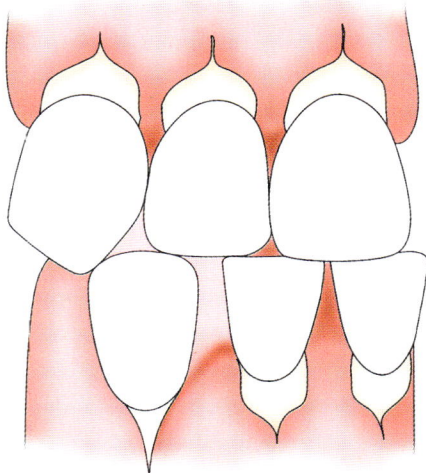

Fig. 18.8: Stillman's clefts

the labial or buccal surfaces **(Fig. 18.7)**. The margins of the cleft are rolled underneath the linear gap in the gingiva and remainder of gingival margin is blunt instead of knife – edge **(Fig. 18.8)**. It was originally described by Stillman, as a result of occlusal trauma. It may be simple – cleavage in a single direction or compound – cleavage in more than one direction.

d. *McCall's festoons*: McCall's festoons are the enlargement of the marginal gingiva with the formation of "life-saver" like gingival prominence in relation to canine and premolar facial surfaces mostly **(Figs 18.9 and 18.10)**. These are semilunar enlargements named after John Opple McCall who

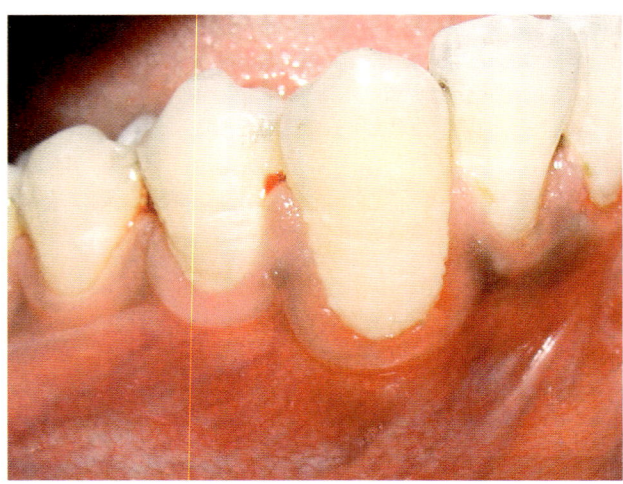

Fig. 18.9: McCall's festoons in relation to canine and premolars

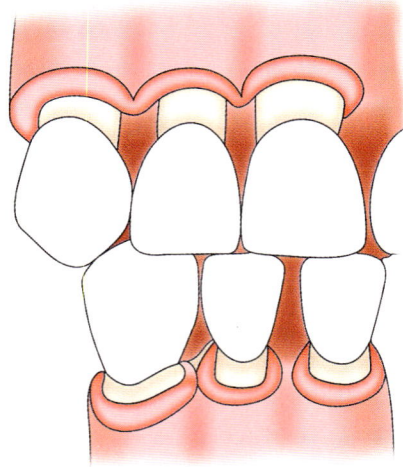

Fig. 18.10: McCall's festoons

along with Paul R Stillman, believed occlusal traumatism to be an etiologic factor.

e. NUG: Papillae may be cratered.

Changes in Gingival Consistency

In acute gingivitis, there is puffiness and softening of the gingiva. In chronic gingivitis, there is soggy puffiness that pits on pressure or firm, leathery consistency. Both destructive (edematous) and reparative (fibrotic) changes coexist in chronic gingivitis and the consistency of the gingiva is determined by their relative predominance. Gingival lump is seen in the following conditions: erupting third molars,

pregnancy gingivitis, fibroepithelial polyp and malignant conditions (Carcinoma, Kaposi's sarcoma, Lymphoma).

Changes in the Surface Texture of Gingiva

Conditions in which there is change in the surface texture of gingiva are:

A. Loss of stippling (smooth, shiny surface) is seen in chronic gingivitis **(Fig. 18.11)**, atrophic gingivitis and chronic desquamative gingivitis.

B. Leathery texture is seen in hyperkeratosis.

C. Nodular surface is seen in drug induced gingival overgrowth **(Fig. 18.12)**.

Changes in the Position of the Gingiva

In fully erupted tooth, position of gingival margin is 1-2 mm above CEJ, at or slightly below the enamel contour. The junctional epithelium is at the CEJ. The actual position is the level of the epithelial attachment on the

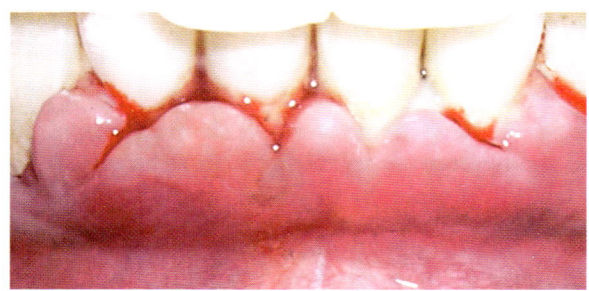

Fig. 18.11: Loss of stippling producing smooth, shiny surface in mandibular anterior region

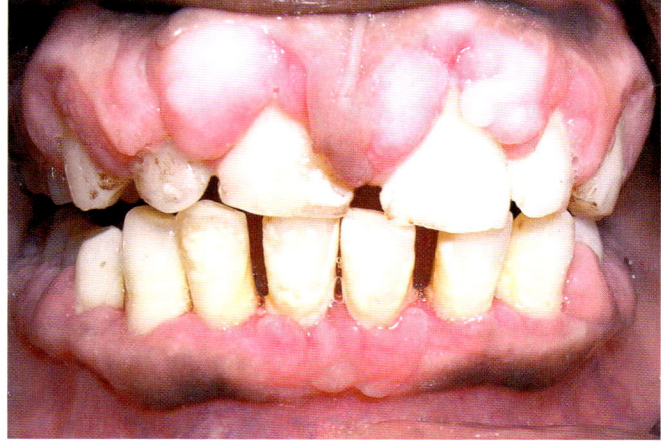

Fig. 18.12: Nodular surface seen in drug induced gingival enlargement

tooth, whereas the apparent position is the level of the crest of the gingival margin which is seen by direct observation. Actual position is not directly visible but can be determined by probing.

A. *Enlargement*: When the gingiva enlarges, the gingival margin may be high on the enamel, partly or nearly covering the anatomic crown **(Fig. 18.13)**.

B. *Recession*: It is exposure of the root surface by an apical shift in the position of the gingiva. The severity of recession is determined by the actual position of the gingiva, not its apparent position **(Fig. 18.14)**.

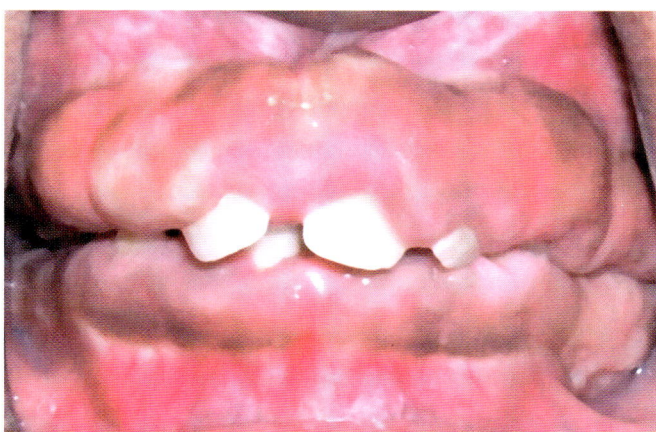

Fig. 18.13: Idiopathic hyperplastic gingival enlargement

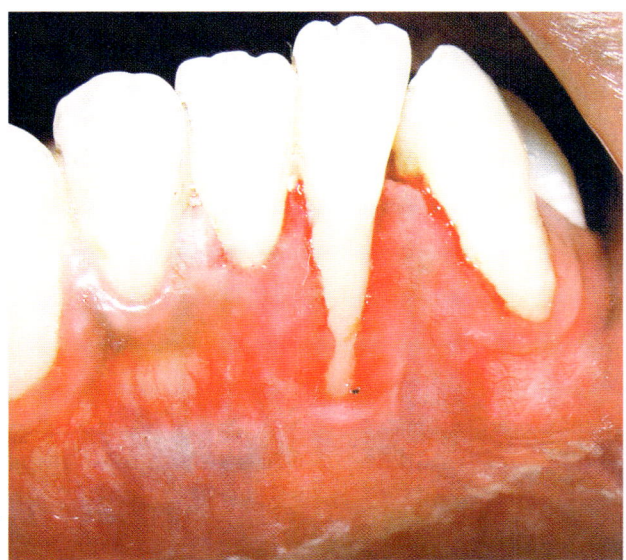

Fig. 18.14: Localized recession around malposed incisor and canine

The characteristics of plaque-induced gingivitis (Mariotti, 1999) are:

- Plaque present in relation to gingival margin
- Disease begins at the gingival margin
- Change in gingival color
- Change in gingival contour
- Sulcular temperature change
- Increased gingival exudates
- Bleeding upon provocation
- Absence of attachment and bone loss
- Histological changes including an inflammatory lesion
- Reversible with plaque removal

POINTS TO PONDER

✓ Gingival conditions/diseases that mainly involve interdental papilla and gingival margin are gingival abscess, necrotizing ulcerative gingivitis, linear gingival erythema and drug induced gingival enlargement.

✓ Gingival ulcers are usually seen in NUG, herpes simplex virus stomatitis, aphthae, self-injury, malignant neoplasms, drugs, dermatoses, systemic diseases (hematological disorders, tuberculosis, syphilis, herpes virus, HIV).

✓ Gingival changes seen in mouth-breathers are erythema, edema, enlargement, diffuse smooth and shiny surface in the exposed gingival area affecting mainly maxillary anterior region.

✓ Gingival red lesions are usually seen in desquamative gingivitis, erythroplasia, hemangiomas, orofacial granulomatosis, Crohn's disease, sarcoidosis, Wegener's granulomatosis, Kaposi's sarcoma and carcinoma.

BIBLIOGRAPHY

1. Carranza FA, Rapley JW, Haake SK. Gingival inflammation. In, Newman, Takei, Carranza. Clinical Periodontology 9th ed WB Saunders 2003;263-68.
2. Carranza FA, Rapley JW. Clinical features of gingivitis. In, Newman, Takei, Carranza. Clinical Periodontology 9th ed WB Saunders 2003;269-78.
3. Carranza FA, Hogan EL. Gingival enlargement. In, Newman, Takei, Carranza. Clinical Periodontology 9th ed WB Saunders 2003;279-96.
4. Claffey N. Plaque Induced Gingival Disease. In, Lindhe J, Karring T, Lang NP. Clinical Periodontology and Implant dentistry. 4th ed Blackwell Munksgaard 2003;198-08.
5. Garant PR, Mulvihill JE. The fine structure of gingivitis in the beagle III Plasma cell infiltration of the subepithelial connective tissue. J Periodontol Res 1972;7:161-72.
6. Grant DA, Stern IB, Listgarten MA. Gingivitis. In, Periodontics. 6th ed CV Mosby Company 1988;315-47.

MCQs

1. The radiographic findings of gingivitis will demonstrate:
   A. Vertical bone loss
   B. Horizontal bone loss
   C. Change in bone trabeculation
   D. Normal bone pattern
2. Gingivitis is initiated MOST often by:
   A. Malocclusion
   B. A hormonal imbalance
   C. Vitamin deficiency
   D. Microorganisms and their products
   E. Psychosocial factors
3. Gingival bleeding on probing appears:
   A. Before the color changes
   B. After the color changes
   C. At the same time as the color changes
   D. Not related with the color changes
4. Junctional epithelium shows formation of rete pegs in:
   A. Stage I gingivitis (Initial)
   B. Stage II gingivitis (Early)
   C. Stage III gingivitis (Established)
   D. Stage IV gingivitis (Advanced)
5. The predominant inflammatory cell in early lesion:
   A. Neutrophil   B. T lymphocytes
   C. Plasma cell   D. Macrophages
6. McCall's festoon is common in:
   A. Incisor area
   B. Canine and premolar area
   C. Molar area
   D. Same in all of the above

7. Crater-like deformities are seen in:
   A. NUG
   B. Aggressive periodontitis
   C. Chronic gingivitis
   D. Chronic periodontitis
8. Which of the following is not a clinical feature of necrotizing ulcerative gingivitis:
   A. Pocket formation
   B. Spontaneous bleeding
   C. Pain
   D. All of the above
9. All of the exogenous factors can cause gingival colour changes *except*:
   A. Coal dust
   B. Alcohol
   C. Tobacco
   D. Amalgam
10. Endogenous gingival pigmentation can be caused by all of the following *except*:
    A. Iron
    B. Melanin
    C. Bilirubin
    D. Metronidazole
11. Burtonian line is a linear pigmentation of gingival margin due to overexposure to:
    A. Bismuth   B. Silver
    C. Lead   D. Arsenic

Answers

1. D	2. D	3. A	4. B	5. B
6. B	7. A	8. A	9. B	10. D
11. C				

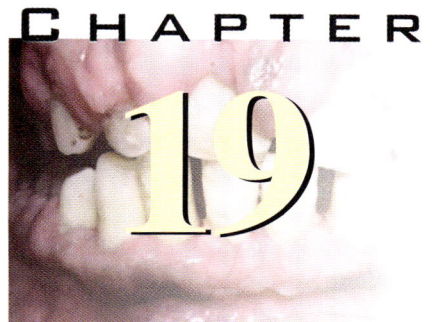

CHAPTER 19

Gingival Enlargement

Shalu Bathla

INTRODUCTION

Gingival enlargement may be viewed as a spectrum extending from idiopathic gingival hyperplasia (fibromatosis), in which inflammatory elements are absent, to phenytoin hyperplasia, where inflammatory elements may be present, to hyperplastic inflammation, seen in mouth breathers, to hormonally conditioned gingivitis in pregnancy.

CLASSIFICATION

Gingival enlargement can be classified as:

According to the etiologic factors and pathologic factors:
I. Inflammatory enlargement
   A. Chronic
   B. Acute
II. Drug induced gingival enlargement
   • Idiopathic gingival fibromatosis
III. Enlargements associated with systemic disease
   A. Conditioned enlargement
      1. Pregnancy
      2. Puberty
      3. Vitamin C deficiency
      4. Plasma cell gingivitis
      5. Nonspecific conditioned enlargement (granulomatous pyogenicum)
   B. Systemic diseases causing gingival enlargement
      1. Leukemia
      2. Granulomatous diseases (Wegener's granulomatosis, sarcoidosis, and so on)
IV. Neoplastic enlargement (gingival tumors)
   A. Benign tumors
   B. Malignant tumors
V. False enlargement

According to location and distribution, gingival enlargement is designated as follows:
1. *Localized*: Limited to the gingiva adjacent to a single tooth or a group of teeth.
2. *Generalized*: Involving the gingiva throughout the mouth.
3. *Marginal*: Confined to the marginal gingiva.
4. *Papillary*: Confined to the interdental papilla.
5. *Diffuse*: Involving the marginal, attached gingiva and papillae.
6. *Discrete*: An isolated sessile or pedunculated tumor like enlargement.

SCORING OF GINGIVAL ENLARGEMENT

The degree of gingival enlargement can be scored as follows:

Grade 0 : No signs of gingival enlargement

Grade I : Enlargement confined to interdental papilla

Grade II : Enlargement involves papilla and marginal gingiva

Grade III : Enlargement covers three quarters or more of the crown.

INFLAMMATORY ENLARGEMENT

Acute Inflammatory Enlargement

Gingival Abscess: A gingival abscess is a localized, painful, rapidly expanding lesion that is usually of sudden onset. It is generally limited to the marginal gingiva or interdental papilla. It results from bacteria carried deep into the tissues when a foreign substance such as a toothbrush bristle, a piece of apple core, or a lobster shell fragment is forcefully embedded into the gingiva. In its early stages, it appears as a red swelling with a smooth, shiny surface. Within 24 to 48 hours, the lesion usually becomes fluctuant and pointed with a surface orifice from which a purulent exudate may be expressed.

Histopathologic features: In connective tissue, purulent foci are present surrounded by diffuse infiltration of PMNs and vascular engorgement. Intra- and extracellular edema is present in the epithelium. Sometimes epithelium is ulcerated and invaded by leukocytes.

Chronic Inflammatory Enlargement

The main etiological factor is prolonged exposure to dental plaque due to poor oral hygiene. Other predisposing factors are anatomic abnormalities, irritation by improper restorative and orthodontic appliances.

Clinical Features:

- It may represent from slight ballooning of the interdental papilla and/or the marginal gingiva to the bulge covering most of the crown **(Figs 19.1 and 19.2)**
- Usually painless and progresses slowly
- The enlargement may be localized or generalized.
- May occur as a discrete sessile or pedunculated mass on the interproximal or marginal or attached gingiva.

Histopathologic features: There is preponderance of inflammatory cells and fluid with vascular engorgement. There is abundance of fibroblasts, collagen fibers and new capillaries in the connective tissue.

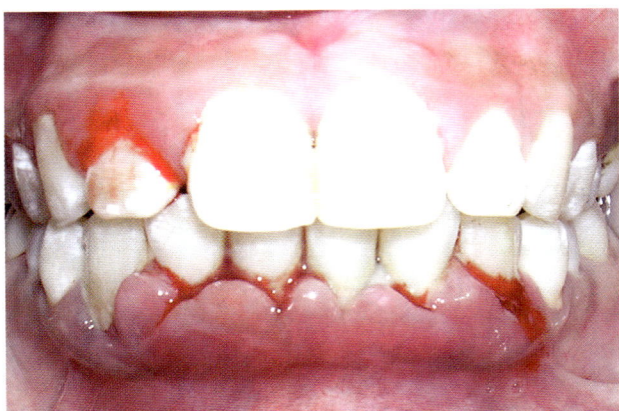

Fig. 19.1: Chronic inflammatory gingival enlargement

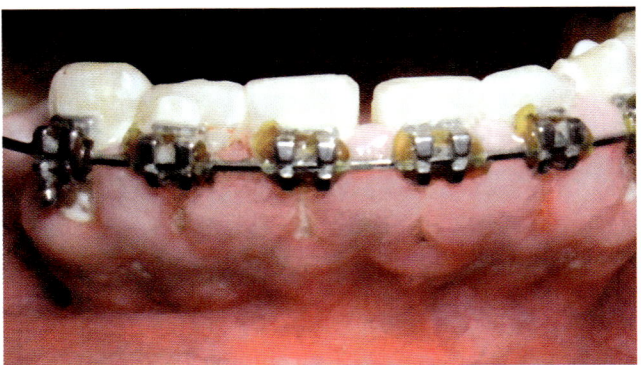

Fig. 19.2: Chronic gingival enlargement around orthodontic appliance

DRUG INDUCED GINGIVAL ENLARGEMENT

It arises most commonly as a result of ingestion of various medications such as anticonvulsants, immunosuppressants and antihypertensives. Anticonvulsant drugs associated with gingival enlargement are: Phenytoin, Phenobarbital, Carbamazepine, Sodium Valproate, Primidone and Felbamate. Antihypertensive drugs associated with gingival enlargement are: Nifedipine, Amlodipine, Nimodipine, Nicardine, Nitrendipine, Diltiazem, Felodipine and Bepridil. The precise mechanism involved is still being investigated, but it appears that these medications modify fibroblast function, either directly or indirectly through altering levels of cytokines/MMP activity within the tissue. Analogs of phenytoin that stimulate proliferation of fibroblast like cells are 1 – allyl - 5 - phenylhydantoinate and 5 – methyl - 5 - phenylhydantoin. Fibroblasts from phenytoin induced gingival overgrowth show increased synthesis of sulfated glycosaminoglycans. Phenytoin may induce decrease in collagen degradation due to the production of an inactive fibroblast collagenase.

Clinical Features:

- Initially the growth is painless, beadlike enlargement of the interdental papilla and extends to the facial and lingual gingival margins (**Fig. 19.3**).
- The marginal and papillary enlargements unite and cover a considerable portion of the crowns, which interfere with occlusion.
- Lesion is mulberry shaped, firm, pale pink and resilient with no tendency to bleed, when uncomplicated by inflammation (**Fig. 19.4**).
- Common and severe in maxillary and mandibular anterior regions.
- Enlargement is chronic and slowly increases in size.

Histological Features

There is acanthosis of epithelium and elongation of rete pegs. In connective tissue, there are foci of chronic inflammatory cells particularly plasma cells and large number of fibroblasts and new blood vessels.

Where overgrowth is already present, the following measures may be taken – Substitution of drugs or the reduction of dosage of phenytoin should be considered by the physician. Rigid oral hygiene practices are instituted. With good oral hygiene, the extent of overgrowth can be minimized or avoided. Hyperplastic tissues are most often removed surgically by gingivectomy or undisplaced flap.

Idiopathic Gingival Fibromatosis

Synonyms of Idiopathic gingival fibromatosis are hereditary gingival hyperplasia, congential familial fibromatosis and elephantiasis. The cause is said to be idiopathic and believed to have hereditary basis. The mode of inheritance is autosomal recessive as well as autosomal dominant. It may be an isolated disease entity or part of a syndrome. It has been described in tuberous sclerosis, which is characterized by a triad of epilepsy, mental retardation and cutaneous angiofibromas.

Clinical features: Affects gingival margin, interdental papillae and attached gingiva of the facial and lingual surfaces of the mandible and maxilla. It presents as large mass of firm, dense, resilient, insensitive fibrous tissue that covers the alveolar ridges and extends over the teeth. Color may be normal or erythematous if inflamed. If the enlargement is present before tooth eruption, dense fibrous tissue may then interfere with or prevent the eruption. Jaw appears distorted because of bulbous enlargement of the gingiva and patient complains of functional and esthetic problems (**Figs 19.5 and 19.6**).

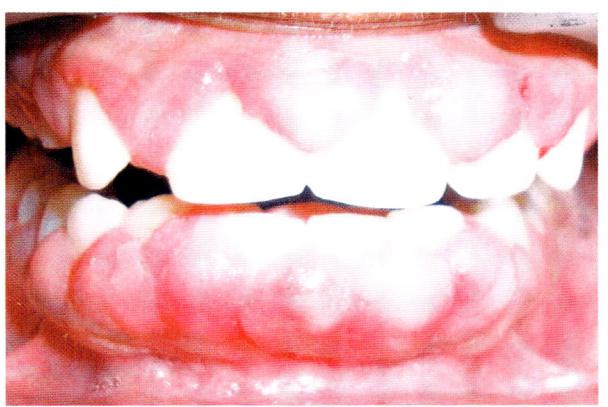

Fig. 19.3: Phenytoin induced gingival enlargement

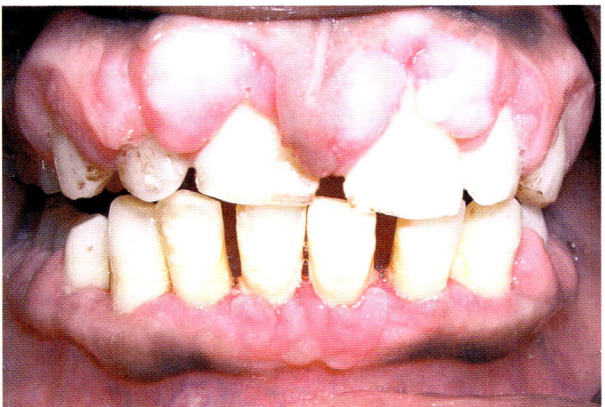

Fig. 19.4: Cyclosporine induced gingival enlargement

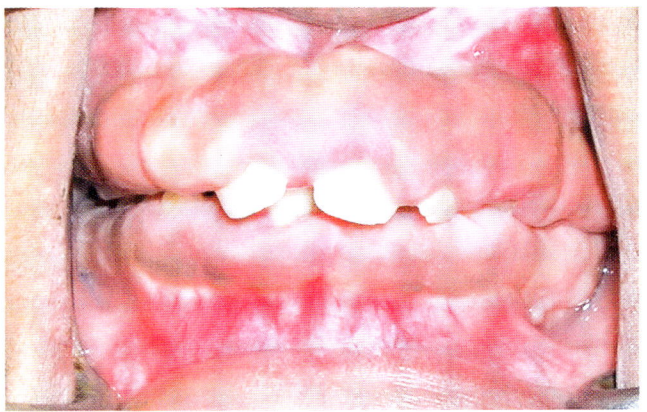

Fig. 19.5: Idiopathic gingival fibromatosis—Advanced gingival enlargement covering most of the crown portion

PERIODONTICS REVISITED

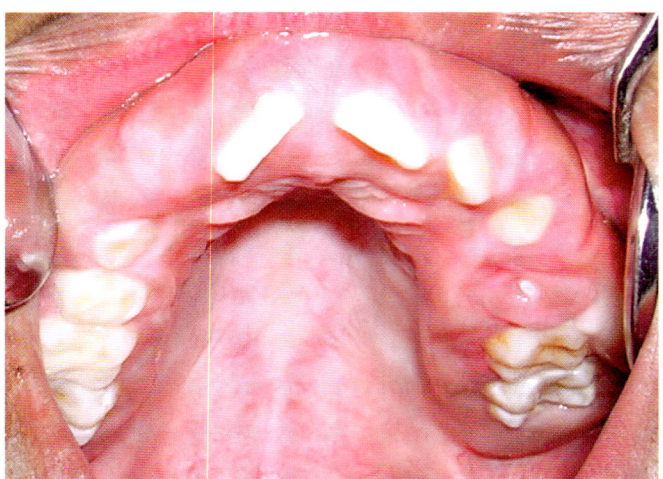

Fig. 19.6: Idiopathic gingival fibromatosis (Occlusal view)—The hyperplastic gingiva deflects the erupting teeth from proper alignment

Histological features: There is moderate hyperplasia of a slightly hyperkeratotic epithelium with acanthosis and elongated rete pegs. There is bulbous increase in the amount of connective tissue due to dense collagen bundle that is relatively avascular.

Differential diagnosis: Idiopathic gingival fibromatosis is different from phenytoin – induced hyperplasia. Idiopathic gingival fibromatosis involves gingival margin, interdental papillae and attached gingiva whereas in phenytoin – induced hyperplasia, only gingival margin and interdental papillae are involved. Histological examination may facilitate the differential diagnosis from other genetically determined gingival enlargement such as Fabry disease which is characterized by telangiectasia.

Treatment involves surgical removal by series of gingivectomies. If the volume of the overgrowth is extensive repositioned flap surgery is done.

ENLARGEMENT ASSOCIATED WITH SYSTEMIC DISEASES

Conditioned Enlargement

In conditioned enlargement, the systemic condition of the patient exaggerates the usual gingival response to dental plaque. Although bacterial plaque is the primary etiological factor for the initiation of this type of enlargement but is not the sole determinant of the nature of enlargement. The types of conditioned gingival enlargement are hormonal (pregnancy, puberty), nutritional (associated with vitamin C deficiency) and allergic.

Enlargement in pregnancy: There are hormonal changes seen during pregnancy which induce changes in vascular permeability and cause increase in *Prevotella intermedia* leading to gingival edema and an increased inflammatory response to dental plaque. Gingival edema may be marginal and generalized or may occur as single or multiple tumor-like masses.

Marginal enlargement: The gingival enlargement does not occur without the presence of bacterial plaque. Usually present on interproximal surfaces. The enlarged gingiva is bright red,soft and friable with smooth, shiny surface **(Fig. 19.7)**. Bleeding occurs spontaneously or on slight provocation.

Tumor like gingival enlargement: It usually appears after the third month of pregnancy but may occur earlier. It appears as dark red or magenta, with smooth, glistening surface that often exhibits numerous deep red, pinpoint markings **(Fig. 19.8)**. The lesion appears as a soft, friable, discrete, mushroomlike, flattened spherical mass that protrudes from the gingival margin or more commonly from the interproximal space and is attached by a sessile or pedunculated base.

Although spontaneous reduction in the size of gingival enlargement commonly follows the termination of pregnancy. Complete elimination of the residual inflammatory lesion requires the removal of all plaque deposits and factors that favor its accumulation.

Enlargement in puberty: Enlargement of the gingiva is sometimes seen in both male and female adolescents and appears in areas of plaque accumulation. It is characterized by prominent bulbous interproximal papillae. Gingival enlargement during puberty has all

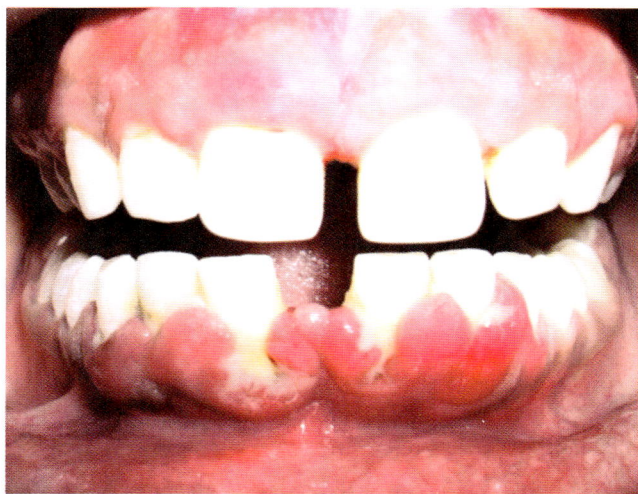

Fig. 19.7: Conditioned gingival enlargement—Pregnancy gingivitis

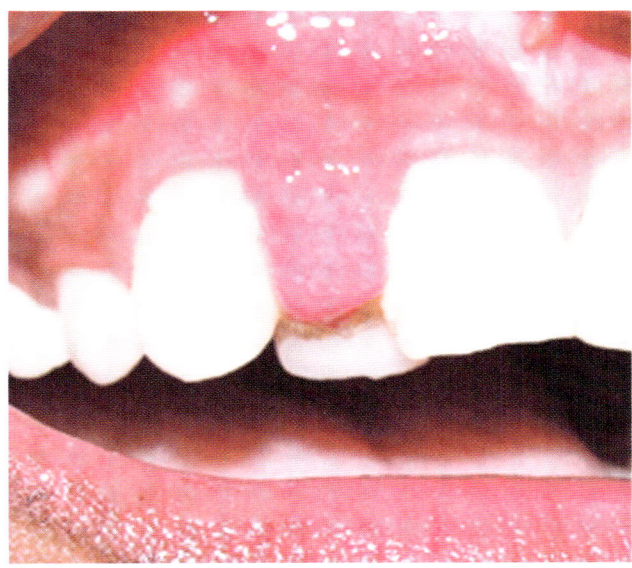

Fig. 19.8: Pregnancy tumor

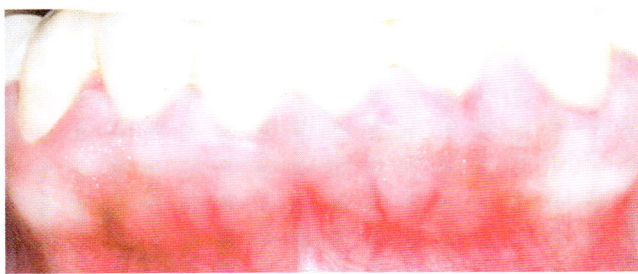

Fig. 19.9: Conditioned gingival enlargement—Puberty gingivitis

the clinical features generally associated with chronic inflammatory gingival disease. It is the degree of enlargement and the tendency to develop massive recurrence in the presence of relatively scanty plaque deposits that distinguish pubertal gingival enlargement from uncomplicated chronic inflammatory gingival enlargement **(Fig. 19.9)**.

After puberty, there is spontaneous reduction of enlargement but it does not disappear until plaque and calculus are removed.

Enlargement in Vitamin C Deficiency (scurvy): It is essentially a conditioned response to bacterial plaque. Acute vitamin C deficiency as such does not cause gingival inflammation itself, but it does cause collagen degeneration, hemorrhage and edema of the gingival connective tissue. These changes modify the response of the gingiva to plaque to the extent that the normal

defensive delimiting reaction is inhibited, and the extent of the inflammation is exaggerated.

Clinical features: There is marginal gingival enlargement. It appears as bluish red, soft, and friable with smooth, shiny surface. There is spontaneous bleeding or on slight provocation. There may be surface necrosis with pseudomembrane formation.

Plasma cell gingivitis: It is also called as atypical gingivitis and plasma cell gingivostomatitis. A localized lesion, referred to as plasma cell granuloma is located in the oral aspect of the attached gingiva and therefore differs from plaque-induced gingivitis. Plasma cell gingivitis is thought to be allergic in origin, possibly related to components of chewing gum, dentifrices, or various diet components. There is mild marginal gingival enlargement that extends to the attached gingiva. The gingiva appears red, friable and sometimes granular which bleeds easily. Cessation of exposure to the allergen resolves the lesion.

Nonspecific conditioned enlargement (Pyogenic Granuloma): Pyogenic granuloma is a tumor like gingival enlargement that is considered as an exaggerated conditioned response to minor trauma. The exact nature of the systemic conditioning factor has not been identified. The lesion varies from a discrete spherical, tumorlike mass with a pedunculated attachment to a flattened, keloid like enlargement with a broad base **(Fig. 19.10)**. It is reddish or bluish, sometimes lobulated, and may be sessile or pedunculated with surface ulceration and purulent exudation. It may develop rapidly and the size varies considerably.

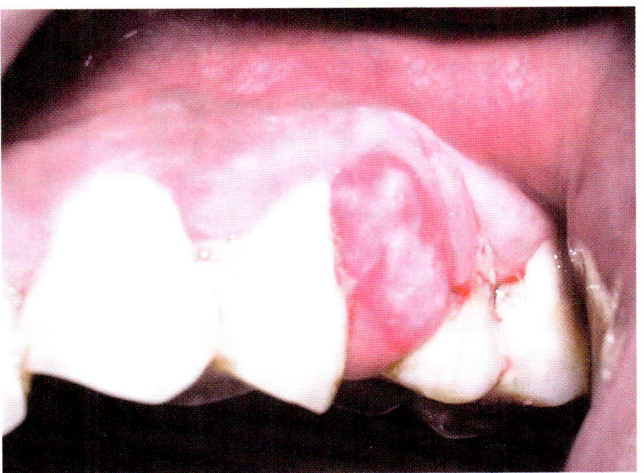

Fig. 19.10: Pyogenic granuloma

Bleeding from the ulcerated lesion is common, but typically it is not painful. Teeth may become separated due to interdental growth of the lesion. Due to its red color, which may sometimes turn to a cyanotic hue, pyogenic granuloma may be mistaken for giant cell granuloma. Treatment consists of surgical excision of the lesion and the elimination of irritating local factors.

Systemic Diseases Causing Gingival Enlargement

Leukemia: Leukemic enlargement may be diffuse or marginal, localized or generalized. It may appear as a diffuse enlargement of the gingival mucosa, an oversized extension of the marginal gingiva, or a discrete tumor like interproximal mass. The gingiva is generally bluish red and has a shiny surface. The consistency is moderately firm, but there is a tendency towards friability. Hemorrhage, occurs either spontaneously or on slight irritation **(Fig. 19.11)**. Patients with leukemia may also have a simple chronic inflammation without the involvement of leukemic cells and may present with the same clinical and microscopic features seen in patients without the disease. Most cases reveal features of both simple chronic inflammation and a leukemic infiltrate.

Granulomatous Diseases: Wegener's granulomatosis: It is a rare disease characterized by acute granulomatous necrotizing lesions of the respiratory tract, including nasal and oral defects. Renal lesions develop, and acute necrotizing vasculitis affects the blood vessels. The initial manifestations of Wegener's granulomatosis may involve the orofacial region and include oral mucosal ulceration, gingival enlargement, abnormal tooth mobility, exfoliation of teeth, and delayed healing response. The cause of Wegener's granulomatosis is

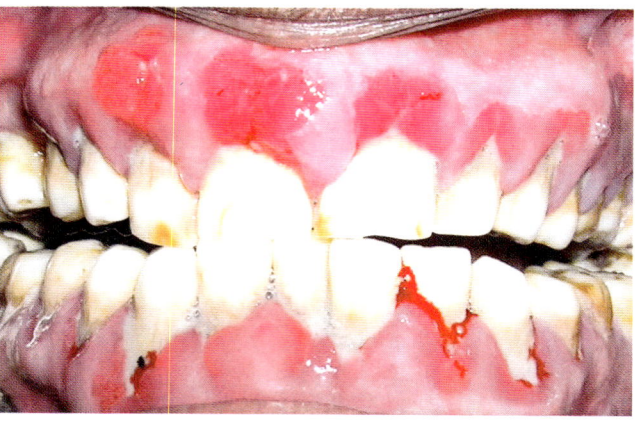

Fig. 19.11: Leukemic gingival enlargement

unknown, but the condition is considered an immunologically mediated tissue injury. The granulomatous papillary enlargement is reddish purple and bleeds easily on stimulation.

Sarcoidosis: Sarcoidosis is a granulomatous disease of unknown etiology. It starts in individuals in their twenties or thirties, affects predominantly blacks. Gingival enlargement may be red, smooth and painless.

NEOPLASTIC ENLARGEMENT

Benign Tumors of the Gingiva

Epulis is a generic term used clinically to designate all discrete tumors and tumorlike masses of the gingiva. It serves to locate the tumor but not to describe it. Most lesions referred to as epulis are inflammatory rather than neoplastic.

Fibroma: Fibromas of the gingiva arise from the gingival connective tissue or from the periodontal ligament. They are slow-growing, spherical tumors that tend to be firm and nodular but may be soft and vascular. Fibromas are usually pedunculated.

Histopathological features: There is hyperkeratinization of epithelium. It consist of scattered angular and multinucleated cells of a different appearance and nature than the giant cells in giant cell granulomas. Connective tissue consist of poor cell and hyperplastic collageneous tissue.

It is managed by complete surgical excision including superficial periodontal ligament fibers from where fibroma originate.

Papilloma: Papillomas are benign proliferations of surface epithelium associated with the human papilloma-virus (HPV). They are mainly seen in the third to fifth decade.

Clinical features: Gingival papillomas appear as reddish/normal or whitish/gray color, solitary, wartlike or cauliflower-like protuberances. They may be small and discrete or broad, hard elevations with minutely irregular surfaces.

Histopathological features: The epithelium is hyperkeratotic stratified squamous with irregular rete ridges. Connective tissue is fibrovascular.

Surgical excision, including the base of lesion is the treatment of choice.

Peripheral Giant Cell Granuloma: These lesions however, occur as response to local injury. The prefix peripheral is needed to differentiate them from comparable lesions that originate within the jaw bone (central giant cell granulomas). It is more frequent in women than in men, and the mandible is more often affected than the maxilla.

Clinical features: Usually occur on interdental or the gingival margin as red or purple ulcers. The lesions are pedunculated or sessile or may be firm or spongy. Local irritation or trauma appears to be important for these lesions to occur. They cause separation of teeth due to the pressure exerted by the growth. They may vary from smooth, regularly outlined masses to irregularly shaped, multilobulated protuberances with surface indentations. Ulceration of the margin is occasionally seen. The lesions are painless, vary in size, and may cover several teeth and the color varies from pink to deep red or purplish blue. In some instances, the giant cell granuloma of the gingiva is locally invasive and causes destruction of the underlying bone.

Histopathological features: There is hyperplasia of epithelium with ulceration at the base. The lesion is characterized by focal collections of multi-nucleated osteoclast-like giant cells with a rich cellular and vascular stroma separated by collageneous septa.

Although not encapsulated these lesions are well delimited and readily excised.

Central Giant Cell Granuloma: These lesions arise within the jaws and produce central cavitation. They occasionally create a deformity of the jaw that makes the gingiva appear enlarged. Mixed tumors, salivary gland type tumors, and plasmacytomas of the gingiva have also been described but are not often seen.

Leukoplakia: World Health Organization defined Leukoplakia, as a white patch or plaque that does not rub off and cannot be diagnosed as any other disease. The cause of leukoplakia remains obscure, although it is associated to the use of tobacco (smoke or smokeless). Other probable factors are Candida albicans, HPV-16 and HPV-18, and trauma.

Clinical features: They appear as solitary or multiple grayish white patches or plaques with distinct or sharply demarcated borders. They may be slightly thickened and smooth or wrinkled and fissured, or they may appear as raised, sometimes corrugated, verrucous plaques.

Gingival cysts: These cysts are of developmental origin. They occur in the mandibular canine and premolar areas, most often on the lingual surface. Gingival cysts appear as localized enlargements that may involve the marginal and attached gingiva. They are painless, but with expansion, they may cause erosion of the surface of the alveolar bone. The cysts develop from odontogenic epithelium or from surface or sulcular epithelium traumatically implanted in the area.

Histopathological features: The gingival cysts are lined by a stratified squamous epithelium with a parakeratotic surface and flat palisading basal cells. The cyst lumen is filled with keratin. The gingival cyst of adults is lined with a thin, non-keratinized squamous epithelium sometimes exhibiting focal thickenings of the epithelial lining.

Gingival cysts of adults are treated by local surgical excision and usually there is no tendency to recur.

Malignant Tumors of the Gingiva

Squamous cell carcinoma: Squamous cell carcinoma is the most common malignant tumor of the gingiva. It may be exophytic, presenting as an irregular outgrowth, or ulcerative, which appears as flat, erosive lesion. It is often symptom free, often going unnoticed until complicated by inflammatory changes that may mask the neoplasm but cause pain and loosening of teeth. It is locally invasive, involving the underlying bone and periodontal ligament of adjoining teeth and the adjacent mucosa. Metastasis is usually confined to the region above the clavicle; however, more extensive involvement may include the lung, liver, or bone.

Histopathological features: Islands and cords of malignant epithelial cells are seen infiltrating the underlying tissues. Varying amounts of 'horn pearls' are formed and usually a strong inflammatory reaction is found in the stroma.

Gingival squamous cell carcinomas are usually treated by surgery, irradiation or combinations of these.

Malignant Melanoma: Usually occurs in the hard palate and maxillary gingiva of older persons. It is usually darkly pigmented which is preceded by the occurrence of localized pigmentation. It may appear as flat or nodular characterized by rapid growth and early metastasis. It arises from melanoblasts in the gingiva, cheek, or palate. Infiltration into the underlying bone and metastasis to cervical and axillary lymph nodes is common.

Malignant lymphoma: It presents as a diffuse swelling which is usually ulcerated. The diagnosis may be quite difficult to arrive at as the first manifestations may resemble a non-specific periodontitis, pyogenic granuloma or pericoronitis. In HIV-infected patients non-Hodgkin's lymphomas occur with increased frequency. Occasionally, a gingival tumor may be the first manifestation of a non-Hodgkin's lymphoma in an HIV-infected patient.

PERIODONTICS REVISITED

Histomorphologic features, immunologic and genetic markers are used to diagnose and classify malignant lymphomas. The lesions contain lymphocytic-appearing cells; in low-grade tumors the cells are well-differentiated small lymphocytes, whereas high-grade tumors contain less differentiated cells. Common to all lymphomas are infiltrative growth as characteristically seen in all malignant tumors.

Depending on the extension and spread of the tumor, surgical removal, irradiation, cytostatics and combinations of these may be the treatment of choice.

Kaposi's sarcoma: Kaposi's sarcoma often occurs in the oral cavity of patients with acquired immunodeficiency syndrome (AIDS), particularly in the palate and the gingiva. Kaposi's sarcoma usually manifests first as skin lesions followed by oral lesions.

They may represent as single or multiple blue, violet or red slightly raised lesions.

Histopathological features: The typical features are a lesion with bundles of spindle- shaped cells and many thin-walled vascular luminae, often lined by plump endothelial cells. There are usually a number of mitotic figures of which some are atypical.

There is no curative treatment but palliative treatment includes both cytostatics and irradiation.

FALSE ENLARGEMENT

False enlargements are not true enlargements of the gingival tissues but may appear as such as a result of increase in size of the underlying osseous or dental tissues **(Fig. 19.12)**.

The gingiva usually presents with no abnormal clinical features except the massive increase in size of the area.

Underlying Osseous Lesions

Enlargement of the bone subjacent to the gingival area occurs in tori, exostoses **(Fig. 19.13)**, fibrous dysplasia, cherubism, central giant cell granuloma, ameloblastoma, osteoma, and osteosarcoma. The gingival tissue can appear normal or may have unrelated inflammatory changes.

Underlying Dental Tissues

During the various stages of eruption, particularly of the primary dentition, the labial gingiva may show a bulbous marginal distortion caused by superimposition of the

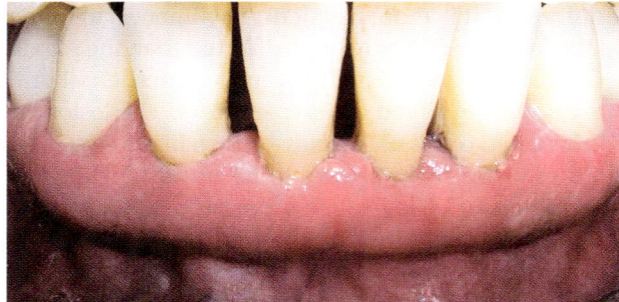

Fig. 19.12: False enlargement

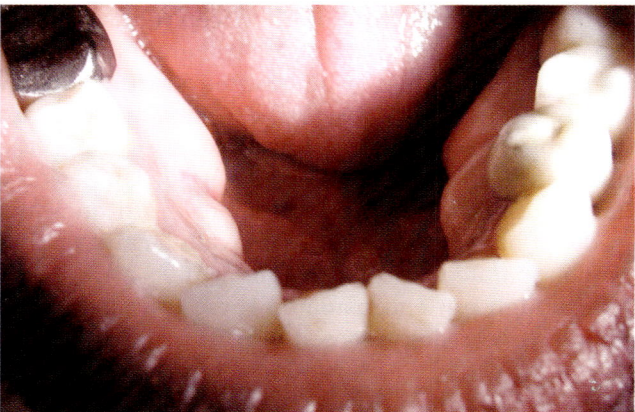

Fig. 19.13: Enlargement due to the presence of bilateral exostoses
(*Courtesy:* Dr SK Salaria)

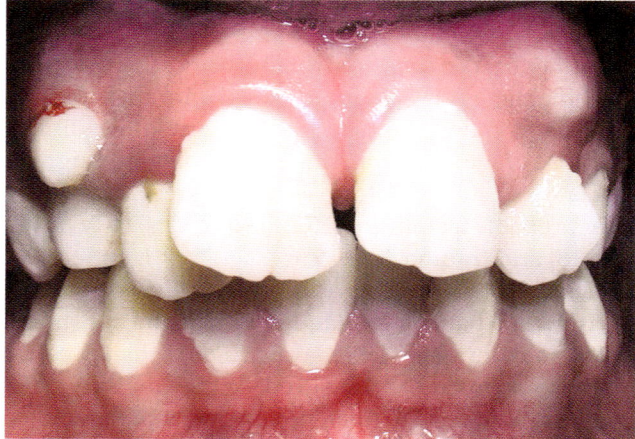

Fig. 19.14: Developmental gingival enlargement

bulk of the gingiva on the normal prominence of the enamel in the gingival half of the crown. This enlargement has been termed developmental enlargement **(Fig. 19.14)** and often persists until the junctional epithelium has migrated from the enamel to the cementoenamel junction. In a strict sense, developmental gingival enlargements are physiologic and ordinarily present no problems.

However, when such enlargement is complicated by marginal inflammation, the composite picture gives the impression of extensive gingival enlargement.

Treatment to alleviate the marginal inflammation, rather than resection of the enlargement, is sufficient in these cases.

POINTS TO PONDER

✓ Hypertrophy is an increase in size of cells causing the increase in the size of the tissues.

✓ Hyperplasia is an increase in number of cells in a tissue thus, contributing to an overall increase in the size. Gingival hyperplasia is caused mainly by an increase in the number of local cellular elements and intercellular fibers.

✓ The clinical features of phenytoin – induced hyperplasia are different from that of idiopathic fibrous hyperplasia. The administration of phenytoin often leads to overgrowth of the papillae, leaving the attached gingiva. Whereas in idiopathic fibrous hyperplasia there is involvement of all marginal, interdental and attached gingiva.

BIBLIOGRAPHY

1. Carranza FA, Hogan EL. Gingival enlargement. In, Newman, Takei, Carranza. Clinical Periodontology 9th ed WB Saunders 2003;279-96.
2. Eley BM, Manson JD. Epulides and tumours of the gingivae and oral mucosa. In, Periodontics 5th ed Wright 2004;358-60.
3. Genco RJ, Goldman HM, Cohen DW. Gingival enlargement: Hyperplastic and inflammatory enlargement. In, Contemporary Periodontics. CV Mosby Company 1990;469-78.
4. Holmstrup P, Reibel J. Differential Diagnoses: Periodontal Tumors and Cysts. In, Lindhe J, Karring T, Lang NP. Clinical Periodontology and Implant dentistry. 4th ed Blackwell Munksgaard 2003;298-317.
5. Ramfjord SP, Ash MM. Gingivitis, Gingivostomatitis and Gingival atrophy. In, Periodontology and Periodontics. Modern Theory and Practice. 1st ed AITBS Publisher and distributor India, 1996;139-61.

MCQs

1. Conditioned Gingival enlargements are usually not due to:
   A. Hormones
   B. Leukemia
   C. Granuloma pyogenicum
   D. Drug induced
2. Drug induced gingival enlargement starts in:
   A. Marginal gingiva
   B. Attached gingiva
   C. Interdental papilla
   D. None of the above
3. Gingival enlargement is caused when the daily dose of cyclosporine is greater than:
   A. 500 mg
   B. 200 mg
   C. 300 mg
   D. 100 mg

Answers

1. B   2. C   3. A

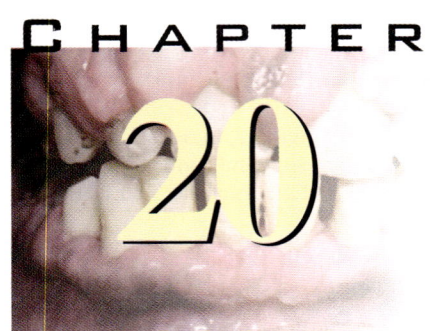

CHAPTER 20

Acute Gingival Conditions

Shalu Bathla

NECROTIZING ULCERATIVE GINGIVITIS

Historical Perspective

Necrotizing ulcerative gingitivitis (NUG) had been recognized in the 4th BC by Xenophon who stated that Greek soldiers were plagued with sore, ulcerated and foul-smelling mouths. In 1778, John Hunter first delineated the clinical differences between NUG, scurvy, and chronic periodontitis. NUG occurred in epidemic form in the 19th century and in 1886 Hersch described that increased salivation, enlarged lymph nodes, fever and malaise had been associated with NUG. Acute necrotizing ulcerative gingitivitis (ANUG), now classified under Necrotizing Periodontal Disease according to the 1999 American Academy of Periodontics classification system, is a distinct and specific disease characterized by rapidly progressive ulceration typically starting at the tip of the interdental papilla, spreading along the gingival margins, and going on to acute destruction of the periodontal tissue.

Synonyms of NUG are Trench mouth, Vincent's gingivostomatitis, Vincent's gingivitis, ulceromembranous gingivitis, acute necrotizing ulcerative gingivitis (ANUG) and fusospirochetal gingivitis. The term "trench mouth" comes from World War I, when many soldiers suffered from the condition as they were stuck in the trenches without the means to take care of their mouth and teeth properly. It was also called Vincent's Stomatitis or Vincent's angina after French bacteriologist Jean Hyacinth Vincent (1862-1950).

Clinical Features

The characteristic features of NUG are:
1. *Rapid onset of gingival pain*: The lesions are extremely sensitive to touch, and the patient often complains of a constant radiating, gnawing pain which is intensified by eating hot and spicy foods.
2. *Interdental gingival necrosis*: Punched out, crater-like depressions at the crest of the interdental papillae, subsequently extending to the marginal gingiva and

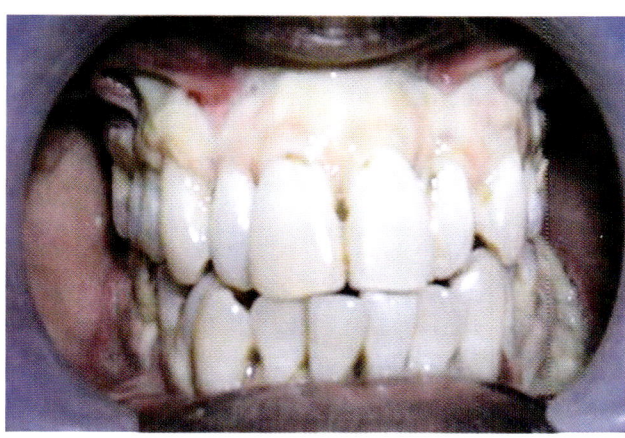

Fig. 20.1: NUG (*Courtesy:* Dr Ambika)

rarely to the attached gingiva and oral mucosa. The ulcers are covered by a yellowish-white or grayish slough, which has been termed "pseudomembrane", demarcated from the remainder of the gingival mucosa by a pronounced linear erythema. However, the sloughed material has no coherence, and bears little resemblance to a membrane **(Fig. 20.1)**. It consists primarily of fibrin and necrotic tissue with leukocytes, erythrocytes and masses of bacteria. Removal of the sloughed material results in bleeding and exposure of ulcerated underlying tissue.

3. *Bleeding*: There is spontaneous gingival hemorrhage or pronounced bleeding on the slightest stimulation due to the acute inflammation and necrosis with exposure of the underlying connective tissue.

Other clinical features are:

1. Fetid odor: A characteristic and pronounced fetor ex ore is often associated with NUG, but can vary in intensity.
2. Increased salivation: There is a metallic foul taste and the patient is conscious of an excessive amount of "pasty" saliva.
3. Site and extent of involvement: The interdental cols and tips of the interdental papillae are characteristically affected first, although the disease may involve the gingival margins. The distribution of the disease does not follow any consistent pattern and may differ from person to person. The reasons for necrotic lesions appearing at the interdental papilla are two fold:
   - The papilla has relatively less vascularity with the tip being supplied by a single vessel arising from the papillary plexus. If the vascularity arising from this vessel is for some reason cut off, the resultant lack of oxygenation leads to the death of the tissues.

- There is an extensive infiltration of spirochetes into the tissues of the gingiva. Among the other vessels, the papillary plexus is affected as well, by spirochetal infiltration. The lack of an alternate supply with the blockage of the existing one leads to tissue necrosis. This manifests clinically as the characteristic punched out crater like lesions at the crest of the papilla.

4. Relation of necrotizing ulcerative periodontal disease (NUP) to pocket—This condition is otherwise termed as atypical periodontitis. The pockets that are a characteristic clinical sign associated with periodontitis are absent in this condition. Pocket formation necessitates apical migration of junctional epithelium and this requires viable epithelial cells. Necrosis of the epithelial cells results in an epithelium that is unable to exhibit any proliferation or migration. Therefore, in necrotizing gingival inflammation, the spread of inflammation does not result in pocket formation.

Extraoral signs and symptoms are local lymphadenopathy, slight elevation in temperature to high fever, increased pulse rate, leukocytosis, loss of appetite and general lassitude.

Etiology

The possible etiological and predisposing factors are explained in **Figure 20.2**.

Bacterial flora–Necrotizing ulcerative gingivitis is an infectious disease. Dramatic resolution of signs and symptoms can be affected by reduction of the microbial plaque either by antibiotic therapy, mechanical debridement, or both. A specific infectious disease should be associated with a specific etiology. The bacterial etiology of NUG provides one of the strongest examples of a primary bacterial etiology in a periodontal disease. This bacterial etiology was first proposed by Plaut in 1894 and Vincent in 1896. Working independently, they both reported that fusiform-spirochete bacterial flora were associated with the lesions of necrotizing ulcerative gingivitis.

Pre-disposing Factors

- *Psychological stress*: Stress could be in the form of emotional stress, which is often seen among military cadets, in harsh physical conditions, in drug addicts during periods of drug withdrawal, in college students during examination and in stressful living endemic contagious diseases, especially measles.

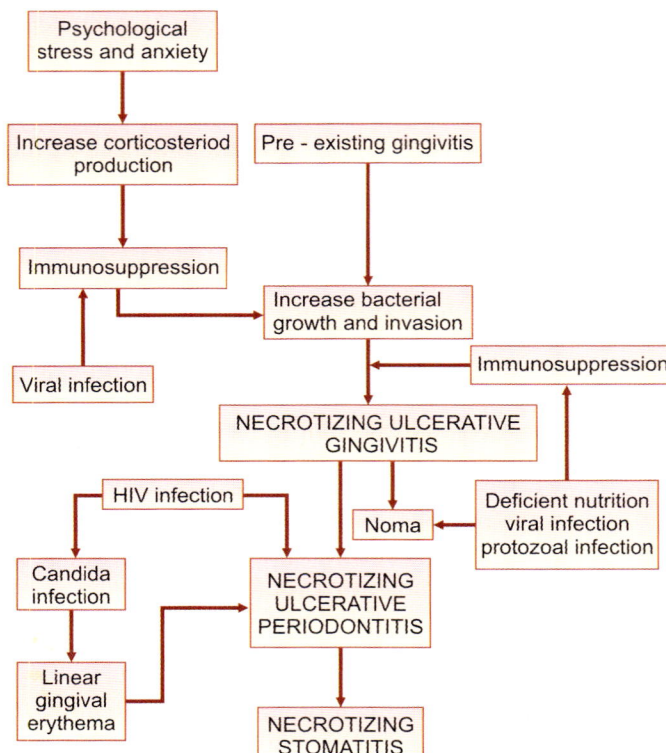

Fig. 20.2: Necrotizing ulcerative gingivitis: Possible mechanisms and sequelae

Synergism between malnutrition and measles, a viral infection, has been reported to promote secondary infection by some resident oral micro-organisms that spreads NUG rapidly. Stress is believed to predispose to NUG by causing an elevation in adrenocortical secretion. It also causes the release of substance P, a peptide hormone which suppresses both specific and nonspecific immunity. It also affects patient's mood resulting in changes in oral hygiene and nutrition.

- Other predisposing factors are immunosuppression, malnutrition, tobacco smoking, pre-existing gingivitis and trauma.

Stages in the progress of NUG

Pindborg and colleagues have described the following stages in the progress of NUG:

Stage I	Only the tip of the interdental papilla is affected;
Stage II	The lesion extends to marginal gingiva and causes punched-out papilla;
Stage III	The attached gingiva is also affected; and
Stage IV	The bone is exposed.

Horning and Cohen extended the staging of these oral necrotizing diseases as follows:

Stage 1:	Necrosis of the tip of the interdental papilla (93%) - NUG
Stage 2:	Necrosis of the entire papilla (19%) – either NUG/ NUP
Stage 3:	Necrosis extending to the gingival margin (21%) - NUP
Stage 4:	Necrosis extending also to the attached gingiva (1%) - NUP
Stage 5:	Necrosis extending into buccal or labial mucosa (6%) - Necrotizing stomatitis
Stage 6:	Necrosis exposing alveolar bone (1%) - Necrotizing stomatitis
Stage 7:	Necrosis perforating skin of cheek (0%) - Noma

Histopathology

The microscopic picture of NUG reveals an acute inflammatory process with ulceration and formation of pseudomembrane on the surface. Epithelium is destroyed and is replaced by a meshwork of fibrin, necrotic epithelial cells, PMNs, and micro-organisms. This is the zone that appear clinically as pseudo-membrane. The connective tissue has numerous engorged capillaries and dense infiltration of PMNs.

Listgarten in 1965 provided electron microscopic data confirming the invasion of non-necrotic gingiva by large- and intermediate-sized spirochetes. He further noted that the invasion of spirochetes in the ulcerated lesions could be broadly grouped into four zones of increasing depth from the tissue surface:

Zone 1:	*Bacterial zone*, the most superficial, consists of varied bacteria, including a few spirochetes of the small, medium, and large types.
Zone 2:	*Neutrophil-rich zone* contains numerous leukocytes, mainly neutrophils, with bacteria, including many spirochetes of various types, between the leukocytes.
Zone 3:	*Necrotic zone* consists of disintegrated tissue cells, fibrillar material, remnants of collagen fibers, and numerous spirochetes of the medium and large types, with few other organisms.
Zone 4:	*Zone of spirochetal infiltration* consists of well preserved tissue infiltrated with medium and large spirochetes, without other organisms.

NUG is clinically diagnosed on the basis of clinical findings:

Gingival pain which is constant radiating, gnawing intensified by eating spicy/ hot food

Ulceration – punched out, crater like depression at the crest of interdental papilla

Spontaneous gingival bleeding.

Diagnosis

Diagnosis is easily made on clinical findings of gingival pain, ulceration, and bleeding. Microscopic examination of a biopsy specimen is not sufficiently specific to be diagnostic. It can be used to differentiate NUG from specific infections such as tuberculosis or from neoplastic disease, but it does not differentiate between NUG and other necrotizing conditions of nonspecific origin, such as those produced by trauma or caustic medications. Thus, it is important to take history to determine the underlying predisposing factors responsible for the disease.

Differential Diagnosis

NUG should be differentiated from other conditions that resemble it in some respects, such as herpetic gingivostomatitis, chronic periodontitis, desquamative gingivitis, streptococcal gingivostomatitis, aphthous stomatitis, diphtheritic and syphilitic lesions, tuberculous gingival lesion, candidiasis, agranulocytosis, pemphigus, erythema multiforme and lichen planus. Perhaps the most important differential diagnosis of NUG is that from primary herpetic gingivostomatitis.

The differentiating features of necrotizing ulcerative gingivitis (NUG) and acute herpetic gingivostomatitis (AHG) are presented in the **Table 20.1**.

Treatment

Treatment of NUG should follow an orderly sequence which is divided mainly into 2 stages:

1. Control of acute phase: a) alleviation of the acute inflammation plus treatment of chronic disease either underlying the acute involvement or else where in the oral cavity, b) alleviation of generalized toxic symptoms such as fever and malaise.
2. Management of the residual condition: a) Elimination of pre-disposing factors, b) Correction of tissue deformities by surgery.

1. Control of acute phase: First Visit - Treatment during this initial visit is confined to the acutely involved areas:

- Isolation: Affected site is isolated with cotton rolls and dried.
- Removal of surface debris: A topical anesthesia is applied, and after 2 or 3 minutes the areas are gently swabbed with a cotton pellet to remove the pseudomembrane and nonattached surface debris. Each cotton pellet is used in a small area and is then discarded; sweeping motions over large areas with a single pellet are not recommended.
- Ultrasonic scaling: After the area is cleansed with warm water, the superficial calculus is removed by ultrasonic scaling. Subgingival scaling and curettage are contraindicated at this time because of the possibility of extending the infection to deeper tissues, and also of causing bacteremia.

TABLE 20.1: Differences between NUG and AHG

		NUG	*AHG*
1	Site of ulcers	Interdental papilla, Marginal gingiva	Gingiva, No predilection for interdental papilla entire oral mucosa
2	Character of ulcers	a. Punched out, crater like depression covered by yellow/ white/gray slough	Multiple vesicles that coalesce and form shallow fibrin-covered regular shaped ulcers.
		b. Bleed readily/ spontaneously	No marked tendency to bleed
		c. Painful on stimulation	Non tender
3	Fever	Doubtful/ slight only	38° C (or more)
4	Symptoms	Painful gums/ dead feeling teeth	Sore mouth
5	Duration of ulcers and discomfort	Short lived (1-3 days), with appropriate therapy	More than 1 week, even with therapy
6	Etiology	Interaction between host and bacteria, most probably fusospirochetes	Specific viral etiology
7	Age	Uncommon in children	More frequently in children
8	Contagious	Non- contagious	Contagious
9	Immunity	No demonstrated immunity	An acute episode results in some degree of immunity.

PERIODONTICS REVISITED

- Following instructions are given to the patient:

Do's:

✓ Rinse with a glassful of an equal mixture of 3% hydrogen peroxide and warm water every 2 hours and/or twice daily with 0.12% chlorhexidine solution.

✓ Pursue usual activities.

✓ Patients with moderate or severe NUG and local lymphadenopathy, Penicillin 500 mg orally every 6 hours and for penicillin-sensitive patients, erythromycin are prescribed. Metronidazole (400 mg tid for 7 days), is also effective. Antibiotics are continued until the systemic complications or the local lymphadenopathy have subsided.

Do not's:

× Avoid tobacco and alcohol.

× Avoid excessive physical exertion or prolonged exposure to the sun as required in golf, tennis, swimming, or sunbathing.

× Avoid overzealous brushing and the use of dental floss or interdental cleaners.

Second Visit—At the second visit, 1 to 2 days later the patients condition is improved then scaling is performed, if sensitivity permits. The instructions to the patient are the same as those given during first visit.

Third Visit—At the next visit, 1 to 2 days after the second visit, the patient should be essentially symptom free.

Scaling and root planing are repeated. The patient is instructed to discontinue hydrogen peroxide rinses but chlorhexidine rinses should be maintained for two or three weeks.

2. *Management of the residual condition*

a. Elimination of pre-disposing factors—In subsequent visits, the tooth surfaces in the involved areas are scaled and smoothed, and plaque control by the patient is checked and corrected, if necessary. Patients without gingival disease other than the treated acute involvement are dismissed for 1 week. If the condition is satisfactory at that time, the patient is dismissed for 1 month, at which time the schedule for subsequent recall visits is determined according to the patient's needs. But if the chronic gingivitis, periodontal pockets, and pericoronal flaps are present then appointments are scheduled for their treatment and elimination of all forms of local irritation.

Antibiotics are administered systemically only in patients with toxic systemic complications or local lymphadenopathy.

Nutritional supplements—Nutritional supplementation may be indicated in rare instances when NUG patients suffer such severe pain that ingestion of normal diet is difficult. Thus, difficulty in chewing raw fruits and vegetables in such painful conditions could lead to the selection of a diet inadequate in vitamins B and C. Standard multivitamin preparation combined with a therapeutic dose of vitamins B and C are recommened which may be discontinued after two months.

Supportive systemic treatment including bed rest, copious fluid consumption and analgesics for relief of pain are prescribed.

b. Correction of gingival tissue deformities by surgery – Remaining gingival interproximal craters increase plaque retention. Such defects are eliminated by reshaping gingiva surgically or with electrosurgery to establish and maintain the normal interproximal gingival contour. If the defects are more severe, flap surgery or periodontal plastic surgery may be required. Surgery should not be attempted until the local etiologic factors have been completely eliminated and inflammation has resolved.

Treatment of NUG includes:
Oral hygiene instructions
Mechanical debridement of the teeth
Systemic antimicrobial therapy
Surgical correction of gingival contour

PRIMARY HERPETIC GINGIVOSTOMATITIS

Primary herpetic gingivostomatitis is the most common viral disease that affects the gingiva. It is caused by the herpes simplex virus type 1 (HSV-1). It occurs most often in infants and children younger than 6 years of age, but it is also seen in adolescents and adults. It occurs with equal frequency in male and female patients. In most persons, however, the primary infection is asymptomatic. After the primary infection, the virus ascends through sensory and autonomic nerves and persists in neuronal ganglia that innervate the site as latent HSV. The virus may be reactivated by various stimuli including ultraviolet light, trauma, fever, stress or immunosuppression. These secondary manifestations include herpes labialis, herpes genitalis, ocular herpes, and herpetic encephalitis.

Clinical Features

Oral Signs: It appears as a diffuse, erythematous, shiny involvement of the gingiva and the adjacent oral mucosa, with varying degrees of edema and gingival bleeding. It is characterized by the presence of discrete, spherical gray vesicles which may occur on the gingiva, labial and buccal mucosa, soft palate, pharynx, sublingual mucosa, and tongue. After approximately 24 hours the vesicles rupture and form painful, small ulcers with a red, elevated, halo-like margin and a depressed, yellowish- or grayish-white central portion **(Fig. 20.3)**. These occur either in widely separated areas or in clusters where confluence occurs. Occasionally, primary herpetic gingivitis may occur without overt vesiculation. Diffuse, erythematous, shiny discoloration and edematous enlargement of the gingiva with a tendency toward bleeding make up the clinical picture. The course of the disease is limited to 7 to 10 days. The diffuse gingival erythema and edema that appear early in the disease persist for several days after the ulcerative lesions have healed. Scarring does not occur in the areas of healed ulcerations.

Oral Symptoms: There is generalized "soreness" of the oral cavity, which interferes with eating and drinking. The ruptured vesicles are the focal sites of pain and are particularly sensitive to touch, thermal changes, foods such as condiments and fruit juices, and the action of coarse foods. In infants the disease is marked by irritability and refusal to take food.

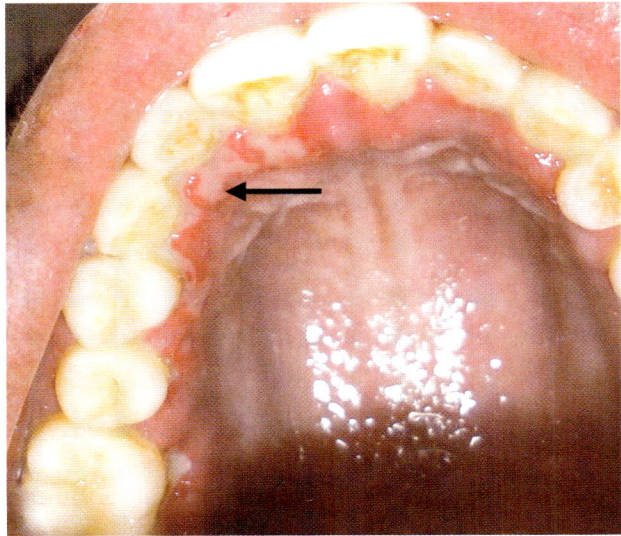

Fig. 20.3: Herpetic gingivostomatitis (*Courtesy:* Dr Gayathri)

Cervical adenitis, fever as high as 101° to 105° F (38.3° to 40.6° C), and generalized malaise are common systemic signs and symptoms.

Histopathology

The virus target the epithelial cells causing acantholysis and nuclear clearing resulting in the formation of Tzanck cells. Intraepithelial vesicles are formed which contain fluid, degenerating cells and herpes virus. Discrete ulcerations resulting from rupture of the vesicles have a central portion of acute inflammation with the varying degree of purulent exduate surrounded by a zone rich in engorged blood vessels.

Diagnosis

The diagnosis is usually established from the patient's history and the clinical findings. The confirmatory diagnosis depends on one or more of the following laboratory tests: a) Inoculation of the virus from a suspected site to tissue culture, this technique takes 3 to 6 days; the virus can be distinguished as type 1 and 2; b) fluorescent monoclonal antibody testing of scraping, this technique requires 15 to 20 minutes; c) serologic studies.

Differential Diagnosis

Primary herpetic gingivostomatitis should be differentiated from the following conditions:

Herpangia is the result of group A coxsackie virus. The lesions in herpes simplex are located predominatly in anterior portion of mouth, whereas those resulting from coxsackie virus are seen in posterior oral pharynx. Also, the duration of illness is longer with herpes simplex virus.

Erythema multiforme can be differentiated because the vesicles in erythema multiforme are generally more extensive than those in primary herpetic gingivos-tomatitis and on rupture demonstrate a tendency toward pseudomembrane formation.

Stevens-Johnson syndrome is a comparatively rare form of erythema multiforme, characterized by vesicular hemorrhagic lesions in the oral cavity, hemorrhagic ocular lesions, and bullous skin lesions.

Bullous lichen planus is a very rare and painful condition. It is characterized by large blisters on the tongue and cheek that rupture and undergo ulceration; it runs a prolonged, indefinite course. Patches of linear, gray, lacelike lesions of lichen planus are often interspersed among the bullous eruptions. Lichen planus involvement of the skin may coexist with the oral lesions and facilitate differential diagnosis.

Treatment

- *Supportive treatment*: Palliative measures make the patient comfortable until the disease runs its course. It runs a 7 to 10-day course and heals without scars. Bland foods and liquid supplements are recommended. If the patient is experiencing pain of longer duration, aspirin or a nonsteroidal anti-inflammatory agent can be given systemically. Plaque, food debris and superficial calculus are removed to reduce gingival inflammation, which complicates the acute herpetic involvement. Extensive periodontal therapy should be postponed until the acute symptoms subside to avoid the possibility of exacerbation.
- *Mucosal ointments*: Mucosal ointments (Orabase) can be applied to lesions with cotton swabs for temporary relief. Especially before meals, topical local anesthetic, such as lidocaine hydrochloride viscous solution can be applied to the affected areas.
- *Antiviral chemotherapy*: Herpes virus-specific drugs, such as acyclovir ointment (apply five times daily for 5 days) are used to lessen the spread and severity of recurrent herpes virus infection. Systemic administration of acyclovir has not demonstrated to alter the clinical course of primary herpes, but it may reduce the duration of viral shedding during which the patient is potentially infectious. Systemically administrated acyclovir (200 mg five times daily for 5 days) may be beneficial for immunocompromised patient.

PERICORONITIS

Definition

Pericoronitis refers to inflammation of the gingiva in relation to the crown of an incompletely erupted tooth. Pericoronitis may be acute, subacute, or chronic. The partially erupted or impacted mandibular third molar is the most common site of pericoronitis. The space between the crown of the tooth and the overlying gingival flap is an ideal area for the accumulation of food debris and bacterial growth **(Fig. 20.4)**. Even in patients with no clinical signs or symptoms, the gingival flap is often chronically inflamed and infected and has varying degrees of ulceration along its inner surface. Acute pericoronitis is identified by varying degrees of inflammatory involvement of the pericoronal flap and adjacent structures as well as systemic complications. The inflammatory fluid and cellular exudate increase the bulk of the flap, which then

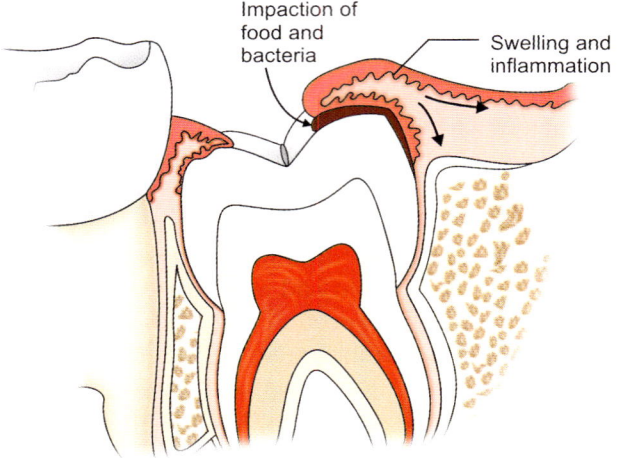

Fig. 20.4: Pericoronitis

may interfere with complete closure of the jaws, and can be traumatized by contact with the opposing jaw, aggravating the inflammatory involvement.

Clinical Features

Symptoms: A patient with pericoronitis may complain of the following symptoms:
- Pain: Pain may be mild but is usually quite intense and may radiate to the external neck, throat, ear, or oral floor.
- Trismus: The patient cannot open the jaw more than few millimeter because of tenderness and extreme pain.
- A bad taste in the mouth caused by pus oozing from beneath the flap
- Swelling in the neck or in the area of the affected tooth
- Fever

Signs: Following are the signs of pericoronitis which are observed during examination:
- A partially erupted tooth
- Markedly red, swollen, suppurating lesion around a partially erupted tooth **(Fig. 20.5)**.
- Pus oozing from under an overlaying tissue flap
- A painful reaction when finger pressure is applied
- Swelling of the cheek (in the region of the angle of the jaw)
- Cervical lymphadenopathy
- The patient may also have toxic systemic complications such as elevated temperature, leukocytosis, malaise and an ipsilateral tonsillitis or upper respiratory infection.

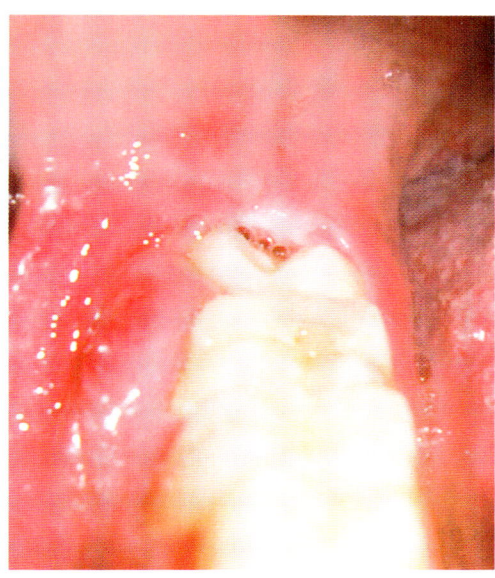

Fig. 20.5: Pericoronitis—Third molar partially covered by infected flap

Complications

- Pericoronal abscess
- Lymphadenopathy – Depending on the severity and extent of the infection, there is involvement of the submaxillary, posterior cervical, deep cervical, and retropharyngeal lymph nodes.
- Peritonsillar abscess formation, cellulitis and Ludwig's angina are infrequent sequelae of acute pericoronitis.

Treatment

In the treatment of pericoronitis, the following emergency procedures are performed:

A. Non surgical therapy: Gently flush the area with warm water and H_2O_2 to remove debris and exudates. Swab with antiseptic after elevating the flap gently from the tooth with a scaler. The underlying debris is removed, and the area is flushed with warm water. Appropriate antibiotics (Amoxicillin and Metronidazole combination) are prescribed, if the patient is febrile or if lymph nodes are palpable.

B. Surgical therapy: After the acute symptoms have subsided, a determination is made as to whether the tooth is to be retained or extracted. The decision as to whether to save the tooth or to extract it depends upon various factors like its position, opposing tooth, chances of eruption to proper occlusion and periodontal status.

Operculectomy: If it is decided to save the tooth an, operculectomy is done. LA is given (usually inferior

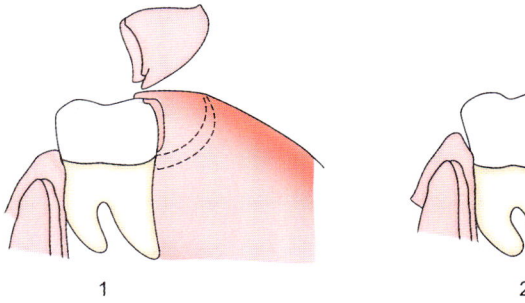

1 Removal of operculum distal to the third molar
2 Appearance of healed area

Fig. 20.6: Operculectomy

alveolar nerve block) for mandibular molar. The pericoronal flap is removed using periodontal knives or electrosurgery. Incision is given anterior to anterior border of ramus and brought downward and forward to the distal surface of the crown as close as possible to the level of CEJ, which will detach a wedge shaped tissue. It is necessary to remove the tissue distal to the tooth, as well as the flap on the occlusal surface **(Fig. 20.6)**. Incising only the occlusal portion of the flap leaves a deep distal pocket, which invites recurrence of acute pericoronal involvement.

Extraction: It is best to extract the tooth after acute symptoms subside if the tooth is not going to serve any purpose. All pericoronal flaps should be viewed with suspicion. Persistent symptom-free pericoronal flaps should be removed as a preventive measure against subsequent acute involvement. Bone loss on the distal surface of the second molars is a hazard following the extraction of partially or completely impacted third molars, and the problem is significantly greater if the third molars are extracted after the roots are formed or in patients older than their early twenties. To reduce the risk of bone loss around second molars, partially or completely impacted third molars should be extracted as early as possible in their development.

POINTS TO PONDER

✓ Necrotizing ulcerative gingivitis is a painful infectious gingival disease primarily of the interdental and marginal gingiva.
✓ In NUG, the zone between the marginal necrosis and the relatively unaffected gingiva usually exhibits a

well-demarcated narrow erythematous zone, sometimes referred to as the linear erythema.

✓ In pericoronitis, the patient is extremely uncomfortable because of a foul taste and an inability to close the jaws, in addition to the pain.

BIBLIOGRAPHY

1. Ammons WF. Jr. Acute lesions of periodontium. Lesions in the oral mucous membranes. In, Wilson TG, Kornman KS. Fundamentals of Periodontics. Quintessence publishing 1996;423-51.
2. Arun KV. Cell cycle. In, Molecular biology of periodontium. 1st ed Jaypee Brothers 2010;70-94.
3. Carranza FA, Klokkevold PR. Acute gingival infections. In, Newman, Takei, Carranza. Clinical Periodontology 9th ed WB Saunders 2003;297-307.
4. Cogen RB. Acute necrotizing ulcerative gingivitis. In, Genco RJ, Goldman HM and Cohen DW. Contemporary Periodontics. CV Mosby Company 1990;459-65.
5. DA, Stern IB, Listgarten MA.Viral infections. In, Grant Periodontics. 6th ed CV Mosby Company 1988;413-20.
6. Eley BM, Manson JD. Acute and infectious lesions of the ginigva. In, Periodontics 5th ed Wright 2004;345-53.
7. Eley BM, Manson JD. Acute Necrotizing Ulcerative Gingivitis. In, Periodontics 5th ed Wright 2004;354-57.
8. Folayan MO. The Epidemiology, Etiology and Pathophysiology of Acute Necrotizing Ulcerative Gingivitis Associated with Malnutrition. J Contemp Dent Pract 2004;5:28-41.
9. Grant DA, Stern IB, Listgarten MA. Necrotizing Ulcerative Gingivitis. In, Periodontics. 6th ed CV Mosby Company 1988;398-12.
10. Grant DA, Stern IB, Listgarten MA. Pericoronitis. In, Periodontics. 6th ed CV Mosby Company 1988;421-24.
11. Holmstrup P, Westergaard J. Necrotizing Periodontal Disease. In, Lindhe J, Karring T, Lang NP. Clinical Periodontology and Implant dentistry. 4th ed Blackwell Munksgaard 2003;243-59.
12. Johnson BD, Engel D. Acute Necrotizing Ulcerative Gingivitis: A Review of Diagnosis, Etiology, and Treatment. J Periodontol 1986; 57:141-50.
13. Klokkevold PR, Takei HH. Treatment of acute gingival disease. In, Newman, Takei, Carranza. Clinical Periodontology 9th ed WB Saunders 2003;622-28.
14. Rose LF. Infective forms of gingivostomatitis. In, Genco RJ, Goldman HM and Cohen DW. Contemporary Periodontics. CV Mosby Company 1990;243-50.
15. Rowland RW. Necrotizing Ulcerative Gingivitis. Ann Periodontol 1999;4:65-73.

MCQs

1. The following may be involved with the etiology of NUG *except*:
   A. AIDS   B. Hypertension
   C. Nutritional deficiency   D. Smoking
2. Lesions in NUG can be described as:
   A. Ulcerative lesions infectious but not contagious
   B. Ulcerative lesions contagious but not infectious
   C. Ulcerative lesions which are contagious
   D. None of the above
3. Laboratory test for NUG is:
   A. Tissue culture
   B. Complement
   C. Dark field examination
   D. None of the above
4. Metronidazole is usually the drug of choice for:
   A. NUG
   B. Primary herptic gingivostomatitis
   C. Chronic periodontitis
   D. Gingivitis
5. Definite treatment for herpetic gingivostomatitis:
   A. Hydrogen peroxide mouthwash
   B. Metronidazole
   C. Corticosteroid
   D. No definite treatment

Answers

1. B   2. A   3. C   4. A   5. D

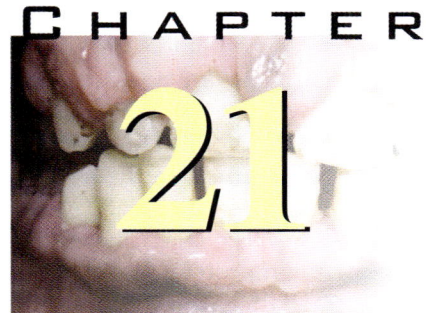

CHAPTER 21

Soft and Hard Tissue Lesions with Periodontal Relevance

Shailja Chatterjee, Shalu Bathla

INTRODUCTION

There are some hard and soft pathological conditions that may affect various parts of the body and oral cavity as well. These lesions are widespread and may affect the periodontium. Some of these lesions involving gingiva and other periodontal tissues are summarized in this chapter.

DESQUAMATIVE GINGIVITIS

Lichen Planus

Lichen planus is a common mucocutaneous disease. It affects about 0.1% to 0.4% of individuals, depending upon the population sampled. Most of the patients with oral lichen planus (OLP) are middle aged and older women (2:1 ratio of females to males), and children are rarely affected.

The clinical lesions of oral lichen planus, include asymptomatic, chronic bilateral interlacing white lines, (Wickham's striae) typically on the posterior buccal mucosa (90% cases), on tongue (30%), or on alveolar ridge/gingiva (13%). Clinical manifestations include white lacy slightly elevated patterns, plaque-type, atrophic, ulcerative or bullous presentations.

The gingival lesions of lichen planus fall into one or more of the following categories:

1. *Keratotic lesions:* These are usually present on the attached gingiva as small raised, round white papules of pinhead size with a flattened surface. These keratotic lesions can be further be classified as papular, plaque-like, linear, reticular or annular.

2. *Vesiculobullous lesions:* These raised, fluid-filled lesions are uncommon and short lived on the gingiva. They quickly rupture and leave ulcerations. These are uncommon on gingiva and can present with difficulties in diagnosis.

3. *Atrophic lesions:* Atrophy of the gingival tissues with ensuing epithelial thinning results in erythema confined to the gingiva. These produce desquamative gingivitis and is the most commonly seen type of gingival lichen planus.

4. *Erosive lesions/Ulcerative lesions:* Erosive form may appear as desquamative gingivitis **(Fig. 21.1)**. These extensive erythematous areas with a patchy distribution may present as focal or diffuse hemorrhagic areas exacerbated by slight trauma (e.g., toothbrushing).

Microscopically, hyperkeratosis, hydropic degeneration of the basal layer, saw – tooth configuration of the rete ridges and a dense band-like infiltrate primarily of T lymphocytes in the lamina propria are observed. Colloid bodies (civatte bodies) may be seen at the epithelium-connective tissue interface.

Treatment—The erosive, bullous, or ulcerative lesions of oral lichen planus are treated with high-potency topical steroids (for example 0.05% fluocinonide ointment applied to lesions three times daily).

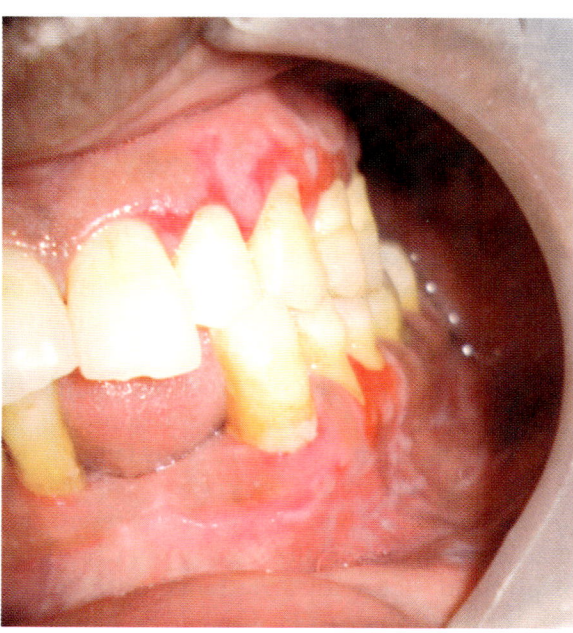

Fig. 21.1: Erosive lichen planus (*Courtesy:* Dr Gayathri)

Cicatrical Pemphigoid

It is also known as mucous membrane pemphigoid (MMP). It is a chronic, scarring vesiculobullous autoimmune disorder. It is closely related to bullous pemphigoid (BP), but unlike BP there are no circulating antibodies. MMP predominantly affects women in their fifth decade of life, and occasionally, young children. The target antigens identified in MMP include the bullous pemphigoid antigens 1 and 2 (BPAg 1 and BPAg 2), laminins 5 (epiligrin) and 6, type VII collagen, β_4 integrin subunit, and additional unknown proteins.

Microscopically, subepithelial clefting occurs with separation of the epithelium from the underlying lamina propria, leaving an intact basal layer. A mixed inflammatory infiltrate consisting of lymphocytes, plasma cells, neutrophils, and scarce eosinophils is observed in the stroma. Direct immunofluorescence reveals deposits of IgG and C3 restricted to the basement membrane.

Treatment includes topical corticosteroid therapy using fluocinonide (0.05%) and clobetasol propionate (0.05%) in an adhesive vehicle which can be used 3 times a day for upto 6 months. When lesions do not respond to steroid, systemic dapsone is given.

Pemphigus

The term being derived from the Greek 'Pemphix' meaning bubble or blister. Pemphigus is a group of potentially life-threatening autoimmune mucocutaneous disease characterized by epithelial blistering affecting cutaneous and/or mucosal surfaces. There is a fairly strong genetic background to pemphigus with linkage to HLA Class II alleles. Certain ethnic groups, such as Ashkenazi Jews and those of Mediteranean origin, are especially predisposed to pemphigus.

Pemphigus Vulgaris

Pemphigus Vulgaris (PV), the most common variant, is an autoimmune blistering disease characterized by the presence of circulating IgG antibodies against the cadherin-type adhesion molecules: desmoglein 3 (Dsg3) and desmoglein 1 (Dsg1).

Oral lesions are the first sign of the disease in approximately 60% of patients and may present one year or more before the cutaneous lesions. Virtually, any region of the oral cavity can be involved, but multiple lesions often develop at sites of irritation or trauma. The soft palate is more often involved (80%), followed by the buccal mucosa (46%), ventral aspect or dorsum of tongue (20%), and lower labial mucosa (10%). The gingiva is not a major intraoral site; however when gingival lesions occur, they are desquamative. These are initially vesiculobullous but readily rupture with ulcer formation.

Diagnosis: The Nikolsky sign is positive in Pemphigus vulgaris. This clinical test is performed by using either an air syringe to blow air on the perilesional tissue or by gently rubbing the perilesional tissue with a finger. If the surface layer of mucosa separates from the underlying tissue, the patient is said to exhibit a positive Nikolsky sign. Biopsy of perilesional tissue, with histological and immunostaining examination is essential for diagnosis. Serum autoantibodies to either Dsg3 or Dsg1 are detected by means of indirect immunofluorescence technique employing monkey oesophagus or by enzyme-linked immunosorbent assay (ELISA).

Microscopically, Pemphigus vulgaris lesions demonstrate a characteristic intraepithelial clefting/ vesiculation above the basal cell layer with a characteristic "tombstone" appearance. Rounded acantholytic *Tzanck cells* are visible in the cleft. The subjacent stroma usually exhibits a mild to moderate chronic inflammatory cells infiltrate **(Fig. 21.2)**.

Paraneoplastic pemphigus: The other important variant of pemphigus affecting the oral cavity is paraneoplastic pemphigus, which is usually associated with lymphoproliferative disease. Sometimes, oral lesions might be the only manifestation. The autoantibodies are IgG or IgA type and are directed against Desmoplakin 1, Desmoplakin 2 and BP230.

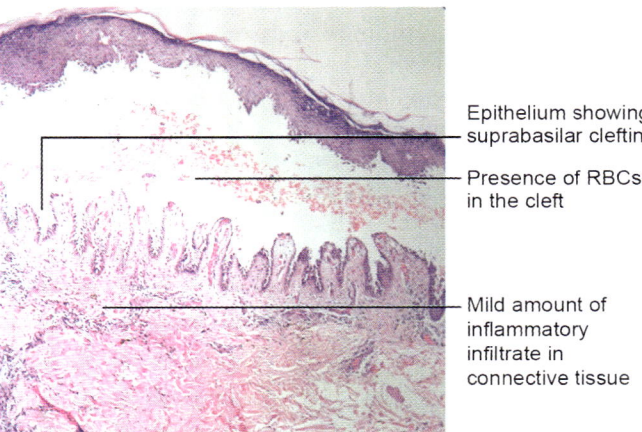

Epithelium showing suprabasilar clefting

Presence of RBCs in the cleft

Mild amount of inflammatory infiltrate in connective tissue

Fig. 21.2: Pemphigus

Treatment: Current treatment is largely based on systemic corticosteroids with or without immunosuppressive agents and tacrolimus. Initially, when only steroids were employed, high initial and maintenance doses of steroids were necessary to control the disease. If the patient responds well to corticosteroids, the dosage can be gradually reduced, but a low-maintenance dosage is usually necessary to prevent or minimize the recurrence of lesions. In patients not responsive to corticosteroids or who gradually adapt to them, steroid-sparing therapies are used. They consist of combinations of steroids plus other medications such as azathioprine, cyclosporine, dapsone, gold, methotrexate. Topical antifungal medication may be needed to eliminate iatrogenic Candidiasis, which often arises when topical steroids are used intraorally. Intravenous administration of immunoglobulins has proved successful and safe in steroid-resistant PV. Plasmaphoresis sometimes with cyclosporin or cyclophosphamide have also been reported to be of benefit.

Meticulous oral hygiene and periodontal care are essential for the overall management of patients with pemphigus. Patients in the maintenance phase may require prednisolone before professional oral prophylaxis and periodontal surgery.

Systemic Lupus Erythematosus

Systemic lupus erythematosus (SLE) is a multisystem autoimmune connective tissue disorder with various clinical presentations. It is prevalent among young women with a peak age of onset between late teens and early 40s with a female to male ratio of 9:1.

SLE is a chronic illness that may be life-threatening when major organs are affected but more commonly results in chronic debilitating ill health. No single cause for SLE has been identified, but precipitating factors include sunlight and drugs, and there is a complex genetic basis. Autoantibodies may be present for many years before the clinical onset of the disease, and there may be increase in numbers of circulating antibodies before manifesting.

Bazin first described oral manifestations of lupus erythematosus in 1861, with a more detailed description in 1901 by Capelle. Oral ulceration is one of the revised diagnostic criteria proposed by the American College of Rheumatology for classification of SLE.

The prevalence of oral lesions is reported to be 7-52% in patients with SLE. A significant proportion of oral lesions are asymptomatic. Clinical presentations are of

PERIODONTICS REVISITED

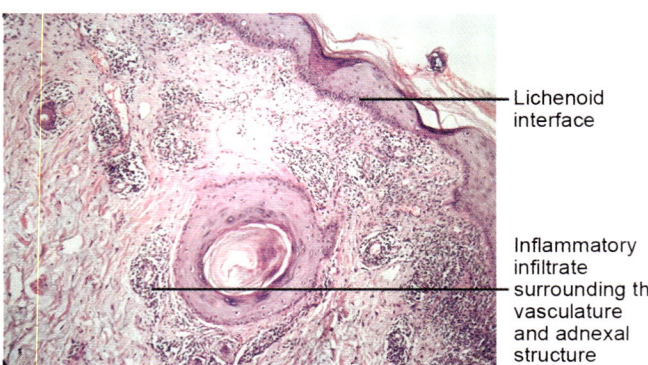

Fig. 21.3: Lupus Erythematosus

three types- *discoid, erythematous and ulcerations*. Discoid lesions appear as central areas of erythema with white spots surrounded by radiating white striae and telangiectasia at the periphery. Erythematous lesions are often accompanied by edema and petechial reddening. Ulcers tend to occur in crops and are shallow, measuring 1-2 cm in diameter.

Antichromatin, anti-DNA and antihistone antibodies are the underlying pathogenic causes.

Histopathologically there is hyperkeratosis, keratotic plugging and liquefactive degeneration of basal layer of epithelium. Lamina propria shows chronic inflammatory perivascular infiltrate (lymphohistiocytic) **(Fig. 21.3)**. Direct immunofluorescence show IgM, IgG, complement and fibrinogen deposits along the dermal-epidermal junction.

The therapy for SLE is dependent on the severity and extent of the disease. Cutaneous rashes are treated with topical steroids, sunscreens, and hydroxychloroquinine. For severe systemic organ involvement, moderate- to-high doses of prednisolone are effective. For severe cases of SLE or when side effects to prednisolone develop, immunosuppressive drugs such as cytotoxic drugs (cyclophosphamide and azathioprine) and plasma-phoresis alone or in conjunction with steroids are useful.

Erythema Multiforme

Erythema multiforme is an acute, self-limiting inflammatory disorder of the skin and mucous membranes with a tendency for recurrence and distinctive clinical appearance. It is considered a hypersensitivity reaction to a variety of precipitating agents, including drugs, neoplasms and infections. Cutaneous involvement exhibits as erythematous papules. Target lesions are distributed symmetrically over the extensor surfaces. Mucosal involvement is in form of ulcerations or papules as in Stevens-Johnson's syndrome.

Circulating immune complexes play an important role in pathogenesis of erythema multiforme. Direct immunofluorescence studies show granular deposits of complement components (C3) and immunoglobulins (IgM) in the superficial dermal vessels or at the dermal-epidermal junction.

Histopathologically, microvascular proliferation is seen in the papillary dermis/lamina propria juxta-epithelially. Perivasculitis is evident.

There is no specific treatment for erythema multiforme. Some cases may even resolve spontaneously, and erythematous lesions may require no treatment. For mild symptoms, systemic and local antihistamines coupled with topical anesthetics and debridement of lesions with an oxygenating agent is adequate. In patients with severe symptoms, corticosteroids are prescribed.

METASTATIC TUMORS IN THE JAWS/SOFT TISSUES

The majority of metatasis to the oral region are intraosseous. The gingiva (including the alveolar mucosa) is most often the seat of soft tissue metastasis in the mouth. In the oral regions, soft tissue metatasis from lung cancer is encountered most frequently in men, while metatasis from breast cancer account for most soft tissue metatasis in women. About 20% of oral soft tissue metatasis were manifested before the primary tumor was diagnosed. Furthermore, in 90% of the cases the clinical manifestation resembled a hyperplastic or reactive lesion. These observations emphasize the need for a histologic examination of all such tumors.

The histopathology resembles the tumor of origin. Most cases are carcinomas and sarcomas that rarely metastasize to the oral region. The histopathologic appearance of metastatic jaw disease often is poorly differentiated, therefore, making it challenging to determine the primary lesion site.

The radiographic appearance of metastatic disease in jaws varies from well to poorly circumscribed radiolucencies. Alveolar bone extensions may be confused with periodontal disease. Metastatic disease of the jaws may extend into the overlying soft tissues, appearing to be a dental or periodontal infection. Alternatively, metastasis may occur directly in the soft tissues, usually the gingiva.

Differential diagnosis of metastatic peripheral lesions on the gingiva or alveolar ridge include- pyogenic granuloma, peripheral giant cell granuloma, peripheral ossifying fibroma or fibroma.

Most of the cases presenting as metastatic lesion to the jaws have an undiagnosed primary malignancy at the time of the presentation of jaw lesion. Patient may present with innocuous dental symptoms, such as pulpal or periodontal pain. Therefore, all tissues excised from the oral cavity should be submitted for pathological evaluation.

MALIGNANT LESIONS OF GINGIVA

Proliferative Verrucous Leukoplakia

The term Proliferative Verrucous Leukoplakia (PVL) was based upon its clinical appearance resembling an expanding verrucal white growth. The early lesions of PVL appear as a deceptive solitary homogenous leukoplakia. Despite its innocuous appearance, the leukoplakia recurs and rapidly spreads over time resulting in diffuse, multifocal, and exophytic or verrucous type of oral lesions. The most common site is buccal mucosa followed by the gingiva and the tongue. However, gingival lesions exhibit the greatest malignant transformation rate, usually 7 years after the initial diagnosis.

Histopathologically, varying grades of epithelial dysplasia can be seen with superficial surface showing verrucal exophytic growth **(Fig. 21.4)**.

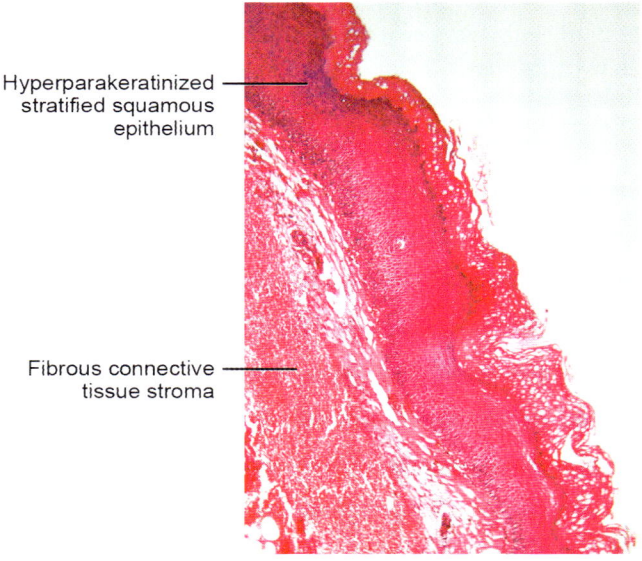

Hyperparakeratinized stratified squamous epithelium

Fibrous connective tissue stroma

Fig. 21.4: Proliferative verrucous leukoplakia

Surgical eradication and laser vaporization of the lesions is difficult due to widespread nature of the condition with disappointing results of repeated recurrences.

Squamous Cell Carcinoma

Squamous cell carcinoma is the most common malignancy of the oral cavity and oropharynx. The gingiva is the third most common site for intraoral squamous cell carcinoma and represents about 15 to 25% of the oral epithelial malignancies. Mandibular gingival squamous cell carcinoma are more common than their maxillary counterparts (2:1 ratio) and characteristically exhibit a wide spectrum of clinical presentations, sometimes deceptively mimicking innocuous inflammatory conditions.

Microscopically, infiltrative cords, islands and sheets of malignant keratinocytes invade the connective tissue and exhibit cellular pleomorphism, hyperchromatism, and aberrant mitosis. The well differentiated squamous cell carcinomas show keratin pearl formation that facilitate their identification, where as the poorly differentiated carcinomas may have to be subjected to immuno-cytochemical examination to be properly diagnosed.

Treatment for gingival squamous cell carcinoma is the surgical resection with or without post operative radiotherapy. When irradiation therapy is required, extraction of involved teeth is often necessary before irradiation is instituted if the teeth suffer from severe periodontitis. This is due to an increased risk of osteoradionecrosis after extraction of teeth situated in irradiated bone as the result of permanently reduced vascularization.

Donor-cell Derived Oral Squamous Cell Carcinoma

Oral squamous cell carcinomas (OSCCs) developing after bone marrow transplantation are rare, occurring in 1 of 500 long-term survivors. The lesion develops on oral mucosa, with a highly aggressive behaviour, leading to death within few months despite early and large surgical removal. Such incidences have been found in patients with chronic graft versus host disease underlying prolonged immunosuppression.

Malignant Melanoma

Melanoma originates from two types of neural crest cells; melanocytes and nevus cells. Melanocytes are dendrites cells that reside in the epithelium and show contact inhibition. In contrast, nevus cells reside in the subjacent

PERIODONTICS REVISITED

connective tissue and tend to aggregate in clusters. Although the most common site for melanoma is the palate (40%), gingiva melanomas represent close to one third of these tumors. Oral melanoma may appear de novo as a rapidly growing mass. Although the presence of pigmentation in a rapidly growing mass is an ominous sign suggestive of melanoma requiring biopsy without delay. Clinically, oral melanoma may exhibit three presentations: a pigmented macula, a pigmented nodule with or without areas of ulceration, or a nodule with similar color to the surrounding oral mucosa (amelanotic melanoma).

Microscopically, the pigmented nodular type of melanoma is the most common, consisting of proliferating atypical, pleomorphic, spindle-shaped, or epitheloid tumor cells containing melanin with frequent mitotic figures.

The treatment of choice for oral melanoma is surgical excision with adequate negative margins. Radiotherapy and chemotherapy are palliative interventions that may be used in addition to the surgical excision.

Sarcomas

Intraoral soft tissue sarcomas (STS) are extremely rare and periodontal tissues are affected the least. Usually, STS are diagnosed in patients older than 20 years with no sex predilection. Clinically, oral STS are exophytic, infiltrative masses that may exhibit rapid growth and may or may not be painful.

The prognosis of a malignant tumor is largely dependent on early diagnosis. Soft tissue sarcomas initially produce a bulging of the mucosa without destroying it but may grow rapidly causing destruction.

REACTIVE LESIONS OF GINGIVA

Pyogenic Granuloma

Pyogenic granuloma is a nodular, purple to red, hemorrhagic circumscribed friable polypoid lesion that bleeds easily and is often ulcerated. Microtrauma from tooth brushing and local irritants such as dental plaque and calculus seem to be the etiologic factors of this condition. Pyogenic granuloma is painless, occurs mainly in women during the second and fifth decades of life. Usual site is the anterior mandibular or maxillary gingiva. The so-called pregnancy tumor is a clinical term used to identify a pyogenic granuloma that occurs in pregnant women.

Microscopically, this lesion exhibits ulceration of the surface epithelium and, characteristically there is

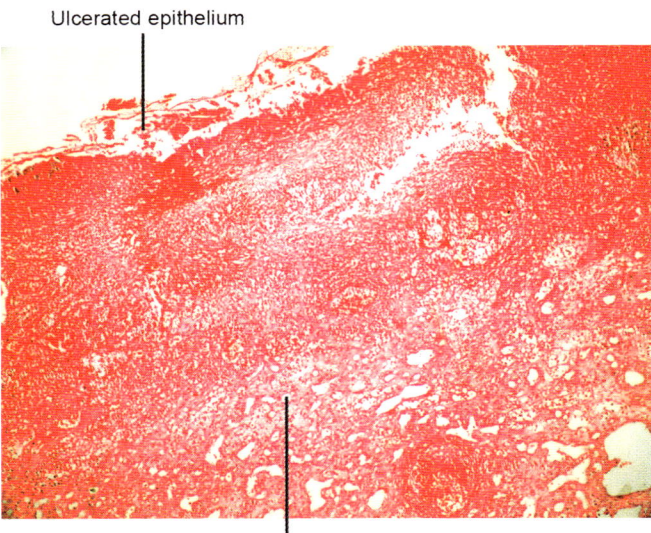

Ulcerated epithelium

Stroma containing numerous blood vessels and extravasated RBCs

Fig. 21.5: Pyogenic granuloma

fibroendothelial proliferation of the stroma surrounded by acute and chronic inflammatory cells **(Fig. 21.5)**.

Surgical excision is the preferred treatment of choice, with removal of local irritants to prevent recurrence. For pregnancy tumor, a conservative approach is recommended. In the absence of significant aesthetic or functional problems, or both, the lesion should not be excised because it may resolve after parturition. Local irritants such as plaque and calculus should be removed. Those lesions failing to resolve should be surgically excised. Follow-up of the patient is needed because pyogenic granuloma exhibits a tendency to recur.

Peripheral Fibroma

Peripharal fibroma is typically an asymptomatic, dome shaped nodule. True fibromas are very less in incidence. Usual site of occurrence is interdental region. These lesions can be sessile as well as pedunculated.

Microscopically, the peripheral fibroma is surfaced by parakeratinized stratified squamous epithelium with or without focal hyperkeratinization. The main feature is the presence of hyperplastic collagen fibers arranged in intersecting fascicles with a varied amount of blood capillaries and occasionally, inflammatory cells **(Fig. 21.6)**. This lesion is managed by surgical excision and has an excellent prognosis with a low recurrence rate.

Peripheral Ossifying Fibroma

Peripheral ossifying fibroma usually presents as a polypoid, pink mass in the interdental papilla **(Fig. 21.7)**.

Hyperplastic epithelium

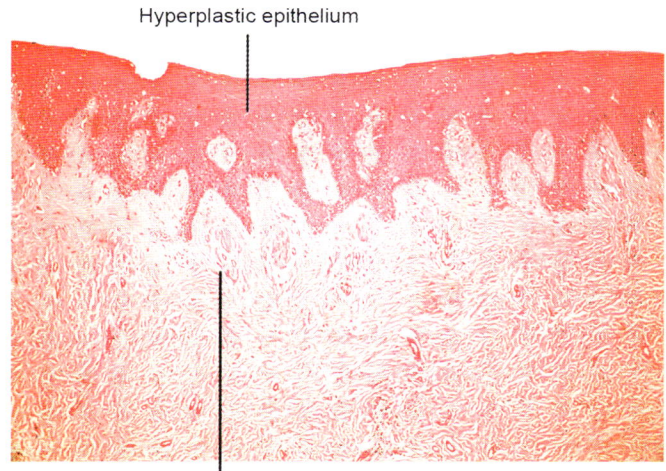

Dense fibrous connective tissue stroma

Fig. 21.6: Peripheral fibroma

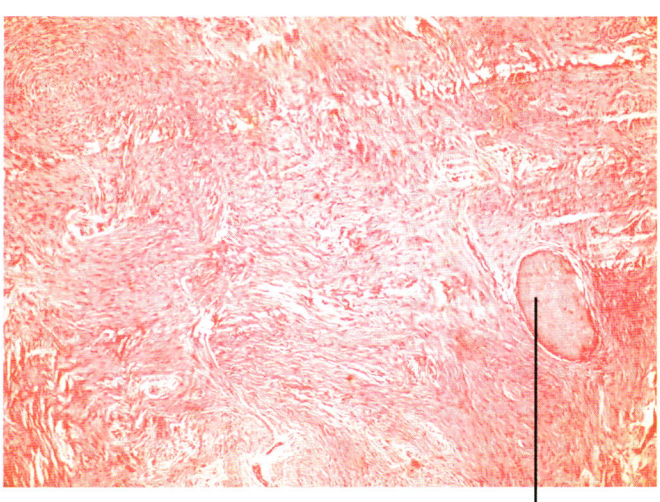

Osseous deposition in fibrocellular connective tissue

Fig. 21.8: Peripheral ossifying fibroma

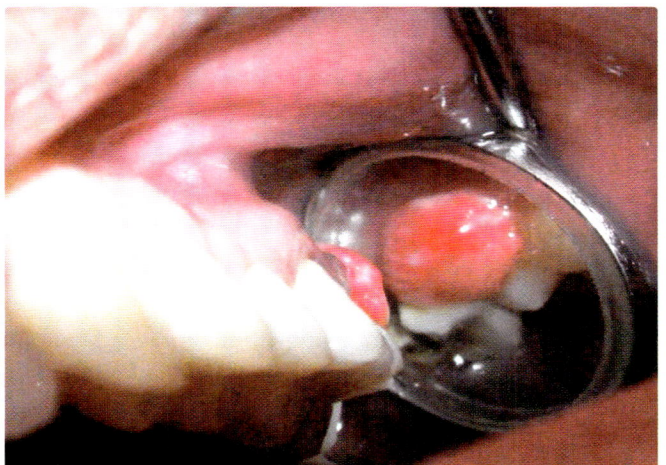

Fig. 21.7: Peripheral ossifying fibroma

Clinically, this lesion may be impossible to distinguish from a pyogenic granuloma. In some cases, clinician may make a clinical diagnosis of peripheral ossifying fibroma by taking a periapical film of the suspicious area that reveals the presence of radiopacities in the gingival lesion. However, calcifications within the lesions may not always be visible radiographically. Peripheral ossifying fibroma may appear from the first to the sixth decade of life with a peak incidence in the second decade of life.

Microscopically, the surface epithelium may or may not be ulcerated, but in presence of ulceration, associated granulation tissue is observed. The main microscopic feature is the presence of either bone metaplasia or dystrophic calcification in the fibrous connective tissue stroma of the lesion **(Fig. 21.8)**. When strands and islands of odontogenic epithelium are found in the stroma of the specimen, the diagnosis of peripheral odontogenic fibroma is appropriate.

Treatment include deep surgical excision upto the periosteum and periodontal ligament with thorough root planing.

Peripheral Giant Cell Tumor

Peripheral giant cell tumor presents as a gingival nodule with a sessile base and a red to purple discoloration that may sometime produce displacement of the teeth. Local etiologic factors such as trauma, calculus, food debris, and ill – fitting dental restorations/prosthesis seem to play a significant role in the development of this lesion. They can occur from the first to the eighth decade of life with a mean age of 35 years. A female-male ratio of 2:1 is routinely observed.

Microscopically, the surface epithelium may or may not show areas of ulceration. The underlying fibrous connective tissue exhibits the presence of conspicuous distinct nodules of multinucleated giant cells between spindle mesenchymal cells and numerous vascular channels. Hemosiderin granules, hemorrhage and, in some occasions, dystrophic calcifications, osteoid and even frank bone metaplasia may also be observed. In those cases, the presence of multinucleated giant cells may be absent, or present only in small numbers.

PERIODONTICS REVISITED

Surgical excision is the treatment of choice for peripheral giant cell lesions.

PERIPHERAL ODONTOGENIC LESIONS

Gingival Cyst

The gingival cyst of adults is a rare odontogenic lesion with a slight predilection for men in their fifth to sixth decade of life. The majority of these lesions (75%) are located in the labial attached or free gingiva of the mandible in the premolar – canine – incisor area.

Clinically, a single, small raised lesion reminiscent of a vesicle shows a bluish discoloration (**Fig. 21.9**). Interestingly, this bluish discoloration with fluid content

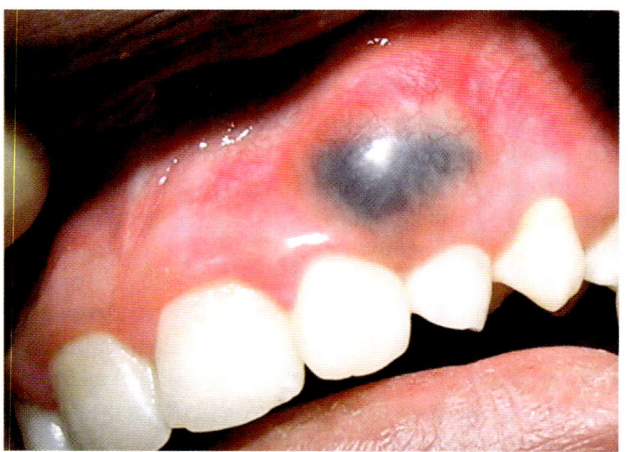

Fig. 21.9: Clinical picture of Gingival cyst

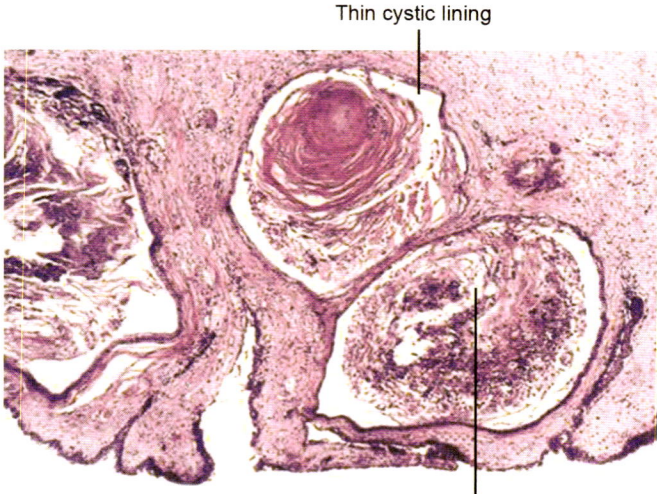

Thin cystic lining

Presence of cystic contents in lumen

Fig. 21.10: Gingival cyst

is suggestive of mucocele. However, gingival tissues do not normally contain minor salivary glands and only rarely are ectopic gingival salivary glands observed. On rare occassions, multiple unilateral or bilateral gingival cysts may be present.

Microscopically, the gingival cyst is typically lined by a thin epithelium with or without focal intraluminal budding and a noninflamed cyst wall (**Fig. 21.10**).

Surgical excision is the preferred treatment, and, in some cases, superficial saucerization of the alveolar bone may be seen during surgery. If incompletely excised, recurrence of the lesion is feasible.

Peripheral Ameloblastoma

Peripheral ameloblastoma is a painless, sessile growth with a firm consistency. The surface is usually smooth and similar in color to the surrounding mucosa, but in some cases it has been described as erythematous, papillary, or even warty. In rare occassions, the lesion is ulcerative rather than exophytic.

The microscopic features of peripheral ameloblastoma are identical to those seen in the central ameloblastoma. The most common histologic patterns are the follicular and acanthomatous patterns.

Surgical excision with adequate margins is the treatment of choice. Recurrence is thought to be caused by incomplete removal.

Peripheral Odontogenic Keratocysts

These have been reported in the 4th to 6th decade of life. Histopathologically, characteristic 7 to 8 layered cystic lining exhibit a tomb-stone appearance in the basal cell layer with parakeratinized surface corrugation. Epithelial-connective tissue interface is flattened and is highly friable. A high recurrence rate has been reported therefore, a conservative surgical treatment is advised.

Epithelial Odontogenic Ghost Cell Tumor

It is an uncommon odontogenic lesion that is closely linked histologically to the calcifying odontogenic cyst. Most investigators today accept that Epithelial odontogenic ghost cell tumor is a neoplastic, solid tumor counterpart of calcifying odontogenic cyst.

Histopathologically, it consists of ameloblastoma-like odontogenic epithelial proliferations infiltrating the bone and connective tissue. Ghost cells are seen with varying amounts of dentinoid. Most islands consist of small basaloid cells having round, hyperchromatic nuclei with scanty cytoplasm and squamous differentiation. Surrounding stroma is fibrous and contains few giant cells.

GRANULOMATOUS GINGIVITIS

Orofacial Granulomatosis (OFG)

The term OFG describes a clinical entity presenting with swelling of the facial and/or oral tissues in association with histologic evidence of noncaseating granulomatous inflammation. This class includes idiopathic disorders such as Melkersson-Rosenthal syndrome and Miescher chronic granulomatous cheilitis, as well as localized orofacial presentations of Crohn's disease and Sarcoidosis. Granulomatous gingivitis may occur in 21 to 26% of patients.

Crohn's disease (regional enteritis, granulomatous enteritis) first described by Crohn and colleagues in 1932, is characterized by a chronic granulomatous, relapsing inflammatory involvement of the gastrointestinal tract, particularly the terminal ileum. The incidence of oral lesions in patients with Crohn's disease ranges from 6 to 20%. These lesions are significant as they precede the intestinal symptoms in up to 60% of cases. Common oral manifestations of Crohn's disease include hypertrophy and swelling of lips, gingival swelling, cobblestone appearance of buccal mucosa and palate and deep ulcers. Microscopic examination reveals an ulcerated, edematous epithelium infiltrated by aggregates of numerous neutrophils and lymphocytes. Numerous granulomas with epithelioid histiocytes intermixed with lymphocytes and Langerhan giant cells in the subjacent connective tissue are seen. Treatment for oral lesions is application of medium to high potency steroids (Clobetasol propionate 0.05% mixed with Benzocaine). Systemic treatment protocols include drugs like cyclosporine and thalidomide as well as steroid-sparing agents such as azathioprne, methotrexate and hydroxychloroquine and fully human immunoglobulin G1 anti-tumor necrosis factor agents and humanized anti-α4-integrin IgG4 antibody.

Orofacial granulomatosis may be a manifestation of Sarcoidosis. The absence of clinical signs suggestive of Sarcoidosis, a normal chest radiograph, and normal levels of serum angiotensin-converting enzymes make Sarcoidosis unlikely.

Tuberculosis and Leprosy should also be considered as possibilities in patients with OFG; however, proper examination is mandatory to establish the diagnosis.

BENIGN NEOPLASMS OF PERIODONTAL HARD TISSUES

Ameloblastoma

Ameloblastoma is the second most common odontogenic tumor and originates from any sort of odontogenic epithelium including dental lamina rests, epithelial rests of Malassez, reduced enamel epithelium and cystic epithelial lining. Ameloblastoma exhibits no sex predilection and occurs in the mandible and the maxilla of adults at about their fourth decade of life. Most ameloblastomas occur in the mandibular molar area, are usually asymptomatic, and are discovered during a routine radiographic examination or during the exploration of a painless jaw swelling.

Histopathological picture shows palisading and nuclear hyperchromatism with reverse polarization and vacuolization of basal cells.

Surgical excision with margins free of tumor is the treatment of choice. Conservative treatments such as enucleation and curettage results in high recurrence rates.

MALIGNANT NEOPLASMS OF PERIODONTAL HARD TISSUES

Osteosarcoma

Osteosarcoma is the most common primary malignant tumor of bone. It is a malignant tumor characterized by the direct formation of bone or osteoid tissue by the tumor cells. The rapidly growing firm or hard tumor may cause loosening and migration of the teeth. Osteosarcoma of the jaws can appear throughout a wide age spectrum, but it is usually diagnosed during the third to fourth decade of life. The maxilla and mandible are affected with equal frequency. Men are affected more commonly than women. Clinically, swelling, pain, mobile teeth, nasal obstruction and paresthesia are the most common signs and symptoms.

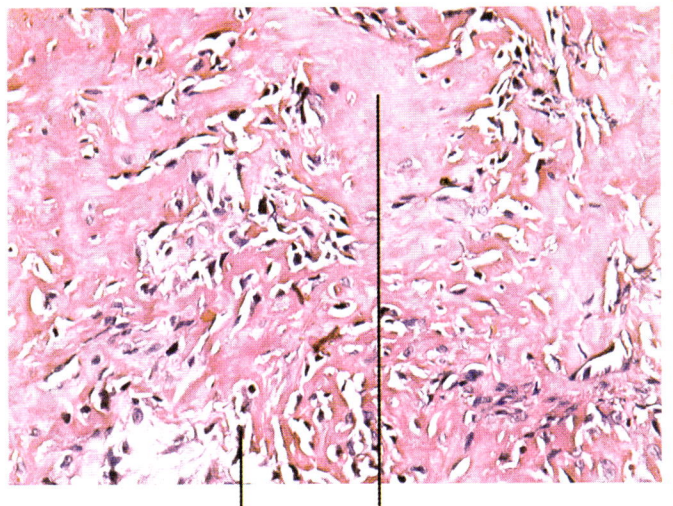

Pleomorphic nuclei   Osteoid deposition in stroma

Fig. 21.11: Osteosarcoma

Radiographically, the neoplasm demonstrates a variety of patterns ranging from radiolucent to radiopaque changes.

Microscopically, osteosarcoma is composed of malignant stromal cells that form osteoid or primitive bone **(Fig. 21.11)**. Sometimes the formation of bony trabeculae results in a sunray appearance in a direction perpendicular to the outer surface called as "sunburst" appearance. A symmetric widening of the periodontal ligament space is a significant feature of osteosarcoma.

Resection of involved and surrounding bone is the common treatment. Sometimes supplementary chemotherapy and/or radiotherapy are used.

BIBLIOGRAPHY

1. Aguirre A, Neiders MF, Nisengard R. Desquamative gingivitis. In, Newman, Takei, Carranza. Clinical Periodontology 9th ed WB Saunders 2003;314-35

2. Aguirre A, Tapia JL. Selected Soft and Hard Tissue Lesions With Periodontal Relevance. In, Rose LF, Mealey BL, Genco RJ, Cohen DW. Periodontics, Medicine, Surgery and Implants. Elsevier Mosby. 2004;879-911.

3. Ahmed AR, Graham J, Jordon RE, Prevost TT. Pemphigus: current concepts. Ann Intern Med 1980;92:396-405.

4. Anhalt GJ, Diaz LA. Prospects for autoimmune disease: research advances in Pemphigus. J Am Med Assoc 2001;285:652-54.

5. Anhalt GJ, Kim SC, Stanley JR, Korman NJ, Jabs DA, Kory M et al. Paraneoplastic Pemphigus. An autoimmune mucocutaneous disease associated with neoplasia. N Engl J Med 1990;323:1729-35.

6. Becker BA, Gaspari AA. Pemphigus vulgaris and vegetans. Dermatol Clin 1993;11:429-53.

7. Cotterill JA, Barker DJ, Millard LG. Plasma exchange in the treatment of Pemphigus vulgaris. Br J Dermatol 1978;98:2-10.

8. Creath CJ, Steinmetz S, Roebuck R. Gingival swelling due to a fingernail-biting habit. JADA 1995;126:1019-21.

9. Curtis RE, Metayer C, Rizzo JD et al. Impact of chronic GVHD therapy on the development of squamous cell cancers after hematopoetic stem-cell transplantation: an international case-control study. Blood 2005;105:3802-11.

10. D'Silva NJ, Summerlin DJ, Cordell KG, Abdelsayed RA, Tomich CE, Hanks CT et al. Metastatic tumors in the jaws: A retrospective study of 114 cases. JADA 2006;137(12):1667-72.

11. Faustino SES, Pereira MC, Rossetto AC, Oliveira DT. Recurrent peripheral odontogenic keratocyst: a case report. Dentomaxillofac Radiol 2008;37:412-14.

12. Franklin MR, Fritzmorris CT. Antibodies against conjunctival basement membrane zone. Occurence in cicatricial pemphigoid. Arch Ophthalmol 1983;101:1611-13.

13. Holmstrup P, Reibel J. Differential Diagnoses: Periodontal Tumors and Cysts. In, Lindhe J, Karring T, Lang NP. Clinical Periodontology and Implant dentistry. 4th ed Blackwell Munksgaard 2003;298-317.

14. Janin A, Murata H, Leboeuf C, Cayuela JM, Gluckman E, Legres L et al. Donor-derived oral squamous cell carcinoma after allogeneic bone marrow transplantation. Blood 2009;113:1834-40.

15. Kim HJ, Choi SK, Lee CJ, Sun CH. Aggressive epithelial odontogenic ghost cell tumor in the mandible CT and MR imaging findings. AJNR Am J Neuroradiol 2001;22:175-79.

16. Kirtschig G, Murrell D, Wojnarowska F, Khumalo N. Interventions for mucous membrane pemphigoid/cicatricial pemphigoid and epidermolysis bullosa acquisita. Arch Dermatol 2002;138:380-4.

17. Lozada F, Spitter L, Silverman S. Results of immunologic testing in patients with erythema multiforme. J Dent Res 1980;59:567-72.

18. Mjor IA. Problems and benefits associated with restorative materials: Side-effects and long-term cost. Adv Dent Res 1992;6:7-16.

19. Mobini N, Sarela A, Ahmed AR. Intravenous immunoglobulin in the therapy of autoimmune and systemic inflammatory disorders. Ann Allergy Asthma Immunol 1995;74:119-28.

20. Porter SR, Kirby A, Olsen I, Barrett W. Immunologic aspects of dermal and oral lichen planus. Oral Surg Oral Med Oral Pathol Oral Radiol Endod 1997;83:358-66.

21. Ramirez-Amador VA, Esquivel-Pedraza L, Orozco-Topete R. Frequency of oral conditions in a dermatology clinic. Int J Dermatol 2000;39:501-5.

22. Scuibba JJ. Autoimmune aspects of Pemphigus vulgaris and mucosal pemphigoid. Adv Dent Res 1996;10(1):52-56.

23. Scully C, Beyli M, Ferreiro MC, Ficarra G, Gill Y, Griffiths M et al. Update on oral lichen planus : Etiopathogenesis and Management. Crit Rev Oral Biol Med 1998;9:86-122.

24. Simon JA, Cablides J, Ortiz E, Alcocer-Varela J, Sanchez-Guerrero J. Anti-nucleosome antibodies in patients with systemic lupus erythematosus of recent onset. Potential utility as a diagnostic tool and disease activity marker. Rheumatology 2004;43:220-24.

25. Stewart DJ, Kernohan DC. Self-inflicted gingival injuries: gingival artefacts, factitial gingivitis. Dent Pract Dent Rec 1972;22:418-26.

26. Sultan SM, Ioannou Y, Isenberg DA. A review of gastrointestinal manifestations of systemic lupus erythematosus. Rheumatology 1999;38:917-32.

27. Torpet LA, Krageland C, Reibel J, Nauntofte B. Oral adverse drug reactions to cardiovascular drugs. Crit Rev Oral Biol Med 2004;15:28-46.

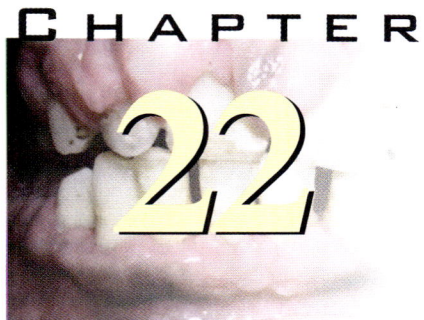

CHAPTER 22

Periodontal Pocket

Shalu Bathla

DEFINITION

Periodontal pocket is pathologically deepened gingival sulcus. It is bordered by the tooth on one side, by ulcerated epithelium on the other and has the junctional epithelium at its base. A periodontal pocket is an area that is inaccessible for plaque removal, resulting in the establishment of the following feedback mechanism for further plaque buildup: plaque → gingival inflammation → periodontal inflammation → periodontal pocket formation → more plaque buildup.

CLASSIFICATION

I. Depending on Morphology:
    A. Gingival/pseudopocket – Deepening of the gingival sulcus, mainly owing to an increase in the size of the gingiva, without any appreciable loss of the underlying tissues or apical migration of the junctional epithelium.
    B. Periodontal pocket **(Fig. 22.1)**
        i.   Suprabony pocket
        ii. Infrabony pocket
    C. Combined pocket
II. Depending on the number of surfaces involved **(Fig. 22.2)**:
    A. Simple - involve one tooth surface.

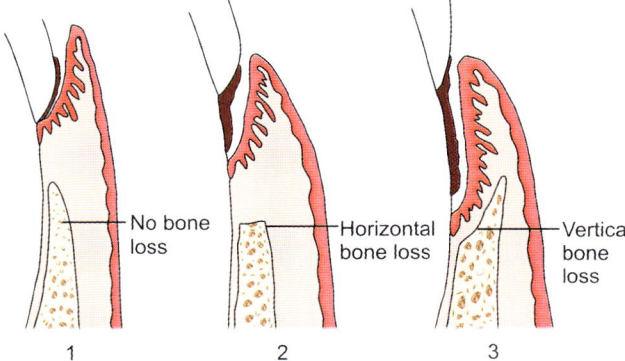

1. Gingival pocket- No destruction of supporting periodontal tissues
2. Suprabony pocket- Base of pocket coronal to alveolar crest
3. Infrabony pocket- Base of pocket apical to alveolar crest.

Fig. 22.1: Different types of pocket

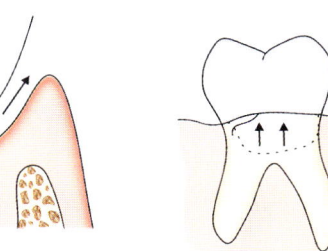
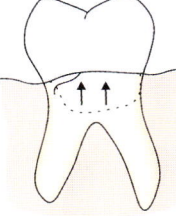
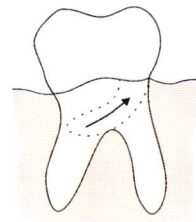
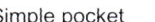

Simple pocket   Compound pocket   Spiral/complex pocket (tortuous)

Fig. 22.2: Classification of pocket according to involved tooth surface

TABLE 22.1: Differences between Suprabony and Infrabony Pocket

		Suprabony pocket	Infrabony pocket
1	Relationship of the soft tissue wall of the pocket to the alveolar bone	Base of the pocket coronal to the level of alveolar bone	Base of the pocket is apical to the crest of the alveolar bone
2	Pattern of bone destruction	Horizontal	Vertical
3	Direction of transseptal fibers interproximally	Horizontal	Oblique
4	Direction of periodontal ligament, on facial and lingual surfaces	Normal horizontal-oblique course between the tooth and the bone	Follows the angular pattern of the adjacent bone. They extend from the cementum beneath the base of the pocket along the bone and over the crest to join with the outer periosteum.

B. Compound - This type of pocket involves two or more tooth surfaces. The base of the pockets is in direct communication with the gingival margin along each of the involved surface.

C. Complex/Spiral- This type of pocket originates on one tooth surface and twists around the tooth to involve one or more additional surfaces. The only communication with gingival margin is at surface where the pocket originates.

III. Depending on disease activity:
  A. Active pocket
  B. Inactive pocket
IV. Depending on the nature of soft tissue wall:
  A. Edematous
  B. Fibrotic
V. Depending on the lateral wall of the pocket:
  A. Suprabony: consist of soft tissue alone
  B. Infrabony: consist of both soft tissue and bone. The alveolar bone becomes a part of the pocket wall.

CLINICAL FEATURES

Symptoms

Following are the symptoms which are suggestive of the presence of periodontal pocket:
• Localized pain or a sensation of pressure after eating, which gradually diminishes
• Radiating pain deep in the bone
• A foul taste in localized areas
• A gnawing feeling or feeling of itching in the gingiva
• Urge to dig with pointed instrument into the gingiva
• A tendency to suck material from the interproximal spaces
• Sensitivity to heat and cold and toothache in the absence of caries.
Clinical signs: Following are the clinical signs which are suggestive of the presence of periodontal pocket:

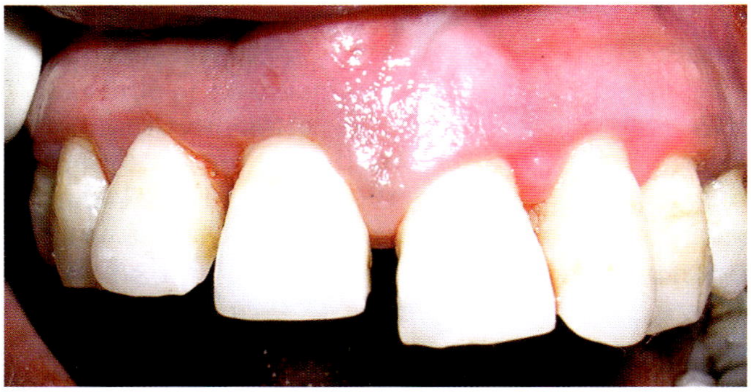

Fig. 22.3: Extrusion and diastema associated with periodontal pocket

• Enlarged, bluish red thickened marginal gingiva with a rolled edge separated from the tooth surface
• Bluish-red vertical zone extending from the gingival margin to the alveolar mucosa
• A break in the faciolingual continuity of the interdental gingiva
• Shiny, discolored and puffy gingiva associated with the exposed root surfaces
• Gingival bleeding and suppuration from the gingival margin
• Extrusion, mobility, diastema and migration of teeth **(Fig. 22.3)**.

PATHOGENESIS

The following old theories related to pathogenesis of periodontal pocket are presented as useful background for the interpretation of current and future concepts:
1. Destruction of gingival fibers is a prerequisite for the initiation of pocket formation— *Fish*
2. The initial change in pocket formation occurs in cementum— *Gottlieb*

3. Stimulation of the epithelial attachment by inflammation rather than destruction of gingival fibers is the prerequisite for the initiation of periodontal pocket— *Aisenberg*
4. Pathologic destruction of the epithelial attachment due to infection or trauma is the initial histologic changes in pocket formation— *Skillen*
5. The periodontal pocket is initiated by invasion of bacteria at the base of the sulcus or the absorption of bacterial toxins through the epithelial lining of the sulcus— *Box*
6. Pocket formation is initiated as a defect in sulcus— *Becks*
7. Proliferation of the epithelium of the lateral wall, rather than epithelium at the base of the sulcus, is the initial change in the formation of periodontal pocket — *Wilkinson*
8. Two stage pocket formation—*James & Counsell*
   a. Proliferation of the subgingival epithelium (epithelial attachment).
   b. Loss of superficial layers of proliferated epithelium, which produces space or pocket.
9. Inflammation is the initial change in the formation of periodontal pocket— *J. Nuckolls*
10. Pathologic epithelial proliferation occurs secondary to non- inflammatory degenerative changes in periodontal membranes.

The most accepted recent concept is that the apical migration of apical cells of junctional epithelium and deattachment of coronal portion of junctional epithelium leads to intraepithelial cleft and pocket formation and deepening. **Figure 22.4** clearly show how the periodontal pocket is formed.

HISTOPATHOLOGY

The soft tissue wall of periodontal pocket presents the following microscopic features: -

The epithelium of the lateral wall of the pocket presents striking proliferative and degenerative changes. Epithelium buds or interlacing cords of epithelial cells project from the lateral wall into the adjacent inflamed connective tissue. These epithelial projections and rest of lateral epithelium are densely infiltrated by leukocytes and edema from the inflamed connective tissue. Epithelial cells undergo vacuolar degeneration and rupture to form vesicles. Progressive degeneration and necrosis of the epithelium leads to ulceration of the lateral wall and exposure of underlying connective tissue.

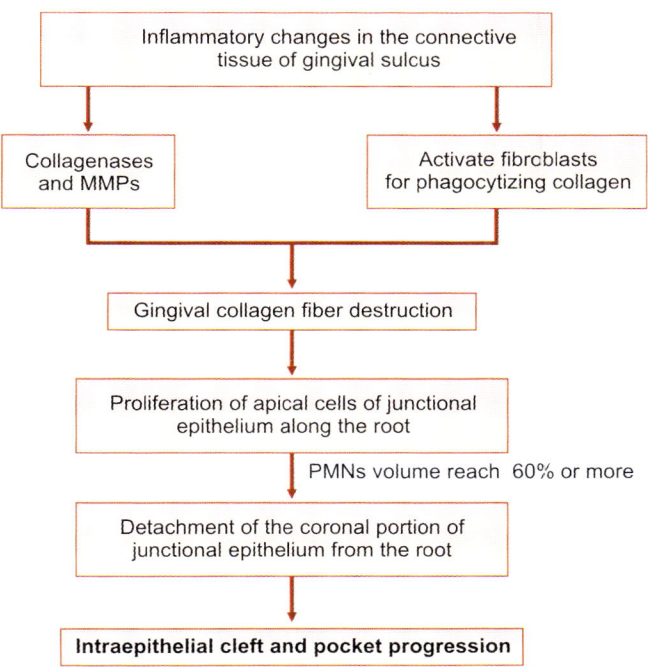

Fig. 22.4: Pathogenesis of periodontal pocket

Junctional epithelium at the base of the pocket is usually shorter than that of normal sulcus. The corono-apical length of junctional epithelium is reduced to only 50 to 100 µm. The epithelium at the gingival crest of a periodontal pocket is generally intact and thickened, with prominent rete pegs.

The connective tissue is edematous and densely infiltrated with approximately 80% of plasma cells, lymphocytes and PMNs. The blood vessels are increased in number, dilated and engorged. The connective tissue presents proliferation of the endothelial cells with newly formed capillaries, fibroblasts and collagen fibers.

Some bacteria may invade the intracellular space and are found between deeper epithelial cells and accumulate on the basement lamina. *P. gingivalis, P. intermedius* and *Aggregatibacter actinomycetemcomitans* traverse the basement lamina and invade the subepithelial connective tissue.

Microtopography of the Gingival Wall of the Pocket: There are different areas showing different type of activity in the soft tissue wall of the pocket due to the host- microbial interactions.

1. Areas of relative quiescence, showing a relatively flat surface with minor depressions and mounds and occasional shedding of cells.

PERIODONTICS REVISITED

2. Areas of bacterial accumulation, which appear as depressions on the epithelial surface, with abundant debris and bacterial clumps penetrating into the enlarged intercellular spaces. These bacteria are mainly cocci, rods, and filaments with a few spirochetes.
3. Areas of emergence of leukocytes, where leukocytes appear in the pocket wall through holes located in the intercellular spaces.
4. Areas of leukocyte-bacteria interaction, where numerous leukocytes are present and covered with bacteria in an apparent process of phagocytosis. Bacterial plaque associated with the epithelium is seen either as an organized matrix covered by a fibrin-like material in contact with the surface of cells or as bacteria penetrating into the intercellular spaces.
5. Areas of intense epithelial desquamation, which consist of semi-attached and folded epithelial squames, sometimes partially covered with bacteria.
6. Areas of ulceration with exposed connective tissue
7. Areas of hemorrhage with numerous erythrocytes.

Pocket contents: Periodontal pockets consist of microorganisms and their products (enzymes, endotoxins and other metoblic products), GCF, salivary mucin, food debris, desquamated epithelial cells and leukocytes. Purulent exduate consist of living, degenerated and necrotic leukocytes, living and dead bacteria, serum and fibrin.

Root surface wall changes:

The root surface wall of periodontal pockets often undergo changes that are significant because they may perpetuate the periodontal infection, cause pain and complicate periodontal treatment. Root surface wall may undergo into structural, chemical and cytotoxic changes.

Structural changes: It include presence of pathologic granules which represent area of collagen degradation. There may be areas of hypermineralization or demineralization causing root caries.

Chemical changes: The mineral content of exposed cementum is increased. Exposed cementum absorbs calcium, phosphorus, and fluorides from its local environment, making it possible to develop a highly calcified layer that appears to be highly resistant to decay. This ability of cementum to absorb from its environment, on the other hand, may be detrimental if these absorbed materials are toxic to the surrounding tissues.

Cytotoxic changes: Endotoxins are found in the cementum of periodontally involved teeth. Endotoxin limits the proliferation and attachment of fibroblasts to the diseased root surfaces.

CLINICAL ASSESSMENT

The only reliable method of locating and determining periodontal pocket extent is careful exploration of the gingival margin along each tooth surface with a periodontal probe. The probe should be inserted parallel to the vertical axis of the tooth (**Fig. 22.5**) and walked circumferentially around each surface of each tooth to detect the areas of deepest penetration. Probe tip penetrates the most coronal intact fibers of the connective tissues attachment and goes about 0.3mm apical to the junctional epithelium in periodontal pocket. The probing forces of about 0.75N have been found to be well tolerated. Probe reading that falls between two calibrated marks on the probe should be rounded

PERIODONTICS REVISITED

TABLE 22.2: Correlation of clinical and histopathologic features of the periodontal pocket

		Clinical features	Histopathologic features
1	Color	The gingival wall of the periodontal pocket is usually bluish-red in color.	The discoloration is caused by circulatory stagnation
2	Surface texture	Smooth, shiny surface which pit on pressure	The smooth, shiny surface is due to the atrophy of the epithelium and edema; the pitting on pressure is because of edema and degeneration.
3	Consistency	Usually flaccid but less frequently, the gingival wall may be pink and firm	Flaccidity is due to destruction of the gingival fibers and surrounding tissues but is firm when fibrotic changes predominate over exudation and degeneration
4	Bleeding	It is elicited by gently probing the soft tissue wall of the pocket	Ease of bleeding results from increased vascularity, thinning and degeneration of the epithelium, and the proximity of the engorged vessels to the inner surface
5	Pain	When explored with a probe, the inner aspect of the periodontal pocket is generally painful.	Pain on tactile stimulation is due to ulceration of the inner aspect of the pocket wall
6	Pus	Sometime pus may be expressed by applying digital pressure	Pus occurs in pockets with suppurative inflammation of the inner wall.

upwards to the next highest millimeter e.g if the probe penetrates far enough to cover the 4mm mark, it should be recorded as 5mm.

Gutta percha points or caliberated silver points can be used with radiograph to assist in determining the level of attachment of periodontal pockets.

Periodontal pocket is pathologically deepened gingival sulcus.
Can be pseudo or true pockets
Simple, compound or complex pockets
Suprabony or infrabony pockets.

LANDMARK STUDIES RELATED

Armitage GC, Svanberg GK, Loe H. Microscopic evaluation of clinical measurements of connective tissue attachment levels. Journal of Clinical Periodontology 1977; 4:173.

Armitage et al evaluated the penetration of a probe in healthy beagle, dog's specimens using a standardized force of 25 grams. They reported that probe penetrated the epithelium to about 2/3rd of its length in heathly specimens, it stopped 0.1mm short of its apical end in gingivitis specimens and in periodontitis specimens probe tips went past the most apical cells of the junctional epithelium. Thus, probe penetration varies depending on the force of introduction and the degree of tissue inflammation.

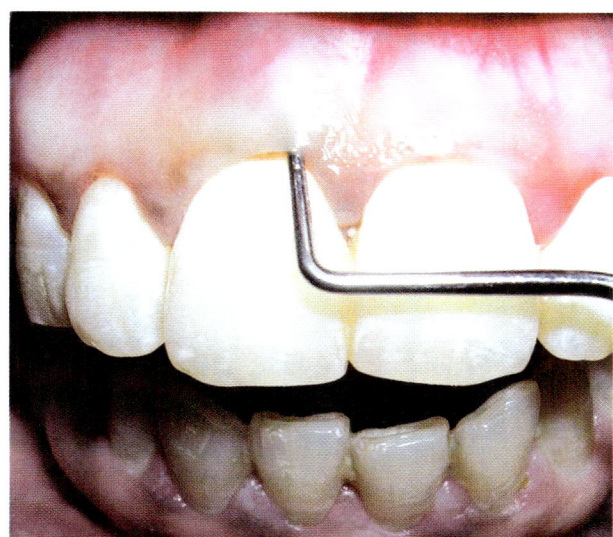

Fig. 22.5: Pocket probing- probe is inserted parallel to the vertical axis of the tooth

Glauser WM, Schroeder HE. The Pocket Epithelium: A Light and Electronmicroscopic Study. Journal of Periodontology 1982; 53: 133 – 144.

The study was conducted on biopsy material of 8 beagle dogs between the age of 1 – 4 years following the application of cotton floss ligatures for periods of 4 to 21 days or up to 5 months, block biopsies comprising dental and gingival tissues were taken on the buccal side. The tissues were processed for light and electronmicroscopic examination. The observation revealed that the pocket epithelium (1) does not attach to the tooth, (2) forms irregular ridges and, over connective tissue papillae, thin coverings which occasionally ulcerate, (3) consists of cells only some of which show a tendency to differentiate, (4) presents a basal lamina complex with discontinuities and multiplications, and (5) is infiltrated mainly by, T and B lymphocytes and plasma cells, and is transmigrated by neutrophilic granulocytes.

POINTS TO PONDER

✓ Periodontal pocket is a soft tissue change thus can be not detected during radiographic examination.
✓ Biologic/histologic depth is the distance between the gingival margin and base of the pocket (coronal end of the junctional epithelium).
✓ Clinical/probing depth is the distance between the gingival margin to the base of the probeable crevice upto which probe penetrates into the pocket.

BIBLIOGRAPHY

1. Aleo JJ, De Renzis FA, Farber PA, et al. The presence and biologic activity of cementum - bound endotoxin. J Periodontol 1974;45: 672.
2. Aleo JJ, Vandersall DC. Cementum - Recent concepts related to Periodontal Disease Therapy. DCNA 1980;24:627-50.
3. Armitage GC, Svanberg GK, Loe H. Microscopic evaluation of clinical measurements of connective tissue attachment levels. J Clin Periodontol 1977; 4:173.
4. Carranza FA, Camargo PM. The periodontal pocket. In, Newman, Takei, Carranza. Clinical Periodontology 9th ed WB Saunders 2003;336-53.
5. Glauser WM, Schroeder HE. The Pocket Epithelium: A Light and Electronmicroscopic Study. J Periodontol 1982;53:133-44.

PERIODONTICS REVISITED

MCQs

1. A pseudopocket (or gingival pocket) is formed by the:
   A. Coronal migration of the gingival margin
   B. Coronal migration of the epithelial attachment
   C. Apical migration of the gingival margin
   D. Apical migration of the epithelial attachment
2. Periodontal pockets can BEST be detected by:
   A. Radiographic detection
   B. The color of the gingival
   C. The contour of the gingival margin
   D. Probing the sulcular area
3. A compound periodontal pocket is:
   A. Spiral type of pocket
   B. Present on two or more tooth surfaces
   C. Infrabony in nature
   D. All of the above
4. Periodontal pocket wall between tooth and bone is:
   A. Infrabony pocket
   B. Suprabony pocket
   C. Gingival pocket
   D. Pseudopocket

Answers

1. A   2. D   3. B   4. A

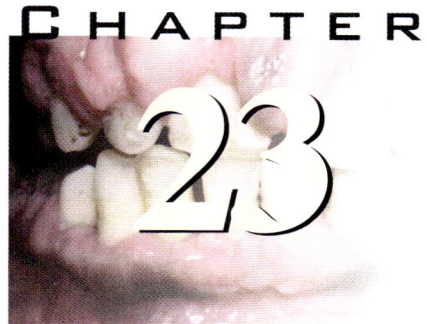
Periodontal Abscess

Shalu Bathla

DEFINITION

A periodontal abscess is defined as suppurative lesion associated with periodontal breakdown and localized accumulation of pus within the gingival wall of a periodontal pocket.

The periodontal abscess has also been defined as a lesion with an expressed periodontal breakdown, occurring during a limited period of time and with easily detectable clinical symptoms, with a localised accumulation of pus, located within the gingival wall of the periodontal pocket.

CLASSIFICATION

A. Depending on the location of the lesion:
  • Periapical abscess
  • Periodontal abscess
  • Pericoronal abscess
B. Depending on the course of lesion:
  • Acute abscess
  • Chronic abscess
C. Depending on the tissue involved:
  • Gingival abscess
  • Periodontal abscess
  • Pericoronal abscess

D. Depending on the cause of the acute infectious process, two types of periodontal abscess may occur:
  • Periodontitis-related abscess
  • Non-periodontitis-related abscess
E. Depending on the number of abscess
  • Single
  • Multiple

CLINICAL FEATURES OF PERIODONTAL ABSCESS

1. Pain of acute periodontal abscess is throbbing and radiating whereas in chronic periodontal abscess pain is dull and gnawing.
2. The gingiva is edematous and red, with a smooth, shiny, ovoid elevation **(Fig. 23.1)**.
3. Suppuration may be spontaneous or occur after putting pressure on the outer surface of the gingiva.
4. Swelling
5. Sensitivity to percussion of the affected tooth
6. Tooth elevation
7. During the periodontal examination, the abscess is usually found at a site with a deep periodontal pocket.
8. Bleeding on probing
9. Pinpoint orifice of sinus may be present. Sinus may be covered by small, pink, bed - like mass of granulation tissue **(Fig. 23.2)**.

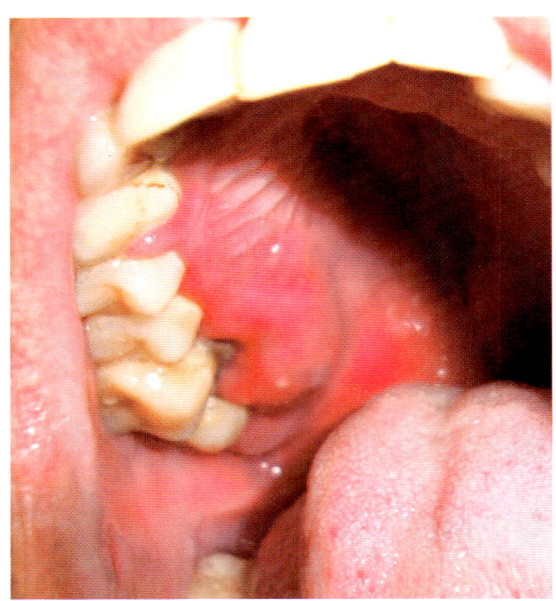

Fig. 23.1: Periodontal abscess associated with palatal surface of upper right molar (*Courtesy:* Dr Vikrender)

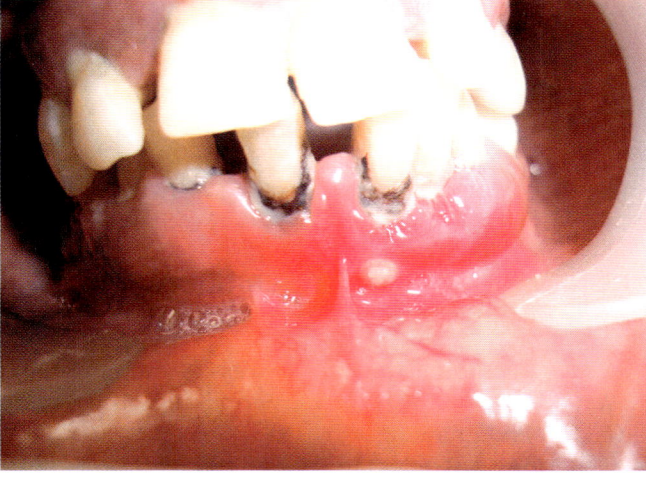

Fig. 23.2: Periodontal abscess associated with lower left central incisor

Extraoral Signs

In some patients the occurrence of a periodontal abscess may be associated with:

- Elevated body temperature
- Malaise
- Regional lymphadenopathy

Acute periodontal abscess is associated with:

Pain
Tenderness
Sensitivity to palpation
Suppuration upon gentle pressure

Chronic abscess is associated with:

Sinus tract
Usually asymptomatic

MICROBIOLOGY

The microflora related with periodontal abscess is complex, dominated by gram-negative, strict anaerobe rods resembling the microbiota of chronic periodontitis lesions. Gram-negative anaerobic species are non-fermentative and display moderate to strong proteolytic activity mainly *Porphyromonas gingivalis, Prevotella intermedia.* Strict anaerobic, gram positive bacterial species in periodontal abscesses include *Peptostreptococcus micros, Actinomyces spp.*

PATHOGENESIS AND HISTOPATHOLOGY

Following are the factors that may provoke the formation of an abscess:

1. Obstruction to the opening of deep pocket, frequently one which is tortuous or associated with furcation defect.
2. Gingival injury with a foreign body, e.g. toothbrush bristle or woodstick, which carries bacteria into the tissues. Careless subgingival scaling may also carry microorganisms into damaged tissue, as can powerful irrigation of a pocket.
3. Incomplete removal of plaque and subgingival calculus from the depths of a pocket. Frequently after scaling there is a tightening of the gingival cuff which occludes a pocket containing bacteria.
4. Infection of tissues damaged by excessive occlusal stress which may be produced by:
   - Bruxism
   - Excessive orthodontic forces.
5. As a consequence of pulp disease:
   - Where a periapical lesion spreads up to the lateral surface of a tooth
   - Where lateral pulp canal links with the periodontal ligament. This is especially common in the furcation.
   - Perforation of the lateral wall of a tooth during endodontics.
6. Altered host response as in diabetes.

The formation of periodontal abscess is initiated by the bacterial invasion of the soft tissue wall of the pocket and then multiply therein. An inflammatory infiltrate is formed followed by destruction of the connective tissues, encapsulation of the bacterial mass and pus formation. The lowered host resistance and the virulence as well as the number of bacteria present determine the course of the infection. Tissue destruction is caused by the extracellular enzymes and inflammatory cells itself. An acidic environment will favor the activity of lysosomal enzymes and promote tissue destruction.

Periodontal abscess contains bacteria, bacterial products, inflammatory cells, tissue breakdown products and serum. Neutrophils are found in the central area of the abscess and close to soft tissue debris **(Fig. 23.3)**. At a

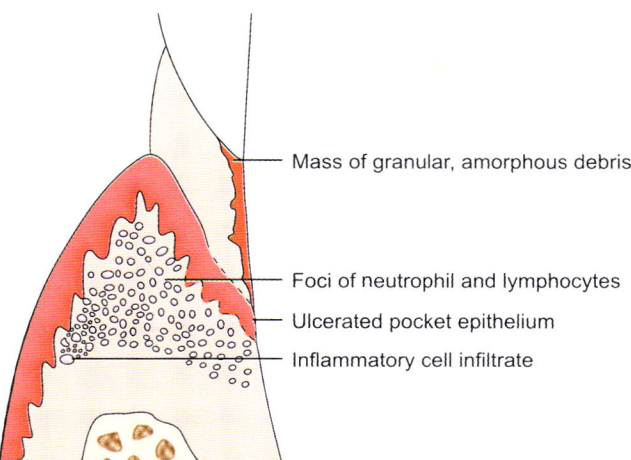

Fig. 23.3: Diagrammatic representation of histopathology of periodontal abscess

- Mass of granular, amorphous debris
- Foci of neutrophil and lymphocytes
- Ulcerated pocket epithelium
- Inflammatory cell infiltrate

later stage, a pyogenic membrane, composed of macrophages and neutrophils, is organized.

DIAGNOSIS

The diagnosis of a periodontal abscess is made by the overall evaluation, interpretation of the patient's chief complaint and the clinical and radiographic findings. The suspected area is probed carefully along the gingival margin in relation to each tooth surface to detect a tract from the marginal area to deeper periodontal tissues. The radiographic examination may either reveal a normal appearance of the interdental bone, or some bone loss, ranging from a widening of the periodontal ligament space to bone loss involving most of the affected tooth. Radiographs taken in the earliest stage of periodontal abscess provide little useful information, but once the lesion is established its position can be identified. Radiolucent area along the lateral surface of the root suggests the presence of periodontal abscess. A radiograph taken with gutta percha point inserted gently into the suspected pocket can help to define the origin of the abscess.

DIFFERENTIAL DIAGNOSIS

The differential diagnosis of periodontal abscess can be made with other abscesses that occur in the oral cavity. Gingival abscess, periapical abscess, endoperiodontal abscess **(Fig. 23.4)**, lateral periapical cysts and vertical root fractures may have a similar appearance. Gingival abscess is a localized painful, rapidly expanding lesion

TABLE 23.1: Differences between periodontal abscesses and periapical abscesses

		Periodontal abscesses	Periapical abscesses
1	History	• Periodontal disease • Periodontal treatment	• Caries, fracture, toothwear • Restorative and endodontic treatment
2	Clinical findings	• Vital pulp responses • Periodontal probing release pus • Periodontal disease evident • Swelling is generalized and located around the involved tooth and gingival margin. Seldom with a fistulous tract • Pain is usually dull, constant and less severe than in a periapical abscess. Pain is localized and patient usually can locate offending tooth	• Questionable/Non responsive pulp tests • Narrow probing defect (May be isolated lesion) • Advanced caries, advanced toothwear, large restoration • Swelling is localized often with fistulous opening in the apical area • Pain is usually severe, throbbing and patient may not be able to locate offending tooth
3	Radiographic findings	• Alveolar crest bone loss, angular bone defects, furcation involvements	• Apical radiolucency **(Fig. 23.5)** • Endodontic or post perforations
4	Response to treatment	• Responds dramatically to release of pus, subgingival debridement	• Responds poorly, or not at all to periodontal treatment

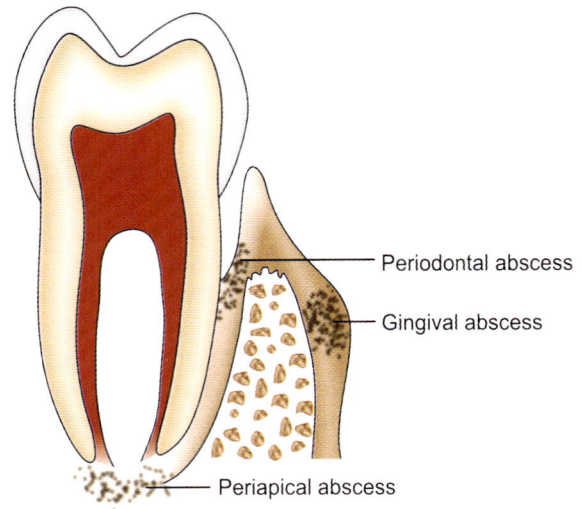

Fig. 23.4: Various abscesses that occur in oral cavity

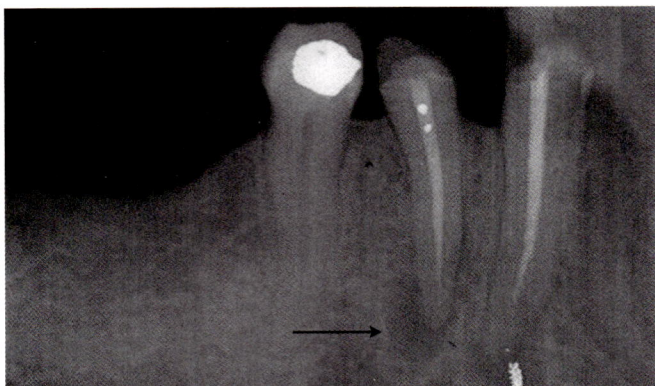

Fig. 23.5: Radiographic appearance of periapical abscess

usually of sudden onset. It is generally limited to the marginal gingiva or interdental papilla. Signs such as lack of pulp vitality, the presence of deep caries lesions, the presence of a sinus tract and findings made in the radiographic examination, will aid in the distinction between abscesses of different etiologies.

TREATMENT

Treatment depends upon the stage of abscess development, amount of bone loss and whether pulp pathology is also involved or not.

Gingival Abscess

After topical anesthesia is applied, the fluctuant area of the lesion is incised with a Bard – Parker handle and surgical blade, and the incision is gently widened to permit drainage. The area is cleansed with warm water and covered with a gauze pad. After bleeding stops, the patient is dismissed for 24 hours and instructed to rinse every 2 hours with a glassful of warm water.

Acute Periodontal Abscess (Incision and Drainage)

Drainage through the pocket: After application of a topical anesthesia flat instrument or a probe is carefully introduced into the pocket in an attempt to distend the pocket wall. A small curette or a Morse scaler can then be gently used to penetrate the tissue and establish drainage.

Drainage through an external incision: After LA is given, with a Bard – Parker handle and blade no. 11, a vertical incision is made through the most fluctuant part of the lesion, extending from the mucogingival fold to the gingival margin **(Fig. 23.6)**. If swelling is on the lingual surface, the incision is started just apical to the swelling extending through the gingival margin. The blade should penetrate to firm tissue to be sure of reaching deep, purulent areas. After initial extravasation of blood and pus, irrigate the area with warm water and gently spread the incision to facilitate drainage. Postoperative instructions are given to rinse hourly with a solution of a teaspoon of salt in a glass of warm water. Antibiotic Penicillin and Metronidazole is prescribed for patient with systemic complications.

Chronic Periodontal Abscess

Treatment by Flap operation: All deposits are scaled from the teeth, and the root surfaces are planed with the hoe scalers and smoothened with curettes. Systemic antibiotics Amoxicillin and Metronidazole are prescribed. To locate the abscess area, probing is done

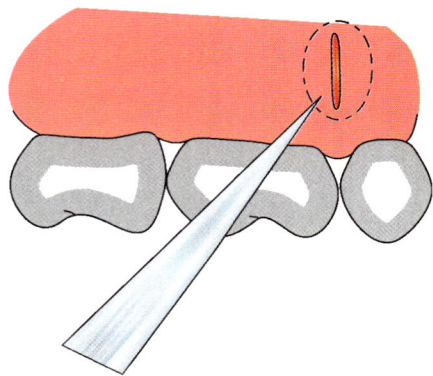

Fig. 23.6: Vertical incision

around the gingival margin, following tortuous pockets to their termination. If a sinus is present, the abscess may be probed through it.

- *Anesthesize:* The area is anesthetized with local infiltration.
- *Incision:* Two vertical incisions are made from the gingival margin to the mucobuccal fold, outlining the field of operation. If the lingual approach is used; the incisions are made from the gingival margin to the level of the root apices. After the vertical incisions are made, a mesiodistal incision is made across the interdental papilla with a knife to facilitate the detachment of the flap **(Fig. 23.7)**.
- *Reflect the flap:* A full thickness flap is raised with a periosteal elevator and held in position with a retractor.
- *Remove granulation tissue:* The granulation tissue is removed with curettes to provide a clear view of the root. If a sinus is present, it is explored and curetted.
- *Control bleeding:* The facial and lingual surfaces are covered with a piece of gauze shaped into a U, which is held in position until the bleeding stops.
- *Suture:* The gauze is then removed, and the flap is sutured and covered with a periodontal pack.

Sorrin's operation—A type of flap approach in the treatment of a periodontal abscess; especially suitable when the marginal gingiva appears well adapted and gives no access to the abscess area. A semilunar incision is made below the involved area in the attached gingiva, leaving gingival margin

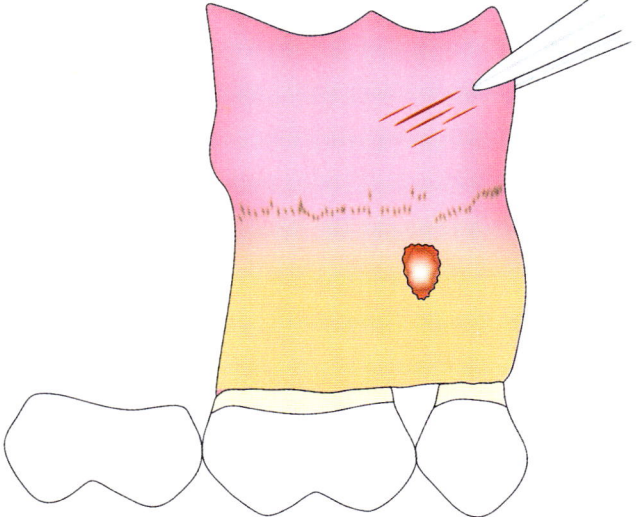

Fig. 23.7: Full thickness flap raised to facilitate removal of granulation tissue

undisturbed. A flap is raised, allowing access to the abscessed area for curettage.

COMPLICATIONS

a. Tooth loss: Periodontal abscesses have been suggested as the main cause for tooth extraction during the phase of supportive periodontal therapy.
b. Dissemination of the infection-Cellulitis, subcutaneous infection, phlegmone and mediastinitis can result from odontogenic infections but are very uncommon with periodontal abscess. Mechanical treatment of a periodontal abscess may result in bacteremia which, in patients with, for example endoprosthesis or in immunocompromised states, can result in nonoral infections. Occasional dissemination of periodontal bacteria can result in brain abscess.

LANDMARK STUDIES RELATED

DeWitt G, Cobb C, Killoy W. The acute periodontal abscess: microbial penetration of the tissue wall. International Journal of Periodontics and Restorative Dentistry 1985;1:39-51.

In this study 12 biopsies punches were taken just apical to the area of major fluctuance and processed for histological examination. Following were the observation from the outside to the inside: (a) a normal oral epithelium and lamina propria; (b) an acute inflammatory infiltrate; (c) an intense foci of inflammation (neutrophil-lymphocyte) with the surrounding connective tissue destroyed and necrotic; (d) a destroyed and ulcerated pocket epithelium; (e) a central region, as a mass of granular, acidophilic, and amorphous debris. In 7 out of 9 specimens evaluated by electron-microscopy, gram-negative bacteria were seen invading the pocket epithelium and altered connective tissue. Bacteria inside the abscess were immersed in tissue exudate and surrounded by necrotic tissues. The presence of fungi inside the abscess was also present.

POINTS TO PONDER

✓ Multiple periodontal abscesses are seen in diabetes mellitus.
✓ Periodontitis related abscess occurs when the acute infection originates from a biofilm present in a deepened periodontal pocket.
✓ Post-scaling periodontal abscess: This type of abscess formation occur when small fragments of calculus

have been forced into the deep, previously non-inflamed portion of the periodontal tissues.

✓ Post-surgery periodontal abscess: It is often the result of an incomplete removal of subgingival calculus or to the presence of foreign bodies in the periodontal tissues, such as sutures, regenerative devices or periodontal pack.

✓ Post-antibiotic periodontal abscess: Treatment with systemic antibiotics without subgingival debridement in patients with advanced periodontitis may cause abscess formation.

BIBLIOGRAPHY

1. DeWitt G, Cobb C, Killoy W. The acute periodontal abscess: microbial penetration of the tissue wall. Int J Periodontics and Restorative Dent 1985;1:39-51.
2. Eley BM, Manson JD. The Periodontal Abscess. In, Periodontics 5th ed Wright 2004;328-31.
3. Herrera D, Roldan S, Sanz M. The periodontal abscess: a review. J Clin Periodontol 2000;27:377-86.
4. Meng HX. Periodontal abscess. Ann Periodontol 1999;4:79-82.
5. Sanz M, Herrera D, Winkelhoff AJ. The Periodontal Abscess. In, Lindhe J, Karring T, Lang NP. Clinical Periodontology and Implant dentistry. 4th ed Blackwell Munksgaard 2003;260-68.
6. Takei HH. Treatment of the periodontal abscess. In, Newman, Takei, Carranza. Clinical Periodontology 9th ed WB Saunders 2003;629-30.

MCQs

1. Most abundant cells in the inflammatory exudates of an acute periodontal abscess are:
   A. Lymphocytes   B. Neutrophils
   C. Monocytes   D. Basophil
2. A young adult shows non-fluctuant, tender and red swelling in the marginal gingiva:
   A. Periapical abscess
   B. Periodontal abscess
   C. Periapical sinus
   D. Gingival abscess

Answers

1. B   2. D

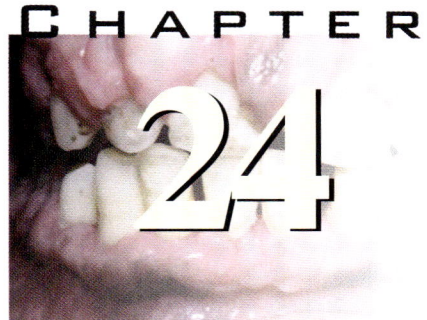

CHAPTER 24

Bone Defects

SK Salaria, Shalu Bathla

INTRODUCTION

Alveolar bone loss is one of the most important and obvious feature of periodontal disease. The height and density of the alveolar bone are normally maintained by an equilibrium, regulated by local and systemic influences between bone formation and bone resorption. When resorption exceeds formation, bone height, density, or both are reduced. The variation is seen in bone loss pattern in between individuals and different sites in the same mouth and even on different aspects of the same tooth.

FACTORS DETERMINING BONE MORPHOLOGY IN PERIODONTAL DISEASES

1. *Normal variation in alveolar bone*: Various anatomic features that influence bone destructive pattern in periodontal disease are: Thickness, width and crestal angulation of the interdental septa, thickness of facial and lingual alveolar plates, presence of fenestration and dehiscence, alignment of teeth, proximity with another tooth surfaces, root and root trunk anatomy and root position within alveolar bone.

2. *Exostoses*: These are outgrowths of bone of varied size and shape. They can occur as small nodules, large nodules, sharp ridges, spike-like projections, or any combination of these.

3. *Trauma from occlusion*: Trauma from occlusion may be a factor in determining the dimension and shape of bone deformities. It may cause a thickening of the cervical margin of alveolar bone or a change in the morphology of the bone angular defects and buttressing bone.

4. *Buttressing bone formation*: Bone formation sometimes occurs in an attempt to buttress bony trabeculae weakened by resorption. When it occurs within the jaw, it is termed central buttressing bone formation. When it occurs on the external surface, it is referred to as peripheral buttressing bone formation. The latter may cause bulging of the bone contour, termed lipping, which sometimes accompanies the production of osseous craters and angular defects.

5. *Food impaction*: Interdental bone defects often occur where proximal contact is abnormal or absent. Pressure from food impaction contributes to the inverted bone architecture.

6. *Aggressive periodontitis:* A vertical or angular pattern of alveolar bone destruction is found around the first molars in aggressive periodontitis.

ETIOLOGY OF BONE LOSS

The various causes of alveolar bone loss are:
  I. Extension of gingival inflammation
 II. Trauma from occlusion
III. Systemic disorders

Extension of Gingival Inflammation

The most common cause of bone destruction in periodontal disease is the extension of inflammation from the marginal gingiva into the deeper periodontal tissues. The inflammatory invasion of the bone surface and the initial bone loss mark the transition from gingivitis to periodontitis.

Histopathology: Interproximally, gingival inflammation spread to the loose connective tissue around the blood vessels, through the fibres and into the bone through vessel channels that perforate the crest of the interdental septum. The inflammation may sometime spreads from the gingiva directly into the periodontal ligament and from there into the interdental septum **(Figs 24.1 and 24.2)**.

Facially and lingually, inflammation from the gingiva spreads along the outer periosteal surface of the bone and penetrates into the marrow spaces through vessels channels in the outer cortex. The gingival and transeptal fibres are destroyed meanwhile. Once the inflammation reaches the bone, it spreads into marrow spaces and replaces the marrow with a leukocytic and fluid exudate, new blood vessels and proliferating fibroblasts. Bone surfaces are lined with multinucleated osteoclasts and howship's lacunae.

In the marrow spaces, resorption proceeds from within, causing a thinning of the surrounding bony trabeculae and enlargement of marrow spaces. This causes, destruction of bone and reduction in bone height.

Radius of action: Garant and Cho were the first to point out that bone resorption stimulators produced by microbial plaque have a finite *radius of action.* Page and Schroeder postulated a range of effectiveness of about 1.5 to 2.5 mm within which bacterial plaque can cause bone destruction. Waerhaug applied this principle to human periodontium by making measurements on radiographs, histologic sections and extracted teeth to determine the distance between microbial plaque and the bone surface. Waerhaug has shown that the bone margin is never

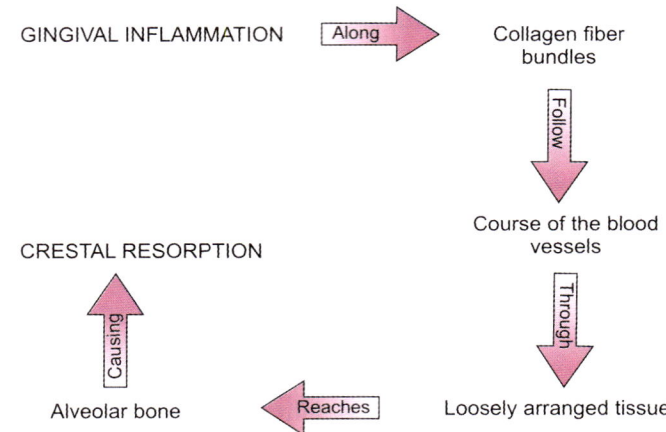

Fig.24.1: Extension of gingival inflammation to alveolar bone

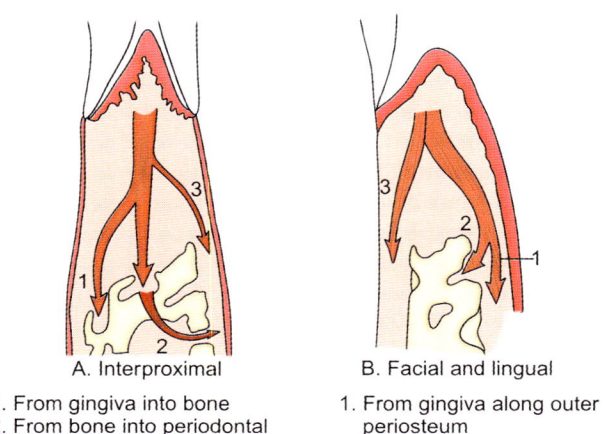

A. Interproximal
1. From gingiva into bone
2. From bone into periodontal ligament

B. Facial and lingual
1. From gingiva along outer periosteum
2. From periosteum into bone

Fig.24.2: Pathways of inflammation from gingiva to periodontal tissues in periodontitis

located closer than 0.5 mm to plaque and not farther than 1.5 to 2.5 mm from plaque.

Mechanisms of bone destruction: Bone resorption occurs in the presence of both osteoblasts and osteoclasts. Stimulators of bone resorption are IL-1, IL-6, PTH, PTHrP, PGE_2, RANK, RANKL and Vitamin D. Inhibitors of bone resorption are IFN-α, Osteoprotegrin (OPG), calcitonin, estrogen and androgen. Systemic and local bone resorbing factors exert their influence by stimulating the osteoblast and this osteoblast is involved in the regulation of osteoclast function at several levels. Osteoblasts stimulated by these factors mediate their response through a series of intracellular secondary messenger systems; one pathway involves cyclic AMP and second involves membrane phospholipids and protein kinase C. Both these mechanism are stimulated by PGE$_2$, prostacyclin (PGI$_2$) and thrombin.

According to Hausmann, following are possible pathways of alveolar bone loss in periodontal diseases:

i. Direct action of plaque products on bone progenitor cells induces the differentiation of these cells into osteoclasts.

ii. Plaque products act directly on bone, destroying it through a noncellular mechanism.

iii. Plaque products stimulate gingival cells, causing them to release mediators, which in turn induce bone progenitor cells to differentiate into osteoclasts.

iv. Plaque products cause gingival cells to release agents that can act as cofactors in bone resorption.

v. Plaque products cause gingival cells to release agents that destroy bone by direct chemical action, without osteoclasts.

Sequence of events in the bone resorptive process are:

1. *Formation of osteoclast*: Osteoclasts are multinucleated giant cells of 50 to 100 µm size derived from circulating blood cells monocytes **(Fig. 24.3)**. Osteoclasts are found in baylike depression in the bone called Howship's lacunae. The part of the cell in contact with bone shows convoluted surface and is called ruffled border.

2. *Osteoblast-osteoclast coupling*: The development of osteoclasts is controlled by the stromal cells through the RANK/ RANKL/OPG axis. RANK is activated through its ligand RANKL. RANKL is produced from the osteoblasts/stromal cells. Upon RANK/RANKL binding, the activation of osteoclasts occurs, that subsequently leads to bone resorption. Osteo-protegrin (OPG) acts as a soluble decoy receptor of RANKL and thus prevents osteoclastogenesis **(Fig. 24.4)**.

3. *Attachment of osteoclasts to the mineralized surface of bone*: The part of the cell in contact with bone shows convoluted surface, the ruffled border which is the

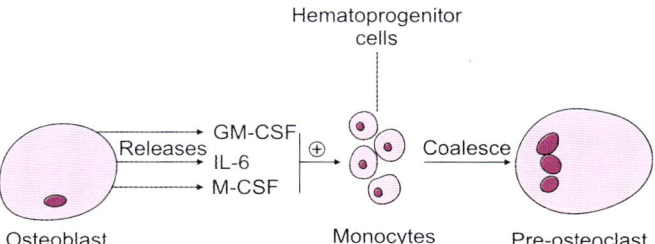

Fig. 24.3: Formation of pre-osteoclast

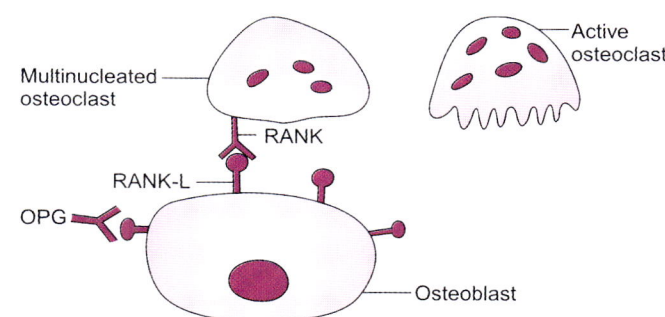

RANK-L is a cell surface protein on osteoblast
RANK is present on osteoclast
OPG block the action of RANK-L by acting as decoy receptor

Fig. 24.4: Activation of osteoclast through RANK/RANKL/OPG axis

site of great activity due to ion transport and protein secretion. Ruffled border is surrounded by a clear zone that has no organelles but only fine granular cytoplasm with microfilaments. Peripheral region of apical membrane is tightly juxtaposed to matrix which is called as sealing zone. Clear zone and sealing zone are responsible for attachment of osteoclast to bone matrix. This contains podosomes which are specialized protrusions of the ventral membrane of the osteoclast which adhere directly to the bone surface being broken down.

4. *Creation of a sealed acidic environment through action of the proton pump, which demineralizes bone and exposes the organic matrix*: The mineral is dissolved by acid secretion, which is brought about by an electrogenic hydrogen ion transporting system. This is an ATP driven proton pump. Intracellular pH regulation is achieved by carbonic anhydrase which is abundant in the osteoclast cytoplasm. Bicarbonate generated by the carbonic anhydrase appears to be secreted from the basal outer membrane, the hydrogen ions are released in the functional extracellular lysosomal compartment and there they dissolve the mineral and expose the organic matrix **(Fig. 24.5)**.

5. *Degradation of the exposed organic matrix to its constituents amino acids*: Stimulated osteoblast also secrete procollagenase and plasminogen activator which generates plasmin from plasminogen and this activates procollagenase for removing the non-mineralized collagenase surface layer **(Fig. 24.6)**.

6. Sequestering of mineral ions and amino acids within the osteoclast.

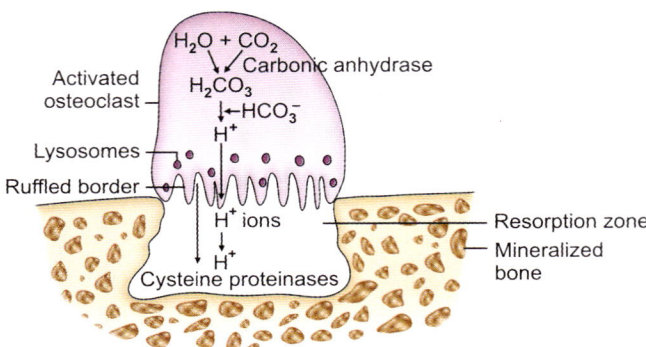

Fig. 24.5: Activated osteoclast causing resorption of mineralized bone matrix

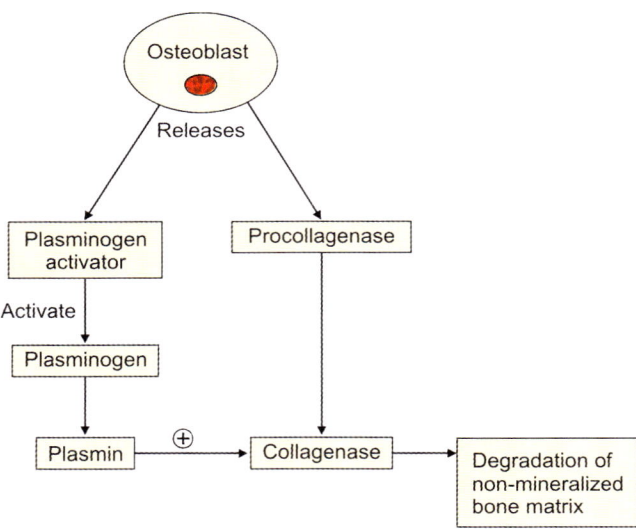

Fig. 24.6: Osteoblast causing degradation of non-mineralized bone matrix

In osteoclastic bone resorption:

First there is the solubilization of the mineral content of bone and then is the dissolution of the organic matrix.

Trauma from Occlusion

Trauma from occlusion can produce bone destruction either in the absence or presence of inflammation. In the absence of inflammation, the changes caused by trauma from occlusion vary from increased compression and tension of the periodontal ligament and increased osteoclasis of alveolar bone, to necrosis of the periodontal ligament and bone and resorption of bone and tooth structure. These changes are reversible in that they can be repaired if the offending forces are removed. However, persistent trauma from occlusion results in funnel shaped widening of the crestal portion of the periodontal ligament, with resorption of the adjacent bone. These changes, which may cause the bony crest to have an angular shape, represent adaptation of the periodontal tissues aimed at cushioning increased occlusal forces, but the modified bone shape may weaken tooth support and cause tooth mobility. When combined with inflammation, trauma from occlusion aggravates the bone destruction caused by the inflammation and causes bizarre bone patterns.

Systemic Disorders

Periodontal bone loss may also occur in generalized skeletal disturbances like hyperparathyroidism, Leukemia or Langerhan's cell histiocytosis. Bone factor concept was given by Irving Glickman in early 1950s. This concept present a clinical guide for determining the diagnosis and prognosis of periodontal disease based upon the response of alveolar bone to local injurious factors. The systemic regulatory influence upon the response of alveolar bone is termed as bone factor in periodontal disease. The individual bone factor affects the severity of bone loss associated with local destructive factors in periodontal disease. The destructive effect of inflammation and trauma from occlusion varies with the status of the individual bone factor. It is less severe in a healthy individual in the presence of positive bone factor.

PATTERN OF BONE DESTRUCTION IN PERIODONTAL DISEASES

The variety of bone defect is infinite, but for the purpose of description they have been classified according to their morphology as marginal defects, intra-alveolar defects, perforation and furcation defects. These are very rough groupings with considerable overlap.

Horizontal bone loss: When the bone loss occurs on a plane that is parallel to a line drawn from the CEJ of a tooth to that of an adjacent tooth, it is called horizontal bone loss. It is one of the common pattern of bone loss in periodontal disease. The bone margin remains roughly perpendicular to the tooth surface **(Fig. 24.7)**.

Vertical or angular defects are those that occur in an oblique direction, leaving a hollowed-out trough in the bone alongside the root; the base of the defect is located apical to the surrounding bone **(Fig. 24.8)**. When there is sufficient volume of bone surrounding the roots of teeth, resorptive bone patterns may take a vertical or funnel form, resulting

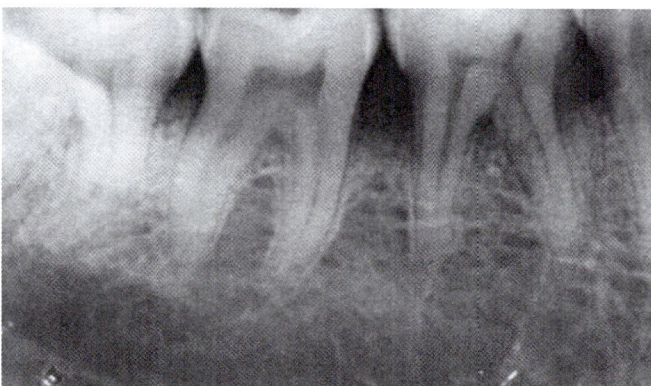

Fig. 24.7: Horizontal bone loss

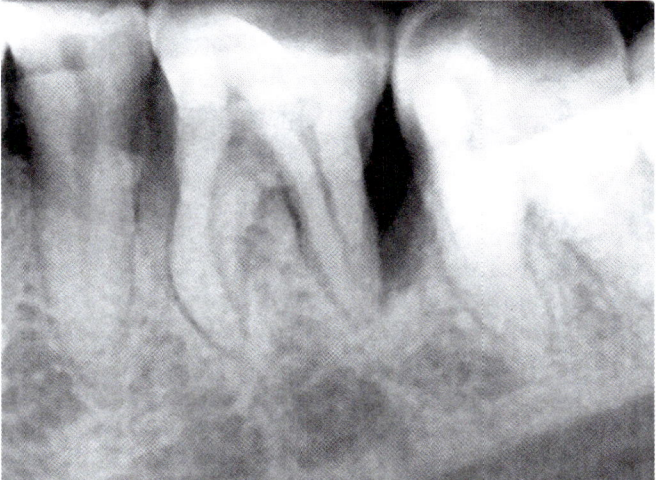

Fig. 24.8: Vertical bone loss

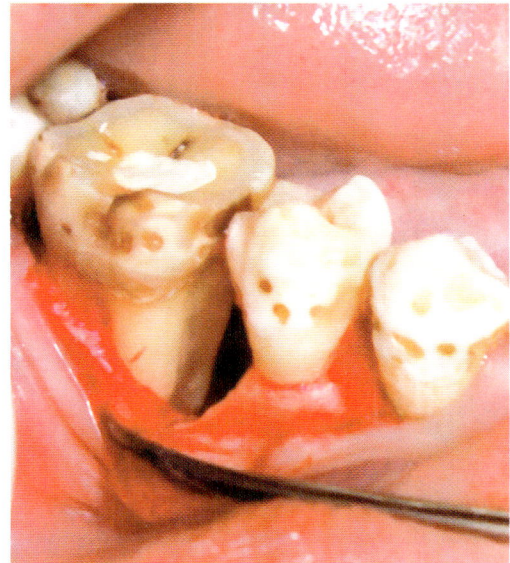

Fig. 24.9: Intrabony defect

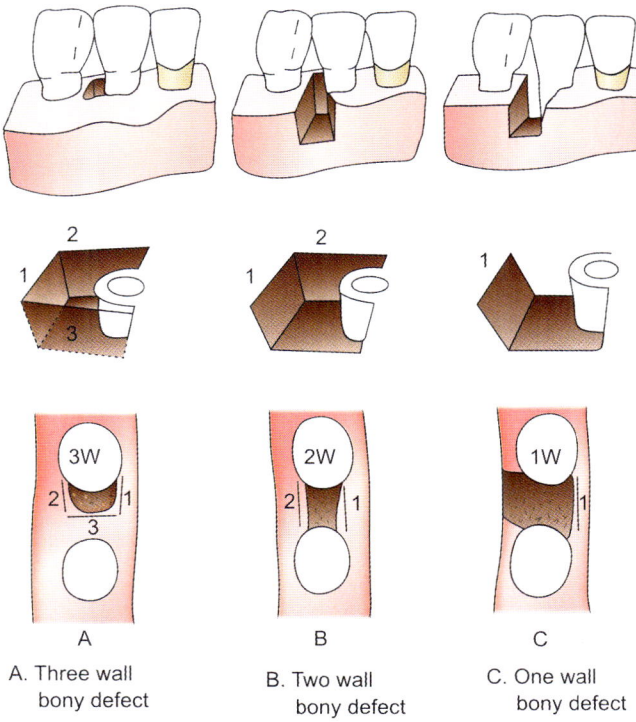

A. Three wall bony defect

B. Two wall bony defect

C. One wall bony defect

Figs 24.10A to C: Various vertical osseous defects

in formation of intrabony defects **(Fig. 24.9)**. Vertical bone loss usually consists of one or many infrabony pockets, because the base of the pocket is usually located apical to the crest of the surrounding bone. Angular defects are classified on the basis of the number of osseous walls **(Figs 24.10A to C)**.

One walled osseous defects where only one wall is present. The one wall vertical defect is called as hemiseptum. Two walled osseous defects where two walls are present. Three walled osseous defects where three walls are present.

Interproximal vertical defects can often be detected radiographically, whereas radicular surface vertical defects are not readily visible.

Interdental osseous craters are concavities in the crest of the alveolar septa centered under the contact point of adjacent teeth. Thus, can be described as a cup or bowl – shaped defect in the interdental alveolar bone **(Fig. 24.11B)**. As cancellous bone is more vascular and less dense than cortical bone it is likely that, the central cancellous part of a broad alveolar septum will resorb more rapidly than the lateral parts made up of cortical bone forming interdental crater. Craters have been found to make up about one third (35.2%) of all maxillary

PERIODONTICS REVISITED

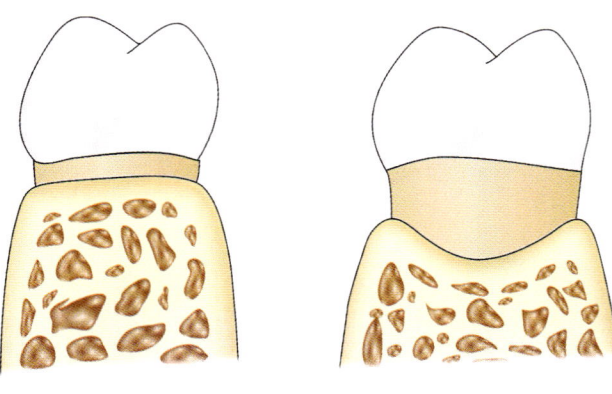

Normal (A)   Crater (B)

Figs 24. 11A and B: Faciolingual longitudinal section showing A. normal bone contour and B. osseous crater

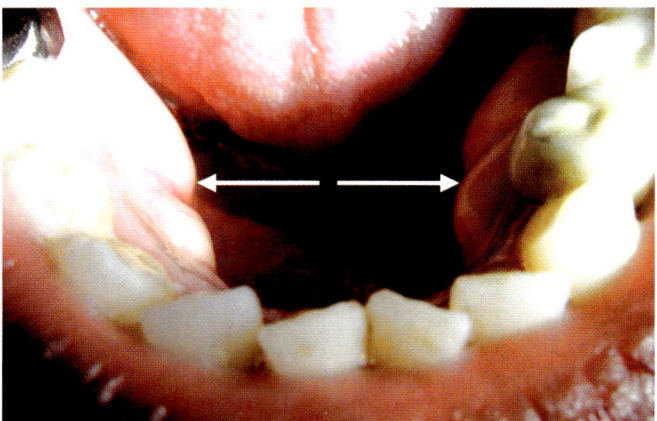

Fig. 24.12: Bilateral mandibular lingual exostosis
(*Courtesy:* Dr SK Salaria)

defects and about two third (62%) of all mandibular defects. They are twice as common in posterior segments as in anterior segments. Ochsenbein divided bony craters into 3 basic types: shallow, medium and deep. Following are the reasons for the high frequency of interdental craters: (a) The interdental area collects plaque and is difficult to clean. (b) The normal flat or even concave faciolingual shape of the interdental septum in lower molars may favor crater formation. (c) Vascular patterns from the gingiva to the center of the crest may provide a pathway for inflammation.

Bulbous bone contours are bony enlargements caused by exostoses, adaptation to function, or buttressing bone formation which are found frequently in the maxilla than in the mandible. Exostosis is a localized harmless idiopathic thickening of bony tissue, whose cause is unknown **(Fig. 24.12)**. Depending on their location in the jaws, they are identified as torus mandibularis (lingual mandibular plate) or torus palatinus (hard palate). Sometimes, several bony overgrowths occur on the vestibular alveolar bone and are simply called multiple exostosis. A peculiar condition consisting of bone exostosis has been reported to occur in some patients after undergoing either a skin graft vestibuloplasty or an autogenous free gingival graft. A slowly growing exostosis develops at the recipient site of the gingival graft. A definitive female sex predilection is characteristic of this condition, which usually presents in the canine-premolar area of the mandible or maxilla.

Reversed architecture forms when the interdental septum resorbs more rapidly than radicular bone **(Fig. 24.13)**.

Ledges are plateau-like bone margins caused by resorption of thickened bony plates **(Fig. 24.14)**.

Furcation involvement refers to the invasion of the bifurcation and trifurcation of multirooted teeth by periodontal disease **(Figs 24.15A and B)**.

Fenestration and dehiscence: Fenestrations are the isolated areas in which root is denuded of bone and marginal bone is intact. Dehiscences are the denuded areas that extend through the marginal bone. Dehiscence and fenestration are both associated with extreme buccal or lingual version of teeth. It occurs in 20% of all teeth. The defects are very important clinically because where they occur the root is covered only by the periosteum and overlying gingiva **(Figs 24.16A and B)**.

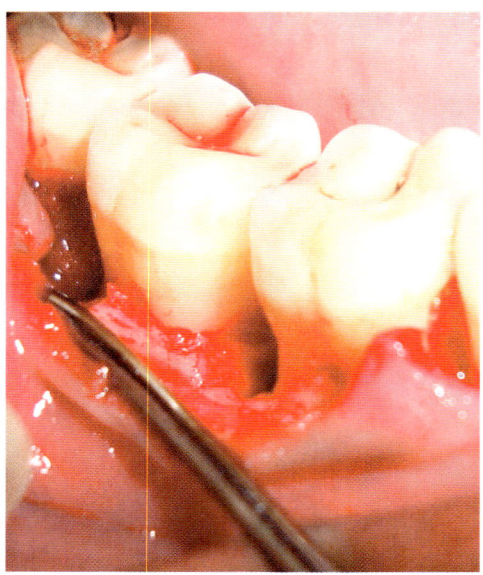

Fig. 24.13: Reversed architecture

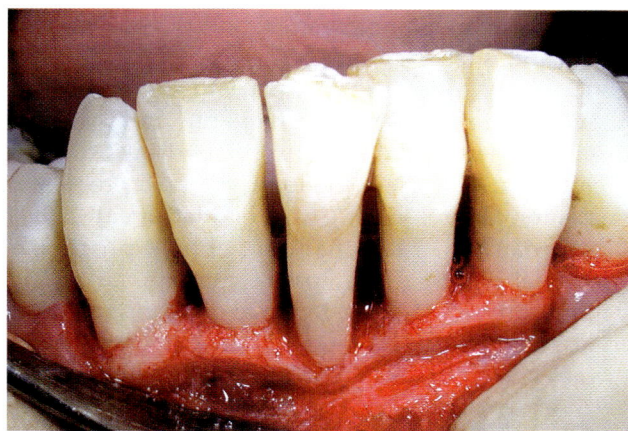

Fig. 24.14: Ledge

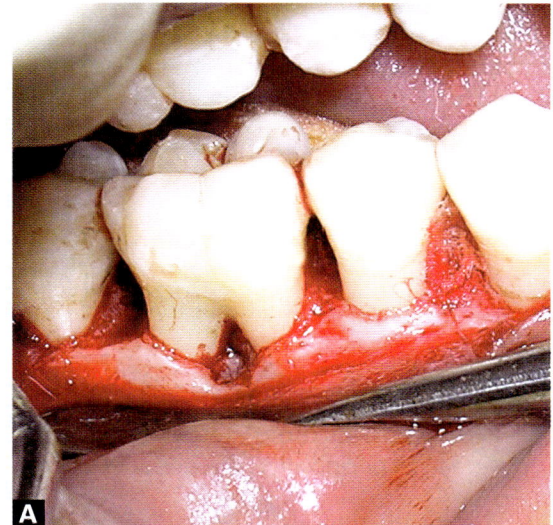

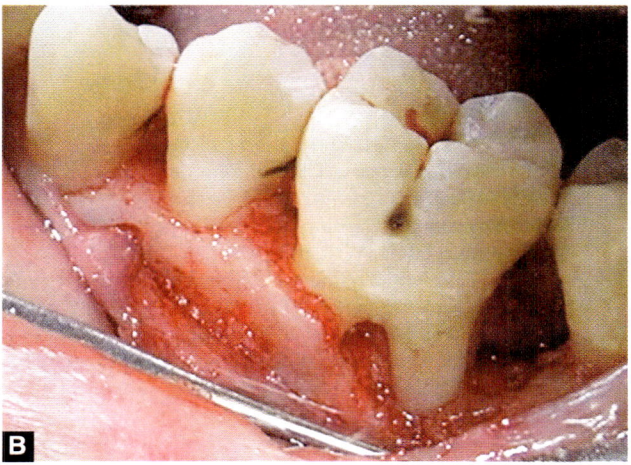

Figs 24.15A and B: Furcation defects

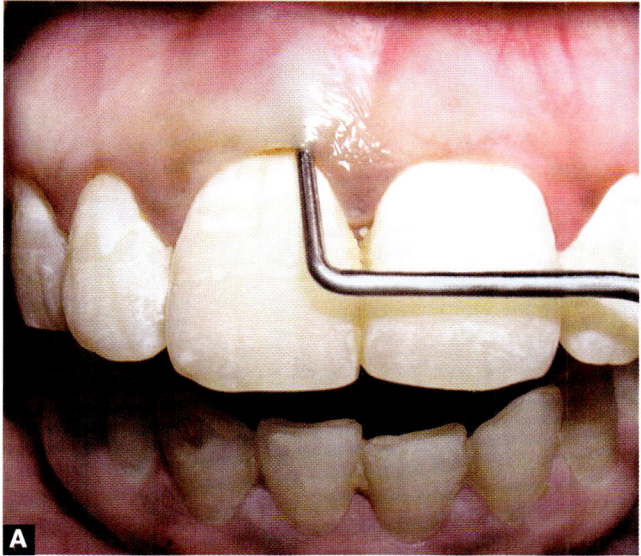

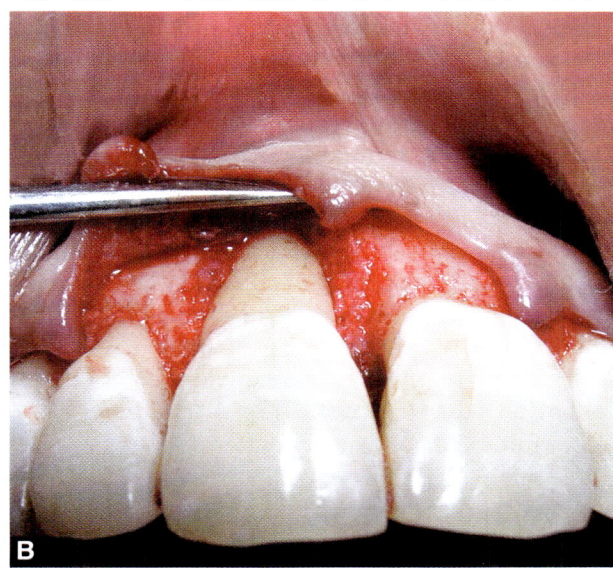

Figs 24.16A and B: (A) Probe in the pocket
(B) After the reflection of flap, dehiscence was found

Marginal gutter is a shallow linear defect between marginal bone of the radical cortical plate or interdental crest, extending the length of one or more root surfaces, usually formed by resorption of the socket side of the plate and deposition of the facial surface.

Irregular bony margins are the abrupt irregularities in the scalloped level of marginal bone and interdental septa.

PERIODONTICS REVISITED

Various bone destructive patterns are:

Horizontal bone loss
Vertical/Angular defects
Osseous craters
Bulbous bone contours
Reversed architecture
Ledges
Furcation involvement
Dehiscence and fenestration
Marginal gutter
Irregular bony margins

DIAGNOSIS OF BONE DEFECTS

1. *Probing*: Probing to determine the presence of these destructive patterns must be done horizontally and vertically around each involved root and in the crater area to establish the depth of the vertical component. The diagnosis of furcation involvement is made by clinical examination and careful probing with one of the specially designed Nabers probe.
2. *Bone sounding*: It is done by anaesthetizing the tissue locally and inserting probe horizontally and walking along the tissue tooth interface, so that the operator can feel the bony topography. It is also called as transgingival probing.
3. *Radiographic examination*: Radiographic examination of the area is helpful, but furcation lesions can be obscured by angulation of the beam and the radiopacity of neighboring structures.
4. *Surgical exposure*: Surgical exposure of bone defect through full thickness flap is the best way to determine the bone defect pattern.

LANDMARK STUDIES RELATED

Loe H, Anerud H, Boyen H, et al. Natural history of periodontal disease in man. Rapid, moderate and no loss of attachment in Sri Lankan tea labourers14 to 46 years of age. Journal of Clinical Periodontology 1986;13:431-45.

This ingeniously designed study was started in 1969 with a group of 565 male students and teachers aged 17 – 31 years in Norway. The next year the same investigators started work with the 480 male tea labourers aged 14 – 31 years in Sri Lanka who gave the study its customary name. Both groups declined in number, respectively to 245 and 161 at their last examinations. In the Sri Lankan group, with the prolonged 15 years period, 32 years progression could be covered.

In 1985, 161 remaining participants of a group of 480 Sri Lankan tea labourers aged 14 – 31 years in 1970 were periodontally examined. Plaque and gingivitis were ubiquitous and calculus was frequently in all subjects. Three subgroups were distinguished according to attachment loss: (a) 8% population had rapid progression of periodontal disease (RP). Loss of attachment of 0.1 to 1.0 mm yearly. (b) 81% had moderately progressive periodontal disease (MP). Loss of attachment of 0.05 to 0.5 mm yearly. (c) 11% had minimal or no progression of periodontal disease (NP). Loss of attachment of 0.05 to 0.09 mm yearly. In the RP subjects, almost all teeth were lost by 45 years; in MP, 7 teeth were lost; in NP virtually no teeth were lost. There were apparent changes in the rates of attachment loss in RP and MP groups; by age 45 years, the mean total loss was respectively, 13 mm and 7 mm. Thus, a clear demonstration of differing patient susceptibility to periodontal attachment loss was found.

POINTS TO PONDER

✓ 1.97mm ± 33.16% is the distance between apical extent of calculus and alveolar crest.
✓ 0.5- 2.7 mm is the distance between attached plaque and alveolar bone.
✓ Rate of bone loss depends upon the type of disease present and tooth surface. An average of 0.2 mm/year on facial surfaces and 0.3 mm/year on proximal surfaces.
✓ The most common bony lesion described and encountered in periodontal disease is the interdental crater.
✓ Approx. 1.5 to 2 mm is the radius of action of bacterial plaque that can induce bone loss.

BIBLIOGRAPHY

1. Carranza FA. Bone Loss and Patterns of Bone Destruction. In, Newman, Takei, Carranza. Clinical Periodontology 9th ed WB Saunders 2003;354-70.
2. Eley BM, Manson JD. The natural history of periodontal disease. In, Periodontics 5th ed Wright 2004;112-19.
3. Hausmann E. Potential pathways for bone resorption in human periodontal disease. Science 1974;45:338.
4. Loe H, Anerud H, Boyen H, et al. Natural history of periodontal disease in man. Rapid, moderate and no loss of attachment in Sri Lankan tea labourers 14 to 46 years of age. J Clin Periodontol 1986;13:431-45.
5. Manson JD. Chronic periodontitis. In, Periodontics 4th ed Wright Henry Kimpton Publishers 1980;97-117.
6. Manson JD, Nicholson K. The distribution of bone defects in chronic periodontitis. J Periodontol 1974;54:88-92.

PERIODONTICS REVISITED

7. Papapanou PN, Tonetti MS. Diagnosis and epidemiology of periodontal osseous lesions. Periodontol 2000 2000;22:8-31.
8. Schwartz,Z Goultschin J, Dean DD, Boyan BD. Mechanisms of alveolar bone destruction in periodontitis. Periodontol 2000 1997;14:158-72.

MCQs

1. Reversed architecture is:
   A. The level of interdental bone is more apical to radicular bone.
   B. The interdental bone is at the same level to that of radicular bone.
   C. The level of radicular bone is apical to the interdental bone
   D. None of the above
2. Mirror image type of bone loss pattern of Arc shaped bone loss around molars is seen in:
   A. Localized aggressive periodontitis
   B. Rapidly progressive periodontitis
   C. Chronic periodontitis
   D. Necrotizing ulcerative periodontitis
3. How many osseous walls are present in one – walled vertical defects?
   A. Two walls present   B. One wall present
   C. Three walls present   D. Four walls present
4. Window - shaped alveolar defect on labial alveolar bone is called:
   A. Dehiscence
   B. Crater
   C. Fenestration
   D. Trough
5. Bony defects which results in plateau – like marginal bone are called:
   A. Bulbous adaptive
   B. Ledges
   C. Craters
   D. Trough
6. The most potent bone resorbing interleukin is:
   A. IL – 8
   B. IL – 1β
   C. IL – 5
   D. IL – 3
7. Bone factor concept was given by:
   A. Schluger   B. Newman
   C. Irving Glickman   D. None of the above

Answers

| 1. A | 2. A | 3. B | 4. C | 5. B |
| 6. B | 7. C | | | |

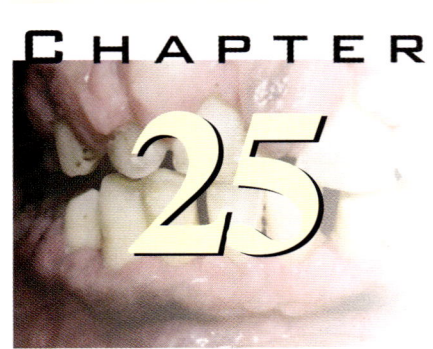

CHAPTER

25

Chronic Periodontitis

Shalu Bathla, Anish Manocha

INTRODUCTION

Chronic periodontitis is the most common form of destructive periodontal disease in adults; it can occur over a wide range of ages. It can occur in both the primary and secondary dentition. It usually has slow to moderate rates of progression, but may have periods of rapid progression. Chronic periodontitis is initiated and sustained by bacterial plaque, but host defense mechanism plays an integral role in its pathogenesis. The progressive nature of the disease can only be confirmed by repeated examinations. It is reasonable to assume that the disease will progress further if treatment is not provided.

Chronic periodontitis is defined as an infectious disease resulting in inflammation within the supporting tissues of the teeth leading to progressive attachment and bone loss. It is also characterized by pocket formation and/or gingival recession. It is recognized as the most frequently occurring form of periodontitis.

CLASSIFICATION

Chronic periodontitis can be further characterized by extent and severity. Extent is the number of sites involved and can be described as localized or generalized.
- Localized if ≤ 30% of the sites are affected **(Fig. 25.1)**
- Generalized if > 30% of the sites are affected **(Fig. 25.2)**

Severity can be described for the entire dentition or for individual teeth and sites. As a general guide, severity can be categorized on the basis of the amount of clinical attachment loss (CAL) as follows:
- Slight = 1 to 2 mm CAL
- Moderate = 3 to 4 mm CAL
- Severe ≥ 5 mm CAL.

CLINICAL FEATURES

1. *Amount of destruction is consistent with the presence of local factors*: Characteristic clinical finding in patient with chronic periodontitis include supragingival and subgingival plaque accumulation that is frequently associated with subgingival calculus formation **(Fig. 25.3)**.
2. *Gingival inflammation*: The gingiva ordinarily is slightly to moderately swollen and exhibits alterations in color ranging from pale red to magenta. Loss of gingival stippling and changes in the surface topography may include blunted or rolled gingival margins and flattened or cratered papillae. Gingival bleeding, either spontaneous or in response to probing, is frequent, and inflammation related exudates of crevicular fluid **(Fig. 25.4)**.
3. *Periodontal pocket formation*: Pocket depths are variable, and suppuration from the pocket can be found.

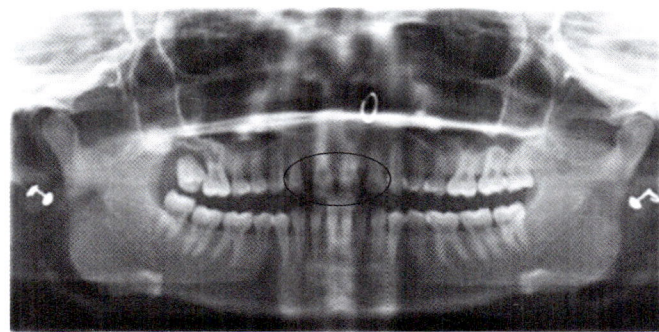

Fig. 25.1: OPG showing localized bone loss in localized chronic periodontitis

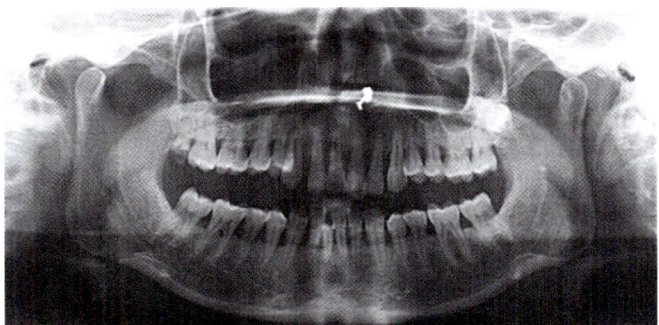

Fig. 25.2: OPG showing generalized bone loss in generalized chronic periodontitis

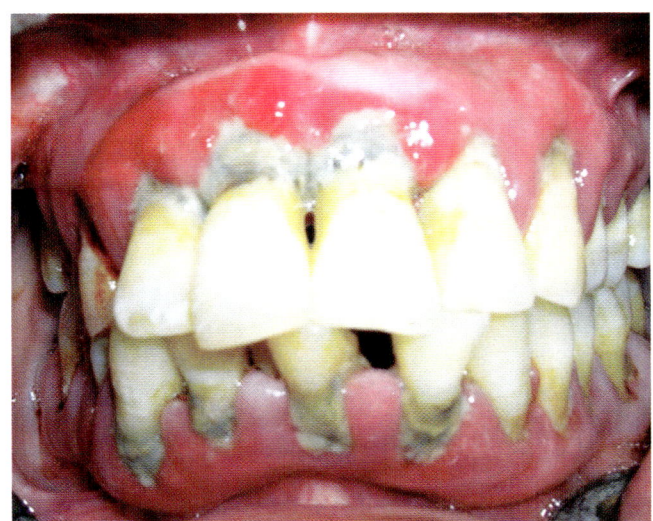

Fig. 25.3: Increased amount of calculus and plaque associated with chronic periodontitis

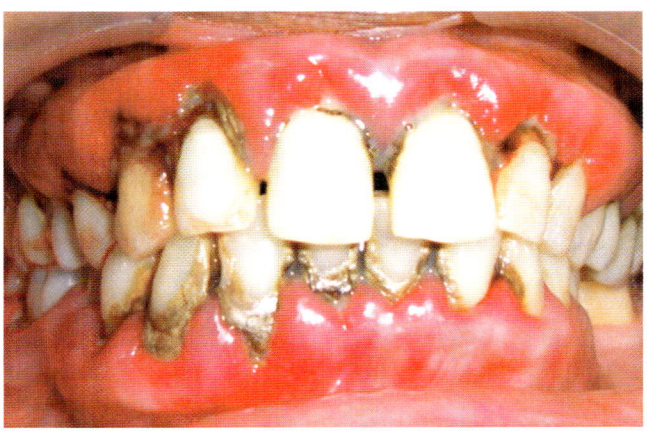

Fig. 25.4: Gingival inflammation associated with chronic periodontitis

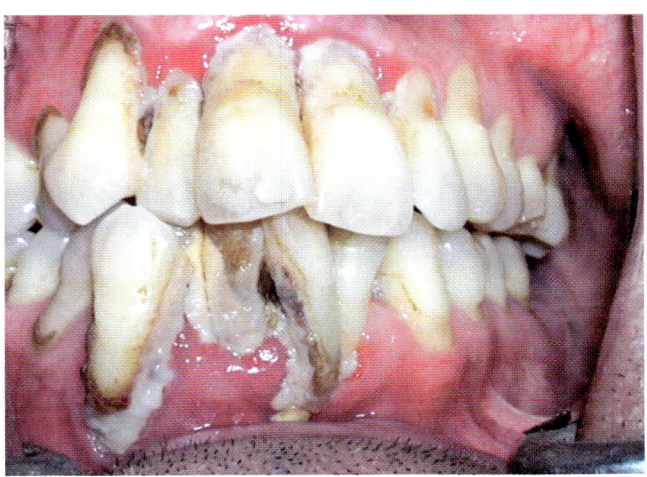

Fig. 25.5: Generalized loss of attachment

4. *Loss of periodontal attachment*: Chronic periodontitis with slight to moderate loss of periodontal supporting tissues may be localized or generalized **(Fig. 25.5)**.

5. *Loss of alveolar bone*: Resorption of alveolar bone in the form of both horizontal and vertical bone loss can be seen. There is considerable variation in both the form, pattern and rate of alveolar bone resorption.

6. *Mobility*: Tooth mobility often appears in advanced cases when bone loss has been considerable.

7. This type of periodontitis can be associated with local predisposing factors (e.g. tooth-related or iatrogenic factors).

8. May be modified by and/or associated with systemic diseases (e.g. diabetes mellitus, HIV); can be modified by factors other than systemic disease such as cigarette smoking and emotional stress.

9. Slow to moderate rate of progression, but may have periods of rapid progression also.

PERIODONTICS REVISITED

RADIOGRAPHIC FEATURES

Radiographic examination is an essential part of periodontal diagnosis and with certain limitations provides evidence of the alveolar bone height, extent, form of bone destruction, and the density of cancellous trabeculation. Various bone loss patterns can be seen in chronic periodontitis patient **(Fig. 25.6)** and is explained in chapter 24 Bone defects. In a marginal periodontitis, bone destruction is indicated first by the loss of the dense margin, which delineates the alveolar process in health. As bone density decreases the bone margins becomes radiolucent and indistinct. With continuing bone resorption the height of the alveolar bone is reduced.

Chronic periodontitis is diagnosed by:

Chronic inflammatory changes in the gingiva
Presence of periodontal pockets
Loss of clinical attachment and
Alveolar bone loss

PROGRESSION OF PERIODONTAL DISEASE

Chronic periodontitis does not progress at an equal rate in all affected sites throughout the mouth. Some involved areas may remain static for long periods of time, whereas others may progress more rapidly. More rapidly progressive lesions occur most frequently in interproximal areas and are usually associated with areas of greater plaque accumulation and inaccessible areas to plaque control measures (furcation areas, overhanging margins, malposed teeth).

Following are the models that describe the rate of disease progression:

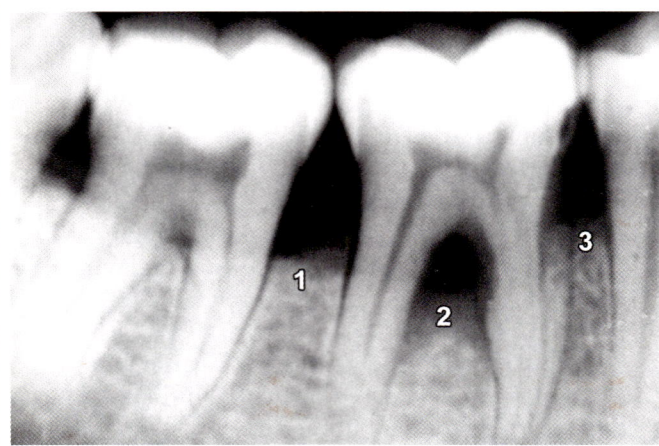

Fig. 25.6: Radiograph of chronic periodontitis showng various pattern of bone loss: 1. Vertical bone loss, 2. Furcation defect, 3. Horizontal bone loss

i. *Continuous disease model*: In this model, loss of attachment has commenced and proceed continuously and slowly until tooth loss eventually results. Linear correlation between age and loss of attachment, supports this concept of gradual destruction **(Fig. 25.7)**.

ii. *Random burst disease model*: In 1982, Goodson et al challenged the continuous disease model and

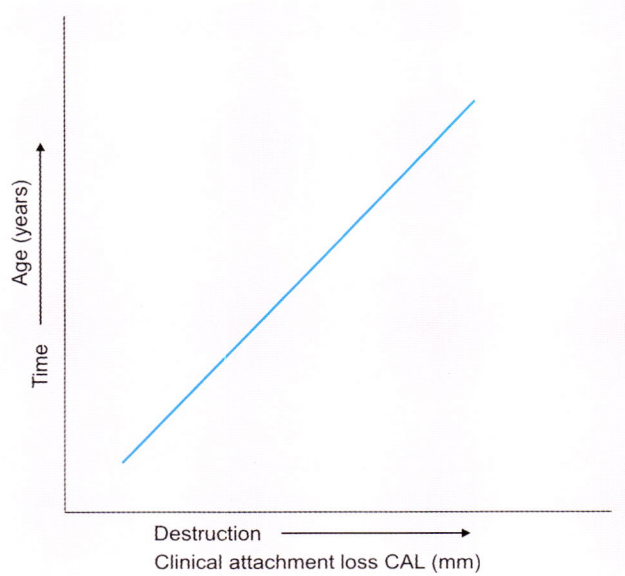

Fig. 25.7: Continuous disease model

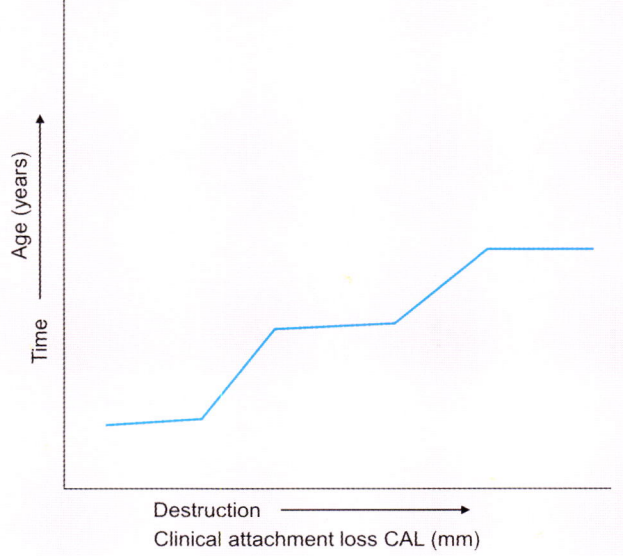

Fig. 25.8: Random burst disease model

proposed that destruction occurs during periods of exacerbation, interjected with intervals of remission. Breakdown occurs in recurrent acute episodes/bursts of activity over a short time span, interspersed with periods of quiescence **(Fig. 25.8)**.

iii. *Stochastic disease model*: In 1989 Manji and Nagelkerke proposed Stochastic model for periodontal breakdown that essentially combines both of the above models. They suggested that, as well as an underlying slow continuous breakdown (the progression rate of which depends on host and sites), some sites of some individuals are also undergoing random bursts of activity as a result of a combination of biological events.

RISK FACTORS OR SUSCEPTIBILITY

Prior History of Periodontitis: Although not a true risk factor for disease but rather a disease predictor, a prior history of periodontitis puts patients at a greater risk for developing further loss of attachment and bone, given a challenge from bacterial plaque accumulation. This means that patient with pocket and attachment and bone loss will continue to lose periodontal support if not successfully treated.

Bacterial risk factors: Plaque accumulation on tooth and gingival surfaces at the dentogingival junction is considered the primary initiating agent in the etiology of chronic periodontitis. Specific microorganisms have been considered as potential periodontal pathogens but it is clear that although pathogens are necessary, their mere presence may not be enough for disease activity to occur. Microbial plaque (biofilm) is a crucial factor in inflammation of the periodontal tissues, but the progression of gingivitis to periodontitis is largely governed by host-based risk factors. Microbial biofilms of particular compositions will initiate chronic periodontitis in certain individuals whose host response and cumulative risk factors predispose them to periodontal destruction rather than to gingivitis.

Systemic Factors: The rate of progression of plaque-induced chronic periodontitis is generally considered to be slow. However, when chronic periodontitis occurs in a patient who also suffers from a systemic disease that influences the effectiveness of the host response, the rate of periodontal destruction may be significantly increased. Diabetes is a systemic condition that can increase the severity and extent of periodontal disease in an affected patient.

Age: Although the prevalence of periodontal disease increases with age it is unlikely that becoming older in itself greatly increases susceptibility to periodontal disease. It is more likely that the cumulative effects of disease over a lifetime, i.e. deposits of plaque and calculus, and the increased number of sites capable of harboring such deposits, as well as attachment and bone loss experience, explain the increased prevalence of disease in older people.

Smoking: It is not only the risk of developing the disease that is enhanced by smoking, but also the response to periodontal therapy is impaired in smokers. A further feature in smokers is that their signs and symptoms of both gingivitis and chronic periodontitis, mainly gingival redness and bleeding on probing, are masked by the dampening of inflammation.

Stress: Stress and other psychosomatic conditions may have direct anti-inflammatory and/or anti-immune effects and/or behavior mediated effects on the body's defenses.

Genetics: There is convincing evidence from twin studies for a genetic predisposition to the periodontal diseases. The twin studies have indicated that risk of chronic periodontitis has a high inherited component. It is likely that chronic periodontitis involves many genes, the composition of which may vary across individuals and races. Much attention has focused on polymorphisms associated with the genes involved in cytokine production. Such polymorphisms have been linked to an increased risk for chronic periodontitis but these findings have yet to be corroborated.

TREATMENT

The goals of periodontal therapy are to alter or eliminate the microbial etiology and contributing risk factors for periodontitis, thereby arresting the progression of the disease and preserving the dentition in a state of health, comfort, and function with appropriate esthetics; and to prevent the recurrence of periodontitis. In addition, regeneration of the periodontal attachment apparatus, where indicated, may be attempted. Clinical judgement is an integral part of the decision making process. Many factors affect the decisions for the appropriate therapy(ies) and the expected therapeutic results. Patient-related factors include systemic health, age, compliance, therapeutic preferences, and patient's ability to control plaque. Other factors include the clinician's ability to remove subgingival deposits, restorative and prosthetic demands, and the presence and treatment of teeth with more advanced chronic periodontitis.

Treatment considerations for patients with slight to moderate loss of periodontal support are described below:

PERIODONTICS REVISITED

1. Contributing systemic risk factors may affect treatment and therapeutic outcomes for chronic periodontitis. These may include diabetes, smoking, certain periodontal bacteria, aging, gender, genetic predisposition, systemic diseases and conditions (immunosuppression), stress, nutrition, pregnancy, HIV infection, substance abuse and medications. Elimination, alteration, or control of risk factors which may contribute to chronic periodontitis should be attempted. Consultation with the patient's physician may be indicated.

2. Instruction, reinforcement and evaluation of the patient's plaque control should be performed.

3. Supragingival and subgingival scaling and root planing should be performed to remove microbial plaque and calculus. To accomplish this, the following procedures may be considered:
   - Removal or reshaping of restorative overhangs and over-contoured crowns
   - Correction of ill-fitting prosthetic appliances
   - Restoration of carious lesions
   - Odontoplasty
   - Tooth movement
   - Restoration of open contacts which have resulted in food impaction
   - Treatment of occlusal trauma.

4. Antimicrobial agents or devices may be used as adjuncts.

5. Evaluation of the initial therapy's outcomes should be performed after an appropriate interval for resolution of inflammation and tissue repair. A periodontal examination and re-evaluation may be performed with the relevant clinical findings documented in the patient's record. These findings may be compared to initial documentation to assist in determining the outcome of initial therapy as well as the need for and the type of further treatment.

6. For reasons of health, lack of effectiveness or non-compliance with plaque control, patient desires, or therapist's decision, appropriate treatment to control the disease may be deferred or declined.

7. If the results of initial therapy res olve the periodontal condition, periodontal maintenance should be scheduled at appropriate intervals.

8. If the results of initial therapy do not resolve the periodontal condition, periodontal surgery should be considered to resolve the disease process and/or correct anatomic defects.

9. Periodontal Surgery: A variety of surgical treatment modalities may be appropriate in managing the patient.

- Gingival augmentation therapy.
- Regenerative therapy: Bone replacement grafts, Guided tissue regeneration and Combined regenerative techniques.
- Resective therapy: Flaps with or without osseous surgery and Gingivectomy.

11. The desired outcome of nonsurgical and surgical periodontal therapy in patients with chronic periodontitis should result in: Significant reduction of clinical signs of gingival inflammation; reduction of probing depths; stabilization or gain of clinical attachment and reduction of clinically detectable plaque to a level compatible with gingival health.

12. Compromised therapy: In certain cases, because of the severity and extent of disease and the age and health of the patient, treatment that is not intended to attain optimal results may be indicated. In these cases, initial therapy may become the end point. This should include timely periodontal maintenance.

BIBLIOGRAPHY

1. Kinane DF and Lindhe J. Chronic Periodontitis. In, Lindhe J, Karring T, Lang NP. Clinical Periodontology and Implant dentistry. 4th ed Blackwell Munksgaard 2003;209-15.
2. Manson JD. Chronic Periodontitis. In, Periodontics 4th ed Wright 1980 Henry Kimpton Publishers; 97-117.
3. Nagy RJ, Novak MJ. Chronic periodontitis. In, Newman, Takei, Carranza. Clinical Periodontology 9th ed WB Saunders 2003;398-402.
4. Grant DA, Stern IB, Listgarten MA. Periodontitis. In, Periodontics. 6th ed CV Mosby Company 1988;348-75.

MCQs

1. To be diagnosed as localized form of chronic periodontitis, the number of sites involved should be less than:
   A. 10%
   B. 20%
   C. 30%
   D. 40%

2. In chronic periodontontitis:
   A. Amount of destruction is consistent with the presence of local factors
   B. Amount of destruction is inconsistent with the presence of local factors
   C. It depends upon age
   D. None of the above

Answers

1. C   2. A

CHAPTER

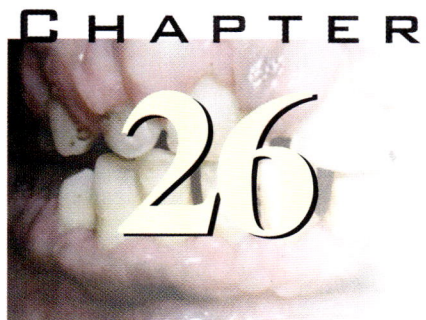

Aggressive Periodontitis

Shalu Bathla

HISTORICAL PERSPECTIVE

A variety of names have been given to a form of periodontal disease characterized by deep pockets and advanced alveolar bone loss in the young children, adolescents and adults, without any associated systemic disease. In 1923, Gottlieb called *diffuse atrophy of the alveolar bone* characterized by loss of collagen fibers in the periodontal ligament and their replacement by loose connective tissue and extensive bone resorption, resulting in a widened periodontal ligament space. In 1928, Gottlieb termed *deep cementopathia* hypothesizing inhibition of continuous cementum formation. In 1938, Wannenmacher described it as *parodontitis marginalis progressiva*. In 1942, Orban and Weinmann introduced the term *periodontosis* and described the development of the disease in three stages. In 1966, the World Workshop in Periodontics concluded the concept of periodontosis. The term *juvenile periodontitis* was introduced by Chaput and colleagues in 1967 and by Butler in 1969. In 1971, Butler defined it as "a disease of the periodontium occurring in an otherwise healthy adolescent which is characterized by a rapid loss of alveolar bone about more than one tooth of the permanent dentition. The amount of destruction manifested is not commensurate with the amount of local irritants." Page and Baab in 1985, suggested that all forms of the disease be designated as *early onset periodontitis* (EOP). In 1989, World Workshop in Clinical Periodontics categorized this disease as *localized juvenile periodontitis* (LJP), a subset of the broad classification of early onset periodontitis (EOP). At the 1999 International Classification Workshop, the different forms of periodontitis were reclassified into chronic, aggressive periodontitis and periodontitis as a manifestations of systemic diseases and it was renamed as *aggressive periodontitis*.

Aggressive periodontitis has been defined, based on the following primary features (Lang, et al 1999):

- Non-contributory medical history.
- Rapid attachment loss and bone destruction.
- Familial aggregation of cases.

Secondary features that are considered to be generally, but not universally present are:

- Amount of microbial deposits inconsistent with the severity of periodontal tissue destruction **(Fig. 26.1)**.
- Elevated proportions of *Aggregatibacter actinomycetemcomitans*
- Phagocyte abnormality
- Hyper – responsive macrophage phenotype, including elevated production of PGE_2 and IL - 1β in response to bacterial endotoxin.
- Progression of attachment loss and bone loss may be self arresting.

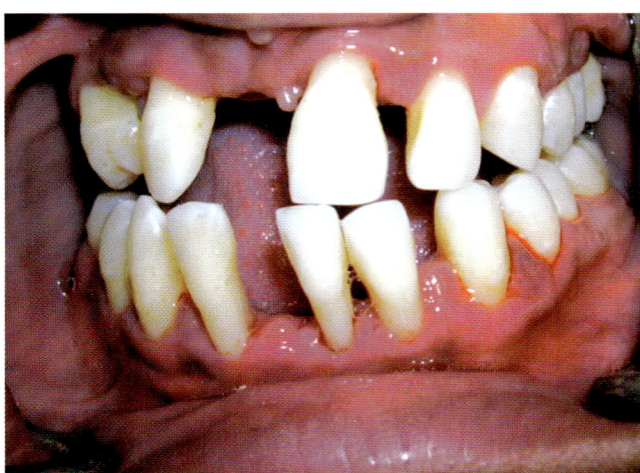

Fig. 26.1: Generalized aggressive periodontitis- amount of plaque is inconsistent with the amount of periodontal destruction

LOCALIZED AGGRESSIVE PERIODONTITIS

Characteristics Features

i. Circumpubertal onset.
ii. Robust serum antibody response to infecting agents.
iii. Localized first molar/incisor presentation with interproximal attachment loss on at least two permanent teeth, one of which is a first molar and involving no more than two teeth other than first molars and incisors. Following are the possible reasons, suggested for the limitation of periodontal destruction to certain teeth:

- After initial colonization on the first erupting permanent teeth (the first molars and incisors), *Aggregatibacter actinomycetemcomitans* evades the host defenses by different mechanisms, including production of polymorphonuclear leukocyte chemotaxis-inhibiting factors, endotoxin, collagenases, leukotoxin, and other factors that allow the bacteria to colonize the pocket and initiate the destruction of the periodontal tissues. After this initial attack, adequate immune defenses are stimulated to produce opsonic antibodies to enhance the clearance and phagocytosis of invading bacteria and neutralize leukotoxic activity. Thus, colonization of other sites is to be prevented. A strong antibody response to infecting agents is one characteristic of localized aggressive periodontitis.
- Bacteria antagonistic to *Aggregatibacter actinomycetemcomitans* may colonize the periodontal tissues and inhibit *Aggregatibacter actinomycetemcomitans*

and localize *Aggregatibacter actinomycetemcomitans* infection and tissue destruction.

- The progression of the disease may become arrested or retarded and colonization of new periodontal sites averted as *Aggregatibacter actinomycetemcomitans* may lose its leukotoxin producing ability for unknown reasons.
- The defect in cementum formation may be responsible for the localization of the lesion.

Radiographic Findings

Vertical loss of alveolar bone around the first molars and incisors, beginning around puberty in otherwise healthy teenagers, is a classic diagnostic sign of localized aggressive periodontitis. There is an *arc-shaped loss of alveolar bone* extending from the distal surface of the second premolar to the mesial surface of the second molar **(Fig. 26.2)**. It is usually bilaterally symmetrical in both the first molars of each jaw.

Clinical findings of aggressive periodontitis
Lack of clinical inflammation
Deep periodontal pockets
Minimal amount of plaque

GENERALIZED AGGRESSIVE PERIODONTITIS

Clinically, generalized aggressive periodontitis is characterized by "generalized interproximal attachment loss affecting at least three permanent teeth other than first molars and incisors".

i. Usually affecting person under 30 years of age, but patients may be older.

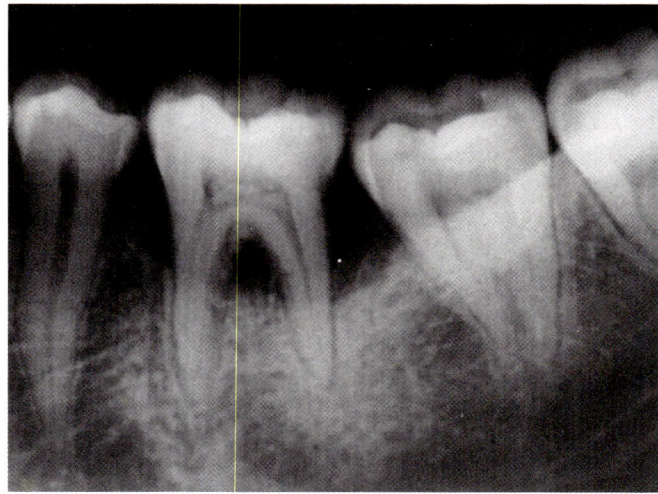

Fig. 26.2: Arc-shaped bone loss around mandibular first molar

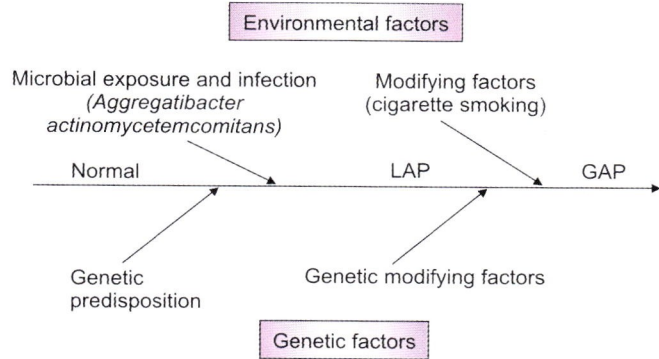

Fig. 26.3: Risk factors associated with aggressive periodontitis

ii. Generalized interproximal attachment loss affecting at least three permanent teeth other than first molars and incisors.

iii. Pronounced episodic nature of the destruction of attachment and alveolar bone.

iv. Poor serum antibody response to infecting agents.

RISK FACTORS

Aggressive forms of periodontitis are currently considered to be multifactorial diseases developing as a result of complex interactions between specific host genes and the environment **(Fig. 26.3)**. Inheritance of aggressive periodontitis susceptibility is probably insufficient for the development of disease. Environmental exposure to potential pathogens endowed with specific virulence factors is also a necessary step. Host inability to effectively deal with the bacterial aggression and to avoid inflammatory tissue damage results in the initiation of the disease process. Interactions between the disease process and environmental (e.g. cigarette smoking) and genetically controlled (e.g. IgG$_2$ response to *Aggregatibacter actinomycetemcomitans*) modifying factors are thought to contribute in determining the specific clinical manifestation of disease.

Microbiologic factors: Although several specific microorganisms frequently are detected in patients with localized aggressive periodontitis (*Aggregatibacter actinomycetemcomitans, Eikenella corrodens, Prevotella intermedia* and *Campylobacter rectus*), *Aggregatibacter actinomycetemcomitans* has been implicated as the primary pathogen associated with this disease.

Immunologic Factors: Several immune defects have been implicated in the pathogenesis of aggressive periodontitis. The human leukocyte antigens (HLA), which regulate immune responses, have been evaluated as candidate markers for aggressive periodontitis. Patients with aggressive periodontitis display functional defects of polymorphonuclear leukocytes (PMNs), monocytes, or both. Patients with localized aggressive periodontitis exhibit a PMN chemotactic defect and depressed phagocytosis in peripheral blood. Neutrophil migration into the gingival crevice is slower. Neutrophils from individuals with classic form of localized aggressive periodontitis are characterized by decrease in chemotactic responses to a variety of chemotactic factors, including C5a, FMLP (a formyl peptide), and leukotriene B$_4$. The neutrophil dysfunction is associated with a functional decrease in chemotaxin receptors on the polymorphonuclear neutrophil surface. The defect has been described as a *pan – receptor defect*, because all chemotaxin receptors appears to be decreased.

Neutrophil defects associated with Aggressive periodontitis are:
- Abnormalities in adherence: LAD – I, LAD – II
- Abnormalities in chemotaxis:
  - Decreased number of several receptors for chemotactic factors – Pan receptor defect.
  - Papillon – Lefevre syndrome
  - Chediak – Higashi syndrome
- Abnormalities in phagocytosis and intercellular killing.

Monocytes show hyperresponsiveness with respect to their production of PGE$_2$ in response to lipopolysaccharide (LPS). This hyperresponsive phenotype could lead to increased connective tissue or bone loss due to excessive production of the catabolic factors.

Genetic factors: All individuals are not equally susceptible to aggressive periodontitis. Currently, specific genes have not been identified that are responsible for these diseases. But some segregational analysis and linkage analysis of families with a genetic predisposition for localized aggressive periodontitis suggest that it is transmitted through an autosomal dominant mode of inheritance.

Environmental Factors: Smoking is considered to be important environmental risk factor for aggressive periodontitis. Patients with generalized aggressive periodontitis who smoke have more affected teeth and more loss of clinical attachment than nonsmoking patients with generalized aggressive periodontitis.

PERIODONTICS REVISITED

TREATMENT MODALITIES

Past treatment modalities for localized aggressive periodontitis are: (a) Extraction: The involved teeth usually the first molars used to be extracted. Transplantation of developing third molars to the sockets of previously extracted first molars has also been attempted; (b) Standard periodontal therapy: It included scaling and root planing, curettage, flap surgery with and without bone grafts, root amputations and hemisections. (c) Antibiotic therapy: Genco and colleagues reported the treatment of localized aggressive periodontitis with scaling and root planing plus tetracycline (250 mg four times daily for 14 days every 8 weeks).

Current treatment modalities for localized aggressive periodontitis: Successful treatment of aggressive periodontitis is considered to be dependent on early diagnosis, directing therapy towards elimination or suppression of the infecting microorganisms and providing an environment conducive to long-term maintenance. The differential element of treatment of aggressive periodontitis, however, relates to specific efforts to affect the composition and not only the quantity of the subgingival microbiota.

Systemic antibiotics should only be administered as an adjunct to mechanical debridement because in undisturbed subgingival plaque, the target organisms are effectively protected from the antibiotic agent due to the biofilm effect. Antibiotics have been used in essentially two ways for the treatment (a) in combination with intensive instrumentation over a short period of time after achievement of adequate plaque control in a pretreatment motivation period; or (b) as a staged approach after completion of the initial therapy.

In almost all cases, systemic tetracycline (250 mg of tetracycline hydrochloride four times daily for at least 1 week) should be given in conjunction with local mechanical therapy. If surgery is indicated, systemic tetracycline should be prescribed, with the patient instructed to take the antibiotic approximately 1 hour before surgery. Doxycycline 100 mg/day may also be used. Chlorhexidine rinses should also be prescribed and continued for several weeks.

Occlusal adjustment: Migration of incisors is a late characteristic of aggressive periodontitis but orthodontic treatment is usually contraindicated. If teeth which are to remain have drifted into premature contact, these should be treated by selective grinding.

Recurrence of disease is an indication for a repetition of microbiologic tests, for re-evaluation of the host immune response, and re-assessment of the local and systemic modifying factors. In refractory cases, tetracycline-resistant Actinobacillus species are suspected and a combination of amoxicillin and metronidazole can be tried.

Microbiologic testing may be repeated 1 to 3 months after completion of therapy to verify the elimination or marked suppression of the putative pathogen. After resolution of the periodontal infection, the patient should be placed on an individually tailored maintenance care programme, including continuous evaluation of the occurrence and of the risk of disease progression.

Treatment modalities for generalized aggressive periodontitis: In general, the treatment of patients with generalized forms of aggressive periodontitis should be very similar to that of patients with refractory forms of the disease.

TABLE 26.1: Comparison between chronic periodontitis, localized aggressive periodontitis and generalized aggressive periodontitis

Chronic periodontitis	Localized aggressive periodontitis	Generalized aggressive periodontitis
1. Most prevalent in adults, can occur in children	Usually occur in adolescents	Usually affects people under 30 yrs. of age, but patients may be older
2. Slow to moderate rate of progression	Rapid rate of progression	Rapid rate of progression (Pronounced episodic periods of progression)
3. Amount of microbial deposits consistent with severity of destruction	Amount of microbial deposits not consistent with severity of destruction	Amount of microbial deposits sometimes, consistent with severity of destruction
4. Variable distribution of periodontal destruction; No discernible pattern.	Periodontal destruction localized to permanent first molars and incisors	Periodontal destruction in addition to first molars and incisors
5. No marked familial aggregation	Familial aggregation	Marked familial aggregation
6. Frequent presence of subgingival calculus	Subgingival calculus usually absent	Subgingival calculus may or may not be present

BIBLIOGRAPHY

1. Eley BM, Manson JD. Early onset periodonititis: Juvenile periodonititis/Aggressive periodonititis. In, Periodontics 5th ed Wright 2004;332-44.
2. Lindhe Tonetti MS, Mombelli A. Aggressive Periodontitis. In, Lindhe J, Karring T, Lang NP. Clinical Periodontology and Implant dentistry 4th ed Blackwell Munksgaard 2003;216-42.
3. Manson JD. Juvenile periodonititis. In, Periodontics 4th ed Wright Henry Kimpton Publishers 1980;244-49.
4. Miyasaki KT. Altered Leukocyte function and periodontal disease. In, Carranza and Newman. Clinical Periodontology 8th ed WB Saunders 1996;132-50.
5. Nagy RJ, Novak KF. Aggressive Periodontitis. In, Newman, Takei, Carranza. Clinical Periodontology 9th ed WB Saunders 2003;409-14.
6. Nagy RJ, Newman MG. Treatment of Refractory Periodontitis, Aggressive Periodontitis, Necrotizing Ulcerative Periodontitis, and Periodontitis Associated with Systemic Diseases. In, Newman, Takei, Carranza. Clinical Periodontology 9th ed WB Saunders 2003;558-66.
7. Wilson TG, Kornman KS. Treating Aggressive forms of periodontal disease. In, Wilson TG, Kornman KS. Fundamentals of Periodontics.Quintessence Publishing Co.1996;389-422.

MCQs

1. Which of the following periodontal diseases is characterized by relative sparse subgingival plaque and bilateral angular bone loss in the first molars and incisors?
   A. Necrotizing ulcerative gingivitis
   B. Chronic periodontitis
   C. Prepubertal periodontitis
   D. Localized aggressive periodontitis
   E. Refractory periodontitis
2. The amount of plaque on the affected teeth is inconsistent with the amount of periodontal destruction in:
   A. Chronic periodontitis
   B. Aggressive periodontitis
   C. Periodontitis as a manifestation of systemic diseases
   D. Chronic gingivitis
3. Periodontitis is more prevalent in:
   A. American whites
   B. American brunnets
   C. Indo-Americans
   D. African Americans
4. Deep pockets without clinical inflammation is a striking feature of:
   A. Chronic periodontitis
   B. Localized aggressive periodontitis
   C. Leukemia
   D. Diabetes

Answers

1. D   2. B   3. D   4. B

CHAPTER

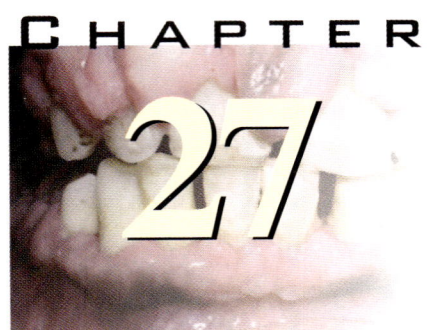

27

AIDS and Periodontium

Amit Aggarwal, Shalu Bathla

INTRODUCTION

The acquired immunodeficiency syndrome (AIDS) is a disabling or a life threatening condition caused by infection with the human immunodeficiency virus. The first case of AIDS was reported by Centers for Disease Control in 1981 in young homosexual men and later in injecting drug users and persons with hemophilia. The virus was first recognized in 1983 and fully recognized coincidently in France by Montagnier et al. in 1984 and in the USA by Gallo et al in the same year who called the virus human T-cell leukemia/lymphoma virus (HTLV-III). The clinical periodontal signs were detected in HIV infected people in 1986. The occurrence of a distinctive form of periodontal disease as a manifestation of HIV infection was first reported in 1987, when Winkler and Murray described an unusual form of gingivitis occurring in HIV seropositive individuals which presented as a distinct erythematous band at the marginal gingiva and was associated with petechiae.

All studied clinical periodontal parameters and microbiological evaluation of the periodonto-pathogens showed that periodontal health of the HIV-positive patients was moderately deteriorated in comparison to the healthy people. The increased periodontal destruction has been considered to be due, at least partly, to atypical microbial infections of the periodontium and to altered host response.

CLASSIFYING PERIODONTAL DISEASES IN AIDS PATIENTS

Severe forms of periodontal diseases have long been known to be associated with immune system defects. Different HIV-related periodontal disease classifications have been presented.

Category A patients have	Category B patients have	Category C patients have
• Asymptomatic HIV-1 infection • Persistent generalized lymphadenopathy • Acute (primary) HIV-1 infection or history of acute HIV-1 infection	• Oropharyngeal candidiasis • Oral hairy leukoplakia • Idiopathic thrombocytopenia • Constitutional symptoms of fever, diarrhea and weight loss During all this period (category A+B): The patients are HIV-positive infected but not yet got AIDS.	• Full blown disseminated life-threatening bacterial viral and protozoal infections • Malignancy • **CD4-T4 lymphocytes level less than 200/mm^3**

According to the CDC Surveillance Case Classification (1993) AIDS patients have been grouped as follows:

Laboratory categories:
Category 1: ≥ 500 CD4 lymphocytes/mm^3
Category 2: 200 to 499 CD4 lymphocytes/mm^3
Category 3: < 200 CD4 lymphocytes/mm^3

HIV associated periodontal diseases are categorized as follow:
1. HIV-associated gingivitis (HIV-G)
2. HIV- associated periodontitis (HIV-P)
3. NUG
4. Necrotizing stomatitis (NS)

In a later classification it was considered important to drop the term HIV, because any of those conditions could also be found in non-HIV-infected subjects. The HIV associated periodontal lesions accepted by the EC-Clearinghouse 1993 includes:
1. Linear gingival erythema (LGE), a non-plaque-induced gingivitis exhibiting a distinct erythematous band of the marginal gingiva, which either diffuses or punctuates erythema of the attached gingiva.
2. Necrotizing periodontal diseases, which are sub-classified as necrotizing ulcerative gingivitis (NUG), necrotizing ulcerative periodontitis (NUP), and necrotizing stomatitis (NS). NUG involves destruction of one or more interdental papillae and is limited to the marginal gingiva. NUP extends beyond the papillae and marginal gingiva, causing loss of periodontal attachment, possibly exposing bone. When the necrosis extends beyond the periodontium into the mucosa and osseous tissue, it results in NS. These three conditions appear to be different stages of the same disease. The only distinction appears to be their severity.

PATHOGENESIS

Periodontitis is a multifactorial disease where environmental, genetic and systemic conditions play a role together with altered host response and this interplay may be even more significant than the microbial challenge. Risk factors for periodontitis in HIV-positive patients are age, smoking, viral load, micro-organisms (*viz. Fusobacterium nucleatum, Prevotella intermedia, Aggregatibacter actinomycetemcomitans*) and enzymes (*viz.* GCF neutrophil elastase and beta glucuronidase).

There may be increased incidences of periodontal disease in patients with more advanced stages of HIV infection, related to the severity of the systemic disease and to the decreasing numbers of CD4+ lymphocytes in peripheral blood leading to immunosuppression, but not to clinical signs or periodontal pathogenic micro-organisms. However, immunosuppression is a risk factor for gingival inflammation. The attachment loss of HIV-positive patients can also be caused by lifestyle factors such as smoking habits and poor oral hygiene rather than HIV infection alone. There are indications that periodontitis progresses more rapidly in HIV-positive patients than in HIV-negative patients. Still, there is generally no difference in periodontopathogens of HIV-positive or HIV-negative patients.

Alterations in local host response could explain the accelerating rate of chronic periodontitis in HIV-positive patients. Both local and systemic host inflammatory and humoral immune responses in HIV infection may play a role in the progression of periodontal disease.

In chronic periodontitis lesions of HIV-positive patients, highly increased numbers of plasma cells, mast cells, macrophages and neutrophils have been found to release proinflammatory cytokines and other mediators leading to periodontal loss.

PERIODONTAL PATHOLOGIES IN HIV INFECTED PATIENTS

Linear gingival erythema (LGE): Linear gingival erythema is defined as a gingival manifestation of immuno-suppressed patients which is characterized by a distinct linear erythema limited to the free gingival margin. The lack of response of linear gingival erythema to conventional periodontal therapy, including plaque control, scaling and root planing is a key diagnostic feature of linear gingival erythema.

Another key feature of LGE is its association with Candida infection (Candida dubliniensis). Linear gingival erythema presents as a red band along the gingival margin and may or may not be accompanied by occasional bleeding and discomfort. It is seen most frequently in association with anterior teeth.

The microbiologic findings are consistent with that of conventional periodontitis rather than gingivitis. It is a potential clinical marker of HIV infection.

Necrotizing ulcerative gingivitis (NUG): It is characterized by ulcerated, necrotic papillae and gingival margins are covered by pseudo-membrane which is associated with intense pain and spontaneous gingival bleeding. It frequently may or may not be associated with depressed CD4+ Tcell count.

PERIODONTICS REVISITED

Necrotizing ulcerative periodontitis (NUP): It is a marker of severe immune suppression. The condition is characterized by severe pain, loosening of teeth, bleeding, fetid odor, ulcerated gingival papilla, and rapid loss of bone and soft tissue. Patients often refer to the pain as deep jaw pain. Other features include oral malodor, lymphadenopathy, fever and malaise. The microbial flora is similar to that of chronic periodontitis, it has same pathogen but at a higher level. There is evidence of increased prevalence of Candida. NUP is a predictive marker for CD4+ lymphocyte count less than $200/mm^3$.

Necrotizing ulcerative stomatitis: A severely destructive, acutely painful necrotizing ulcerative stomatitis (NUS) has occasionally been reported in HIV-positive patients. It is characterized by necrosis of significant areas of oral soft tissue and underlying bone. It may occur separately or as an extension of NUP and is commonly associated with severe depression of CD4 immune cells. The condition appears to be identical to cancrum oris (noma), a rare destructive process reported in nutritionally deprived individuals, especially those in Africa. NUS may be associated with severe immunodeficiency regardless of the cause of onset.

DIAGNOSIS OF PERIODONTITIS IN HIV PATIENTS

A diagnosis is derived from the information obtained from the patient's medical and dental history, combined with findings from thorough oral examination. The entire constellation of signs and symptoms associated with the disease or condition is taken into account before a diagnosis is reached. The clinical presentation of periodontitis is due to inflammation and the pathology that results from the inflammation. Injury mediated by inflammation is due to the inability of the host to resolve the inflammation. The altered immune response in HIV-positive patients is only a varied presentation of the normal, but is not in itself diagnostic. Moreover, there are no specific criteria to distinguish periodontal diseases occurring in HIV-positive from those in HIV-negative patients. It is now known that the lesions of NUP are commonly observed in individuals with systemic conditions including, but not limited to, HIV infection, severe malnutrition and immmunosuppression.

Seven oral cardinal lesions strongly associated with HIV infection are:
Oral candidiasis
Hairy leukoplakia
Kaposi's sarcoma
Linear gingival erythema
Necrotizing ulcerative gingivitis
Necrotizing ulcerative periodontitis
Non-Hodgkin's lymphoma

TREATMENT OF PERIODONTAL DISEASES IN HIV PATIENTS

Goals of Treatment in HIV Patients

i. Reduce HIV related morbidity and mortality, improve the quality of life.
ii. Restore and preserve immunologic function.
iii. Suppress viral load maximally and durably.

Chemotherapeutic Agents Used in Treatment of HIV

Valid anti-viral HIV medication since the mid 1990s is HAART (Highly Active Anti-Retroviral Therapy), a combination of drugs:
A. Nucleoside reverse transcriptase inhibitors (NRTI)—AZT (azidothymidine), zalcitabine (ddC), lamivudine (3TC), stavudine (d4T)
B. Non-nucleoside reverse transcriptase inhibitors (NNRTI)—delaviradine and nevirapine
C. Protease inhibitors (PI)—saquinavir, indinavir, ritonavir, nelfinavir
D. Entry (Fusion) inhibitors.

These drugs act at various points in the lifecycle of the virus and are administered with the aim of reducing the viral load to undetectable levels to allow immune restoration. HAART significantly increases absolute CD4+ lymphocyte counts, reduces HIV viral load and improves survival, even in patients with very low absolute CD4+ lymphocyte counts.

Timely referral to primary care is indicated to rule out other systemic opportunistic infections. An emphasis on nutrition is critical as the painful nature of this condition limits food choices. Thus, nutritional supplements are required. Clinicians are advised to optimize oral hygiene, establish regular review periods, screen for HIV-related oral lesions and treat them, if necessary.

PERIODONTICS REVISITED

Treatment of Linear gingival erythema (LGE):
- Meticulous oral hygiene (severe oral hygiene instructions)
- Scaling, subgingival irrigation with chlorhexidine.
- Chlorhexidine digluconate 0.12% mouth wash.
- If persists, evaluate for candidiasis and retreat if necessary

Treatment of Necrotizing ulcerative gingivitis (NUG):
- Debridement of necrotic lesion and light scaling
- Scaling and root planing
- Chlorhexidine digluconate 0.12% mouth wash.
- Meticulous oral hygiene.
- Antibiotic: Metronidazole 400 mg b.i.d for 5-7 days

Treatment of Necrotizing ulcerative periodontitis (NUP):
- Scaling, root planing and subgingival irrigation.
- Removal of necrotic soft tissues utilizing a 0.12% chlorhexidine digluconate or 10% povidone-iodine lavage
- Antibiotic: Metronidazole 400 mg b.i.d for a week
- Prophylactic systemic antifungal agent.
- Frequent follow-up visits.

BIBLIOGRAPHY

1. Coogan MM, Greenspan J, Challacombe SJ. Oral lesions in infection with human immunodeficiency virus. Bull World Health Organ 2005;83:700-06.
2. Doshi D, Ramapuram J, Anup N. Periodontal status of HIV-positive patients. Med Oral Patol Oral Cir Bucal 2009;14:384-87.
3. Eley BM, Manson JD. Acquired immunodeficiency syndrome. In, Periodontics 5th ed Wright 2004;108-12.
4. Mellanen L. The influence of HIV infection to the periodontium-a clinical, microbiological, and enzymological study. Academic dissertation. Department of Oral and Maxillofacial Diseases, Helsinki University Central Hospital (HUCH), Helsinki, Finland. 2006.
5. Rees TD. AIDS and the periodontium. In, Newman, Takei, Carranza. Clinical Periodontology 9th ed WB Saunders 2003; 415-31.
6. Reznik DA. Oral manifestations of HIV Disease. International AIDS society-USA, Topics in HIV medicine 2005;13:143-48.
7. Umadevi M, Adeyem O, Patel M, Reichart PA, Robinson PG. Periodontal Diseases and Other Microbial Infections. Adv Dent Res 2006;19:139-45.
8. Van Dyke TE, Serhan CN. Resolution of inflammation: a new paradigm for the pathogenesis of periodontal diseases. J Dent Res 2003;82:82-90.

MCQs

1. NUP occurs in HIV patients when:
   A. CD4+count <500/mm^3
   B. CD4+ count < 1000/mm^3
   C. CD4+ count < 200/mm^3
   D. CD4+ count <150/mm^3
2. Distinctive form of periodontal disease as a manifestation of HIV infection was first reported in:
   A. 1982
   B. 1986
   C. 1987
   D. 1990
3. HAART Therapy:
   A. Increases CD4+ counts
   B. Increases HIV viral load
   C. Reduces pain
   D. Decreases CD4+ counts
4. Key diagnostic feature of linear gingival erythema is:
   A. Discomfort
   B. Lack of response to conventional periodontal therapy
   C. Bleeding from gums
   D. Association with anterior teeth
5. Most common form of periodontal disease associated with HIV is:
   A. HIV-Associated Gingivitis
   B. HIV- Associated Periodontitis
   C. NUG
   D. Necrotizing Stomatitis
6. Risk factors for periodontitis in HIV-positive patients are:
   A. Age
   B. Smoking
   C. Viral load
   D. Microorganisms
   E. All of the above

Answers

1. C	2. C	3. A	4. B	5. A
6. E				

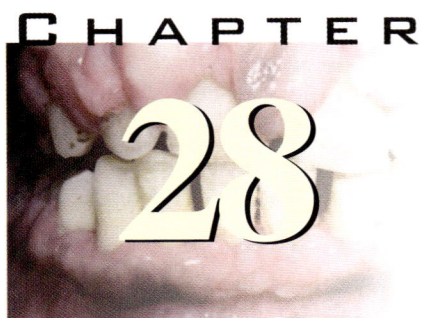

28

Trauma from Occlusion and Pathologic Tooth Migration

Shalu Bathla

DEFINITIONS

When occlusal forces exceed the adaptive capacity of the tissues, tissue injury results. The resultant injury is termed trauma from occlusion. Thus, trauma from occlusion refers to the tissue injury, not the occlusal force. An occlusion that produces such injury is called a traumatic occlusion.

Trauma from occlusion was defined by Stillman (1917) *as a condition where injury results to the supporting structures of the teeth by the act of bringing the jaws into a closed position.*

In Glossary of Periodontics Terms (AAP 1986), Occlusal trauma was defined as *an injury to the attachment apparatus as a result of excessive occlusal forces.*

PRIMARY AND SECONDARY TRAUMA FROM OCCLUSION

Primary trauma from occlusion: When trauma from occlusion is the result of alterations in occlusal forces, it is called primary trauma from occlusion. Examples are: (i) placement of a high restoration (ii) insertion of a fixed bridge or partial denture that places excessive force on the abutment teeth and (iii) the drifting movement or extrusion of teeth into spaces created by unreplaced missing teeth. Primary trauma from occlusion occurs if trauma from occlusion is considered the primary etiologic factor in periodontal destruction and if the only local alteration to which a tooth is subjected is from occlusion **(Fig. 28.1A)**.

Secondary trauma from occlusion: When trauma from occlusion results from reduced ability of the tissues to resist the occlusal forces, it is known as secondary trauma from occlusion. It occurs when the adaptive capacity of the tissues to withstand occlusal forces is impaired by bone loss resulting from marginal inflammation **(Fig. 28.1B)**. The periodontium becomes more vulnerable to injury and previously well tolerated occlusal forces become traumatic.

CONCEPTS REGARDING TRAUMA FROM OCCLUSION

Glickman's Concept

According to Glickman (1965), the pathway of the spread of a plaque associated gingival lesion can be changed if forces of an abnormal magnitude are acting on teeth harboring subgingival plaque.

The periodontal structures can be divided into two zones according to Glickman regarding the effect of

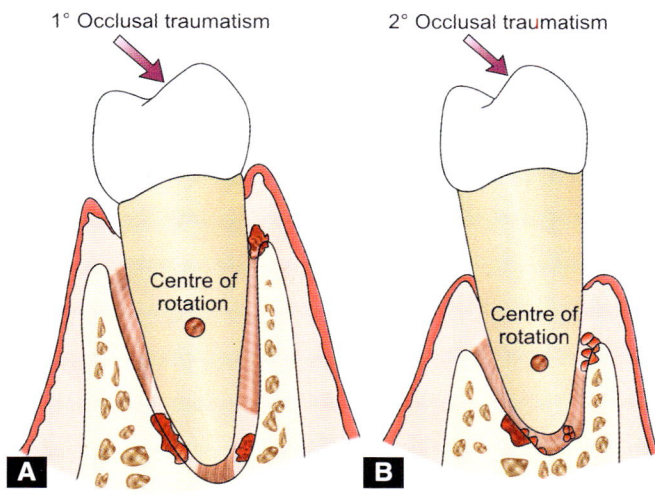

Figs 28.1A and B: Primary and secondary trauma from occlusion

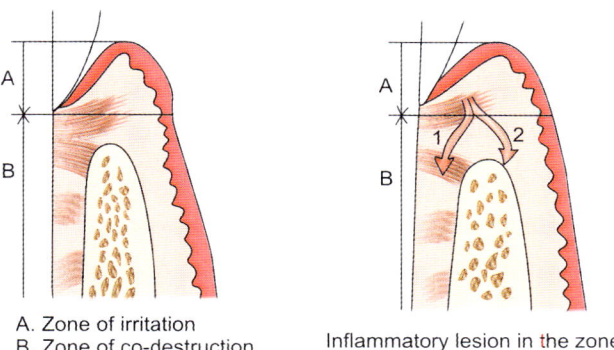

A. Zone of irritation
B. Zone of co-destruction

Inflammatory lesion in the zone of irritation propagate into:
1. Periodontal ligament when teeth are subjected to trauma from occlusion and into
2. Alveolar bone when teeth not subjected to trauma from occlusion

Fig. 28.2: Glickman's concept

trauma from occlusion on the spread of the plaque associated lesion:
1. The zone of irritation
2. The zone of co-destruction

The zone of irritation includes the marginal and interdental gingiva. The soft tissue of this zone is bordered by hard tissue (the tooth) only on one side and is not affected by forces of occlusion. This means that gingival inflammation cannot be induced by trauma from occlusion but is the result of irritation from microbial plaque. The plaque – associated lesion at a non – traumatized tooth propagates in apical direction by first involving the alveolar bone and later the periodontal ligament area. The progression of this lesion results in an even (horizontal) bone destruction **(Fig. 28.2)**.

The zone of co-destruction includes the periodontal ligament, the root cementum and the alveolar bone and is coronally demarcated by the transseptal (interdental) and the dentoalveolar collagen fiber bundles. The tissue in this zone may become the seat of a lesion caused by trauma from occlusion. The spread of the inflammatory lesion from the zone of irritation directly down into the periodontal ligament (i.e. not via the interdental bone) may hereby be facilitated. This alteration of the normal pathway of spread of the plaque – associated inflammatory lesion results in the development of angular bony defects. Glickman (1967) in a review paper stated that trauma from occlusion is an etiologic factor (co-destructive factor) of importance in situations where angular bony defects combined with infrabony pockets are found at one or several teeth.

Waerhaug's Concept

According to Waerhaug, the loss of connective tissue attachment and the resorption of bone around teeth are exclusively the result of inflammatory lesions associated with subgingival plaque. Waerhaug concluded that angular bony defects and infrabony pockets occur when the subgingival plaque of one tooth has reached a more apical level than the microbiota on the neighbouring tooth and when the volume of the alveolar bone surrounding the roots is comparatively large.

Glickman's conclusion was that trauma from occlusion is an aggravating factor in periodontal disease and Waerhaug's concept was that there is no relationship between occlusal trauma and the degree of periodontal tissue breakdown.

TISSUE RESPONSE TO INCREASED OCCLUSAL FORCES

Tissue response occurs in three stages: injury, repair and adaptive remodeling of the periodontium **(Fig. 28.3)**.

Stage I: Injury

Slightly excessive pressure stimulates resorption of the alveolar bone, with a resultant widening of the periodontal ligament space whereas slightly excessive tension causes elongation of the periodontal ligament fibers and apposition of alveolar bone. Greater pressure produces compression of periodontal fibers, which produces area of hyalinization and increased resorption of alveolar bone and tooth surface whereas severe tension causes widening and tearing of periodontal ligament fibers and increased resorption of alveolar bone. The areas of the periodontium most susceptible to injury from excessive occlusal forces are the furcations.

PERIODONTICS REVISITED

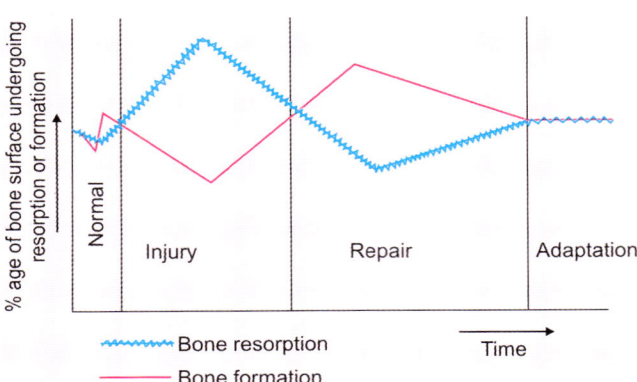

Fig. 28.3: Stages of tissue response to increased occlusal forces

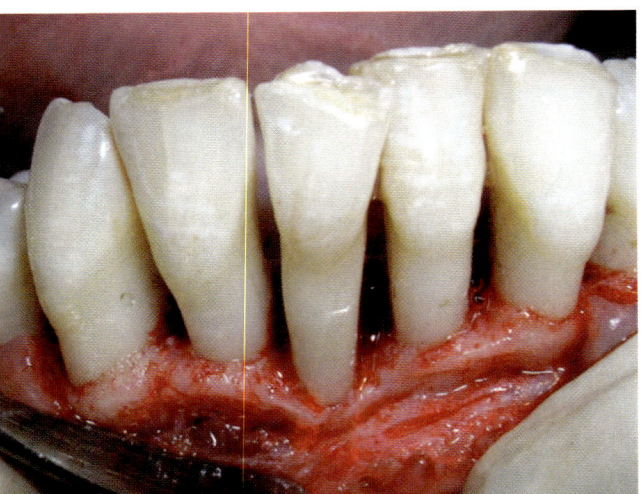

Fig. 28.4: Lipping of alveolar bone

Stage II: Repair

When bone is resorbed by excessive occlusal forces, the body attempts to reinforce the thinned bony trabeculae with new bone. This attempt to compensate for lost bone is called buttressing bone formation and is an important feature of the reparative process associated with trauma from occlusion. Buttressing bone formation occurs within the jaw i.e central buttressing and on the bone surface i.e peripheral buttressing. In central buttressing, the endosteal cells deposit new bone, which restores the bony trabeculae and reduces the size of the marrow spaces. Peripheral buttressing occurs on the facial and lingual surfaces of the alveolar plate. Depending on its severity, peripheral buttressing may produce a shelf – like thickening of the alveolar margin, referred to as lipping **(Fig. 28.4)**, or a pronounced bulge in the contour of the facial and lingual bone.

Stage III: Adaptive Remodeling of the Periodontium

If the repair process cannot keep pace with the destruction caused by the occlusion, the periodontium is remodeled in an effort to create a structural relationship in which the forces are no longer injurious to the tissues. This results in a thickened periodontal ligament, which is funnel shaped at the crest, and angular defects in the bone, with no pocket formation. The involved teeth become mobile.

Tissue response to increased occlusal forces

Injury phase—increased resorption and decreased bone formation

Repair phase—decreased resorption and increased bone formation

Adaptive remodeling phase—bone resorption and formation return to normal.

CLINICAL FEATURES OF TRAUMA FROM OCCLUSION

Increased tooth mobility: In the injury stage of trauma from occlusion, destruction of periodontal fibers occurs, which increases the mobility of the tooth. In the final stage, the accommodation of the periodontium to increased forces entails a widening of the periodontal ligament, which also leads to increased tooth mobility. Although this tooth mobility is greater than the so-called normal mobility, it cannot be considered pathologic because it is an adaptation and not a disease process. When it becomes progressively worse, it can be considered pathologic.

RADIOGRAPHIC FEATURES OF TRAUMA FROM OCCLUSION ALONE

- Increased width of the periodontal space, often with thickening of the lamina dura along the lateral aspect of the root, in the apical region, and in bifurcation areas **(Fig. 28.5)**.
- Usually there is vertical rather than horizontal bone loss.
- Radiolucency and condensation of the alveolar bone with root resorption is sometimes seen **(Fig. 28.6)**.

PATHOLOGIC TOOTH MIGRATION

Definition

Pathologic tooth migration is defined as a change in tooth position that occurs when there is disruption of forces that

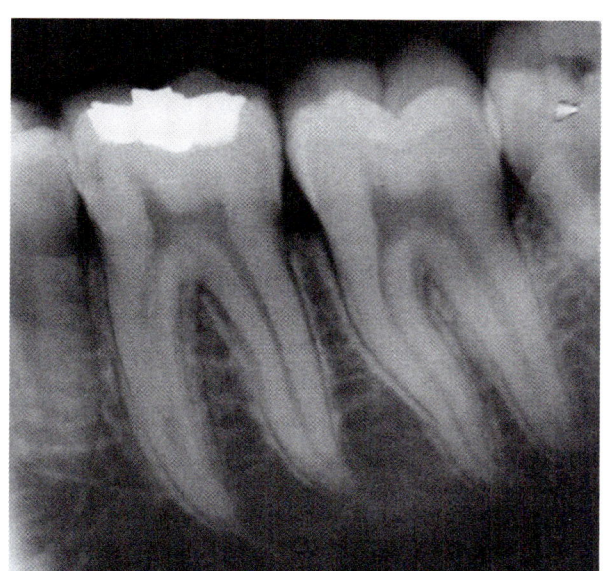

Fig. 28.5: Radiographic features of trauma from occlusion (Discontinuity and thickening of lamina dura)

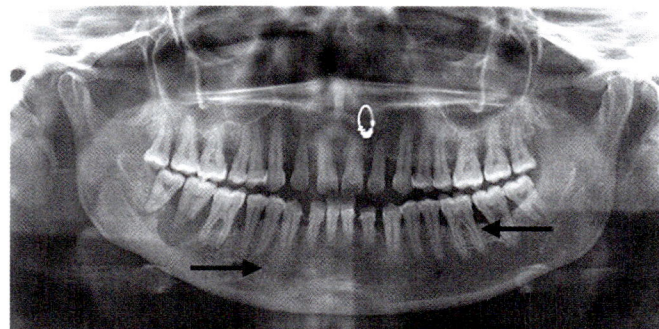

Fig. 28.6: OPG showing trauma from occlusion

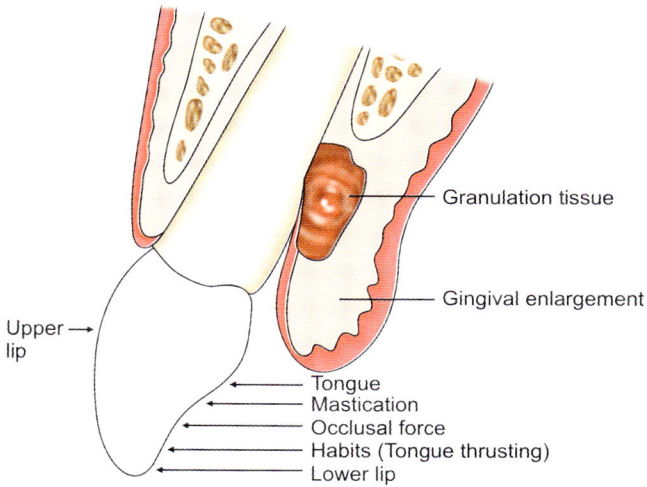

Fig. 28.7: Factors influencing tooth position

maintain teeth in a normal relationship. Thus, there is tooth displacement that results when the balance among the factors that maintain physiologic tooth position is disturbed by periodontal disease. Pathologic migration is relatively common and may be an early sign of disease, or it may occur in association with gingival inflammation and pocket formation as the disease progresses.

Etiology

Many factors influence tooth position and, therefore, there are many possible etiologic factors for pathologic tooth migration. The multiple causes of incisor flaring emphasize the complexity of differential diagnosis. The main factors known to influence tooth position are tissues of the periodontium; soft tissue pressures of the cheek, tongue and lips; and a variety of oral habits **(Fig. 28.7)**.

Periodontal inflammation and eruptive forces also influence tooth position.

1. *Destruction of periodontal supporting tissues*: Destruction of periodontal tissues plays a significant role in the etiology of pathologic tooth migration. The transseptal fibers may play important role in pathologic tooth migration. They form a chain from tooth to tooth and are thought to maintain contacts between teeth throughout the arch. It has been suggested that if the continuity of this chain is broken or weakened by periodontal disease, the balance of forces is upset and displacement of the teeth can occur. The contractile force observed in the transseptal fiber is thought to originate from gingival fibroblasts which are known to produce collagen contraction.

2. *Occlusal factors*: Occlusal factors connected to the etiology of pathologic tooth migration include posterior bite collapse from loss of posterior teeth, Class II malocclusion, occlusal interferences, the anterior component of force, protrusive functional patterns of mastication, bruxism, and shortened dental arches. Posterior bite collapse is a pattern of unfavourable occlusal change that occur most frequently after first molar teeth are lost and not replaced.

    Following are the consequences of failure to replace first molars:
    • The second and third molars tilt, resulting in a decrease in vertical dimension.
    • The premolars move distally, and the mandibular incisors tilt or drift lingually.
    • Anterior overbite is increased.

PERIODONTICS REVISITED

- The mandibular incisors strike the maxillary incisors near the gingiva and traumatize the gingiva.
- The maxillary incisors are pushed labially and laterally.
- The anterior teeth extrude because the incisal apposition has largely disappeared.
- Diastema are created by the separation of the anterior teeth.

Closely related to posterior bite collapse is arch integrity. Occlusal forces are related to teeth in the arch through interproximal contacts. If these contacts are destroyed, tooth migration can occur. Besides tooth loss, other factors that can destroy interproximal contacts include dental caries, faulty restorations, and severe attrition.

3. *Soft tissue pressure of the tongue, cheek and lips*: Orthodontic research has confirmed that soft tissue forces of the tongue, cheek and lips can move teeth, especially after loss of periodontal support. Because of their long duration, these very light forces are thought to be more important than the relative short duration of occlusal contacts during speech, swallowing, and mastication.

4. *Periodontal and periapical inflammation*: In 1933, Hirschfeld described pathologic drifting of the teeth resulting from pressure of inflammatory tissue in periodontal pockets. Scientific support for these observations was provided by recent animal research showing that inflamed gingiva displays an increase in interstitial fluid pressure, due to an increase in capillary filtration. The extravasation of fluid into the interstitial tissue causes a rise in interstitial hydraulic pressure. When gingival inflammation is controlled then, there is spontaneous correction of migration.

5. *Habits*: Oral habits of patients may affect tooth position and have been associated with pathologic tooth migration. Habits that have been associated are lip and tongue thrusting habits **(Fig. 28.8)**, fingernail biting, thumb sucking, pipe smoking, bruxism and playing wind instruments. Duration of force in tooth movement is more important than force magnitude. The greater the duration of the habit, the greater potential to move teeth.

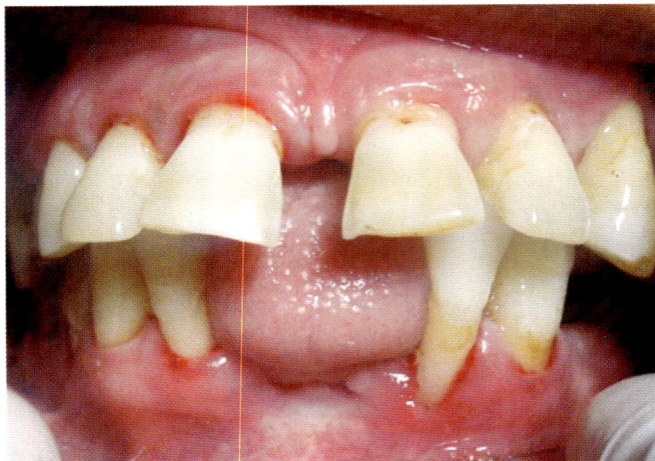

Fig. 28.8: Pathologic migration associated with tongue thrusting habit

Treatment

Treatment of severe pathologic tooth migration often involves orthodontic therapy that is preceded by non – surgical and surgical periodontal therapy and prosthodontic treatment. Selecting a method to manage pathologic tooth migration is usually based on an interdisciplinary approach.

Correction of pathologic tooth migration can be divided into four categories:

1. Extraction and replacement of migrated teeth when migration is very severe.
2. Spontaneous correction of the early stages of pathologic tooth migration following periodontal therapy.
3. Limited or adjunctive orthodontic therapy.
4. Conventional orthodontic treatment.

Many patient factors enter into the decision for the best treatment of pathologic tooth migration. These include patient compliance and cooperation, motivation to keep the natural teeth, skeletal factors, economic factors, availability for treatment, systemic health, and acceptance of surgical periodontal treatment, if necessary.

There may be reactive positioning or spontaneous correction of pathologic migration following periodontal treatment. Migrated teeth sometimes move back to their normal position following non-surgical periodontal treatment alone or in some instances when combined with surgical methods.

POINTS TO PONDER

✓ *Karolyi Effect*: An effect named after Moritz Karolyi, a Viennese dentist who described the possible role of hyperfunction of the masticatory muscles in eliciting traumatic occlusion as a cause of periodontitis. He recommended its correction by grinding the occlusal surfaces and the use of bite planes at night. Karolyi introduced the current concept of bruxism but never used the term.

BIBLIOGRAPHY

1. Brunsvold MA. Pathologic Tooth Migration. J Periodontol 2005; 76:859-66.
2. Carranza FA, Camargo PM. Periodontal Response to External Forces. In, Newman, Takei, Carranza. Clinical Periodontology 9th ed WB Saunders 2003;371-83.
3. Lindhe J, Nyman S, Ericsson I. Trauma from occlusion. In, Lindhe J, Karring T, Lang NP. Clinical Periodontology and Implant dentistry 4th ed Blackwell Munksgaard 2003;352-65.
4. Lindhe J, Nyman S. Occlusal therapy. In, Lindhe J, Karring T, Lang NP. Clinical Periodontology and Implant dentistry 4th ed Blackwell Munksgaard 2003;731-43.
5. Moxham BJ, Berkovitz BKB. The effects of External forces on the periodontal ligament. In, Berkovitz BKB, Moxham BJ, Newman HN. The Periodontal Ligament in Health and Disease 2nd ed Mosby – Wolfe 1995;215-41.
6. Newman HN. Trauma and the periodontal ligament. In, Berkovitz BKB, Moxham BJ, Newman HN. The Periodontal Ligament in Health and Disease 2nd ed Mosby – Wolfe 1995;315-40.

MCQs

1. Radiographic features of trauma from occlusion include all of the following *expect*:
   A. Thickening of lamina dura
   B. Angular bone loss
   C. Increase in the width of periodontal ligament space
   D. Hyalinization of periodontal ligament space
2. Trauma from occlusion does not produce:
   A. Tooth mobility
   B. Widening of periodontal spaces
   C. Angular bone loss
   D. Periodontal pockets

Answers

1. D   2. D

CHAPTER 29

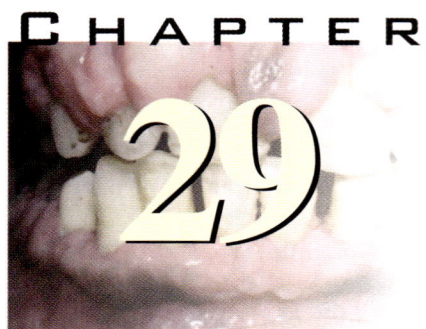

Female Sex Hormones and Periodontium

Shalu Bathla

INTRODUCTION

Sex hormones have been considered to play an influential role on periodontal tissues, bone turnover rate, wound healing and periodontal disease progression. Gingival inflammation and hyperplasia are frequently seen in puberty, pregnancy and menstrual cycle which is induced by increased concentrations of female sex hormones in the circulation. Throughout a woman's life cycle, hormonal influences affect therapeutic decision making in periodontics.

EFFECT OF SEX HORMONES ON PERIODONTIUM

Sex hormones namely estrogens, progesterone, and testosterone have been linked with periodontal disease pathogenesis **(Fig. 29.1)**.

Estrogen

Estrogen is a steroid sex hormone which is responsible for physiological changes in women at specific phases of their life starting in puberty.

Estradiol in the plasma may reach 30 times higher levels than during the reproductive cycle.

Effects of increased estrogen on the periodontium during pregnancy:
- Decreases keratinization, while increasing epithelial glycogen
- Increases cellular proliferation in blood vessels
- Inhibits proinflammatory cytokines release
- Inhibits PMN chemotaxis
- Estrogens influence the cytodifferentiation of stratified squamous epithelium as well as the synthesis and maintenance of fibrous collagen.

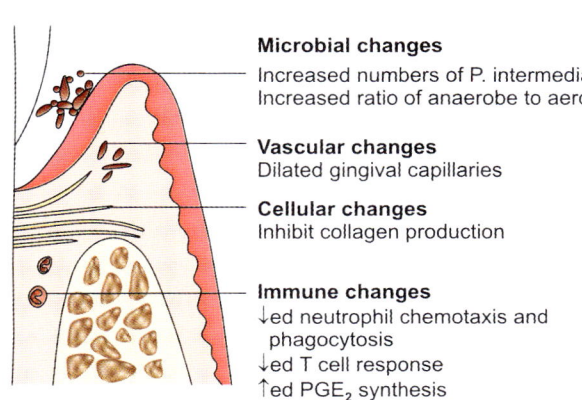

Microbial changes
Increased numbers of P. intermedia
Increased ratio of anaerobe to aerobe

Vascular changes
Dilated gingival capillaries

Cellular changes
Inhibit collagen production

Immune changes
↓ed neutrophil chemotaxis and
  phagocytosis
↓ed T cell response
↑ed PGE$_2$ synthesis

Fig.29.1: Effect of increased sex hormones on periodontium

Progesterone

Progesterone is another sex hormone that has direct effects on the periodontium. Progesterone is active in bone metabolism and plays an important role in the coupling of bone resorption and bone formation. In pregnancy, progesterone reaches levels of 100 ng/ml, 10 times the peak luteal phase of menses. Progesterone shows a significant impact on the gingival vascular system, causing increased exudation, as well as affecting the integrity of the capillary endothelial cells.

Effects of increased progesterone level on the periodontium during pregnancy:

- Increases production of prostaglandins
- Increases PMN and PGE$_2$ in the GCF
- Reduces glucocorticoid anti-inflammatory effect
- Increases vascular permeability
- Alter collagen and noncollagenous protein synthesis
- Alter periodontal fibroblast metabolism

Androgens

These are hormones responsible for masculinization. Testosterone has been associated with bone metabolism. Effects of androgens on the periodontium:

- Stimulate matrix synthesis by osteoblasts and periodontal ligament fibroblasts
- Inhibit prostaglandin secretion
- Reduce IL-6 production during inflammation
- Stimulate osteoblast proliferation and differentiation.

PUBERTY

It is a complex process of sexual maturation resulting in an individual capable of reproduction. It is also responsible for changes in physical appearance and behavior that are related with increased levels of the steroid sex hormones, testosterone in males and estrogens in females. Puberty occurs between the average ages of 11 to 14 years in most women. The production of sex hormones (estrogen and progesterone) increases, then remains relatively constant during the remainder of the reproductive phase. During puberty, periodontal tissues may have an exaggerated response to local factors.

Periodontal Manifestations

1. *Gingivitis*: The inflamed tissues become erythematous, lobulated and retractable (**Fig. 29.2**). Bleeding on probing may occur easily.
2. *Subgingival microflora*: Puberty is usually associated with higher bacterial counts especially of *P. intermedia*. Kornman and Loesche postulated that this anaerobic organism may use ovarian hormone as a substitute for vitamin K growth factor.
3. *Perimolysis*, i.e. smooth erosion of the enamel and dentin due to eating disorders, bulimia and anorexia nervosa occurs typically on the lingual surfaces of maxillary anterior teeth.

Management

Preventive care including a vigorous program of oral hygiene is required. During puberty oral health education is given to the parents also. Only scaling and root planing with frequent oral hygiene reinforcement is required in milder gingivitis. Severe cases of gingivitis may require antimicrobial mouthwashes, local site drug delivery or antibiotic therapy.

MENSTRUAL CYCLE

Under the influence of FSH (follicle stimulating hormone) and LH (luteinizing hormone), estrogen and progesterone

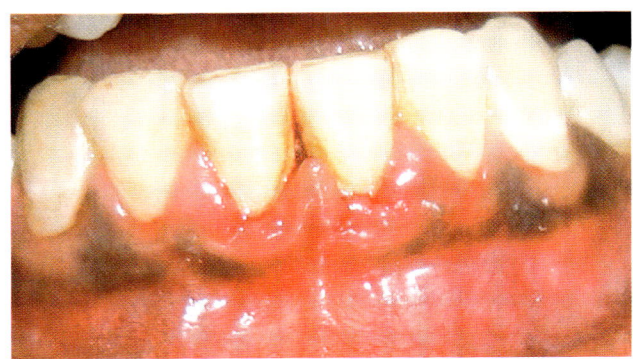

Fig.29.2: Puberty gingivitis

PERIODONTICS REVISITED

are the steroid hormones produced by the ovaries during the menstrual cycle. During menses, progesterone increases from the second week, peaks at approximately 10 days, and dramatically drops before menstruation. During the peak level of progesterone (about 7 to 10 days before menstruation), premenstrual syndrome (PMS) may also occur.

Periodontal Manifestations

1. Gingival bleeding: Gingival inflammation seems to be aggravated by an imbalance and/or increase in sex hormones.
2. Gingival tissues appear to be more edematous during menses and erythematous preceding the onset of menses in some individuals. There is increased production of gingival exudates **(Fig. 29.3)**.
3. There is alteration in the production rate and pattern of gingival collagen.
4. The menstrual period is sometimes associated with a minor increase in tooth mobility.
5. The incidence of postextraction osteitis has also been reported to be higher during the initiation of menses.
6. Intraoral recurrent apthous ulcers, herpes labialis lesions, and candida infections occur in some women as a cyclic pattern.

Management

Emphasis should be placed on oral hygiene. An antimicrobial mouthrinse before cyclic inflammation may be indicated. The gingival and oral mucosal tissues should be treated gently. Careful retraction of the oral mucosa, cheeks, and lips is necessary in both the apthous and herpetic prone patient. Avoid prescribing nonsteroidal anti-inflammatory medications and high alcohol content mouthwashes. Acidic foods exacerbate gastrooesophageal reflux disease (GERD). PMS is often treated by selective serotonin reuptake inhibitor (SSRI) antidepressants.

PREGNANCY

During this period, both progesterone and estrogen are elevated due to continuous production of these hormones by the corpus luteum. Hormonal influences associated with the reproductive process alter periodontal and oral tissue responses to local factors creating diagnostic and therapeutic dilemmas.

Periodontal Manifestations

1. *Pregnancy gingivitis*: The occurrence of pregnancy gingivitis is extremely common, occurring in approximately 30 to 100% of all pregnant women. Gingivitis becomes more severe by the eighth month and decreases during the ninth month. It usually presents on marginal gingiva and interdental papilla which is characterized by erythema, edema and hyperplasia **(Fig. 29.4)**. Bleeding occur spontaneously or on slight provocation. The gingiva appears smooth and shiny giving raspberry-like appearance. Tooth mobility, pocket depth, and gingival fluid are also increased in pregnancy.

   The microscopic picture of gingival disease in pregnancy is one of nonspecific, vascularizing and proliferative inflammation. There is marked inflammatory cellular infiltration with edema and degeneration of the gingival epithelium and connective tissue. The epithelium is hyperplastic,

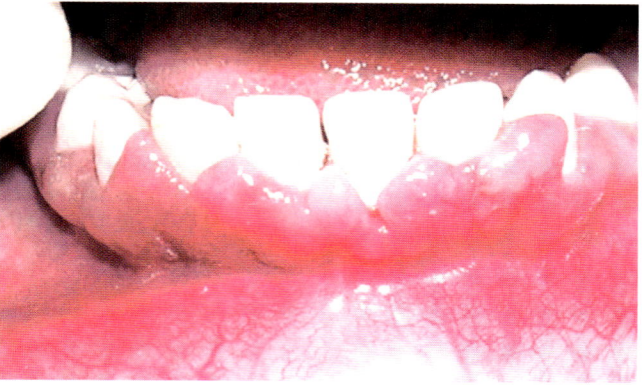

Fig.29.3: Gingivitis seen during menstrual cycle

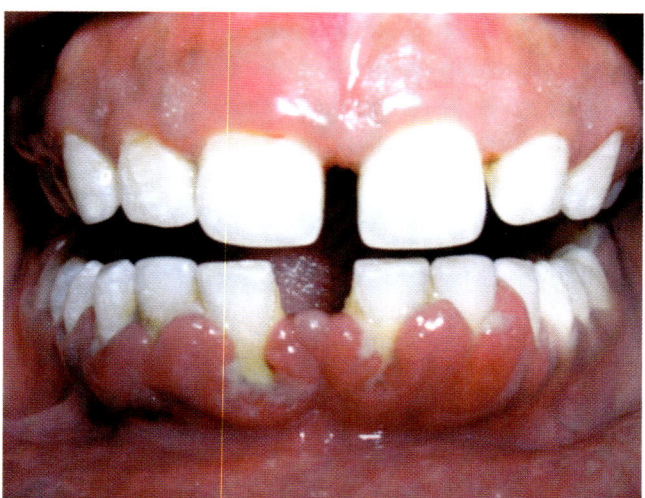

Fig.29.4: Severe pregnancy gingivitis in lower anterior teeth

with accentuated rete pegs, reduced surface keratinization, and various degrees of intracellular and extracellular edema and infiltration by leukocytes. Newly formed engorged capillaries are present in abundance.

2. *Pregnancy tumors*: Usually appears during the second trimester in the interproximal areas of anterior teeth. The lesion appears as an isolated, hyperplastic, protruding, bright red growth with a mulberry–like surface. It is a superficial lesion which does not invade the underlying bone. The consistency varies from semifirm to soft and friable. Gingiva bleeds on slightest provocation **(Fig. 29.5)**. The tissue growth may cause migration and increased mobility of the adjacent teeth.

Gingival changes seen during pregnancy are:
Erythema
Edema
Smooth and shiny surface
Raspberry-like appearance
Increased tendency to bleed
Effecting mainly anterior region.

Maternal Immunoresponse

In pregnancy, there is decreased neutrophil chemotaxis, phagocytosis and depressed antibody production. Destruction of gingival mast cells by the increased sex hormones and the resultant release of histamine and proteolytic enzymes also contribute to the exaggerated inflammatory response to local factors. There is increased number of periodontopathogens especially *P. gingivalis* and *P. intermedia* because these microbes use estrogen and progesterone as a substitute for Menadione (Vitamin K growth factor). PGE_2 synthesis is increased during pregnancy.

Management

Following precautions should be taken during treatment of a pregnant patient:
1. Short appointments, served in series because patient fatigues easily.
2. Gently lower and straighten the chair for pregnant patient because of genuine awkwardness due to new shape and weight gain.
3. Place the patient on left side or elevate the right hip 5 to 6 inches by placing pillow or blanket roll underneath. Supine position allows the weight of developing fetus to bear down directly on vena cava, aorta and major vessels. The reduction in return cardiac blood supply may cause supine hypotensive syndrome with decreased placental perfusion.
4. Advice non-alcoholic mouthwash and neutral sodium fluoride rinse.
5. Advice not to brush right after vomiting to prevent erosion as nausea and vomiting are common in first trimester.
6. Recommend less strong flavored dentifrice because of adverse reaction to strong smells and flavor to the pregnant patient.
7. Recommend a small toothbrush; take care in instrument and radiographic film placement to prevent gagging.
8. Ideally, no medications should be prescribed because of toxic or teratogenic effects of therapy on the fetus.

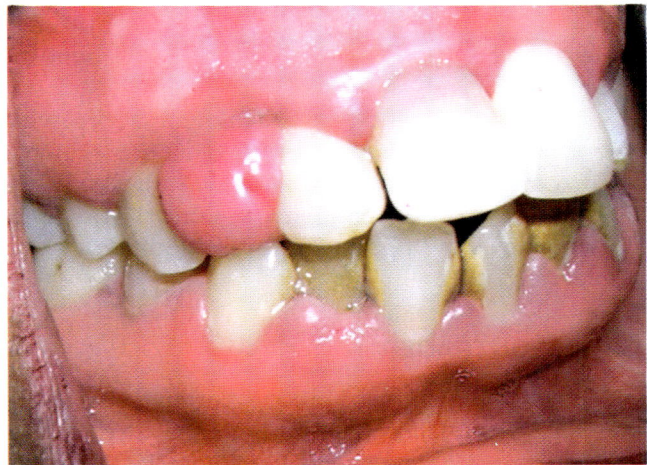

Fig. 29.5: Pregnancy tumor in between right maxillary lateral incisor and canine

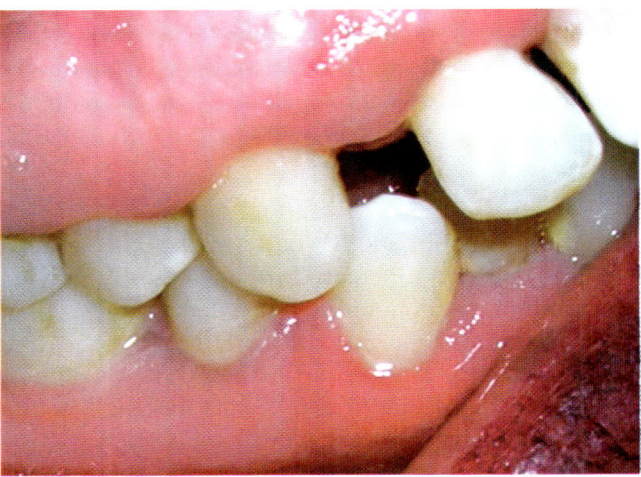

Fig. 29.6: Pregnancy tumor excised

PERIODONTICS REVISITED

9. Use of dental radiographs during pregnancy should be kept to a minimum. When they are required during pregnancy, patient is covered with a lead apron, thyroid collar and a second apron for the back to prevent secondary radiations from reaching the abdomen.

10. The mother should take prescribed drugs just after breastfeeding and then avoid nursing for 4 hours or more, if possible to markedly decrease the drug concentration in breast milk.

11. Plaque control: Establishment of a healthy oral environment and optimal oral hygiene levels are primary objectives in the pregnant patient. A preventive periodontal program consisting of nutritional counselling and rigorous plaque control measures in the dental office and at home should be reinforced. Scaling, polishing, and root planing may be performed whenever necessary throughout the pregnancy.

12. Generally, pregnancy tumor will regress somewhat postpartum but surgical excision is often required for complete resolution **(Fig. 29.6)**. Tumor is surgically removed in pregnancy only if it is being traumatized by opposing teeth or restoration causing bleeding.

ORAL CONTRACEPTIVES (OC)

Hormonal contraceptives induce a hormonal condition that stimulates a state of pregnancy to prevent ovulation by the use of gestational hormones. Synthetic hormones which mimic the effects of the endogenous female hormones are used as oral contraceptives. These hormonal oral contraceptives contain progesterone, often combined with estrogen. As pregnancy hormonal level changes, do not affect healthy tissues in a clean mouth but exaggerate a preexisting gingivitis and is secondary to bacterial plaque, same is with oral contraceptives.

Periodontal Manifestations

1. Gingival inflammation: Women taking oral contraceptives shows an increased prevalence of gingivitis. Inflammation ranges from mild edema and erythema to severe inflammation with hemorrhagic or hyperplastic gingival tissues. The degree of inflammation seems to be related to the length of time the woman is taking the pill.
2. There is increase in the amount of gingival exudates.
3. Higher gingival index scores.
4. More loss of attachment
5. Subgingival microflora: A 16-fold increase in *Bacteroides* species was noted in the OC group versus the nonpregnant group. Increased female sex hormones substitute the napthaquinone requirement of certain *Bacteroides* species which is most likely responsible for this increase.
6. Sometime the use of oral contraceptive therapy causes the gingival melanosis in light complexion individuals.

Management

The dental management of patient taking OC should include the establishment of a plaque control program and the elimination of all local predisposing factors. Antibiotics such as tetracycline shoud be avoided, as these antibiotics may lead to failure of the oral contraceptive therapy.

MENOPAUSE

Menopausal gingivostomatitis occurs during menopause or in the postmenopausal period. As the women approach menopause, the levels of estrogens begin to drop mainly during the late follicular and luteal phase of the menstrual cycle. The effects of estrogen are reduced and thus, compromising the anti-inflammatory effect of this hormone on the periodontium. Osteopenia and Osteoporosis have been associated with the menopausal patient.

Periodontal Manifestations

1. The gingiva appears dry, vary in color from abnormal paleness to redness and bleeds easily.
2. Fissuring occurs in the mucobuccal fold.
3. The patient complains of a dry, burning sensation throughout the oral cavity, associated with extreme sensitivity to thermal changes.
4. Alveolar bone loss and alveolar ridge resorption
5. Altered taste sensation
   Microscopically, the gingiva exhibits atrophy of the germinal and prickle cell layers of the epithelium and, in some instances, areas of ulceration.

Management

Advice to use extra soft toothbrush and dentifrices with minimal abrasive particles. Mouth rinses should have low alcohol concentration. Root surfaces should be debrided gently with minimal soft tissue trauma. Hormone replacement therapy (HRT) or estrogen replacement therapy (ERT) should be advised. If patient is osteoporotic, advice bisphosphonates or selective estrogen receptor modulators after consulting physician.

EFFECT OF SEX HORMONES ON PERIODONTAL/IMPLANT WOUND HEALING

Sex hormones have a regulatory effect on growth factors involved in the wound healing, such as keratinocytes growth factor. These growth factors cause stimulation proliferation and morphogenesis of pleuripotent cells. Lack of sex hormones often causes the reduction of bone density. Osteoporosis is considered as a risk factor for implant success.

LANDMARK STUDIES RELATED

Mombelli A, Gusberti FA, Van Oosten MA and Lang NP. Gingival health and gingivitis development during puberty. A 4 years longitudinal study. Journal of Clinical Periodontology 1989;16:451-456.

Twenty two (22) boys and 20 girls from a suburban elementary school, Switzerland, between the age of 11 and 15 years were taken. Pubertal and skeletal development as well as Plaque index (PI) and gingival index (GI) was monitored at 12 months interval for 4 years. Ten times during the 4 years of the observation period, the Papillary bleeding index (PBI) was assessed after interdental stimulation with a toothpick in all interdental spaces of the dentition. 35% of the children reached a mean PBI peak value within 1.5 years after the initiation of puberty. PI and GI which were recorded annually did not show a significant trend of increase or decrease. The highly significant trends of increase in bleeding scores both in boys and girls indicate clear changes in the gingival conditions taking place during puberty and suggest an important impact of hormonal changes both on host tissues and on oral microbiota.

Jensen J, Liljemark W, Bloomquist C. The Effect of female sex hormones on subgingival plaque. Journal of Periodontology 1981;52:599-602.

One hundred and four (104) women, aged 18 to 40 years were taken for study. Of this group 54 were pregnant (P), 27 were non pregnant (NP) and 23 were nonpregnant but were taking oral contraceptives (NPP). They were evaluated clinically and microbiologically for changes in their gingiva and subgingival microbial plaque, specifically the percentage of Fusobacterium species and Bacteroides species. Statistically significant increased scores were observed in the gingival index and the GCF flow in P group compared with NP group. In P group, there was 55 fold increases in the recovery of Bacteroides as compared to 16 fold increase in NPP group over the NP group. The marked increase in proportions of Bacteroides species seen during pregnancy seems to be associated with increased serum levels of circulating sex hormones, i.e. progesterone and estrogens; both have been shown to substitute for the naphthaquinone requirement of *B. melaninogenicus* and *B. intermedius*.

POINTS TO PONDER

✓ *Prevotella intermedia* is increased in puberty and pregnancy gingivitis because it uses estrogen and progesterone as a substitute for Menadione (Vitamin K growth factor), which increases with increased level of gonadotrophic hormone in puberty and pregnancy.

BIBLIOGRAPHY

1. Corgel JO. Periodontal therapy in female patient (Puberty, menses, pregnancy, menopause). In, Newman, Takei, Carranza. Clinical Periodontology 9th ed WB Saunders 2003;513-26.
2. Jensen J, Lilijmack W, Blookquist C. The effect of female sex hormones on subgingival plaque. J Periodontol 1981;52(10):599.
3. Kornman K, Loseche JF: Direct interaction of estradiol and progesterone with Bacteroides melaninogenicus. J Dent Res 1979;58A:10.
4. Manson JD, Eley BM. The effect of systemic factors on the periodontal tissues. In, Periodontics 5th ed Wright 2004;90-107.
5. Mascarenhas P, Gapski R, Al-shammari K, Wang HL. Influence of sex hormones on the periodontium. J Clin Periodontol 2003;30:671-81.
6. Mealey BL, Klokkevold PR, Corgel JO Periodontal treatment of medically compromised patients. In, Newman, Takei, Carranza. Clinical Periodontology 9th ed WB Saunders 2003;527-50.
7. Palmer R, Soory M. Modifying factors: Diabetes, Puberty, Pregnancy and the Menopause and Tobacco Smoking. In, Lindhe J, Karring T, Lang NP. Clinical Periodontology and Implant dentistry. 4th ed Blackwell Munksgaard 2003;179-97.
8. Roberts WE, Simmons KE, Garetto LP and Decastro RA. Bone physiology and metabolism in dental implantology: risk factors for osteoporosis and other metabolic bone diseases. Implant dentistry 1992;1:11-21.
9. Rose LF. Sex hormonal imbalances, oral manifestations and dental treatment. In, Genco RJ, Goldman HM and Cohen DW. Contemporary Periodontics CV Mosby Company 1990;221-27.

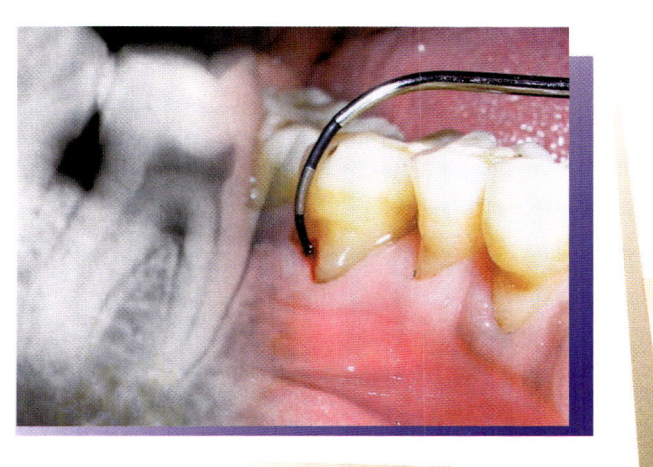

SECTION

FIVE

DIAGNOSIS

CHAPTER 30

Clinical Diagnosis

Shalu Bathla

INTRODUCTION

Diagnosis may be defined as identifying disease from an evaluation of the history, signs and symptoms, laboratory tests and procedures.

An accurate diagnosis can only be made by a thorough evaluation of data that have been systematically collected by: 1. patient interview, 2. medical consultation as indicated, 3. clinical periodontal examination, 4. radiographic examination and 5. laboratory tests as needed. From this information, the clinician has to distinguish between normal and abnormal findings. Periodontal diagnosis should first determine whether disease is present; then identify its type, extent, distribution, and severity; and finally provide an understanding of the underlying pathologic processes and its cause.

PATIENT INTERVIEW

The patient interview includes information concerning the source of referral, chief complaint, symptoms and medical and dental history. The source of referral may be important if another dentist or physician referred the patient and may be a valuable asset in diagnosis **(Fig. 30.1)**.

Vital statistics include the patient's name, age, sex, home and business address, phone number, marital and family status and occupation. These are all significant.

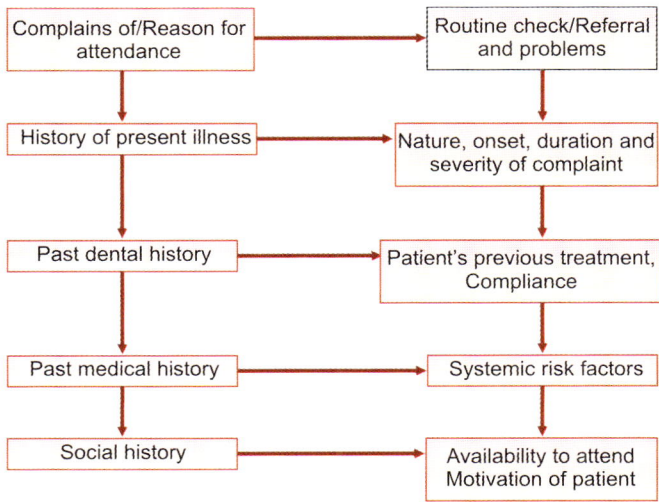

Fig. 30.1: Key stages in history taking for periodontal patient

Importance of Name: Aids in establishing rapport with patient.

Importance of Age: Certain diseases have a predilection at certain age groups, e.g. Herpetic gingivostomatitis is common in children below 6 years. Age also has effect on dental procedures and personal care.

Importance of Sex: Certain diseases are common in either males or females, e.g. Desquamative gingivitis is more common in females.

Importance of Address: Various conditions are endemic to certain areas. Address tells about the presence of fluoride in drinking water.

Importance of Telephone no: For change of appointment. Immediate consultation may be needed so that urgent treatment may proceed.

Importance of Occupation: May be a factor in the etiology of certain occupational diseases like asbestosis and erosion.

Economic and social status: People who are under stress are more likely to suffer from psychosomatic diseases like lichen planus and ANUG.

MEDICAL AND DENTAL HISTORY

Objectives of medical history:
1. To identify systemic factors which may help to account for the periodontal condition. Debilitating diseases like diabetes can influence periodontal health.
2. To note the existence of systemic conditions for which special precautions, e.g. antibiotic prophylaxis are required to safeguard the patient during periodontal therapy.
3. To note the existence of any transmissible disease which may present a hazard to the clinician, dental staff or other patients.

The dental history should include reference to the frequency, date of the most recent visit, nature of the treatment and oral prophylaxis or cleaning by a dentist. The patient's oral hygiene regimen should be noted, including tooth brushing frequency, time of day, method, type of toothbrush and dentifrice, and interval at which brushes are replaced. History of previous periodontal problems should also be noted, including the nature of the condition and, if previously treated, the type of treatment received and approximate period of termination of previous treatment.

CLINICAL EXAMINATION

Subjective sensations resulting from the disease that are reported by the patient are called symptoms. Signs of illness are objective findings that are observed by the clinician. The clinical examination should include an examination of the extra oral, parafunctional habits and intraoral tissues including teeth, gingiva and the periodontal tissues. Any abnormal findings should be recorded and used to develop a definitive diagnosis or further investigated by referral or biopsy.

I. **Extraoral examination:** Observe patient during reception and seating to note physical characteristics and abnormalities and makes an overall appraisal. Inspection includes evaluation of bilateral symmetry, the comparison of the anatomy of one side of the head, face, and neck to the opposite side. Palpation is used to determine the texture, size and consistency by the sense of touch. Palpation may be accomplished by using both hands, comparing one side of the head, face and neck with the other side. This is called bimanual palpation. The clinician may palpate the structures of the neck, lymph nodes, and salivary glands. The clinician may use auscultation to listen to the TMJ for crepitus. The temporomandibular joint (TMJ) is found just in front of the ear. The TMJ may be examined by palpation and auscultation. Palpating with the index and middle finger over the head of the condyle, or a finger just inside the external auditory meatus, allows the clincian to evaluate the function of TMJ **(Fig. 30.2)**. Auscultation for joint sounds may be accomplished by listening with the unaided ear or with a stethoscope placed over the TMJ.

II. **Oral examination:** The cleanliness of the oral cavity is appraised in terms of the extent of accumulated food debris, plaque, materia alba, and tooth surface stains. Disclosing solution may be used to detect plaque that would otherwise be unnoticed.

Halitosis is foul or offensive odor emanating from the oral cavity. Mouth odors may be of diagnostic significance, and their origin may be either oral or extraoral. More is explained in chapter no.33 Halitosis.

Lymph nodes may become enlarged in certain gingival and periodontal diseases like necrotizing ulcerative gingivitis, primary herpetic gingivostomatitis and acute periodontal abscesses. The clinician palpates

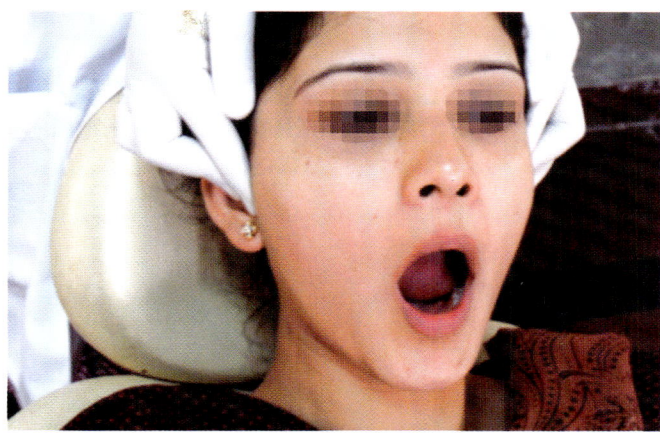

Fig. 30.2: Palpating TMJ

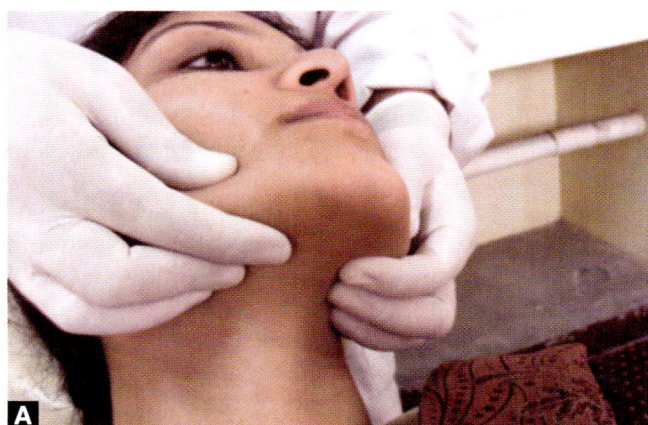

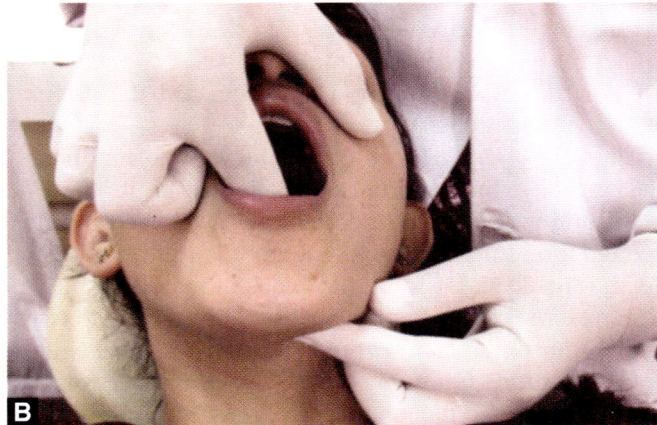

Figs 30.3A and B: Palpating submandibular and sublingual lymph nodes

under the chin and along the mandible. With one digit compressing the floor of the mouth and another digit placed medially to the inferior border of the mandible, the clinician palpates the submandibular gland and the submandibular lymph nodes **(Figs 30.3A and B)**.

Parafunctional habits means abnormal, altered or deviated functions. Classified according to the cause in three ways:

- Tooth to tooth function, e.g. bruxism
- Tooth to soft tissue, e.g. thumb– sucking
- Tooth to foreign object, e.g. chewing of pens and pencils.

Bruxism means a constant or intermittent occlusal contact of the teeth, aside from mastication, swallowing/speech. It is the term for abnormal grinding of the teeth. Bruxism may cause excessive tooth wear characterized by facets on tooth surfaces and widening of the occlusal surfaces. Bruxism may also lead to reduction in vertical dimension.

Tongue thrusting is the persistent, forceful wedging of the tongue against the teeth, especially in anterior region. It is a habit in which patient instead of placing the dorsum of the tongue against the palate with the tip behind the maxillary teeth during swallowing, the tongue is thrust forward against the mandibular anterior teeth which tilt and also spread laterally. Tongue thrusting causes excessive lateral pressure leading to pathologic migration. It may cause spreading and tilting of the anterior teeth and open bite.

Various Tools for Gingival and Periodontal Examination and Assessment (Table 30.1)

Inspection: Gingiva is examined for changes in color, contour, surface texture and size. It tells about the position of frenal attachment.

Exploration: Exploration helps to diagnose bleeding on probing, pocket depth, whether pocket is true/pseudo, suprabony/infrabony, about subgingival calculus and gingival recession.

Percussion: Helps to diagnose healthy or ankylosed tooth and inflamed tissue. A healthy tooth percussed with a metallic instrument gives metallic sound while teeth embedded in inflamed tissue gives dull sound. In periapical abscess tooth will be tender.

Palpation: Helps to diagnose whether gingiva is normal, i.e. firm and resilient or fibrosed or edematous. It also helps to test the degree of mobility. Gentle pressure with the finger can elicit tenderness in inflamed areas. It helps to diagnose exudation or suppuration present or absent. Certain gingival or periodontal diseases in which lymph nodes are enlarged, can be diagnosed through palpation like necrotizing ulcerative gingivitis, primary herpetic gingivostomatitis and acute periodontal abscesses.

PERIODONTICS REVISITED

TABLE 30.1: Various examination tools

Tools	Assessment: Natural Dentition	Assessment: Dental Implants
1 Visual inspection	Gingival color, contour, tone and Calculus detection	Same
2 Compressed air	Gingival tone Calculus detection	Same
3 Calibrated probe	Using metal/ plastic probe: Gingival tone Clinical attachment level Bleeding points Exudate Mucogingival examination Measuring of oral deviations	Using plastic probe: Gingival tone Clinical attachment level Bleeding points Exudate
4 Furcation probe	Furcation involvement	Not applicable
5 Instrument handle	Mobility	Same, using plastic handles
6 Explorer	Calculus detection Detection of plaque retentive factors and subgingival calculus	Not applicable
7 Radiographic	Bone height and density	Same

Examination of Teeth

The teeth are examined for caries, failing restorations, evidence of food impaction, wasting diseases, hypersenstivity, mobility, trauma from occlusion, pathologic migration and occlusal relationships.

Caries: Carious lesions provide a rough surface for plaque and food debris retention. They leave open contact areas that permit food impaction **(Fig. 30.4)**.

Restorations: Characteristics of restorations that leave effect on periodontium are margin of restoration, contour and overhang, material, occlusion, design of removable partial prosthesis and restorative procedure. Overhanging margin contributes to periodontal diseases by providing ideal niches for the accumulation of plaque and by changing the ecological balance of the gingival sulcus from gram positive facultative species to gram negative anaerobic species. Overhanging makes the area inaccessible for the direct application of toothbrush and other plaque removal interdental aids. Overhangs catch and tear dental floss. Overcontoured crown and restorations contributes to periodontal diseases by

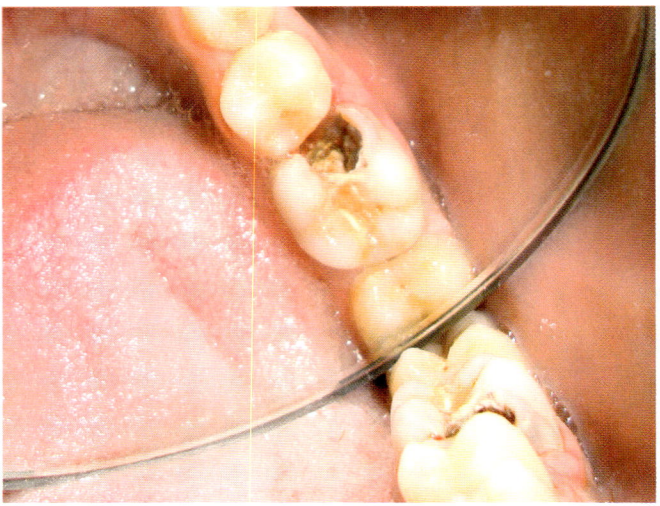

Fig. 30.4: Dental caries acting as plaque retentive area

providing ideal locations for accumulation of plaque and by preventing self cleansing mechanisms of adjacent cheek, lips and tongue.

Proximal Contact Relations: Slightly open contacts permit food impaction. The tightness of contacts should be checked by means of clinical observation and with dental floss.

Food Impaction: It is the forceful wedging of food into the periodontium by occlusal forces.

Hirschfeld in 1930, classified vertical food impaction relative to etiologic factors as:

Class I   - Occlusal wear
Class II - Loss of proximal support
Class III - Extrusion of a tooth beyond the occlusal plane
Class IV - Congenital morphologic abnormalities
Class V   - Improperly constructed restorations

Plunger cusps are the cusps that tend to forcibly wedge food into interproximal embrasures of opposing teeth **(Fig. 30.5)**. Distolingual cusps of maxillary molars are the most common plunger cusp. Plunger cusp effect may occur with wear or it may be the result of a shift in tooth positions following the failure to replace missing tooth.

Wasting diseases: Wasting disease of tooth is defined as any gradual loss of tooth substance characterized by the formation of smooth, polished surfaces, without regard to the possible mechanism of this loss. The various form of wasting diseases are attrition, erosion, abrasion and abfraction.

Attrition is an occlusal wear resulting from functional contacts with opposing teeth. Flat occlusal or incisal

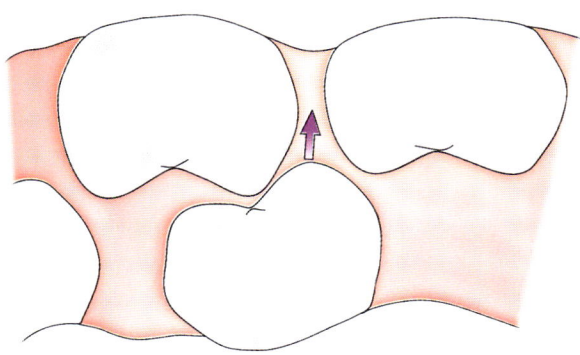

Fig. 30.5: Plunger cusp

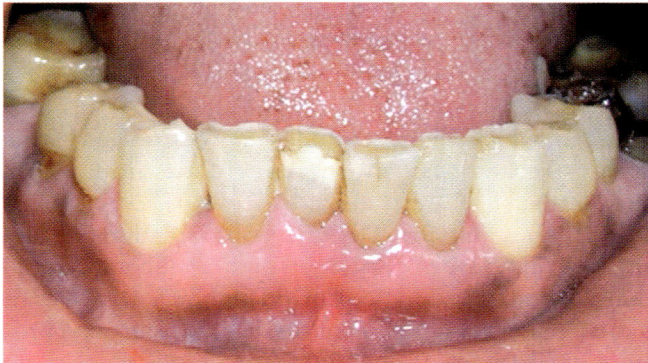

Fig. 30.6: Attrition seen on the incisal edges of incisors

surfaces/ facets with accurate interdigitation of upper and lower teeth are found in attrition **(Fig. 30.6)**. There is hypertrophy of masseter muscle.

Erosion is a wear to the non-occluding tooth surfaces, which is sharply, defined wedge shaped depression in the crevical area of the facial tooth surface. The long axis of the eroded area is perpendicular to the vertical axis. Erosion affects buccal and lingual surfaces of anteriors which appear smooth and shiny with a generated loss of anatomy. On the palatal surface of the upper incisors the exposed dentin is smooth often with a halo of enamel surrounding the lesion.

The various causes of erosion are:
i. Vomiting associated with eating disorders like anorexia nervosa, bulimia nervosa and rumination
ii. Reflux or chronic regurgitation associated with gastrointestinal problems
iii. Regular and high intake of acidic medication (chewable acetylsalicylic acid tablets)
iv. Regular intake of chewable vitamin C tablets
v. High consumption of acidic drinks and foods
vi. Professional wine tasting
vii. Field of occupation — acid battery worker
viii. Pregnancy

Smooth, clean surfaces and presence of dentin hypersensitivity suggest that the process of erosion is active whereas stained teeth, suggest its inactivity. If the erosion is existing around tooth with the restoration, the restoration being resistant to acid remains unchanged but the tooth is gradually dissolved. Comparison of dated study casts to the clinical condition of the teeth over time also suggest whether the erosion lesion is active or inactive.

Erosion can be prevented by the following measures:
i. Reduce the frequency and amount of consumption of acidic drinks and food, especially at bedtime.
ii. If soft drinks are consumed, should be chilled and consumed in one sitting at meal time.
iii. Avoid sipping the acidic drink or swishing it around the mouth before swallowing.
iv. Consume neutralizing food such as cheese after the intake of an acidic drink or food.
v. Encourage the consumption of water and nutritious beverages such as milk.

Abrasion: It is referred to the loss of tooth substance induced by mechanical wear other than that of mastication **(Fig. 30.7)**. It may manifest as rounded blunted or worn flat cusp tip/ incisal edge exposing the dentin, causing a "scooped out" appearance that is softer and more porous than enamel. It is usually caused by foreign substances.

When erosion and attrition occur together there is cupping or undermining of occlusal surfaces, the dentin is less mineralized than enamel and that's why wear preferentially result in occulsal cupping **(Fig. 30.8)**. Causes of abrasion are:
i. Hard-bristle toothbrush.
ii. Coarse abrasive tooth powder.

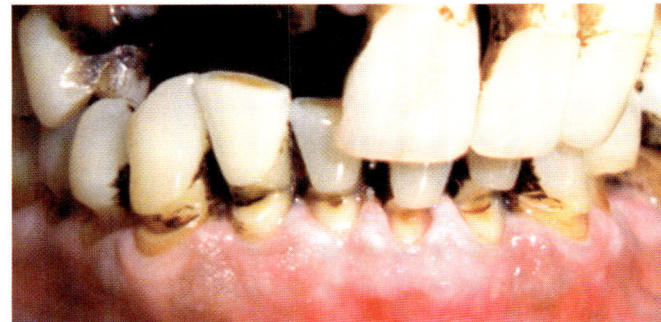

Fig. 30.7: Abrasion attributed to aggressive toothbrushing (V-shaped notches)

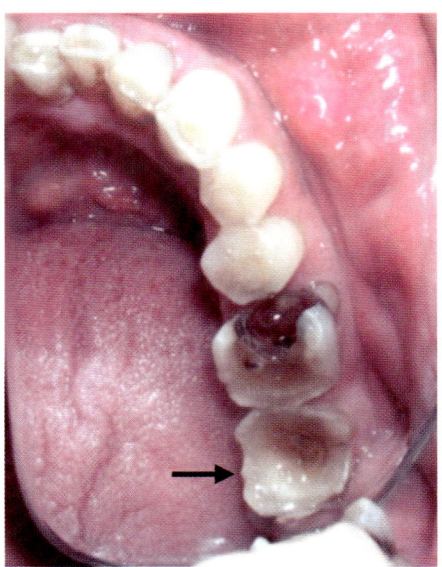

Fig. 30.8: Attrition and erosion causing occlusal cupping of molar

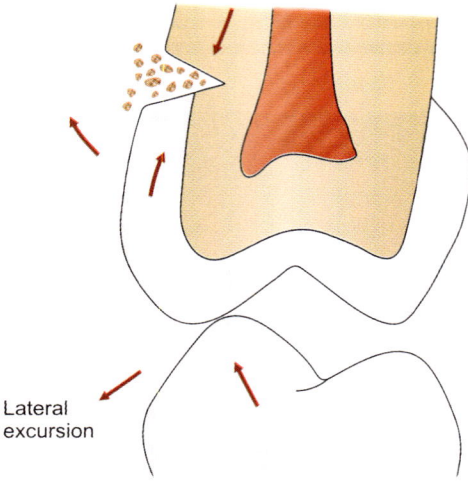

Fig. 30.10: Abfraction

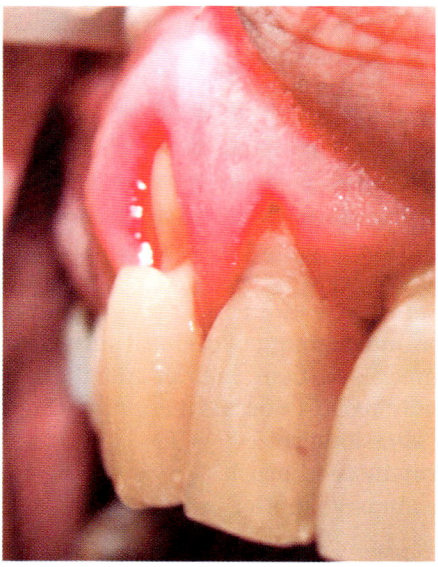

Fig. 30.9: Abrasion due to horizontal toothbrushing

iii. Horizontal tooth brushing technique at right angles to the vertical axis of teeth **(Fig. 30.9)**.
iv. Action of clasps.
v. Abrasion of incisal edges due to habits such as opening bobby pins, nails held by carpenters, pins by dressmakers.
vi. Pipe held between teeth.

Abfraction: It is the flexure of a tooth under heavy lateral load, which may lead to displacement/fracture of enamel rods at the CEJ. The lost enamel exposes more dentin, in which dentinal tubules may be crushed by the same stresses and more readily demineralized **(Fig.30.10)**.

Frictional ablation/Dentoalveolar ablations: It is a process caused by juxtaposition of natural and artificial dental surfaces and hyper functional oral soft tissues. It is caused by the action of soft tissues and saliva against the dentition due to vestibular pressures of suction, swallowing, tongue motions and the intervening forced flow of saliva.

Occlusal relationship: The occlusion is examined for centric, working, non-working and protrusive interferences. Evidence of possible occlusal trauma as indicated by fremitus (mobility in function) is recorded. Effect of malocclusion on periodontium:

Excessive overbite causes impingement of the teeth on gingiva, food impaction, gingival inflammation, gingival enlargement and pocket formation **(Fig. 30.11)**. Open bite causes reduced mechanical cleansing by the passage of food leading to accumulation of debris, calculus formation and extrusion of teeth. Cross bite causes trauma from occlusion, food impaction and spreading of mandibular teeth **(Fig. 30.12)**.

Dental stains: These are pigmented deposits on the teeth. They should be carefully examined to determine their origin. More is explained in chapter no 9. Dental Plaque.

Trauma from occlusion: When occlusal forces exceeds the adaptive capacity of the tissues, tissue injury results, this resultant injury is termed trauma from occlusion. An occlusion that produces such injury is called a

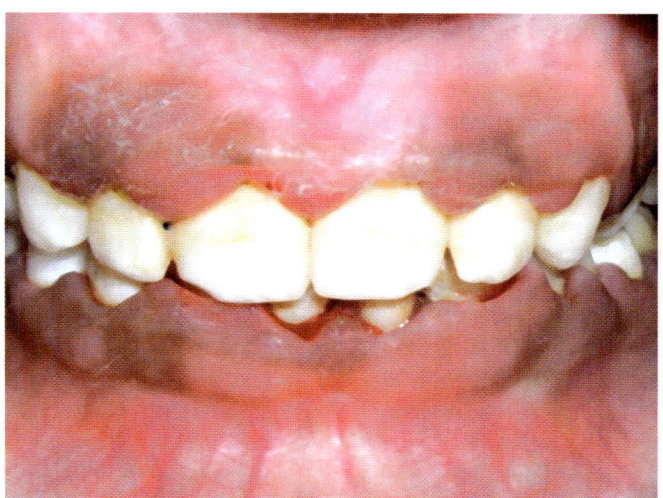

Fig. 30.11: Deep bite causing impingement of maxillary teeth on mandibular gingiva

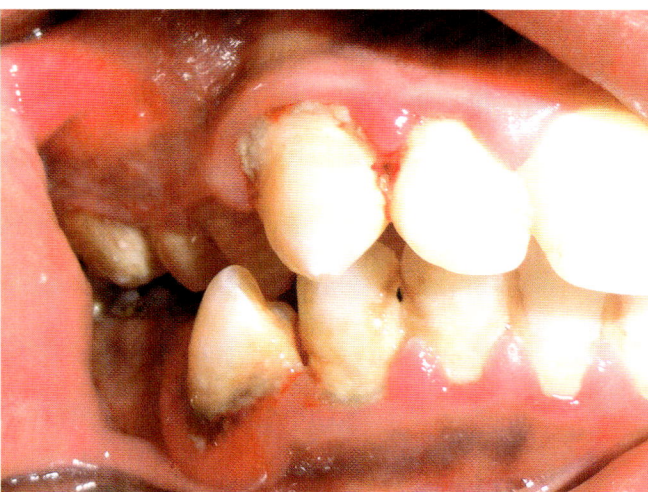

Fig. 30.12: Crossbite

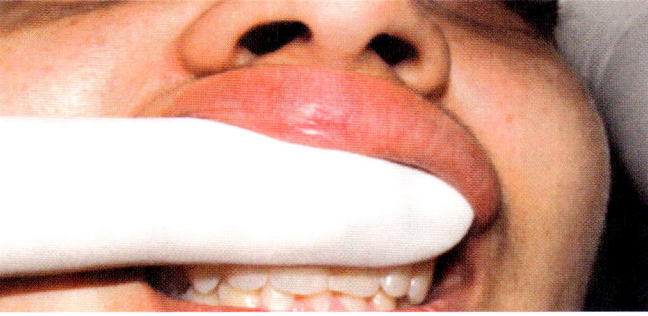

Fig. 30.13: Fremitus test

traumatic occlusion. Trauma from occlusion refers to the tissue injury and not the occlusal force. The main clinical finding associated with trauma from occlusion is progressively increasing tooth mobility. Rest is explained in chapter no. 28. Trauma from occlusion and Pathologic Tooth migration.

Fremitus test: Dampen index finger and place along the buccal and labial surfaces of maxillary teeth. The patient is then asked to tap the teeth together in the maximum intercuspation and to do lateral, protrusive movements **(Fig. 30.13)**.

- Class I   : Mild vibration detected, first degree is recorded as "+"
- Class II : Easily palpable vibration, recorded as "++"
- Class III : Movements visible with naked eye recorded as "+++".

It is a test used to diagnose a case of trauma from occlusion, by measuring the vibratory pattern of teeth, when teeth are placed in contacting positions.

Rationale behind fremitus test: Periodontal fremitus occurs in either of the alveolar bones when an individual sustains trauma from occlusion. It is a result of teeth exhibiting at least slight mobility rubbing against the adjacent walls of their sockets, the volume of which has been expanded ever so slight by inflammatory responses, bone resorption or both. As a test to determine the severity of periodontal disease a patient is told to close his or her mouth into maximum intercuspation and is asked to grind his or her teeth. Finger placed in the labial vestibule against the alveolar bone can detect fremitus. Fremitus is tooth displacement which is created by patient's own occlusal force. Therefore, the amount of force varies greatly from patient to patient, whereas in mobility the force with which it is measured tends to be the same for each examiner. Fremitus is a guide to the ability of the patient to displace and traumatize the teeth.

Pathologic migration of the teeth: Alterations in tooth position should be carefully noted, particularly with a view towards identifying abnormal forces, tongue-thrusting habit, or other habits that may be the contributing factors **(Fig. 30.14)**. Pathologic migration of anterior teeth may be a sign of localized aggressive periodontitis.

Examination of Gingiva

The gingiva must be dried before accurate observations can be made. Light reflection from moist gingiva obscures detail. The architecture of the gingiva should

PERIODONTICS REVISITED

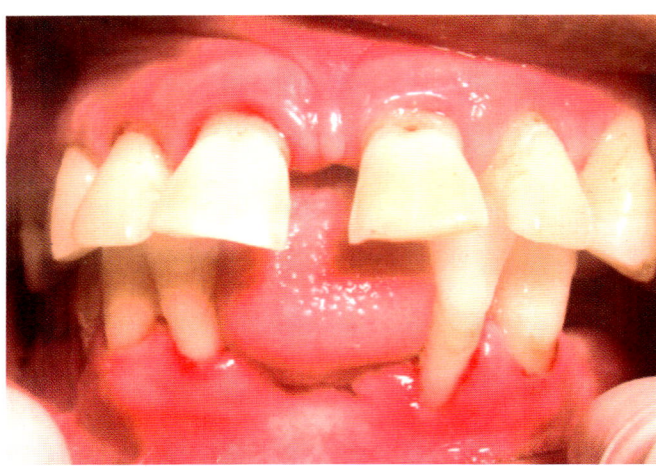

Fig. 30.14: Pathologic migration associated with tongue thrusting habit

be examined for changes in the normal knife-edged appearance of the free gingival margin and interdental papilla as it meets the teeth. In the absence of systemic disease or drug-associated gingival enlargement, any swelling or an enlarged appearance of the marginal gingiva is a sign of inflammation. The consistency of any gingival enlargement should be evaluated with the side of a periodontal probe to determine whether it is edematous or fibrotic. Any significant lack of attached gingiva, especially if it is associated with gingival recession or a high frenum attachment, should be noted and recorded in the dental record. Evidence of interdental cratering is especially important if it is accompanied by necrosis of the gingiva with or without exposure of the underlying bone. Interdental necrosis may be a clinical sign of necrotizing ulcerative gingivitis or necrotizing ulcerative periodontitis. It may also be a clinical sign that is associated with immuno-compromised patients with AIDS. The various mucogingival problems are inadequate width of attached gingiva, abnormal frenum attachment, gingival recession, and decreased vestibular depth, pockets extending upto mucogingival junction, gingival excess (pseudopocket), inconsistent gingival margin, excessive gingival display and abnormal color of gingiva. Inadequate attached gingiva zone would facilitate subgingival plaque formation because of improper closure of the pocket resulting from movability of the marginal tissue and favor attachment loss and soft tissue recession due to the less resistance of the tissue. Inadequate attached gingiva zone would also facilitate accumulation of food particles during mastication and impede proper oral hygiene measures.

Measurement of width of attached gingiva:

i. *Anatomically*: Stretch the lip/cheek to demarcate the mucogingival line while pocket is being probed. Measure the total width of gingiva (gingival margin to mucogingival line) and subtract the sulcus/pocket depth from it to determine width of attached gingiva.

ii. *Functionally*:

a. *Tension test*: Stretch the lip or cheek outward and forward to demarcate the mucogingival line and to see for any movement of free gingival margin. Measure the total width of gingiva (gingival margin to mucogingival line) and subtract the sulcus/pocket depth from it to determine width of attached gingiva.

b. *Roll test*: Push the adjacent mucosa coronally with a dull instrument to mark mucogingival line. Measure the total width of gingiva (gingival margin to mucogingival line) and subtract the sulcus/pocket depth from it to determine width of attached gingiva.

iii. *Histochemically*: Staining test – Paint the gingiva and oral mucosa with Schiller's or Lugol solution (iodine and potassium iodide solution). The alveolar mucosa takes on a brown color owing to its glycogen content, while the glycogen free, attached gingiva remains unstained. Measure the total width of the unstained gingiva and subtract the sulcus/pocket depth from it to determine width of attached gingiva.

Measurement of thickness of gingiva

Earlier the thickness of gingiva were measured using traumatic techniques like probes and injection needle. But now it can be measured atraumatically using the newer ultrasonic device called 'KRUPP SDM'. This uses a pulse echo principle. With the aid of a pulse generator and a measurement frequency of 5 MHz, a piezo crystal is allowed to oscillate. Ultrasonic pulses are transmitted at an interval through the sound permeable gingiva. When it reaches the bone or tooth surface its starts being reflected due to difference in acoustic impedence. A transducer probe of 4 mm diameter is moistened with saliva and applied to the measurement site with slight pressure to produce acoustic coupling. By timing the received echo with respect to transmission of pulse, the thickness of mucosa is determined within seconds and is digitally displayed with a resolution of 0.1mm.

Abnormal frenum: Abnormal frenum jeopardize gingival health as it interfere with proper placement of a toothbrush and open gingival crevice by muscle pull. Frenum is judged abnormal when the frenum is unusually broad or there is no apparent attached gingiva

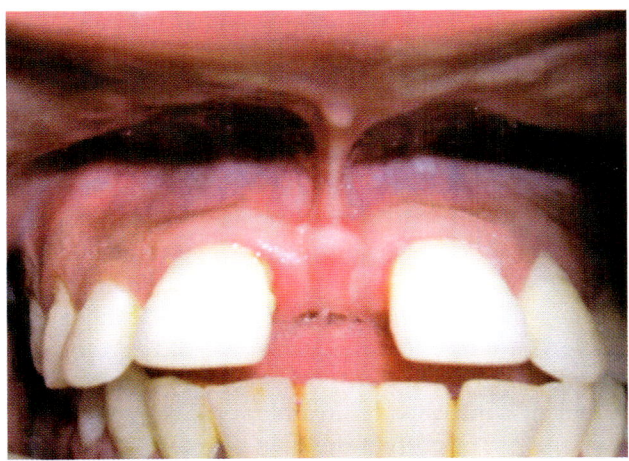

Fig. 30.15: Papillary frenum

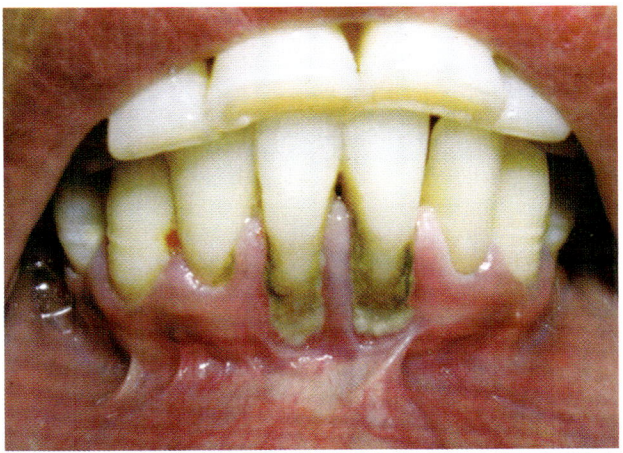

Fig. 30.17: Grade III marginal tissue recession

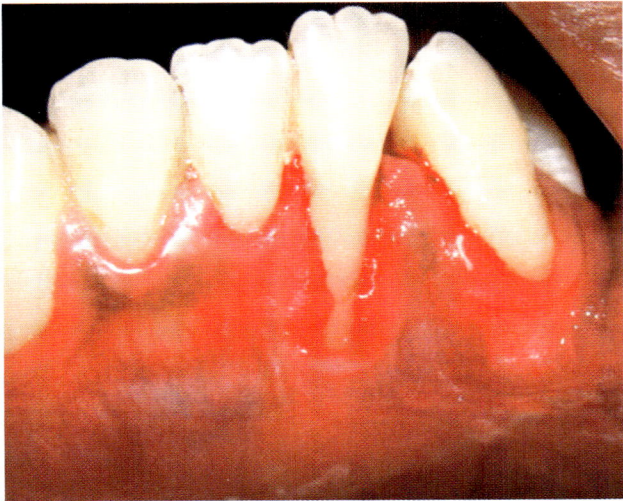

Fig. 30.16: Localized recession on malposed teeth

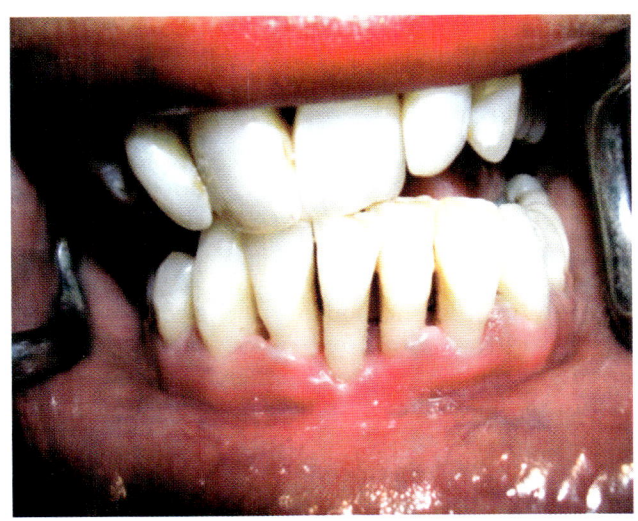

Fig. 30.18: Grade IV marginal tissue recession

in the midline or interdental papilla moves by stretching the frenum **(Fig. 30.15)**. Tension test is done to detect any abnormal frenum attachment (explained earlier in this chapter).

Measurement of gingival recession: Gingival recession can be seen on malposed teeth **(Fig. 30.16)**. It is recorded during periodontal probing as the distance of the free gingival margin to the cementoenamel junction. In 1985, Miller classified marginal tissue recession into four classes:

Class I : Marginal tissue recession not extending to the mucogingival junction. No loss of interdental bone/soft tissue.

Class II : Marginal tissue recession extends to or beyond the mucogingival junction. No loss of interdental bone/soft tissue.

Class III : Marginal tissue recession extends to or beyond the mucogingival junction. Loss of interdental bone/soft tissue or there is malpositioning of the tooth **(Fig. 30.17)**.

Class IV : Marginal tissue recession extends beyond the mucogingival junction. Loss of interdental bone and soft tissue loss interdentally and/or severe tooth malposition **(Fig. 30.18)**.

Bleeding on probing: The insertion of a probe to the bottom of the pocket elicits bleeding if the gingiva is inflamed and the pocket epithelium is atrophic or ulcerated. Bleeding on probing is an earlier sign of inflammation than gingival color changes. To test for bleeding after probing, the probe is carefully introduced to the bottom of the pocket and gently moved laterally

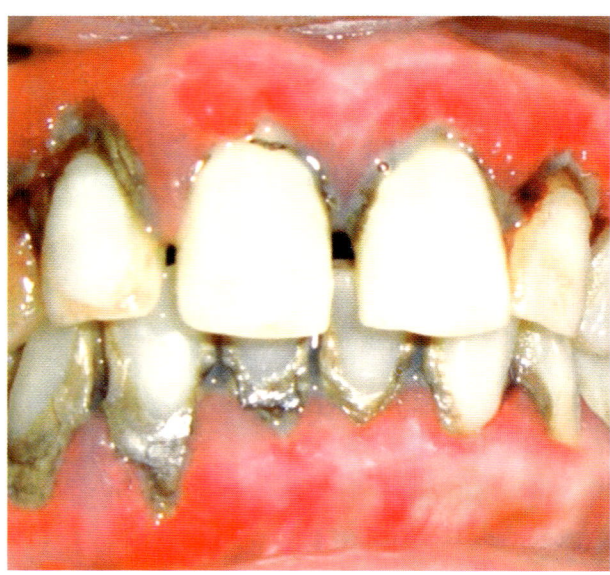

Fig. 30.19: Pus discharge

along the pocket wall. Bleeding may appear immediately after removal of the probe, or delayed by few seconds. Bleeding is checked after 30 to 60 seconds of probing. As a single test, bleeding on probing is not a good predictor of progressive attachment loss; however, its absence is an excellent predictor of periodontal stability.

Suppuration: Clinically, the presence of pus in a periodontal pocket is determined by placing the ball of the index finger along the lateral aspect of the marginal gingiva and applying pressure in a rolling motion toward the crown. Visual examination without digital pressure is not enough **(Fig. 30.19)**.

Examination of Periodontal Tissues

The periodontal tissues are routinely examined in all oral examinations. The periodontal examination consists of a visual inspection of the gingiva, dental plaque and calculus deposition, assessment of mobility, periodontal pocket depth, level of attachment, alveolar bone loss, furcation lesion and abscesses.

Plaque and Calculus: There are many methods for assessing plaque and calculus accumulation. The presence of supragingival plaque and calculus can be directly observed and the amount measured with a calibrated probe. For the detection of subgingival calculus, each tooth surface is carefully checked to the level of the gingival attachment with a sharp no. 17 or no. 3A explorer. Warm air may be used to deflect the gingiva and aid in visualization of the calculus. Although

the radiograph may sometimes reveal heavy calculus deposits interproximally.

Mobility: Tooth mobility should be recorded because teeth that are mobile have been shown to have a poorer prognosis and increased attachment loss after periodontal therapy. Mobility is recorded by moving the teeth in a buccolingual and occlusoapical direction between the blunt handle ends of two instruments or between the finger and instrument handle **(Figs 30.20A to C)**. But the method of detecting mobility with an instrument and finger is not reliable. The degree of movement is observed by comparsion with adjacent teeth that are not being moved. The degree of movement is indicated on an arbitrary scale 0 to 3.

Grade I   : Slightly more than normal.

Grade II   : Moderately more than normal.

Grade III : Severe mobility faciolingually and/or mesiodistally, combined with vertical displacement.

Mobility beyond the physiologic range is termed abnormal or pathologic. It is pathologic in that it exceeds the limits of normal mobility values; the periodontium is not necessarily diseased at the time of examination.

Etiology: Increased mobility is caused by one or more of the following factors:

A. Local Factors: Bone loss or loss of tooth support, trauma from occlusion, hypofunction, periapical pathology, after periodontal surgery, parafunctional habits, pathology of jaws like tumors, traumatic injuries to dentoalveolar unit.

B. Systemic Factors: Menstrual cycle, oral contraceptives, pregnancy, systemic diseases (Papillon-Lefevre syndrome, Down's syndrome, neutropenia, Chediak-Higashi syndrome, hypophosphatasia, hyperparathyroidism, acute leukemia, Pagets disease).

Periodontal pocket depth: Examination for periodontal pockets must include consideration of the following: Presence and distribution on each tooth surface, pocket depth, level of attachment on the root, and type of pocket (suprabony or intrabony). The only accurate method of detecting and measuring periodontal pocket is careful exploration with a periodontal probe. Periodontal probing is done on all surfaces of every tooth in the dentition. Pockets are not detected by radiographic examination. The periodontal pocket is a soft tissue change. Radiographs indicate areas of bone loss where pockets may be suspected; they do not show pocket presence or depth. Gutta percha points or calibrated silver points can be used with the radiograph to assist in determining the level of attachment of periodontal pockets.

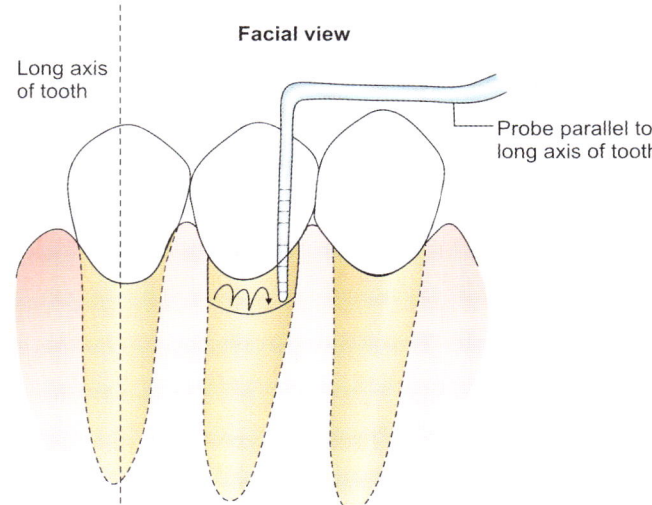

Facial view

Long axis of tooth

Probe parallel to long axis of tooth

Periodontal probing involves walking stroke

Fig. 30.21: Walking stroke

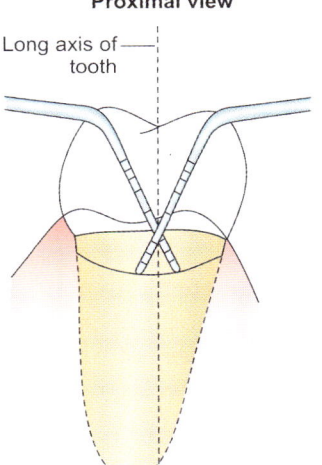

Proximal view

Long axis of tooth

(Area under contact area should be probed from both facial and lingual aspects)

Fig. 30.22: Probing in interproximal area

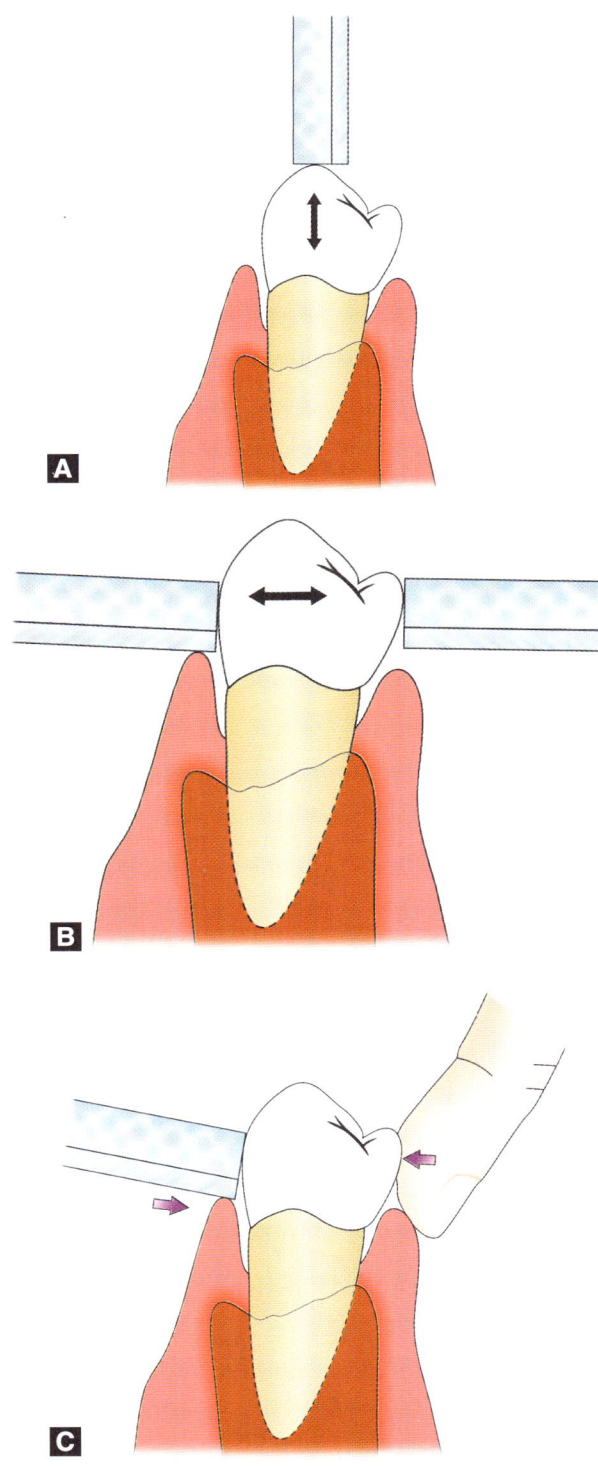

Figs 30.20A to C: A. Tooth mobility checked with one instrument in vertical direction; B. Tooth mobility checked with two instruments in buccolingual direction; C. Tooth mobility checked with one metal instrument and one finger in buccolingual direction (Not reliable method)

The probe should be inserted parallel to the vertical axis of the tooth and "walked" circumferentially around each surface of each tooth without taking out the probe completely from the gingival sulcus to detect the areas of deepest penetration **(Fig. 30.21)**. For the interproximal pocket, it is necessary to angulate the probe beneath the contact area, from both the facial and lingual areas **(Fig. 30.22)**.

Probing of pockets is done at various times for diagnosis, and for monitoring the course of treatment

PERIODONTICS REVISITED

and maintenance. The initial probing of moderate or advanced cases is usually hampered by the presence of heavy inflammation and abundant calculus and cannot be done very accurately. The purpose of this initial probing, together with the clinical and radiographic examination is to determine whether the tooth can be saved or should be extracted. Once the patient has performed an adequate plaque and calculus control, the major inflammatory changes disappears, and a more accurate probing of the pockets can be performed. This second probing is for the purpose of accurately establishing the level of attachment and degree of involvement of roots and furcations.

Various periodontal probes are available to measure pocket depth around natural dentition. To prevent scratching of the implant surface, plastic periodontal probes should be used instead of the usual steel probes used for the natural dentition.

Level of attachment: It is the distance between the base of the pocket and the fixed reference point such as cementoenamel junction (CEJ) on the crown, margin of a permanent restoration; for animal research a notch made in the tooth; in human research studies template/ splint may be made for each patient **(Fig. 30.23)**. There may be gain or loss of attachment. The clinical attachment loss reveals the approximate extent of root surface that is devoid of periodontal ligament.

Limitation:

i.   It is used as an indicator of the amount of periodontal support at a specific location on the tooth, this measurement clearly does not provide an accurate assessment of support in terms of three dimensions/ root surface area.

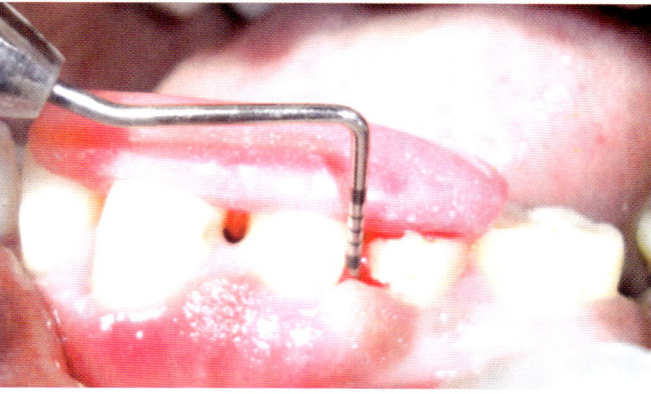

Fig. 30.23: Template/ splint is made to determine level of attachment (Groove acrylic stent to standardize the direction of probe *Courtesy: Dr Nitika*)

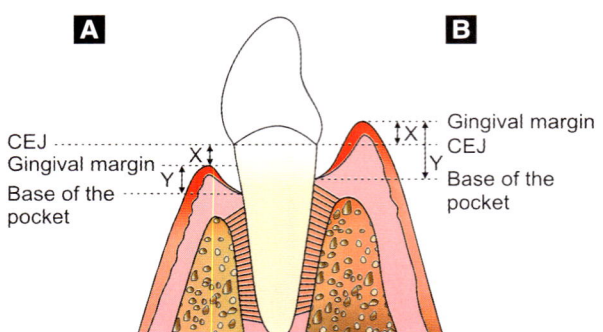

Fig. 30.24: Calculation of CAL in different situations.
A. When gingival margin is below CEJ (Clinical gingival recession). Clinical attachment loss is calculated by ADDING the probing depth (Y) to the distance between CEJ and gingival margin (X).
B. When gingival margin cover the CEJ, locating on anatomic crown. Clinical attachment loss is calculated by SUBSTRACTING the probing depth (Y) to the distance between CEJ and gingival margin (X).

ii. Apical extent of periodontal probe penetration and depth measurement is dependent on degree of inflammation, probing force, probe tip thickness, angulation and position of probing and root anatomy, particularly in furcation areas.

Determining the level of attachment**(Fig. 30.24)**: When the gingival margin is located on the anatomic crown, the level of attachment is determined by subtracting the distance from the gingival margin to the cementoenamel junction to the depth of the pocket. If both are the same, the loss of attachment is zero. When the gingival margin coincides with the cementoenamel junction, the loss of attachment equals the pocket depth.

When the gingival margin is located apical to the cementoenamel junction, the loss of attachment is greater than the pocket depth, and therefore the distance between the cementoenamel junction and the gingival margin should be added to the pocket depth.

Various tests used during periodontal examination:
Tension test is used to detect – Abnormal frenum
Fremitus test is used to detect – Trauma from occlusion
Transgingival probing is used to determine – Alveolar bone loss

Alveolar bone loss: It is evaluated by clinical and radiographic examination. Bone sounding is done by anaesthetizing the tissue locally and inserting probe horizontally and walking along the tissue tooth interface, so that the operator can feel the bony topography. It gives three-dimensional information regarding bone contour. It is also called as transgingival probing. It helps to determine the height and contour of facial and lingual bone; the architecture of the interdental bone; the extent

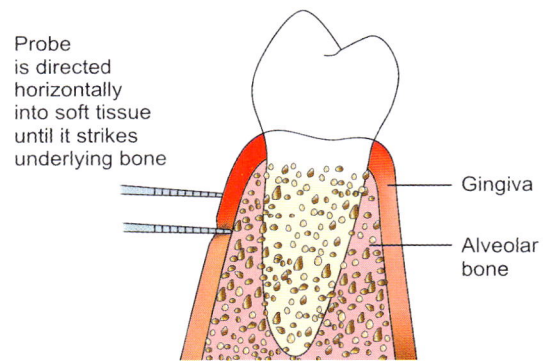

Probe is directed horizontally into soft tissue until it strikes underlying bone

Gingiva

Alveolar bone

Fig. 30.25: Transgingival probing/bone sounding

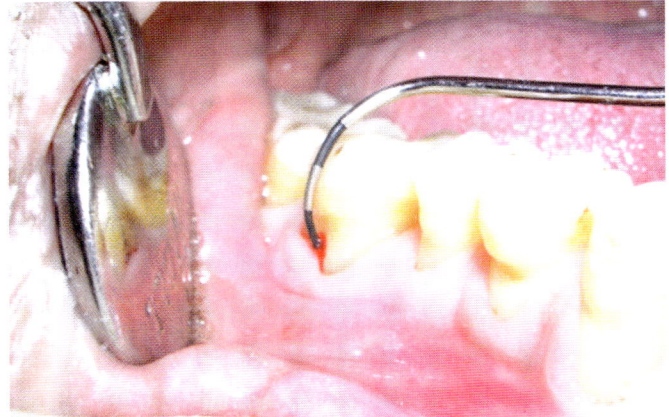

Fig. 30.26: Grade II furcation defect (Cul-de-sac)

and configuration of intrabony component of the pocket **(Fig. 30.25)**.

Furcation lesion: The furcation lesions can be determined by Cowhorn explorer or *Naber's* probe. The probe is directed beneath the gingival margin. At the base of pocket, rotate the probe tip toward the tooth to fit the tip into the entrance of the furcation **(Fig. 30.26)**. Terminal shank of Naber's probe is positioned parallel to the long axis of tooth surface being examined. Distal furcation of maxillary molar can be probed from either buccal or palatal aspect but mesial furcation of maxillary molar is easily probed from the palatal aspect. Radiographs are useful in assessing root morphology and apicocoronal position of the furcation but do not allow the clinician to determine attachment loss in the furcation. It appears that radiographs alone do not detect the furcation lesion with any predictable accuracy and that probing the furcation areas is necessary to confirm the presence and severity of furcation defect.

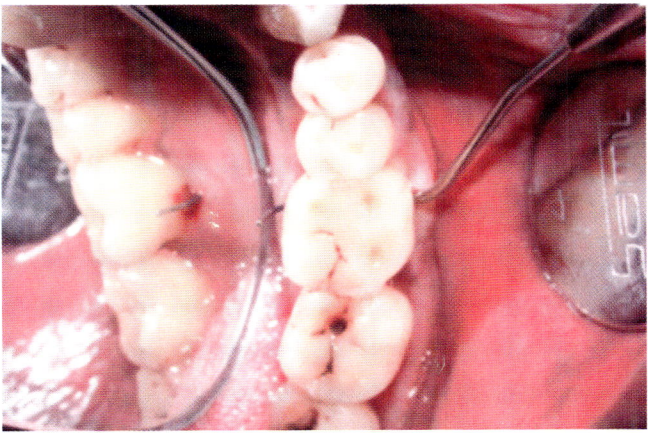

Fig. 30.27: Grade III furcation defect (Through and through)

In 1953, Glickman classified furcation defect into four grades.

Grade I : It is the incipient stage of furcation involvement, but radiographically changes are not usually found.

Grade II : The furcation lesion is a cul-de-sac with a definite horizontal component. Radiographs may or may not depict the furcation involvement.

Grade III : The bone is not attached to the dome of the furcation. Class III furcations display the defect as a radiolucent area in the crotch of the tooth **(Fig. 30.27)**.

Grade IV : The interdental bone is destroyed and soft tissues have receded apically so that the furcation opening is clinically visible.

Determination of disease activity: The determination of pocket depth or attachment levels does not provide information on whether the lesion is in an active or inactive state.

Inactive lesion: There is little or no bleeding and minimal amounts of gingival fluid. It is characterized by greater number of coccoid cells and intact pocket epithelium.

Active lesion: Readily bleed on probing and large amounts of gingival fluid and exudate is present. It is characterized by greater number of spirochetes and motile bacteria. Pocket epithelium is ulcerated and infiltrated mainly by plasma cells and PMNs.

Abscesses

Gingival abscess is a localized painful, rapidly expanding lesion usually of sudden onset. It is generally limited to the marginal gingiva or interdental papilla. It may be due to irritation from foreign substances, toothbrush

PERIODONTICS REVISITED

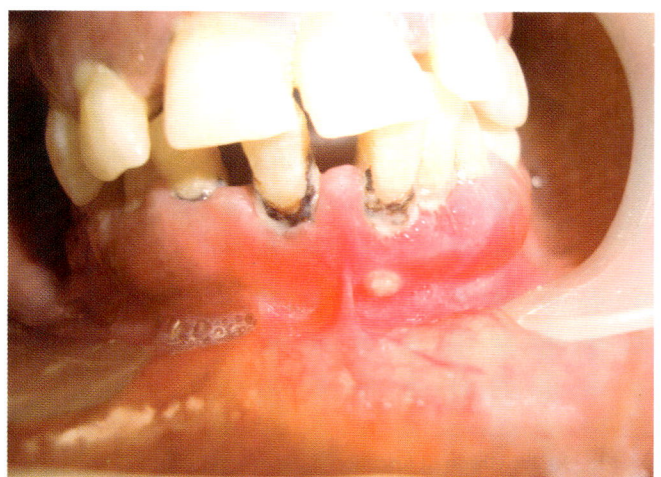

Fig. 30.28: Periodontal abscess

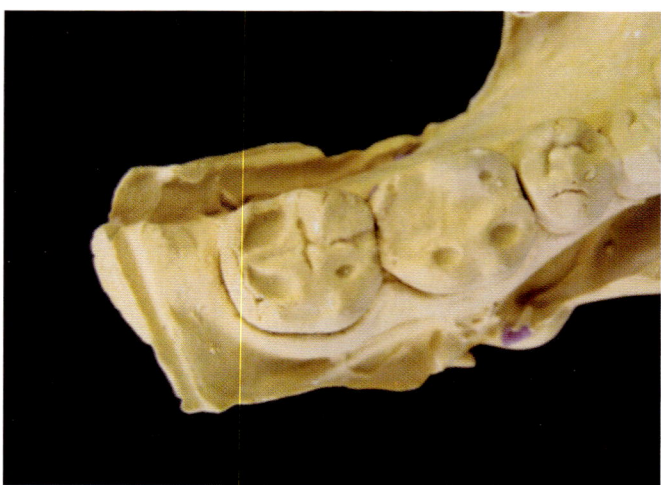

Fig. 30.29: Cast showing attrition

bristle, applecore or lobster shell forcefully embedded into the gingiva.

Several characteristics can be used as guidelines in differentiating a periodontal abscess from a periapical abscess. If the tooth is nonvital, the lesion is most likely periapical. When the apex and lateral surface of a root are involved by a single lesion that can be probed directly from the gingival margin, the lesion is more likely to have originated in a periodontal abscess **(Fig. 30.28)**. More is explained in chapter no. 23—Periodontal Abscess.

RADIOGRAPHIC EXAMINATION

Radiographs are essential adjuncts to other means of assessment when planning the complete care program for the patient. The radiographic survey of full mouth should consist of a minimum of 14 intraoral films and four posterior bitewing films. Rest is explained in chapter no. 31—Radiographic Diagnostic aids.

LABORATORY INVESTIGATIONS

Medical laboratory tests are indicated when more information is needed about the patient's medical status or to help the dentist more precisely to determine the cause or prognosis of periodontal disease.

Blood tests, urine tests, blood smears and biopsies are indicated to identify the systemic factors that might affect or modify periodontal treatment. Analysis of blood smears, red and white blood cell counts, white blood cell differential counts and erythrocyte sedimentation rates are used to evaluate the presence of blood dyscrasias and generalized infections. Determination of coagulation time, bleeding time, clot retraction time, prothrombin time, capillary fragility test and international normalized ratio (INR) may be required at times.

Microbiological testing: Although microbiological testing is not indicated for the majority of periodontal patients, it may help the dentist to more precisely define the cause of periodontal disease and guide therapy for specific patients. It is important to know whether such patients have persistent periodontal infections with these organisms and to know whether the organisms are sensitive to specific antibiotics. This allows the dentist to control or treat disease by combining mechanical debridement with appropriate antimicrobial chemotherapy. There are a variety of methods of assessing the bacterial flora of patients with periodontal disease. Typically, plaque samples are collected with a curette or a paper point. These samples can be analyzed using phase-contrast or dark-field microscopy, bacterial enzyme analysis, immunoassay, DNA probes, polymerase chain reaction or traditional microbiological culturing and sensitivity.

Others

Casts indicate the position of the gingival margins and the position and inclination of the teeth, proximal contact relationships, wasting diseases **(Fig. 30.29)**, food impaction areas and lingual-cuspal relationships. Casts also serve as visual aids in discussions with the patient and are useful for pre- and post-treatment comparisons, as well as for reference at check-up visits.

Color photographs are useful for recording the appearance of the tissue before and after treatment.

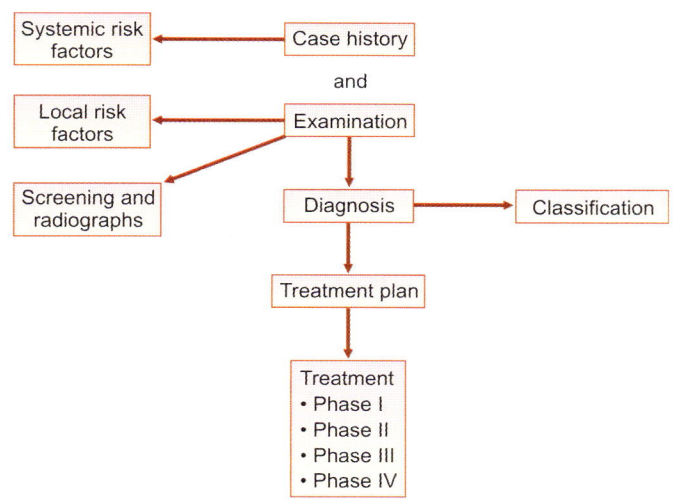

Fig. 30.30: Key stages of management of periodontal patient

Thus, periodontal patients can be well managed after taking proper history, examination and diagnosis **(Fig. 30.30).**

POINTS TO PONDER

✓ Gingivitis toxica is a specific type of gingivitis in which there is destruction of gingiva and the underlying bone due to the chewing of tobacco.

✓ INR, i.e. international normalized ratio is usually 0.9-1.3 for healthy person. An INR of 2.0-3.0 is recommended for people on warfarin therapy except prosthetic mechanical heart valves and prophylaxis of recurrent MI, for which higher intensity warfarin therapy (INR 2.5 to 3.5) is suggested.

✓ Infrabony pocket can be differentiated clinically from suprabony pocket by inserting the probe parallel to the long axis of the tooth and pulling it towards the gingiva, if bony resistance is felt the pocket is said to be infrabony. Bony resistance felt is the bony wall of the infrabony pocket, as the base of the pocket is apical to the alveolar crest.

BIBLIOGRAPHY

1. Armitage GC. Clinical periodontal examination. In, Genco RJ, Goldman HM Cohen DW (Eds). Contemporary Periodontics CV Mosby Company 1990;339-47.
2. Armitage GC. Clinical periodontal examination. In, Rose LF, Mealey BL, Genco RJ, Cohen DW (Eds). Periodontics, Medicine, surgery and implants. Elsevier Mosby 2004;134-45.
3. Carranza FA. Clinical diagnosis. In, Newman, Takei, Carranza. Clinical periodontology 9th ed WB Saunders 2003;432-53.
4. Genco RJ. Periodontal diagnosis, prognosis and treatment planning. In, Genco RJ, Goldman HM, and Cohen DW. Contemporary Periodontics CV Mosby Company 1990;348-60.
5. Lindhe J, Karring T, Lang NP. Examination of patients with Periodontal Disease. In, Clinical periodontology and implant dentistry 4th ed Blackwell Munksgaard 2003;403-13.
6. Pihlstrom BL. Periodontal risk assessment, diagnosis and treatment planning. Periodontol 2000 2001;25:37-58
7. Rhodus NL, Taybos GM. Physical and extraoral examination. In, Daniel SJ, Harfst SA. Dental Hygiene - Concepts, Cases and Competencies. Mosby's 2004;214-27.
8. Serio FG, Stilley KR. Periodontal examination. In, Daniel SJ, Harfst SA. Dental Hygiene - Concepts, Cases and Competencies Mosby's 2004;282-308.
9. Wilkins EM (Eds). Examination procedures. In, Clinical practice of the dental hygienist. Lippincott Williams and Wilkins; 201-23.
10. Wilkins EM. Extraoral and Intraoral examination. In, Clinical practice of the dental hygienist. Lippincott Williams and Wilkins; 116-33.

MCQs

1. Lymph node enlargement is usually not seen in:
   A. NUG
   B. Herpetic gingivostomatitis
   C. Pericoronitis
   D. Plaque-induced gingivitis

2. Bruxism is associated with:
   A. Advanced attrition
   B. Increased tooth mobility pattern
   C. Hypertonicity of the muscles of mastication
   D. Temporomandibular joint discomfort
   E. All of the above

3. When evaluating the col area with a periodontal probe, the clinician should:
   A. Position the length of the probe parallel to the CEJ
   B. Position the length of the probe parallel to the long axis of the tooth
   C. Slant the probe so that the tip of the probe reaches under the contact area
   D. Use a furcation probe instead of a calibrated periodontal probe

4. Moderate furcation involvement with bone destruction to the extent that a probe can enter the furcation area but not pass through and through the furcation is classified as:
   A. Class I   B. Class II
   C. Class III   D. Class IV

5. Which gingival condition usually is MOST characteristic of phenytoin-induced gingival overgrowth (PIGO):
   A. Bulbous and fibrous interdental papillae
   B. Bulbous and erythematous attached gingiva
   C. Festooned margins
   D. Cratered interdental papillae with exudate
   E. Pink tight gingiva with clefting

6. Abnormal tooth mobility may be initiated by each of the following *except*:
   A. Hyperparathyroidism
   B. Traumatic occlusion
   C. Resorption of alveolar bone
   D. Diabetes

7. If the probing pocket depth is 6 mm and gingival recession is 2 mm then the total clinical attachment loss is:
   A. 8 mm
   B. 2 mm
   C. 6 mm
   D. 4 mm

8. The best way to detect bony defects is:
   A. Surgical exposure
   B. Careful history taking
   C. Radiograph at different angulations
   D. Careful probing and measuring pocket depth

9. Which of the following statement best describes the process of attrition:
   A. The wearing of tooth substance by exogenous material forced over the surface by incisive, masticatory, or tooth-cleaning functions
   B. The superficial loss of dental hard tissue due to a chemical process not involving bacteria
   C. Tooth wear caused by tooth-to-tooth contact without the presence of exogenous material
   D. "Flexure" at the cervical region of the tooth, causing loss of mineral
   E. None of the above

10. Which of the following statement best describes the process of abrasion:
    A. The wearing of tooth substance by exogenous material forced over the surface by incisive, masticatory, or tooth - cleaning functions
    B. The superficial loss of dental hard tissue due to a chemical process not involving bacteria
    C. Tooth wear caused by tooth-to-tooth contact without the presence of exogenous material
    D. "Flexure" at the cervical region of the tooth, causing loss of mineral

11. Tension test is done to:
    A. Locate frenal attachment
    B. Detects the adequacy of the width of attached gingiva.
    C. Trauma from occlusion
    D. A and B both

Answers

1. D	2. E	3. C	4. B	5. A
6. D	7. A	8. A	9. C	10. A
11. D				

CHAPTER 31

Radiographic Diagnostic Aids

Shalu Bathla, Amit Aggarwal

INTRODUCTION

Radiographs are an integral component of a periodontal assessment for those with clinical evidence of periodontal destruction. A close consideration of the current approach to periodontal diagnosis compatible with the current classification of periodontal diseases reveals that radiographs provide information with respect to diagnosis of various periodontal diseases. Both clinical and radiographic data are essential for diagnosing the presence and extent of periodontal disease.

Radiographs are considered as a valuable adjunct to the clinical examination, because essential information is provided about the bony tissues covered by the gingiva that cannot be diagnosed by clinical inspection alone. Radiographic image formation is based on the principle of projecting a three-dimensional object onto a two-dimensional image plane, and therefore this technique also has limitations. The radiographic image, in principle, lacks information about the third dimension, at least in a way that is easily perceptible by the human visual system.

DIAGNOSTIC REQUIREMENTS OF RADIOGRAPHS

In order to be useful for the purpose of diagnosis, radiographs have to satisfy the requirements of standardization and reproducibility. The ideal radiographic procedure should also facilitate the collection of quantitative data with regard to the condition of lesion areas and should provide sufficient information about the shape and the extent of the lesion in three dimensions. These requirements are even more important in the radiographic diagnosis of periodontal disease. Following points should also be kept in mind:
1. Radiographs should only be considered following a full clinical examination.
2. A provisional diagnosis should be made with the choice of radiographs based on the type, severity and distribution of disease.
3. Radiographs taken for reasons other than periodontal disease (e.g. horizontal bitewings for caries diagnosis) will often provide useful information and should be examined before further radiographs are requested.

4. Prichard established the following four criteria to determine the adequate angulation of periapical radiographs:
- The radiographs should show the tips of molar cusps with little or none of the occlusal surface
- Enamel caps and pulp chambers should be distinct
- Interproximal spaces should be open
- Proximal contacts should not overlap unless teeth are out of line anatomically.

RADIOGRAPHIC TECHNIQUES FOR ASSESSING PERIODONTAL DISEASES

A variety of radiographic exposure types assist in the development of periodontal treatment plans.

Panoramic radiographs: Panoramic radiographs provide a general view of the oral structures, and are useful for screening bone loss patterns in general. They are not suitable for accurate assessment of the degree of bone loss associated with individual teeth, as there is severe distortion and the outline of the bone margin is often unclear due to superimposition of intervening structures. Panoramic view is useful when assessing generalized periodontitis, where large areas of jaws have to be viewed **(Fig. 31.1)**. Panoramic oral radiographs can be supplemented by intraoral views.

Periapical radiographs: Periapical radiographs are frequently used not only to aid the differential diagnosis of patient's presenting symptoms, but also to screen for otherwise undetected pathological processes of the teeth and surrounding alveolar bone. In the diagnosis of periodontal diseases, periapical radiographs can provide useful information that cannot be obtained through examination of the soft tissues alone **(Fig. 31.2)**.

Bitewing radiographs: These are taken to show the proximal surfaces of the teeth and the crest of the alveolar bone of both the maxilla and the mandible on the same film **(Fig. 31.3)**. While they are used primarily to detect interproximal decay, they can also provide some information on the patient's periodontal status. The height of the interproximal alveolar bone margin relative to the cementoenamel junction can be observed. Also, deposits of subgingival calculus may be detected. However, the value of bitewing radiographs in the diagnosis of periodontal diseases is limited by the fact that only the coronal sections of the roots of the teeth are observed, and they are limited to the molar-premolar

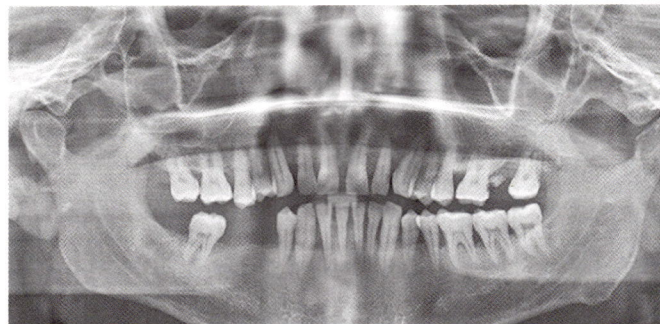

Fig. 31.1: Panoramic oral radiograph (OPG)

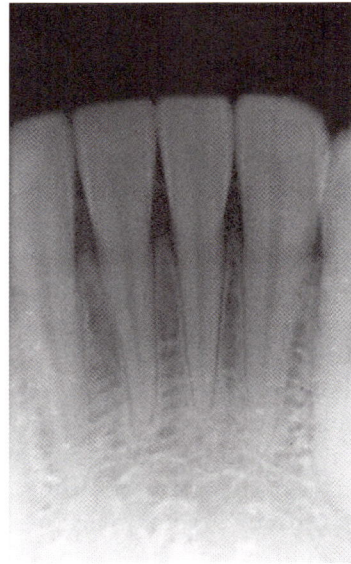

Fig. 31.2: Intraoral periapical radiograph (IOPA)

TABLE 31.1. Types of radiographs required in various periodontal diseases

Gingivitis		No radiographs are indicated
Localized Periodontitis		
Posterior teeth	Mild	Radiographs not usually indicated
	Moderate	Bitewings or periapical if furcation involvement
	Severe	Periapical radiographs of affected teeth or Panoramic +/- Periapical
Anterior teeth	Mild	Radiographs not usually indicated
	Moderate	Periapical radiographs
	Severe	Periapical radiographs
Generalized Periodontitis		
	Mild	Radiographs not usually indicated
	Moderate	Panoramic + periapical or bitewings of specific areas
	Severe	Panoramic or periapical of standing teeth

regions. The posterior bitewing projection offers both optimal geometry and the fine detail of intraoral radiography for patients with small amounts of uniform bone loss.

RADIOGRAPHIC FEATURES OF HEALTHY PERIODONTIUM

Alveolar Bone

In an individual, the dense cortical alveolar bone forming the wall of the socket of tooth appears radiographically as a distinct, opaque, uninterrupted, white line parallel

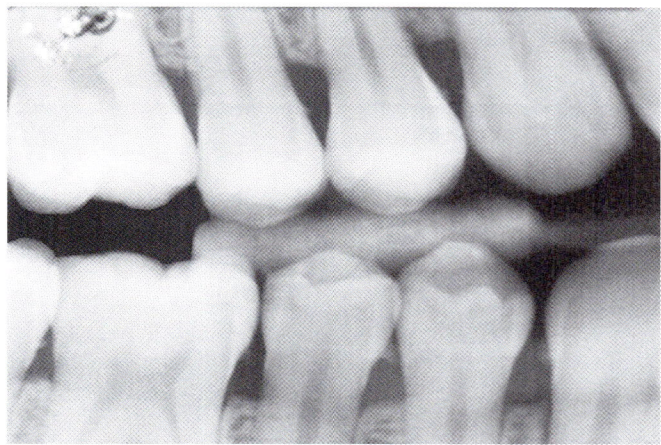

Fig. 31.3: Bitewing radiograph

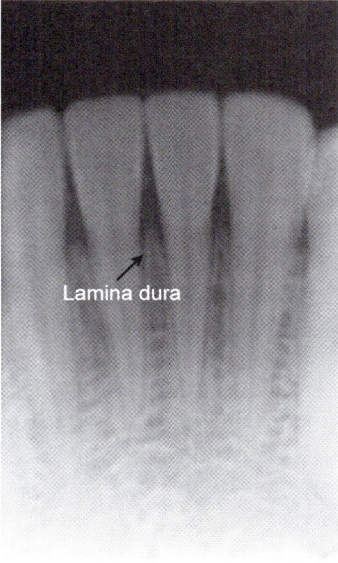

Lamina dura

Fig. 31.4: Ideal IOPA

to the tooth root. This is known as the *lamina dura* **(Fig. 31.4)**. The lamina dura is a continuation of the jawbone cortex, which encases the root in a socket of cortical bone.

Normal, healthy alveolar bone has characteristic appearance on radiograph. The alveolar crest in a young individual is close to the cementoenamel junction. The alveolar crests are situated approximately 2 to 3 mm apical to the cementoenamel junction of the teeth. The shape of the alveolar crest may vary from rounded to flat.

Between incisor teeth, the alveolar crest will usually appear pointed. Between premolar and molar teeth the alveolar crest will be parallel to a line between the adjacent CEJs, where the enamel thins and disappears. The alveolar crest will be continuous with the lamina dura of the adjacent teeth. When viewing the lamina dura and the periodontal ligament, only the interproximal portions are visible. The buccal and lingual areas are not seen in the radiograph. Widening of the periodontal ligament space and loss of lamina dura can be interpreted as resorption of the alveolar bone. The trabecular pattern of interdental bone is distinct and fills the inter-radicular space.

Although these are the usual features of healthy periodontium, they are not always evident. Their absence from radiographs does not necessarily mean that periodontal disease is present. Failure to see these features may be due to technical error, overexposure or normal anatomic variation in alveolar bone shape and density.

Interdental Septa

The interdental septum, or septal bone, is located between the roots of adjacent teeth. It is therefore more clearly visualized than bone that is located on the buccal or lingual aspect of the tooth (the latter being partially obscured by the superimposed image of the root). The shape of the interdental septum is a function of the morphology of the contiguous teeth.

Periodontal Ligament Space

The periodontal ligament is composed of connective tissue which appears as a fine, black, radiolucent line next to the root surface. The radiolucent image between the lamina dura and tooth is the periodontal space and is known radiographically as the *lamina lucida*. With disease, the periodontal ligament space may appear at varying thicknesses. A widened

PERIODONTICS REVISITED

TABLE 31.2. Uses of radiographic assessment in periodontal tissues

Radiographs are helpful in evaluation of the following:
Amount of bone present
Condition of the alveolar crests
Bone loss in the furcation areas
Width of the periodontal ligament

periodontal space is considered to be a sign of chronic inflammation. On the other hand, the periodontal ligament space may vary in width from patient to patient, from tooth to tooth in the individual and even from location to location around one tooth.

RADIOGRAPHIC CHANGES IN VARIOUS PERIODONTAL CONDITIONS

Osseous Defects

- *Horizontal bone loss*: Clinically, horizontal bone loss is seen in suprabony pocket. Radiographically, horizontal bone loss appears as decreased alveolar marginal bone around adjacent teeth. Normally, the crestal bone is located 1-2 mm apical to the cementoenamel junction. With horizontal bone loss, both the buccal and lingual plates of bone, as well as interdental bone resorbs. The remaining bone margin is roughly perpendicular to long axis of tooth, which occurs when the epithelial attachment is coronal to the bony defect **(Fig. 31.5)**.
- *Vertical bone loss*: Clinically, vertical bone loss is seen in infrabony pocket which occurs when the walls of the pocket are within a bony housing. Radio-

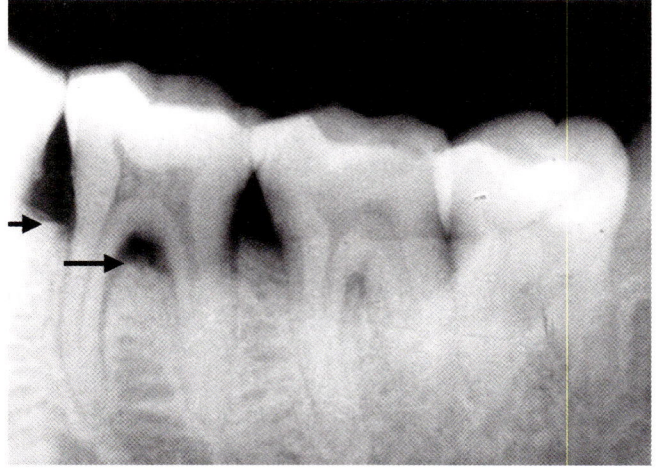

Fig. 31.5: IOPA showing horizontal bone loss and furcation defect

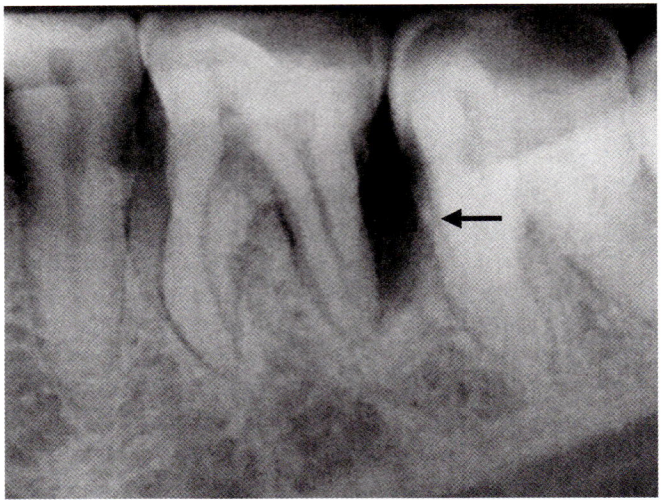

Fig. 31.6: IOPA showing vertical bone loss

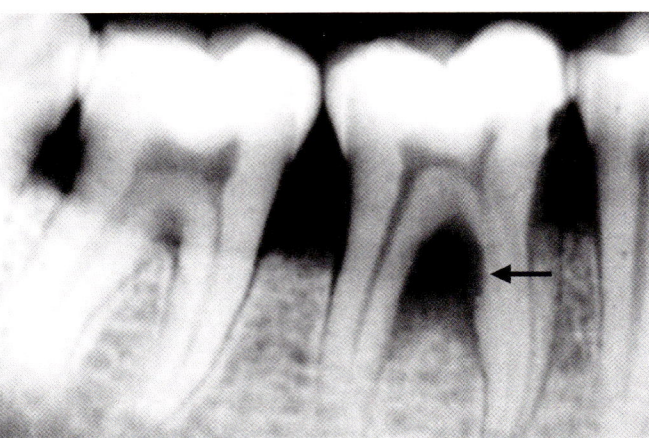

Fig. 31.7: IOPA showing furcation involvement of mandibular first molar

graphically, vertical bone defects are generally V-shaped and are sharply outlined **(Fig. 31.6)**.

- *Furcation defects*: The furcation is where multiple tooth roots divide at the trunk of the tooth. The furcation is a normal structure usually filled with bone. Furcation exposure results from intra-radicular bone loss due to advanced periodontal disease. In Class I (incipient) furcation involvement there is a decreased density of the bone at the furcation. Bone loss at the furcation may or may not be seen in Class II furcation defect. But in Class III (through and through) there will be an area of complete bone loss visible radiographically. Advanced furcation exposures, where both cortical plates are resorbed, are easily recognized on radiographs **(Fig. 31.7)**. Because most maxillary molars have three roots, early change in their furcation areas are more difficult to assess. Bone loss in the facial furcation may occasionally be detected on radiographs, but the superimposition of the palatal root makes such detection difficult. Defects occurring between the mesiobuccal and palatal roots and between the distobuccal and palatal roots often are easier to detect radiographically. Lesions involving these mesial and distal furcations often are manifested by the presence of furcation "arrows". The slightest radiographic change in the furcation area should be investigated clinically, especially if there is bone loss on adjacent roots. Diminished radiodensity in the furcation area in which outlines of bony trabeculae are visible suggests furcation involvement. Whenever there is marked bone loss in relation to a single molar root, it may be assumed that the furcation is also involved.

• *Interdental craters*: Interdental craters are seen as irregular areas of reduced radiopacity on the alveolar bone crests. They are generally not sharply demarcated from the rest of the bone, with which they blend gradually. Radiographs do not accurately depict the morphology or depth of interdental craters, which sometimes appear as vertical defects. Like the two-walled crater, this defect may be difficult to visualize on the radiograph, because the buccal and lingual walls remain intact and obscure the radiographic image of the defect.

Chronic Periodontitis

Following is the sequence of radiographic changes in periodontitis and the tissue changes that produce them:

i. There is fuzziness and break in the continuity of the lamina dura at the mesial or distal aspect of the crest of the interdental septum. These result from the extension of gingival inflammation into the bone causing widening of the vessel channels and a reduction in calcified tissue at the septal margin.

ii. Triangulation (Funnelling): Triangulation is the widening of the periodontal ligament space by the resorption of bone along either the mesial or distal aspect of the interdental (interseptal) crestal bone. The sides of the triangle are formed by the alveolar bone and root surfaces, the base is towards the tooth crown, and the apex of the triangle is pointed towards the root. This is an early sign of bone degeneration and necessitates a search for possible etiologic factors, such as plaque, calculus, gingivitis, or food impaction.

iii. The destructive process extends across the crest of the interdental septum and the height is reduced.

Fingerlike radiolucent projections extend from the crest into the septum. The radiolucent projections into the interdental septum are the result of the deeper extension of the inflammation into the bone.

iv. The height of the interdental septum is progressively reduced by the extension of inflammation and the resorption of bone.

Aggressive Periodontitis

The radiographic appearance is typically that of deep vertical bone loss with a marked predilection for the first molar and central incisor regions with relative sparing of other segments of the dentition. There is an *arc-shaped loss of alveolar bone* extending from the distal surface of the second premolar to the mesial surface of the second molar. It is usually bilaterally symmetrical in both the first molars of each jaw.

Periodontal Abscesses

The typical radiographic appearance of the periodontal abscess is that of a discrete area of radiolucency along the lateral aspect of the root. However, the radiographic picture is often not typical therefore, it cannot be relied upon for the diagnosis of a periodontal abscess.

Conditions Associated with Periodontal Diseases

Various changes in teeth and its supporting structures are associated with periodontal diseases. These include occlusal trauma and local irritants.

Trauma from occlusion: Traumatic occlusion by itself does not cause periodontitis but can result in some traumatic lesion in response to occlusal pressures which are greater than the physiological tolerances of the tooth's supporting structures. In addition to clinical features, trauma from occlusion can produce radiographically detectable changes in the lamina dura, morphology of the alveolar crest, width of the periodontal ligament space, and density of the surrounding cancellous bone. The injury phase of trauma from occlusion produces a loss of the lamina dura at apices, furcations, and/or marginal areas. This loss of lamina dura results in widening of the periodontal ligament space. The repair phase of trauma from occlusion radiographically show widening of the periodontal ligament space, which may be generalized or localized. More advanced traumatic lesions may result in deep angular bone loss, which, when combined with marginal inflammation, may lead to intrabony pocket formation. In terminal stages these lesions extend around the root apex, producing a wide radiolucent periapical image.

PERIODONTICS REVISITED

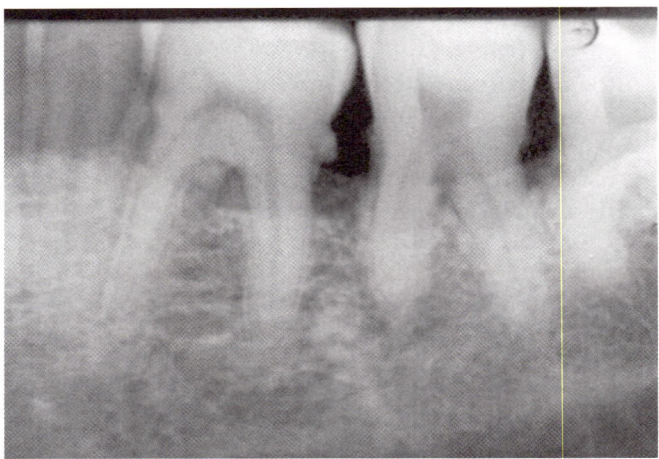

Fig. 31.8: IOPA showing subgingival calculus around mandibular first molar

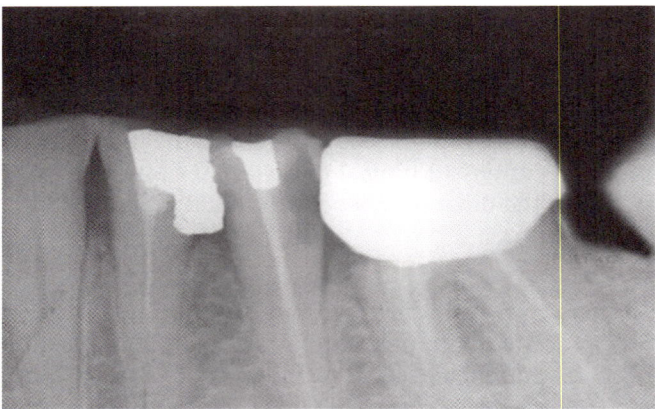

Fig. 31.9: IOPA showing overhanging restorations in mandibular first premolar and molar

Local irritating factors: Many local factors contribute towards periodontal disease. Some of these factors can be visualised on the radiographs. These include calculus deposits **(Fig. 31.8)**, overhanging restorations **(Fig. 31.9)**, lack of local contact points, malposed teeth, partial dentures, faulty restorations and caries. The clinician should not interpret the absence of radiographic calculus as indicative of an absence of calculus clinically, because most subgingival calculus deposits will not be present radiographically.

SKELETAL DISTURBANCES MANIFESTED IN THE JAWS

Skeletal disturbances sometime produce changes in the jaws that affect the interpretation of radiographs from the periodontal perspective.

In scleroderma, the periodontal ligament is uniformly widened at the expense of the surrounding alveolar bone.

In Osteitis fibrosa cystica (Von Recklinghausen's disease of bone) there is osteoclastic resorption of bone creating a mass known as brown tumor. There is generalized disappearance of the lamina dura.

In Paget's disease, the normal trabecular pattern is replaced by a hazy, diffuse meshwork of closely knit, fine trabecular markings. The lamina dura is absent in it.

In Fibrous dysplasia, there is small radiolucent area at a root apex or an extensive radiolucent area with irregularly arranged trabecular markings. There may be enlargement of the cancellous spaces, with distortion of the normal trabecular pattern giving a ground glass appearance and obliteration of the lamina dura.

In osteopetrosis, the outlines of the roots may be obscured by diffuse radiopacity of the jaws.

LIMITATIONS OF CONVENTIONAL RADIOGRAPHS

1. Conventional radiographs provide a two dimensional image of complex, three dimensional anatomy, which may result in following problems in periodontal assessment:
   - Difficult to differentiate between buccal and lingual crestal bone levels.
   - One wall defects may obscure the rest of the defects.
   - Tooth or restoration shadows may obscure bone defects and resorption in furcation area.
2. Due to superimposition, the details of the bony architecture may be lost.
3. Radiographs do not demonstrate incipient disease, as a minimum of 55-60% demineralization must occur before radiographic changes are apparent.
4. Radiographs do not reliably demonstrate soft tissue contours, and do not record changes in the soft tissues of the periodontium.
5. Technique variations can affect the appearance of the periodontal tissues.
6. Overexposure may lead to false interpretations – 'burn-out' phenomenon.
7. Panoramic radiographs cannot be completely relied upon although they do provide a reasonable overview of periodontal status.

ADVANCED RADIOGRAPHIC AIDS

Many clinicians are adopting digital X-ray systems to replace conventional film-based images because more than

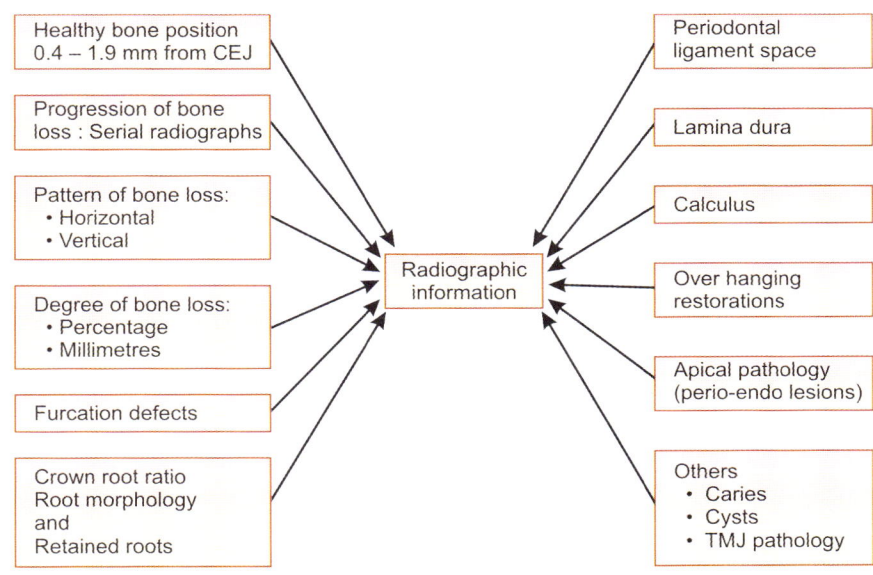

Fig. 31.10: Key aspects of a radiographic periodontal assessment

30% of the bone mass at the alveolar crest must be lost for a change in bone height to be recognized on radiographs. Therefore, conventional radiographs are very specific but lack sensitivity. Because periodontal bone change can be subtle, digital subtraction radiography (DSR) techniques (software algorithms) have been developed.

Digital radiography enables the use of computerized images, which can be stored, manipulated, and corrected for under- and overexposures. There is an important dose reduction obtained with this technique (between 1/3 to 1/2 of dose reduction compared with conventional radiographs). Two digital radiography systems rely on the sensor–the direct and indirect methods. The direct method uses a charge coupled device (CCD) sensor linked with a fiber optic or other wire to the computer system. This direct digital radiography obtains real-time imaging, offering both the clinician and the patient an improved visualization of the periodontium by image manipulation and comparison with previously stored images. The indirect method (Digora System) uses a phosphor luminescence plate, which is a flexible filmlike radiation energy sensor placed intraorally and exposed to conventional X-ray tubes. A laser scanner reads the exposed plates offline and reveals digital image data, which can be enhanced, stored and compared with previous images.

Subtraction Radiography: This technique relies on the conversion of serial radiographs into digital images. The serially obtained digital images can then be superimposed and the resultant composite viewed on a video screen. Changes in the density and/or volume of bone can be detected as lighter areas (bone gain) or dark areas (bone loss). In the DSR technique, a second image is taken at some point after the initial image. The images are then compared after normalization and image alignment. The elements that remain unchanged are subtracted from the two images and the remaining image information is displayed. Using pseudocolorization techniques, only the areas that changes are visible to the dentist.

Computer Assisted Densitometric Image Analysis System (CADIA): In this system, a video camera measures the light transmitted through a radiograph, and the signals from the camera are converted into gray-scale images. The camera is interfaced with an image processor and a computer that allow the storage and mathematical manipulation of the images.

POINTS TO PONDER

✓ Because of the improper vertical angulation or orientation of the tipped tooth, the CEJ is positioned inferiorly relative to the adjacent tooth. This creates the impression of a vertical bony defect when in reality there is no bony defect.

BIBLIOGRAPHY

1. Carranza FA, Takei HH. Radiographic aids in the diagnosis of periodontal disease. In, Newman, Takei, Carranza. Clinical Periodontology 9th ed WB Saunders 2003;454-68.

PERIODONTICS REVISITED

2. Eric Whaites. Periodontal tissues and Periodontal diseases. In, Essentials of Dental Radiography and Radiology 3rd ed Churchill Livingstone, Elsevier 2003;241-52.

3. Heitor C, Moreira C, Fiorini T, Ferreira E, Antoniazzi R, Cassiano. Use of Radiographs for Periodontal Diagnosis in Private Practice. Acta Odontol Latinoam 2007;20:33-37.

4. Karjodkar FR. Periodontal tissues and Periodontal diseases. In, Textbook of Dental and Maxillofacial Radiology. 2nd ed Jaypee Brothers 2009;419-32.

5. Khocht A, Janal M, Harasty L, Chang KM. Comparison of direct digital and conventional intraoral radiographs in detecting alveolar bone loss. JADA 2003;134:1468-75.

6. Lanning SK, Best AM, Temple HJ, Richards PS, Carey A, McCauley LK. Accuracy and Consistency of Radiographic Interpretation among Clinical Instructors Using Two Viewing Systems. J Dent Educ. 2006;70(2):149-59.

7. Miles DA, Thomas MV. Radiography for the periodontal examination. In, Rose LF, Mealey BL, Genco RJ, Cohen DW. Periodontics, Medicine, Surgery and Implants. Elsevier Mosby 2004;146-61.

8. Nyman S, Lindhe J. Examination of Patients with Periodontal Disease. In, Lindhe J, Karring T, Lang NP. Clinical Periodontology and Implant dentistry. 4th ed Blackwell Munksgaard 2003;403-13.

9. Reddy MS. Radiographic methods in the evaluation of periodontal therapy. J Periodontol 1992;63:1078-84.

10. Sanz M, Newman MG. Advanced Diagnostic Techniques. In, Newman, Takei, Carranza. Clinical Periodontology 9th ed WB Saunders 2003;487-502.

11. The use of Dental Radiographs–update and recommendations. American Dental Association Council on Scientific Affairs. JADA 2006;137:1304-12.

12. White SC, Pharoah MJ. Periodontal tissues and Periodontal diseases. In, Oral Radiology-Principles and Interpretation 5th ed Mosby 2000;314-29.

MCQs

1. Triangulation or Funnelling is:
   A. Indistinctness of continuity of lamina dura on mesial or distal aspect of tooth.
   B. Widening of periodontal ligament space by resorption of bone along either mesial or distal aspect of crestal bone.
   C. Interseptal bone changes
   D. Vertical bone loss.

2. The bone loss in aggressive periodontitis is usually:
   A. Vertical (angular) bone loss
   B. Horizontal bone loss
   C. Interdental crater
   D. None of the above

Answers

   1. B   2. A

CHAPTER 32

Microbiological and Immunological Diagnostic Aids

Shalu Bathla

INTRODUCTION

Subgingival oral bacteria are the main initiating agents in the development of periodontal diseases, thus it is logical to look for specific bacteria through the various microbiological methods. These, microbiologic tests have potential relevance to both diagnosis and treatment because current clinical diagnostic methods are not precisely accurate and only allow retrospective diagnosis of attachment and bone loss. Thus, diagnostic tests would need to be predictive of disease activity rather than just correlate with its occurrence.

INDICATIONS OF MICROBIOLOGIC ASSAYS

1. During initial diagnosis and treatment planning: Clinical studies show that most chronic periodontitis patients can be successfully treated by thorough mechanical debridement of the root surface or by means of topical adjunctive antimicrobials applied at the time of scaling and root planing. There are certain patients, however who do not respond well to this local therapy. These patients include those with refractory periodontitis, recurrent periodontitis and aggressive periodontitis. Microbiological assays are

often indicated in these patients as an adjunct to the usual clinical and radiographic examinations in the formulation of an etiology based diagnosis.

2. To monitor treatment efficacy: Microbiologic assays can tell the clinician if the mechanical, surgical and chemotherapeutic approach has been effective in eliminating the microbial etiology identified initially.

3. To select an appropriate recall interval: After periodontal therapy has been completed, microbiologic tests using pooled plaque samples can be useful in determining the rate of reinfection, if any, by periodontal pathogens as an additional parameter to be assessed in determining an individual patient's optimum recall interval.

4. To determine sites of "active" tissue destruction: Related to the selection of an appropriate treatment or recall interval is the determination of which sites are subject to "active" tissue destruction. Clinically, these are determined by changes in probing attachment level measured. Appropriate samples for analysis of site – specific tissue destruction include subgingival plaque from the site or tooth in question, and these can be analyzed by rapid tests targeted to specific periodontal pathogens.

5. To identify antibiotic susceptibility of infecting organisms colonizing diseased sites.

6. For prevention of periodontitis in persons "at risk" for either the initial onset of periodontal disease or for recurrent disease.

SAMPLING DENTAL PLAQUE FOR MICROBIOLOGIC ANALYSIS

In the case of plaque samples, subgingival plaque is the most appropriate for analysis, since it is in close contact with the gingiva and epithelial attachment and is more likely to contain higher numbers and proportions of those microorganisms than supragingival plaque. Other materials that have been used as patient samples in determining periodontal status include supragingival dental plaque, scrappings from oral soft tissue surfaces, saliva, and gingival crevicular fluid.

Subgingival dental plaque can be sampled in several ways. One really expeditious and noninvasive method for sampling subgingival dental plaque involves the use of sterile endodontic paper points. A site or sites of interest is selected and isolated with cotton rolls to prevent contamination of the sample with bacteria in saliva and then air dried. Supragingival plaque is removed using either a sterile cotton pellet or a sterile curette. The instrument is moved in a coronal direction to avoid pushing supragingival plaque into subgingival space. Subgingival plaque can be sampled using a sterile curette. Again, after the sample site has been isolated and the supragingival dental plaque removed as described above, a curette is placed to the depth of the gingival sulcus/periodontal pocket and moved coronally with firm lateral pressure against the root surface. The material is then dislodged from the curette tip into the transport medium, sterilized in a salt sterilizer, and then used to sample the next site. Some investigators advocate the use of nickel – plated curettes as a means of avoiding oxidation within the sample and the death of oxygen-intolerant anaerobic microorganisms.

CANDIDATES FOR BIOMARKERS

The main candidates in the search for biomarkers are:
1. Micro-organisms (Bacteria)
2. Bacterial products (Enzymes)
3. Inflammatory and immune products
4. Enzymes released from dead cells
5. Connective tissue degradation products
6. Products of bone resorption and formation

Microorganisms (Bacteria)

Bacterial plaque plays a primary role in the initiation and progression of periodontal diseases but the composition of the subgingival flora is complex and may vary from patient to patient and site to site. Samples from the oral mucosa or saliva are obtained with sterile paper points or swabs and then transferred directly into an appropriate anaerobic transport medium.

The various diagnostic aids for detecting bacteria are: Culture techniques, dark field microscopy, immuno-diagnostic method, DNA probes, restriction endonuclease analysis and polymerase chain reaction (PCR).

***Culture techniques*:** Culture methods aims at characterizing the composition of the subgingival microflora and are still considered the reference method (gold standard) when determining the performance of new microbial diagnostic methods.

Advantages
i. Can obtain relative and absolute count of the cultured species.
ii. Able to assess for antibiotic susceptibility of microbes.

Disadvantages
i. Putative pathogens such as *Treponemas* and *Tannerella forsythia* are fastidious and difficult to culture
ii. Strict sampling and transport conditions are essential
iii. Time consuming and expensive
iv. Sophisticated equipments and experienced personnel are required
v. Can only grow live bacteria

***Dark field microscopy*:** Darkfield or phase contrast microscopy has been suggested as an alternative to culture methods on the basis of its ability to directly and rapidly assess the morphology and motility of bacteria in a plaque sample.

Advantages
i. Through it, motile spirochetes are seen.
ii. Assessment can be done during the progression and treatment

Disadvantages
i. Unable to identify non-motile species
ii. Unable to differentiate among the various species of Treponema.
iii. Inability to determine their relative susceptibility to antimicrobial agent.

***Immunodiagnostic Methods*:** Immunologic assays employ antibodies that recognized specific bacterial antigens to detect target microorganisms. The various immunodiagnostic procedures, are direct and indirect immunofluorescent microscopy assays (IFA), flow cytometry and latex agglutination.

Immunofluorescent microscopy assays: Direct IFA employs both monoclonal and polyclonal antibodies conjugated to a fluorescein marker that binds with the bacterial antigen to form a fluorescent immune-complex detectable under a microscope. Indirect IFA employs a secondary fluorescein-conjugated antibody that reacts with the primary antigen-antibody complex. Both direct and indirect immunofluorescence assays are able to identify the pathogen and quantify the percentage of the pathogen directly using a plaque smear.

Flow cytometry: It involves labelling bacterial cells from a patient plaque sample with both species-specific antibody and a second fluorescein-conjugated antibody. The suspension is then introduced into the flow cytometer, which separates the bacterial cells into an almost single-cell suspension by means of a laminar flow through a narrow tube. The disadvantages associated with it is the sophistication and procedure cost.

Latex agglutination: It is a simple immunological assay based on the binding of protein to latex. Latex beads are coated with the species-specific antibody, and when these beads come in contact with the microbial cell surface antigens or antigen extracts, cross-linking occurs; its agglutination or clumping is then visible usually in 2 to 5 minutes.

Commercial diagnostic test kits
Evalusite is a chairside kit consisting of enzyme-linked immunosorbent assays (ELISA) using antibodies to detect antigens. It is used to detect *A.actinomy-cetemcomitans, P.gingivalis* and *P.intermedius.*

Advantages
• Identify dead target cells, thus not requiring stringent sampling and transport methodology.

Disadvantages
• Local sampling cannot be done, so site - specific disease parameters cannot be assessed.
• Immunoassays cannot be used to determine bacterial virulence.
• Cannot be used to determine antibiotic susceptibility.

Deoxyribonucleic Acid Probes: DNA probes have been developed to identify nucleotide sequences that are specific for bacteria believed to be of diagnostic significance including suspected periodontal pathogens. Deoxyribonucleic acid (DNA) probes entail segments of single-stranded nucleic acid, labelled with an enzyme or radioisotope, that can locate and bind to their complementary nucleic acid sequences with low cross-reactivity to nontarget organisms. DNA probe may target whole genomic DNA or individual genes. To prepare the probe, specific pathogens used as marker organisms are lysed to remove their DNA. Their double helix is denatured, creating single strands that are individually labeled with a radioactive isotope. Subsequently, when a plaque sample is sent for analysis, it undergoes lysis and denaturation. Single strands are chemically treated, attached to a special filter paper, and then exposed to the DNA library. If complementary base pairs hybridize (cross-link), the radiolabeled strands will also be fixed to the filter paper. After the filter is washed to remove any unhybridized strands, it is covered with a radiographic plate. The radioactive labels create spots on the film, which are read with a densitometer. The darkness and size of the spots indicate the concentration of the organisms present in the given plaque sample. The assay can rapidly test for multiple bacteria, including *A. actinomycetemcomitans, P. gingivalis, B. intermedius, C. rectus, E. corrodens, Fusobacterium nucleatum* and *T. denticola* in multiple clinical plaque samples. The probes are able to detect as few as 10^2 to 10^4 bacteria.

Commercial diagnostic test kits
Omnigene: It is DNA probe system for a number of subgingival bacteria. A paper point sample of subgingival plaque is placed in the container provided and mailed off to the company for assay. Microorganisms detected through DNA probe are *Aggregatibacter actinomycetemcomitans, P.gingivalis, B.intermedius, C.rectus, E.corrodens, T. denticola* and *Fusobacterium nucleatum.*

A commercial PCR-based method for the detection of periodontopathic species in subgingival plaque samples (MicroDent test) has been shown to be quicker, easier to use and much more sensitive than culture methods.

Bacterial Products

Enzymatic method of bacterial identification (BANA test):

Trypsin like enzyme is produced by *B. forsythus, P. gingivalis,* the small spirochete *Treponema denticola,* and *Capnocytophaga* species. The activity of this enzyme can be measured with the hydrolysis of the colorless substrate N-benzoyl-dl-arginine-2-naphthylamide (BANA). When the hydrolysis takes place, it releases the chromophore ß-naphthylamide, which turns orange red when a drop of fast garnet is added to the solution.

Disadvantages
i. Lack of quantitative data
ii. Inability to determine which of three bacteria is responsible for the enzyme production.
iii. BANA system does not include inhibitors of host proteinases, which could cleave this substrate and could also contaminate the bacterial sample tested.
iv. Cannot identify the presence of other pathogens that do not produce trypsin like enzymes.

Commercial diagnostic test kit
Perioscan is a chair side diagnostic test kit system, which utilizes the BANA test for detection of bacteria producing trypsin - like proteases **(Fig. 32.1)**. The bacteria detected through Perioscan are *Treponema denticola, P. gingivalis, Tannerella forsythia* and *Capnocytophaga* microorganisms.

Volatile sulphur compounds: Gram-negative bacteria *Porphyromonas gingivalis, Prevotella intermedia, Prevotella melaninogenica, Bacteroides forsythus, Treponema denticola* and *Fusobacterium nucleatum* have been shown to be capable of producing hydrogen sulphide (H_2S), methyl mercaptan (CH_3SH), dimethyl sulphide ($(CH_3)_2S_2$) through their metabolic pathways.

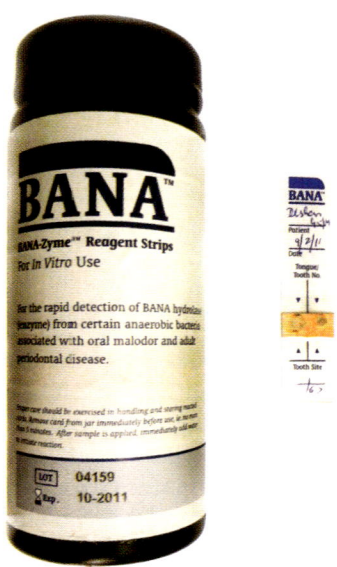

Fig.32.1: BANA chairside kit

Commercial diagnostic test kit
Diamond probe is a recently developed instrument, which combines the features of a periodontal probe with the Silver sulfide sensor for detection of volatile sulphur compounds.

Inflammatory and Immune Products

The microorganisms also trigger inflammatory and immune host response which, along with the direct effects of the bacteria, cause most of the tissue destruction. A number of substances are released from inflammatory and immune cells into the tissues and many of these pass into GCF and are thus, easily available for analysis. Samples of these substances can usually be obtained from GCF through paper strips.

Immune response: Patients with various forms of periodontal disease produce antibodies to antigens from periodontopathogens. These antibodies, total IgG and IgG subgroups and complement component can be detected in serum, saliva, gingival tissue and GCF.

Inflammatory mediators: Arachidonic acid derivatives: Prostaglandin E_2 is a product of the cyclooxygenase pathway of the metabolism of arachidonic acid. It is a potent mediator of inflammation and induces bone resorption. The concentration of prostaglandin E_2 found in GCF is increased during active phases of periodontal destruction whereas levels are low in health.

Cytokines: These are best described as cell to cell messengers or local hormones. They are all small proteins or peptides which are produced and released by one cell type so they can link onto a specific receptor on the cell membrane of another cell(s) of either the same type or another type(s). The best known examples of cytokines are the interleukins (IL) which pass messages between the leukocytes. IL - α and β are present in inflamed gingiva. They are also present in GCF of patients with periodontitis with extremely low concentrations at healthy sites. IL - 8 is secreted by monocytes, macrophages and vascular endothelial cells and mediates chemotaxis and activation of neutrophils. Their levels are reduced in periodontal destruction.

Commercial Diagnostic Test Kits
Periocheck: These commercial kits detects the presence of neutral proteinase such as collagenase in GCF. The GCF sample is collected by paper strip and is placed in contact with a collagen gel to which a blue dye has been covalently bonded. It is then incubated at 43^0C. If the

neutral proteinase is present in the sample, then they will attack the collagen gel and release the blue dye producing blue colour in the strip. The intensity of the colour is proportional to the amount of enzyme present in the sample. The intensity and the area of the blue colour is then scored on a scale of 0 to 2 by comparing it with three standards on a colour card which is provided with the test kit.

Host-derived Enzymes: Various enzymes are released from host cells during the initiation and progression of periodontal disease. The enzymes which are used as markers of active periodontal destruction are asparate aminotransferase, elastase, β-glucuronidase, alkaline phosphatase, arylsulphatase, neutral proteases, cathepsins, lactate dehydrogenase, matrix metalloproteinases and myeloperoxidase.

Cathepsins: These enzymes are a group of acidic lysosomal enzymes that play an important role in intracellular protein degradation.

Alkaline Phosphatase: It is a glycoprotein and membrane bound enzyme. It hydrolyzes monophosphate ester bonds at alkaline pH, increasing local concentrations of phosphate ions. It is produced by many cells, including fibroblasts, osteoblasts and osteoclasts, but the main source of alkaline phosphatase in gingival crevice fluid is neutrophils. Bacteria present in the sulcus or pocket also produce alkaline phosphatase levels in gingival crevice fluid. Alkaline phosphatase in gingival crevice fluid has been suggested as a potential diagnostic marker for periodontitis. Elevated levels have also been found in naturally occurring and experimental gingivitis compared with gingival health.

β-Glucuronidase: It is a lysosomal enzyme found in the primary granules of neutrophil which hydrolyze the glycosyl bonds of intercellular ground substance.

Cathepsin B: It is an enzyme active in proteolysis; it belongs to the class of cysteine proteinases. The cellular source of Cathepsin-B in gingival crevice fluid seems to be mainly macrophages. Cathepsin-B activity has been found in GCF in adult periodontitis. It seems to be increased in periodontitis but is not increased in gingivitis.

Myeloperoxidase (MPO): It is a potent antibacterial enzyme produced by PMNs. Salivary MPO levels are significantly higher in untreated chronic periodontitis patients compared with healthy control subjects.

Lysozyme: It is an antibacterial enzyme found in body secretions. Their level are reduced in chronic periodontitis patient.

Elastase: Neutrophil elastase, sometimes referred to as granulocyte elastase, is an abundant proteinase released from the azurophilic granules of neutrophils, and as such is an indicator of neutrophil activity. Neutrophil elastase is a serine proteinase, active in the degradation of microbiological components in conjunctions with, or without, phagocytosis. This enzyme can degrade host intercellular matrix components, including elastin, fibronectin and collagen. Macrophage elastase, also called MMP-12, may have the same activities as neutrophil elastase. Elastase has been observed in GCF from periodontitis patients at elevated levels.

Enzymes Released by Dead Cells

Enzymes released from dead cells are Aspartate aminotransferase and Lactate dehydrogenase (LDH).

Aspartate aminotransferase (AST) is an enzyme released from dead cells from a variety of tissues throughout the body, including the heart (after myocardial infarction) and the liver (during hepatitis).

Commercial Diagnostic Test Kits
Periogard: It is a rapid chairside test kit for AST. The test involves collection of GCF with a filter paper strip, which is then placed in tromethamine hydrochloride buffer. A substrate reaction mixture containing L-aspartic and α-ketoglutaric acids are added and allowed to react for 10 minutes. In the presence of AST, the aspartate and α-glutarate are catalyzed to oxalacetate and glutamate. The addition of a dye, such as fast red, results in a color product, the intensity of which is proportional to the AST activity in the GCF sample.

Connective Tissue Degradation Products

In periodontitis there is destruction of collagen and extracellular matrix. GCF obtained from sites with periodontitis shows elevated levels of following breakdown products- a) Collagen (Hydroxyproline, Collagen cross links and N-peptide); b) Proteoglycans (Glycosaminoglycans, Heparan sulphate, Chondroitin 6 – sulphate, Chondroitin 4 – sulphate) and c) Fibronectin.

Products of Bone Resorption and Formation

Some possible markers of bone resorption and hence periodontal diseases activity are- Pyridinium cross-link collagen peptide fragment, Tartrate-resistant acid phosphatase (TRAP), Galactosyl hydroxylysine (GHYL), Hydroxyproline, N-terminal osteocalcin fragment and Glycosaminoglycans (GAGs). Pyridinoline cross links of the carboxy terminal telopeptide of type I collagen is a good marker of bone collagen degradation. This degradation product of bone has been preliminary examined as a GCF marker for the progression of periodontitis.

Bone formation markers are Type I procollagen propeptide, Alkaline phosphatase, Osteocalcin and bone Gla protein mineralization (BGP).

Various commercial diagnostic kits are:

Perioscan-BANA test kit
Omnigene-DNA probe system
Periogard-Aspartate aminotransferase (AST) kit
Evalusite-ELISA kit

LIMITATIONS OF MICROBIOLOGICAL AIDS

The various limitations and inconsistency of microbiologic aids are due to:

i.   Technical problems: It includes sample collection and difficulties in cultivation of plaque micro-organisms and identification of isolates.
ii. Conceptual problems: There is complexity of the periodontal microbiota. Periodontal infections are mixed infections, in which it is difficult to distinguish secondary invaders from true pathogens.
iii. Problems associated with the nature of periodontal diseases: Differentiation between active and inactive sites for sampling are difficult as periodontal diseases appears to be episodic in nature.

POINTS TO PONDER

✓ Biomarker is a substance that is measured objectively and evaluated as an indicator of normal biologic processes, pathogenic processes, or pharmacological responses to a therapeutic intervention.
✓ DNA probe is not an instrument but an agent that binds directly to a predefined sequence of nucleic acids. These are synthesized in the laboratory, with a sequence complementary to the target DNA sequence.

BIBLIOGRAPHY

1. Eley BM, Manson JD. Diagnostic tests of periodontal disease activity. In, Periodontics 5th ed Wright 2004;161-88.
2. Emberg G, Waddington JR, Hall RC, Last KS. Connective tissues elements as diagnostic aids in periodontology. Periodontol 2000 2000;24:193-214.
3. Sanz M, Newman MG. Advanced Diagnostic Techniques. In, Newman, Takei, Carranza. Clinical Periodontology 9th ed WB Saunders 2003;487-502.
4. Taba M, Kinney J, Kim AS, Gianobile WV. Diagnostic Biomarkers for Oral and Periodontal Diseases. Dent Clin North Am 2005;49:551-71.
5. Zambon JJ. Microbial diagnosis in periodontal therapy. In, Genco RJ, Goldman HM and Cohen DW. Contemporary Periodontics. CV Mosby Company 1990;449-58.

MCQs

1. Perioscan is:
   A. DNA probe
   B. Rapid chairside test kit for AST
   C. Commercial kits to detect neutral proteinase
   D. Diagnostic test kit to detect bacterial trypsin - like proteases
2. Candidates for biomarker are:
   A. Microorganisms (bacteria)
   B. Bacterial products (enzymes)
   C. Inflammatory and immune products
   D. Enzymes released from dead cells
   E. All of the above
3. Motile spirochetes can be best seen through:
   A. Culture techniques
   B. Dark field microscopy
   C. Periogard
   D. None of the above

Answers

1. D   2. E   3. B

CHAPTER

33

Halitosis

Shalu Bathla

INTRODUCTION

Halitosis or more simply bad breath is derived from the latin words *Halitus* (Breath) + *Osis* (Bad). Indeed, bad breath has been observed for thousands of years. The problem is addressed in Jewish Talmud as well as by Greek and Roman writers. Mohammed is said to have thrown a congregant from mosque for having the smell of garlic in his breath. Islamic teaching stresses the use of a special wooden stick, the siwak for cleaning the teeth and preventing bad breath. Modern literature on bad breath dates to a monograph published in 1874 by Joseph Howe.

Halitosis is also called as bad breath, fetor ex ore, fetor oris. Bad breath can be detrimental to one's self-image and confidence causing social, emotional, and psychological anxiety. With the majority of breath problems having an oral origin, the dental office is the most logical place for patients to seek treatment.

CLASSIFICATION

1. Genuine halitosis
   A. Physiologic halitosis: TN-1 Malodor arises through putrefactive processes within the oral cavity. Neither a specific disease nor a pathologic condition that could cause halitosis is found. Origin is mainly the dorsoposterior region of the tongue.

   B. Pathologic halitosis:
      i. Oral TN-2 Halitosis caused by disease, pathologic condition or malfunction of oral tissues. Halitosis derived from tongue coating, modified by pathologic condition (e.g. periodontal disease, xerostomia) is included in this subdivision.

      ii. Extraoral TN-3 Malodor originates from nasal, paranasal and or laryngeal region, pulmonary tract or upper digestive tract, diabetes mellitus, hepatic cirrhosis, uremia, internal bleeding.

2. Pseudohalitosis | TN-4 | Obvious malodor is not perceived by others although the patient stubbornly complains of its existence.

3. Halitophobia | TN-5 | After treatment for genuine halitosis or pseudohalitosis, the patient persists in believing that he/she has halitosis.

Treatment needs (TN) for breath malodor are:

Category	Description
TN-1	Explanation of halitosis and instructions for oral hygiene.
TN-2	Oral prophylaxis, professional cleaning and treatment for oral diseases, especially periodontal diseases.
TN-3	Referral to a physician or medical specialist
TN-4	Explanation of examination data, further professional instruction education and reassurance.
TN-5	Referral to a clinical psychologist or psychiatrist.

ETIOLOGY

There are various physiologic and pathologic causes of halitosis which may be extraoral or intraoral **(Fig. 33.1)**.

Physiologic

Food containing lactose (dairy products like milk, cheese, yoghurt, icecream), food containing sulphur (onion, garlic), lack of salivary flow during sleep, menstruation, smoking and alcoholic drinks.

Pathologic

A. Intraoral

Disorders of the oral cavity: Poor oral hygiene, dental caries, dental plaque, gingivitis, periodontitis, stomatitis, fissured and hairy tongue, acute primary herpetic gingivostomatitis, oral carcinoma, NUG, open gangrenous pulp and pericoronitis.

B. Extraoral

1. *Disorders of the upper respiratory tract*: Mouth breathing due to upper respiratory tract blockade, chronic sinusitis, foreign bodies, wegener's

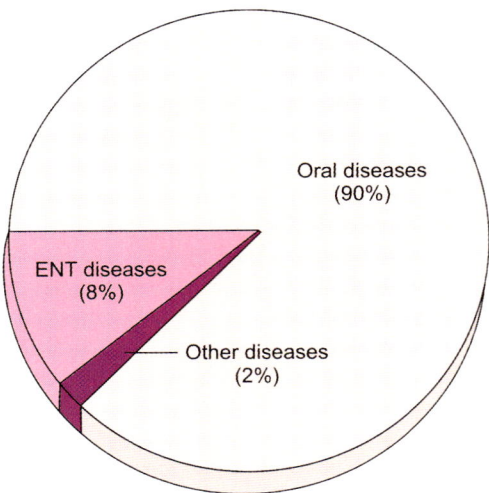

Fig. 33.1: Causes of halitosis

granulomatosis, tuberculosis, adenoiditis, syphilis, nasopharyngeal abscess, carcinoma of larynx and laryngoscleroma.

2. *Disorders of the lower respiratory tract*: Pulmonary abscess, bronchiectasis, chronic fetid bronchitis, pulmonary tuberculosis, carcinoma of the lung, necrotizing pneumonitis and empyema.

3. *Gastrointestinal conditions*: Salivary gland dysfunction, peritonsillar abscess, retropharyngeal abscess, cryptic tonsillopathy, vincent's angina, pharyngitis sicca, carcinoma of tonsils or pharynx, gangrenous angina, Zenker's diverticulum and congenital bronchoesophageal fistula.

4. *Disorders of lower gastrointestinal tract*: Gastric carcinoma, hiatus hernia, pyloric stenosis and enteric infections.

5. *Neurologic disorders*: Dysosmia, Dysgeusia and Zinc deficiency.

6. *Systemic administration of drugs*: Lithium salts, Penicillamine, Griseofulvin, Thiocarbamide, Chloral hydrate, Amphetamine, Antihypertensives, Antihistamines, Disulfiram, Dimethylsulfoxide (used in intersititial cystitis) and Cysteamine (used in nephropathic cystinosis).

7. *Systemic causes*: Hepatic failure (mousy odour, sweetish), Azotemia/kidney failure (uremic/fishy odor), Diabetic ketoacidosis (acetone, fruity odor), Chronic glomerulonephritis, lung abscess (foul, putrefactive) and Sjögren's syndrome (fetid).

8. *Functional disorders*: Psychosis and depression.

PATHOGENESIS (FIG. 33.2)

Role of bacteria: The common microorganisms involved are anaerobic *Streptococci, Peptostreptcoccus, Bacteriodes, Fusobacterium, Veillonella, Eubacterium, Enterococci, Pseudomonas, Campylobacter, Actinomyces, Enterobacter, Klebsiella* and *Aggregatibacter actinomycetemcomitans.*

Their main nutrient sources are proteins, peptides, or amino acids that are degraded to volatile sulfur compounds and other odoriferous substances. The most common intraoral sites of malodor production is tongue. Others are interdental and subgingival areas, denture, overhanging restorations, leaking crowns, large carious lesions, sites of food impaction and abscess. Tongue is the primary source of oral malodor because of large surface area of the tongue exposed to the expired air and availability of substrates that can be degraded to malodorous molecules by the tongue flora. The dorsal tongue mucosa with an area of 25 cm^2 shows a very irregular surface topography with innumerable depressions, which are ideal niche for bacterial adhesion and growth and sheltered for cleaning actions.

Role of Volatile organic compounds: Halitosis is due to the presence of odorous gases in the air expelled from the oral cavity. For the compound to be odoriferous it must be volatile. Volatile sulfur compounds are mainly produced through putrefactive activities of bacteria present on the tongue surfaces, in the saliva, gingival sulcus and other areas. Volatile sulfur compounds increases the permeability of oral mucosa and crevicular epithelium. Proteoglycans and glycoproteins in the extracellular matrix are held together by disulphide bonds and volatile sulfur compounds break this disulphide bonds. It impairs oxygen utilization by host cells, and reacts with cellular proteins, and interferes with collagen maturation. It also increases the collagen solubility. It decrease the DNA synthesis and proline transport reduction of total protein content and collagen synthesis of fibroblasts. It increases the secretion of collagenases, prostaglandins from fibroblasts, ultimately leading to conversion of mature collagen to a product susceptible for enzymatic degradation. Volatile sulfur compounds reduce the intracellular pH, inhibit cell growth, and periodontal cell migration.

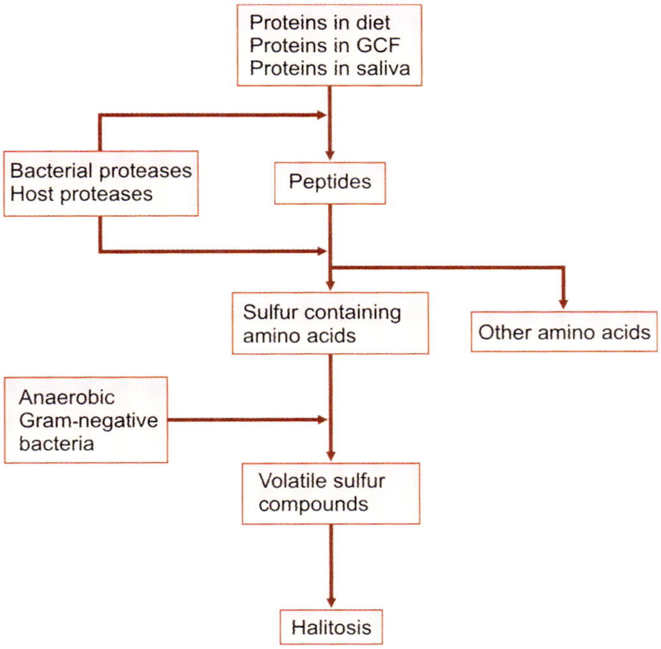

Volatile organic compounds are:

Sulfur compounds: Hydrogen sulphide, Methyl mercaptan and Dimethyl sulphide
Short chain fatty acids: Propionic acid, Butyric acid and Valeric acid
Polyamines: Cadaverine and Putrescine
Alcohols: 1- propoxy-2-propanol
Phenyl compounds: Indole, Skatole and Pyridine
Alkanines: 2-methyl-propane
Ketones :
Nitrogen containing compounds: Urea and Ammonia

Role of saliva: Saliva has dual action of inhibiting and favoring malodour formation. When the salivary flow rates is slow and oxygen availability is low, saliva favors the malodor formation and when the flow of saliva is rapid and there is greater availability of oxygen, the inhibitory property of saliva dominates.

Role of pH: Acidic pH inhibits whereas neutral and alkaline pH favor malodour production.

Role of Oxygen: Low pO$_2$ helps in the proliferation and growth of gram-negative anaerobic odoriferous bacteria.

DIAGNOSIS

Medical history: Ask about the relevant pathologies for breath malodor. "Listen to the patient, and the patient will tell you the diagnosis." Thus, proper questioning about medical history will help to achieve a proper differential diagnosis.

Examination:

A. Clinical Examination:

   a. Self Examination:

Fig.33.2: Production of volatile sulfur compounds causing halitosis

PERIODONTICS REVISITED

The following self testing can be used:

a. Smelling a metallic/nonodorous plastic spoon after scraping the back of the tongue.

b. Smelling a toothpick after introducing it in an interdental area.

c. Smelling saliva spit in a small cup/spoon.

d. Licking the wrist and allowing it to dry (reflects the saliva contribution to malodor).

b. **Organoleptic Measurement:** It is a sensory test scored on the basis of the examiner's perception of the subject's oral malodor. A straw or a plastic tube (24 mm in diameter and 10 cm in length) is inserted into the patient's mouth. While the patient is exhaling slowly, the examiner judges the odor at the other end of the tube. A privacy screen of 50 cm × 70 cm is used to prevent the patient from seeing the examiner sniffing the tube. For the first 1 to 2 seconds, the judge smells the patient's breath. After taking his/ her nose away from the tube for 3 to 4 seconds, the judge re-examines the patient's breath. Lung air should be examined after tongue cleaning and mouth rinsing with 0.75% hydrogen peroxide or 0.12% chlorhexidine. Nasal breath odor is examined using a tube 3 to 5 mm in diameter and 10 cm in length. The tube is inserted into one of the nostrils and the other nostril is pushed closed by a finger.

Instructions to patient:

* Patients are instructed to abstein from taking antibiotics three weeks before the assessment.
* Stop eating foods that contain garlic, onion and spices 48 hours prior to the assessment day.
* Avoid eating, drinking, smoking, oral hygiene practices and breath freshners for 12 hours prior to the assessment.

Instructions to examiner:

* Should have normal sense of smell.
* Refrain from alcohol drinking and using scented cosmetics before the assessment.
* Not to wear gloves, odour of which may interfere with organoleptic assessment.

Assessments should be performed at several appointments on different days, since breath odor fluctuates dramatically from one day to the next. The judge will smell a series of different air samples.

Organoleptic scoring scale:

0 – Absence of odor	- Odor can't be detected
1 – Questionable odor	- Odor is detectable, although the examiners could not recognize it as malodor.
2 – Slight odor	- Odour is deemed to exceed the threshold of malodor recognition
3 – Moderate odor	- Malodor is definitely detected.
4 – Strong odor	- Strong malodor which can be tolerated.
5 – Severe malodor	- Malodor is detected which cannot be tolerated.

The advantage associated with organoleptic measurement is that there is no dilution of malodor with room air. But the objectivity and reproducibility of organoleptic measurements are poor.

B. Laboratory Examination:

a. Sulfide monitor:

Halimeter: Disposable plastic straw was inserted into the air inlet and patients were instructed to place their slightly opened mouth over the straw so that it would extend approximately 4 cm into the mouth during the measurement. Three measurements were taken and the mean of these values were determined in parts per billion sulfide equivalents. The portable sulfidemeter uses electrochemical, voltametric zinc oxide thin film semiconductor sensors which generate a signal on exposure to sulfide and mercaptan gases. It analyzes the concentration of hydrogen sulfide (H_2S) and methyl mercaptan (CH_3SH), without discriminating between the two. It needs regular calibration.

Advantages:

* No need for skilled personnel
* Portability
* Noninvasive
* Low likelihood of cross-infection
* Relatively inexpensive
* Rapid turn around time of one to two minutes between measurements

Disadvantages:

* Inability to distinguish between individual sulphides
* Instrument show slight loss of sensitivity with time, necessitating periodic recalibration
* Measurement cannot be made in the presence of high levels of ethanol or essential oils

b. **Gas Chromatography:** Tonzetich and coworkers developed instrumental analysis of oral malodor using gas chromatography coupled with flame photometric detection.

Advantages:
- Separation and quantitative measurement of individual gases
- Ability to measure extremely low concentrations of gases

Disadvantages:
- Relatively high cost
- Skilled personnel required
- Cumbersome and lack of portability
- More time is required for detection and measurement

c. Dark – Field/Phase contrast Microscopy

d. Saliva Incubation test

e. BANA test- An alternative strategy is to detect in plaque or in the tongue coating taken from individuals with oral malodor, those bacteria or their enzymes that can produce volatile sulfur compounds. Three species associated with periodontal diseases, *Treponema denticola, P. gingivalis, Tannerella forsythia* produces both volatile sulfur compounds and volatile fatty acids. These organisms can be detected in plaque samples.

f. Diamond probe is recently developed instrument in which sensors are integrated into the periodontal probe. Probe is placed directly into the periodontal pocket or tongue. It has an electrical control unit and a disposable sensor tip that combines a standard Michigan 0 Style dental probe with a sulphide sensor which responds to the sulfides present in the periodontal pocket. The control unit reports the sulfide level at each site in a digital score from 0.0 to 5.0.

TREATMENT STRATEGIES TO CONTROL HALITOSIS

Folk remedies for bad breath abound and many are still in use. The Bible (Genesis) mention Labdanum (Mastic), a resin that has been used in Mediterranean countries for breath freshening for thousands of years, it may be the original chewing gum. Other folk cures include parsley (Italy), cloves (Iraq), guava peels (Thailand) and egg shells (China).

Treatment needs (TN) for halitosis in the dental practice have been categorized into 5 classes in order to provide guidelines for clinicians in treating halitosis patients. Treatment of physiologic halitosis (TN-1), oral pathologic halitosis (TN-1 and TN-2), and pseudo-halitosis (TN-1 and TN-4) should be the responsibility of a dentist, however, treatment of extraoral pathologic halitosis (TN-3) or halitophobia (TN-5) should be undertaken by a physician or medical specialist such as a psychiatrist or psychologist.

The management of halitosis depends largely on the cause:

1. Mechanical reduction of intraoral nutrients and microorganisms: Scaling, root planing is done and oral hygiene instructions are given to the patient. Tongue cleaning is done by either a brush or a tongue scraper. Small tongue scrapers are used with light pressure designed to reach as far back on tongue as possible. Rinse and clean the tongue scraper well after each use. This is done to dislodge the trapped food and bacteria in between the filiform papillae, thus decreasing the concentration of volatile sulphur compound.

2. Chemical reduction of oral microorganisms: Chlorhexidine, Listerine, Cetylpyridium chloride and Zinc chloride are common mouthwashes used in cases of halitosis. Zinc is incorporated into various mouthrinses because of strong affinity of zinc ions to thiol groups present in volatile sulfur compound, which would convert volatile H_2S and $CH_3 SH$ to nonvolatile sulfides. Penicillins, Metronidazole, Tetracyclines, Ciprofloxacin and Tinidazole are commonly used antimicrobials/antibiotics for halitosis.

3. Baking soda dentifrices and Zinc salt solutions render malodorous gases nonvolatile.

4. Masking the malodor: Antimalodor effect of oxidising lozenges is because of the activity of dehydroascorbic acid, which is generated by the peroxide- mediated oxidation of ascorbate present in the lozenges. Beneficial effect of chewing gum is due to tea extracts present in it, for its deodorizing mechanism. Epigallocatechin gallate (EGCg) is the main deodorizing agent present in green tea. The chemical reaction between EGCg and CH_3SH results in nonvolatile product.

5. Dietary recommendations: Advice to drink plenty of liquids, eat fresh, fibrous vegetables and rinse their mouth after eating or consuming milk products, fish and meat. Avoid coffee, smoking, drugs and foods that might be responsible for halitosis.

6. Consultation of physician: Bad breath may indicate the presence of an underlying systemic condition. Therefore, whenever local measures prove ineffective, the consultation of physician is indicated for systemic cause. Pseudo-halitosis almost always requires referral to clinical psychologist for management.

PERIODONTICS REVISITED

POINTS TO PONDER

✓ At least 90% of all malodor originates from the oral cavity, whereas, the remaining 10% has systemic or extraoral cause.

✓ The fetid odor is characteristic of NUG which is easily identified.

✓ Tea catechin EGCg suppresses the mgl gene, the gene encoding L-methionine α-deamino γ-mercapto-methanelyase, responsible for methyl mercaptan production by oral anaerobes.

BIBLIOGRAPHY

1. De Boever EH, Loesche WJ. Assessing the contribution of anaerobic microflora of the tongue to oral malodor. J Am Dent Assoc 1995;126:1384-93.
2. Delanghe G, Ghyselen J, Bollen C, et al. An inventory of patients' response to treatment at a multidisciplinary breath odor clinic. Quintessence Int 1999;30:307-10.
3. Grant DA, Stern IB, Listgarten MA. Plaque control, root sensitivity and halitosis. In, Periodontics. 6th ed CV Mosby Company 1988;611-45.
4. Greenstein RB, Goldberg S, Marku-Cohen S, Stere N, Rosenberg M. Reduction of oral malodor by oxidizing lozenges. J Periodontol 1997;68:1176-81.
5. Kim DJ, Lee JY, Kho HS, Chung JW, Hee-Kyung Park, Kim YK. A New Organoleptic Testing Method for Evaluating Halitosis. J Periodontol 2009;80:93-97.
6. Loesche WJ, Kazor C. Microbiology and treatment of halitosis. Periodontol 2000 2002;28:256-79.
7. Rosenberg M. First international workshop on oral malodor. J Dent Res 1994;7:586-9.
8. Rosenberg M, McCulloch CAG. Measurement of oral malodor: Current methods and future prospects. J Periodontol 1992;63;776-82.
9. Sanz M, Roldan S, Herrera D. Fundamentals of breath malodor. J Contemp Dent Pract 2001;2:1-17.
10. Scully C, Greenman J. Halitosis (breath odor). Periodontol 2000 2008;40:66-75.
11. Steenberghe DV, Quirynen M. Breath Malodor. In, Lindhe J, Karring T, Lang NP. Clinical Periodontology and Implant dentistry. 4th ed Blackwell Munksgaard 2003;512-18.
12. Tonzetich J. Production and origin of oral malodor: A review of mechanisms and methods of analysis. J Periodontol 1977;48:13-20.

MCQs

1. Probe used to detect volatile sulfhur compounds:
   A. Diamond probe
   B. DNA probe
   C. Williams probe
   D. Periostat
2. Usually, in NUG the odor is:
   A. Mousy
   B. Fetid
   C. Uremic odor
   D. None of the above
3. Following is true about organoleptic measurement of halitosis:
   A. Sensory test which is scored on the basis of examiner's perception to subject's oral malodor
   B. Patient is asked to perform oral hygiene practice just before the assessment
   C. Examiner should wear gloves during assessment
   D. None of the above
4. Halitosis is primarily because of:
   A. Collagenase enzymes
   B. Alkaline phosphatase
   C. Trypsin like enzymes
   D. Hydrogen sulphide

Answers

1. A   2. B   3. A   4. D

Dentin Hypersensitivity

Shalu Bathla

DEFINITION

Dentin hypersensitivity is an exaggerated response to nonnoxious stimuli. It is characterized by short, sharp pain arising from exposed dentin in response to stimuli typically thermal, evaporative, tactile, osmotic/chemical and which cannot be ascribed to any other form of dental defect/pathology.

ETIOLOGY AND PREDISPOSING FACTORS

Essentially exposure of the dentin may result from one of these processes: either removal of the enamel covering the crown or denudation of the root surface by loss of cementum and overlying periodontal tissues.

A. Removal of the enamel may result from tooth wasting diseases, i.e. attrition, abrasion, erosion or combination. Loss of enamel occurs by attrition associated with occlusal function and may be exaggerated by habits or parafunctional activity such as bruxism; by abrasion from dietary components or habits such as toothbrushing; or by erosion associated with environmental or dietary components, particularly acids.

B. Loss of covering periodontal structures: Denudation of the root surface is multifactorial. Acute and chronic periodontal diseases, incorrect toothbrushing or

chronic trauma from other habits and some forms of periodontal surgery are important casual factors. Factors such as method and frequency of brushing, the brush type, the dentifrice used all relate to the effects produced on soft and hard tissues. Erosive agents primarily acids, environmental, dietary or endogenous are known to cause the damage, e.g. workers exposed to fumes of hydrochloric, sulfuric, nitric and tartaric acids.

The prevalence and distribution of recession and dentin hypersensitivity strongly implicate toothbrushing as an etiologic factor, particularly in the localization of lesions. The buccal cervical site predilection for dentin exposure and sensitivity is consistent with the toothbrushing practices, with lingual sites receiving little attention during brushing. The left sided shift to increased recession and sensitivity but decreased plaque scores in preponderantly right handed toothbrushing groups supports the relevance of tooth cleaning to condition. Interestingly, the finding that females are more commonly affected by dentin hypersensitivity than males, if actually correct, would also relate in part to oral hygiene practices. Females have increased grooming behavior compared with males and this is associated with better oral hygiene.

The role of plaque as an etiologic factor in dentin hypersensitivity would appear to be an area of controversy. Thorough, over enthusiastic toothbrushing has long been associated with gingival recession and sensitivity.

More rapid response to stimuli or the persistence of pain after removal of stimuli applied to dentin have been ascribed to inflammatory changes in the pulp. Such pulpal changes may be due to bacteria or their toxins. Bacteria do penetrate into tubules of dentin left open to the oral environment and their toxins may diffuse to the pulp. This diffusion would have to occur over relatively large distances and against the outward flow of dentinal fluid.

THEORIES RELATED TO DENTINAL HYPERSENSITIVITY

Three major theories described for activation of dental nerve fibers by applying stimuli to enamel or dentin are **(Fig. 34.1)**:

i. *Neural theory*: The neural theory advocates that thermal or mechanical stimuli, directly excite nerve endings which are within the dentinal tubules. These nerve signals are then conducted along the parent primary afferent nerve fibers in the pulp into the dental nerve branches and then into the brain.

ii. *Odontoblastic transduction theory*: This theory proposes that the stimuli initially excite the process of the odontoblast, the membrane of which may come into closer apposition with that of nerve endings in the pulp or in the dentinal tubule. The odontoblast then transmits the excitation to these associated nerve endings.

iii. *Hydrodynamic theory*: Brannstrom (1963) stated that when the fluids within dentinal tubules are subjected to temperatue changes or physical osmotic changes, the movement stimulates nerve receptor sensitive to pressure, which leads to the transmission of the stimuli.

DIAGNOSIS

The diagnosis of dentin hypersensitivity can be made by visual examination of the teeth, detailed dietary history, occlusion assessment and diagnostic tools. The various diagnostic tools are:

Air Syringe

A burst of air (temperature between 65° and 70° F and a pressure 60 psi) from a dental syringe when directed at right angles on to the cut dentin causes evaporative fluid movement across the dentin. The evaporation of fluid occur from the dentin when relatively dry 25°C air is directed at a 32°C tooth, which occurs very quickly (within 1 second). If longer blasts of air are used, one begins to cool the tooth, and the stimulus becomes complex owing to addition of a thermal stimulus with an evaporative stimulus. Air blasts are useful stimuli during patient screening. They quickly identify individual sensitive teeth but they are not useful at identifying sensitive tooth surfaces. The exact location of dentin sensitivity is important because it often dictates the type of therapy that might be employed. Air blasts are too diffuse to permit identification and quantitation of specific sites of sensitivity.

   0 - No discomfort
   1 - Discomfort but no severe pain
   2 - Severe pain during application
   3 - Pain persists even after removal of stimuli.

Osmotic Method

This method is based on the principle of osmosis, i.e. movement of fluid from higher concentration to lower concentration. An osmotic method consisting of the subjective pain response to a sweet stimulus was used by Mcfall and Hamrick in 1987 to measure the effect of several test dentifrices on dentinal sensitivity. After isolation of the test tooth with cotton rolls, a cotton applicator saturated with sucrose solution is applied to the root surface of the tooth and allowed to remain in place for 10 seconds or until discomfort was perceived.

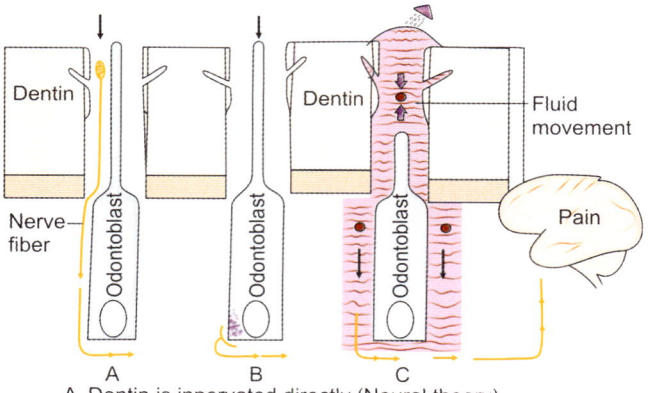

A Dentin is innervated directly (Neural theory)
B Odontoblast act as a receptor (Transduction theory)
C Receptors are in the pulp and are stimulated by fluid movement through the tubules (Hydrodynamic theory)

Fig. 34.1: Theories of dentin sensitivity

Tactile Method

Dental explorer is used to identify regions of sensitive dentin. It is simple yet effective. The movement of explorer across dentin produces hydrodynamic stimulus causing displacement of fluid inwardly at a rapid rate, which activates mechanoreceptors. The amount of displacement is presumably proportional to the depth of the scratch and the volume of surrounding dentin that is compressed. There may be a recoil and outward movement of fluid when the pressure is taken off.

Thermal Test

Thermoelectric devices are useful for delivering cold or warm stimuli in a controlled quantitative manner. Because patients are generally more sensitive to cold than to hot stimuli. In using cold water, each tooth to be tested is isolated with a rubber dam. Water at a known temperature is slowly flowed on the exposed dentin surface for a maximum of 3 seconds from a disposable plastic syringe. The patient is asked whether that temperature causes pain or not and then the next lower temperature is tried until the patient responds unequivocally. Thermal stimuli are effective hydrodynamics stimuli because of differences in thermal conductivity and coefficient of expansion or contraction of pulpal/dentinal fluids, enamel and dentin. Application of cold causes a more rapid volumetric contraction of dentinal fluid than of dentin. This mismatch of volumetric changes produce negative intrapulpal pressures that displace mechanoreceptors and cause pain. Thermal stimuli to vital dentin causes sharp, well – localized pain (that is, activation of A-δ fibers) before there is a change in dentin temperature near the pulp where the nerves are located.

Dentin hypersensitivity pain is:

Rapid in onset
Sharp in nature
Short in duration
Produced by stimuli such as tactile, cold and heat on exposed dentin.

Differential Diagnosis

Dentin hypersensitivity can be differentiated by crack tooth syndrome, chipped teeth, dental caries, post-restorative sensitivity and irreversible pulpitis. Incomplete tooth fracture can be associated with a number of symptoms ranging from mild discomfort to severe pain. The most common complaint is pain on pressure. Tapping the teeth or having the patient bite down on an orangewood stick almost invariably evokes a sharp pain in the affected tooth. Exposure of dentin due to chipped enamel is obvious. Differentiating dentinal hypersensitivity from caries is relatively easy, particularly in the case of a deep carious lesion. New amalgam or crown that has been placed without proper adjustment of the occlusion can cause post-restorative sensitivity. Pain in irreversible pulpitis frequently occurs without provocation. In the case of thermal test, the intense pain persists after stimulus has been removed. Thus, it is important to determine chronology, nature, location, radiation, aggravating and alleviating factors that influence the pain.

HYPERSENSITIVITY MEASUREMENT

Verbal Rating Scale (VRS)

Given by Kanapka and Colucci (1986) and Gillman and Newman (1993). This scale records the response of the patient after scratching and doing air-cold tests on a severity scale. The investigator should test all sensitive areas on all teeth of all subjects with the same tactile pressure. Immediately after the cold air blast, the subject usually reports the level of sensitivity via VRS.

0 – No response
1 – Slight response but no pain
2 – Pain only when stimulus is applied
3 – Severe, sudden and lasting pain
Score: 0 and 1 – Classified as nonsensitive teeth
2 and 3 – Classified as hypersensitive teeth

Visual Analog Scale (VAS)

The VAS would be a more appropriate device than the VRS for measuring levels of sensitivity pain during subject assessment, and for measuring tactile and thermal stimuli of hypersensitivity. The VRS offers a restrictive choice of words that may not represent pain experience with sufficient precision for all subjects. It is a scale of 10 cm which is used to grade sensitivity, labeled at the extremes with no pain at the zero cm end of the scale and severe pain at the 10 cm end of the scale **(Fig. 34.2)**. Subjects are asked to place a mark on the 10 cm line at a location between no pain and severe pain ends. Measurements from the scale were made in mm giving a scoring range of 0 to 100.

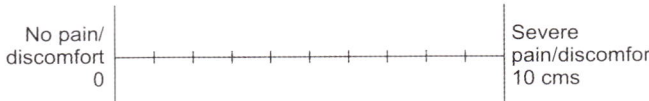

Fig. 34.2: VAS-visual analog scale

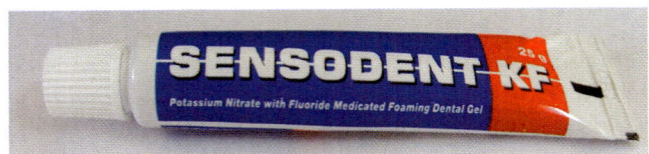

Fig. 34.3: Desensitizing agent

MANAGEMENT OF DENTIN HYPERSENSITIVITY

Historical Perspective

Hippocrates (460 to 355 BC) was perhaps the first to recommend regular use of a dentifrice based on carbonate of lime or chalk, and a mouthwash based on vinegar. Pliny recommended salt as a cleansing agent and mouthwash. He also suggested the use of charcoal and ashes of various types of oral hygiene. Opium therapy, the earliest recorded treatment method, dates to 400 BC and was still advocated as late as 1000 AD. A wide variety of treatments such as henbane plant and crushed beetles were recommended until the late 1800s. In 1855, JD White referred that escharotics are more effective than opium or morphine. Cocaine was introduced in 1859 and other medicaments such as creosate and tannic acid and arsenic were used at the turn of the century.

In the 1920s, aqueous solutions of iodine with silver iodide were reported to be effective for relieving dentinal sensitivity. In 1935, Grossman suggested the criteria for the ideal desensitizing agent. Desensitizing agents should be:

- Nonirritating to the pulp,
- Relatively painless on application,
- Easily applied,
- Rapid in action
- Permanently effective
- Not discolor tooth structure

Hot olive oil, formaldehyde, silver nitrate, zinc chloride, sodium carbonate, and sodium fluoride were used in the 1950s, many of these materials are used to stimulate the formation of secondary dentin, and some are adhesive and used for covering the sensitive areas. Currently, the treatment of choice for the chronic management of dentinal hypersensitivity is the use of dentifrices.

Treatment Approaches for Dentinal Hypersensitivity

1. Patient counseling:
   i. Oral hygiene practices
   ii. Dietary factors
   iii. Remove risk factors by educating
2. Interventional treatment:

i. At home treatment options: Home use applications of desensitizing agents **(Fig. 34.3)** to occlude dentinal tubules; there by blocking hydrodynamic mechanism of dentinal sensitivity. Potassium nitrate decreases fluid flow through the tubules by occluding them. Potassium ions of KNO_3 diffuse through the dentinal tubules and reach the pulp sensory complex and form a region of greatly increased concentration (K^+ ions) which depolarizes the pulpal sensory complex and reduces pain transmission.

ii. In office treatment options:
   a. Noninvasive methods:

   Oxalates: Oxalates have been used popularly as desensitizing agent, they are relatively inexpensive, easy to apply and well tolerated by the patients. 6% ferric oxalate, 30% potassium oxalate and 3% monohydrogen monopotassium oxalate solutions are used as desensitizing agents. The oxalate ions react with calcium ions in the dentinal fluid to form insoluble calcium oxalate crystals that are deposited within the apertures of dentinal tubules.

   Cavity Varnishes: When using desensitizing agents that have a caustic effect on the soft tissue, care must be exercised to prevent them from contacting the alveolar mucosa. The teeth should be isolated and dried with warm air. Dentin often becomes insensitive when open tubules are covered with a thin film of varnish. This may be an effective means of providing temporary relief.

   Strontium Chloride: Topical application of concentrated strontium chloride ($SrCl_2$) on an abraded dentin surface produced a deposit of strontium that penetrated to a depth of approx 20μm and extends into the dentinal tubules.

   Composite resins: The objective of employing composite resin is to seal the dentinal tubules to prevent pain producing stimuli from reaching the pulp.

   GLUMA: It is a dentin bonding system that includes 5% glutaraldehyde primer and 35%

HEMA (hydroxyethyl methacrylate). It provides an attachment to dentin that is immediate and strong.

Calcium hydroxide: Ca(OH)$_2$ has been a popular agent for the treatment of dentin hypersensitivity for many years, particularly after root planing. The exact mechanism of action is unknown, but evidence suggests that it may block dentinal tubules or promote peritubular dentin formation.

Argon, CO$_2$, Ho:YAG, Nd:YAG, erbium YAG are the LASERS types used for desensitizing. These systems have become available which are tailored specifically for dental surgery using fibre optic delivery to a hand piece, smaller than a conventional rotary dental instrument. The availability of laser would potentially satisfy all the requirements of a desensitizing agent. They blocks the tubules probably by fusion of crystals (Hydroxyapatite), as low intensity defocused beam is used.

Iontophoresis: Fluoride Iontophoresis is a mean to drive fluoride ions more deeply into dentinal tubules. It involves the placement of a negative electrode to dentin and a positive electrode to the patient's face or arm. Saliva becomes medium in which ions commence their selective motion. Negative ions flows through the positive charged teeth and positive ions to the negatively charged bristles. Iontophoresis devices are expensive and somewhat difficult to use.

TABLE 34.1: Various desensitizing agents

Trade name	Agents
Sensodyne	10% Strontium chloride and Sodium fluoride
Thermodent	10% Strontium chloride
Protect	2% Dibasic Sodium citrate in a pleuronic gel
Promise	5% Potassium nitrate, Dicalcium phosphate and Sodium monofluorophosphate
Denquel	5% Potassium nitrate
Isodan	Potassium nitrate, Sodium fluoride, HEMA
Sensodyne F^R	KCl and Sodium monofluorophosphate
Colgate Sensitive Care	Potassium citrate and Sodium monofluorophosphate
Macleans Sensitive	Strontium acetate and Sodium monofluorophosphate

b. Invasive methods:
  • Pulpectomy
  • Class V restorations
  • Gingival graft surgery
3. To block neural transmission of the pulp:
  i. By endodontics
  ii. Tooth extraction

PREVENTION OF DENTIN HYPERSENSITIVITY

Patient education and dietary counseling: Dietary acids are capable of causing erosive loss of tooth structure, thereby removing cementum and opening dentinal tubules. Consequently, dietary counseling should focus on the quantity and frequency of acid intake, and intake occurring in relation to toothbrushing. Any treatment may fail if these factors are not controlled. A written diet history should be obtained by the patients with dentinal hypersensitivity in order to advice them concerning eating habits. Red and white wine, citrus fruit juices, apple juice, and yogurt are capable of dissolving the smear layer *in vitro.*

Toothbrushing Techniques: Toothbrushing in combination with decalcification of superficial dentin is capable of accelerating the loss of tooth structure. Because loss of dentin is greatly increased when brushing is performed immediately after exposure of tooth surface to dietary acids. Thus, patients should be cautioned against brushing their teeth soon after ingestion of citrus food. Because incorrect tooth brushing appears to be an etiologic factor in dentin hypersensitivity, instructions for proper brushing techniques can prevent further loss of dentin and resulting hypersensitivity.

Avoid hard bristled toothbrushes without rounded end bristles
Avoid brushing teeth immediately following ingestion of acidic food or beverages
Avoid over brushing and flossing with excessive pressure for prolonged period of time.
Avoid over instrumentation of the root surfaces during calculus removal.
Avoid over polishing of exposed roots during stain removal.
Avoid violating the biologic width when placing crown margins.

POINTS TO PONDER

✓ Robinson's Remedy consist of equal parts of carbolic acid and caustic potash.
✓ Desensitizing agents should be used continuously for at least 2 weeks, to show effective response.

PERIODONTICS REVISITED

BIBLIOGRAPHY

1. Addy M. Etiology and clinical implications of Dentin Hypersensitivity. Dent Clin North Am 1990;34:503-12.
2. Clark GE, Trosllos ES. Designing Hypersensitivity Clinical Studies. Dent Clin North Am 1990;34:531-44.
3. Kanapka JA. Over the Counter Dentifrices in the Treatment of Tooth Hypersensitivity. Review of Clinical Studies. Dent Clin North Am 1990;34:545-60.
4. Kleinberg I, Kaufman HW, Confessore F. Methods of Measuring Tooth Hypersensitivity. Dent Clin North Am 1990;34:515-30.
5. Klokkevold PR, Carranza FA, Takei HH. General principles of periodontal surgery. In, Newman, Takei, Carranza. Clinical Periodontology 9th ed WB Saunders 2003;725-36.
6. Pashley DH. Mechanisms of Dentin Hypersensitivity. Dent Clin North Am 1990;34:449-74.
7. Trowbridge HO, Silver DR. A review of Current Approaches to In – Office Management of Tooth Hypersensitivity. Dent Clin North Am 1990;34:561-82.

MCQs

1. Which of the following areas of the tooth are considered most sensitive from various stimuli?
   A. Occlusal, incisal
   B. Cervical, proximal
   C. Lingual, cervical
   D. Facial, cervical

2. Dentinal sensitivity can be caused by all of the following professional procedures *except*:
   A. Periodontal instrumentation
   B. Periodontal surgery
   C. Cosmetic polishing
   D. None of the above

3. Dentinal sensitivity is a multifactorial condition. Stimuli of thermal, tactile, chemical, or osmotic nature can result in dentinal pain.
   A. The first statement is true; the second is false
   B. The first statement is false; the second is true
   C. Both statements are true
   D. Both statements are false

4. KNO_3 desensitizing agents primarily work by:
   A. Occluding the dentinal tubules by precipitating proteins
   B. Changing the surface ions
   C. Interfering with the neurological responses
   D. Inhibiting the osmotic pressure between membranes

Answers

1. D   2. D   3. C   4. A

CHAPTER 35

Prognosis

Shalu Bathla

DEFINITION

It is a greek word, *pro* means before and *gignoskein* means to fore know or to know. *Prognosis is a predilection of the probable course, duration and outcome of a disease based on a general knowledge of the pathogenesis of the disease and the presence of risk factors for the disease.*

TYPES/RANGE OF DIAGNOSTIC PROGNOSIS

Between the extremes of hopeless and excellent is an entire range of gradations. Careful analysis of prognostic factors allows the clinician to establish one of the following prognosis:

i. *Excellent prognosis*: No bone loss, excellent gingival condition, good patient cooperation, no systemic/environmental factors.

ii. *Good prognosis*: One or more of the following condition: Adequate remaining bone support, adequate possibilities to control etiologic factors and establish a maintainable dentition, adequate patient co-operation, no systemic/environmental factors or if systemic factors are present they are well controlled.

iii. *Fair prognosis*: One or more of the following condition: Less than adequate remaining bone support, some tooth mobility, grade I furcation involvement, adequate maintenance possible, acceptable patient

cooperation, presence of limited systemic/environmental factors.

iv. *Poor prognosis:* One or more of the following condition: moderate to advanced bone loss, tooth mobility, grade I and II furcation involvements, difficult to maintain areas and/or doubtful patient cooperation, presence of systemic/environmental factors.

v. *Questionable prognosis:* One or more of the following condition: advanced bone loss, grade II and III furcation involvements, tooth mobility, inaccessible areas, presence of systemic/environmental factors.

vi. *Hopeless prognosis*: One or more of the following condition: advanced bone loss, non maintainable areas, extraction indicated, presence of uncontrolled systemic/environmental factors.

PROGNOSTIC FACTORS

The factors that predicts the outcome of a disease once the disease is present are known as prognostic factors. Prognosis assessment is the process of using prognostic factors to predict the course of a disease.

Overall Factors Affecting the Prognosis

i. *Patient's age:* Of two patients with equally advanced bone loss, one of whom is 25 and the other 70 years old, the younger will have the poorer prognosis. The prognosis is not good for younger patient because the rate of progression was more rapid in shorter time frame for the younger patient as compared to the older patient.

ii. *Disease severity and distribution*: The severity of the disease might be slight, moderate or severe. Severity depends on pockets depth, level of attachment, bone loss and osseous defect. The distribution of disease may be localized or generalized.

   Pocket depth: Shallower pockets have a better prognosis than do deep pockets. Deep pockets have a favorable prognosis if attachment and bone levels are high.

   Level of attachment: The determination of the level of clinical attachment reveals the approximate extent of root surface that is devoid of periodontal ligament. Pocket depth is less important than level of attachment, because it is not necessarily related to bone loss. Tooth with deep pockets and little attachment and bone loss has a better prognosis than one with shallow pockets and severe attachment and bone loss.

   Bone loss and osseous defect: Greater the bone loss, poorer is the prognosis. Three - walled osseous defect provides a scaffold for repair and good regenerative potential. Two - walled osseous lesion has poorer and one - walled the poorest, prognosis for bone regeneration. Thus, prognosis is related to the height of remaining bone.

iii. *Plaque control*: Patient cooperation is essential for satisfactory plaque control, but is also necessary for the control of predisposing and aggravating etiological factors.

iv. *Patient compliance*: The prognosis for patients with gingival and periodontal disease is dependent on the patient's attitude, motivation and dexterity to keep good oral hygiene. Patient cooperation is more likely to be forthcoming after the patient has been given information about the nature of the problem. Time spent in providing such information and in explaining the rationale behind the treatment plan will improve the chances of achieving a good prognosis.

v. *Smoking*: Smoking affects the severity of periodontal destruction as well as the healing potential of the periodontal tissues. The prognosis in patients who smoke and have slight to moderate periodontitis is generally fair to poor. In patients with severe periodontitis, the prognosis may be poor to hopeless.

vi. *Systemic disease*: Patient's health and associated capacity for repair are important factors to consider in developing the treatment plan and prognosis.

vii. *Genetic factors*: Genetic factors play an important role in determining the nature of the the host response.

viii. *Stress*: Any emotional condition will interfere with the patient's oral hygiene regime.

Local Factors Affecting the Prognosis

i. *Plaque/calculus*: The patient who shows a severe response to minimal amounts of plaque has poorer prognosis than does the patient who exhibits a resistant response in the presence of a considerable amount of plaque. The microbial challenge presented by plaque and calculus is the most important local factor in periodontal disease. Thus, good prognosis is dependent on the ability of the patient and clinician to remove plaque. But when the teeth are drifted or rotated, oral hygiene may be more difficult, in such case the prognosis is poorer.

ii. *Subgingival restorations*: Tooth with overhangs or subgingival margin discrepancies has a poorer prognosis than a tooth with well-contoured, supragingival margins.

iii. *Anatomic factors*:
   • Short, tapered roots: Teeth with short, tapering roots have a poorer prognosis than do those with long and broad roots. The more favorable the crown-root ratio, the better the prognosis. An upper molar with widespread roots and therefore a large root base has a much better prognosis than a conical - rooted premolar or incisor with the same amount of bone loss.
   • CEPs and enamel pearls: These enamel projections on the root surface have a negative effect on the prognosis.
   • Root concavities: Prominent root proximal concavities are present on maxillary first premolars, mesiobuccal root of maxillary first molar, both roots of mandibular first molars and mandibular incisors. These are the areas that can be difficult for the therapist and patient to clean and thus, these worsen the prognosis.
   • Developmental grooves: Grooves on the root are an invagination resulting from incorrect formation of the root. The grooves often begin at the cingulum and extend a variable distance apically on the root - surface between the midpalatal line and the line angle, that is why called as cinguloradicular groove **(Fig. 35.1)**. These grooves are found on maxillary lateral incisors (5.6%) and maxillary central incisors (3.4%) which act as plaque - retentive area that are difficult to instrument.

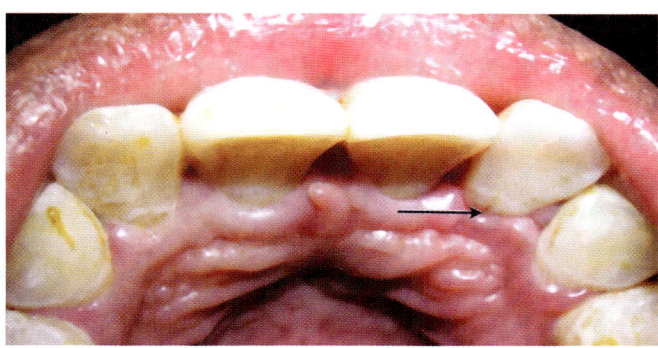

Fig. 35.1: Cinguloradicular/ Palatogingival groove

- Root proximity
- Furcation involvement: Maxillary first premolars offer the greatest difficulties, and therefore their prognosis is usually unfavorable when the lesion reaches the mesial-distal furcation. Maxillary molars also offer some degree of difficulty; sometimes their prognosis can be improved by resecting one of the buccal roots thereby improving access to the area. When mandibular first molars or buccal furcations of maxillary molars offer good access to the furcation area, their prognosis is usually better.
- Tooth mobility: If the cause of tooth mobility can be eliminated, and if the mobility can be controlled or eliminated, the prognosis is better. Tooth mobility caused by inflammation and trauma from occlusion may be corrected but tooth mobility caused by loss of alveolar bone is not likely to be corrected. Thus, prognosis is poor in the presence of advanced bone loss. A tooth that can be rotated or depressed has poorer prognosis than a tooth that has horizontal mobility. Mobility must be correlated with other clinical and radiographic findings in determining prognosis.

RELATIONSHIP BETWEEN DIAGNOSIS AND PROGNOSIS

Many of the criteria used in the diagnosis and classification of the different forms of periodontal disease are also used in developing a prognosis. Factors such as patient's age, severity of disease, genetic susceptibility, and presence of systemic disease are important criteria in the diagnosis of the condition. These are also important in developing a prognosis. These common factors suggest that for any given diagnosis, there should be an expected prognosis under ideal conditions.

Factors common for both prognosis and diagnosis of the disease
Patient's age
Severity of disease
Genetic susceptibility and
Presence of systemic disease.

PROGNOSIS OF PATIENTS WITH GINGIVAL AND PERIODONTAL DISEASES

Prognosis of Patients with Gingival Diseases

Gingivitis associated with dental plaque only: Prognosis for patients with gingivitis associated with dental plaque only is good, provided all local irritants and other local factors contributing to plaque retention are also eliminated.

Plaque-induced gingival diseases modified by systemic factors: Long-term prognosis for these patients depends not only on control of bacterial plaque, but also on control or correction of systemic factors.

Plaque-induced gingival diseases modified by medications: The severity of drug induced gingival enlargement can be limited by controlling the plaque. Surgical intervention is usually necessary to correct the alterations in gingival contour. Continued use of the drug results in recurrence of the enlargement, even following surgical intervention. Long term prognosis is dependent on whether the patient's systemic problem can be treated with an alternative medication that does not have gingival enlargement as a side effect.

Gingival diseases modified by malnutrition: The prognosis in these patients may depend on the severity and duration of the deficiency and on the likelihood of reversing the deficiency through dietary supplementation.

Non-Plaque-induced gingival lesions: Prognosis depends on elimination of the source of the infectious agent. In patients with atypical gingivitis seen in dermatologic disorders, prognosis is linked to management of the associated dermatologic disorder. Prognosis of patients with allergic, toxic, and foreign body reactions, as well as mechanical and thermal trauma, depends on elimination of the causative agent.

Prognosis of Patients with Periodontitis

Chronic Periodontitis: In cases where the clinical attachment loss and bone loss are not very advanced (slight to moderate periodontitis), the prognosis is generally good, provided the inflammation can be controlled through good oral hygiene and the removal of local plaque-retentive factors. In patients with more severe disease, as evidenced by furcation involvement and increasing tooth mobility, or noncompliant patients prognosis may be downgraded from fair to poor.

Aggressive Periodontitis: The clinical, microbiologic, and immunologic features suggest that patients with aggressive periodontitis would have a poor prognosis. However, in cases of localized aggressive periodontitis, the patients often exhibits a strong serum antibody response to the infecting agents, which may contribute to localization of the lesions. When diagnosed early, conservative therapy with oral hygiene instruction and systemic antibiotic therapy, can result in an excellent prognosis.

Periodontitis as a Manifestation of Systemic Diseases: Systemic diseases alter the ability of the host to respond to the microbial challenge presented and this may affect the progression of disease and therefore the prognosis. Unless the systemic disease can be corrected, these patients present with a fair to poor prognosis. In case of genetic disorders that alters the host response, prognosis is generally fair to poor.

Necrotizing Periodontal Diseases: With control of both the bacterial plaque and the secondary factors, such as acute psychologic stress, tobacco smoking, and poor nutrition, the prognosis for a patient with NUG is good. With repeated episodes of NUG, the prognosis may be downgraded to fair. In patients with NUP the prognosis depends on not only reducing the local and secondary factors, but also on dealing with the systemic problem.

LANDMARK STUDIES RELATED

McGuire MK. Prognosis versus actual outcome: a long-term survey of 100 treated periodontal patients under maintenance care. Journal of Periodontology 1991;62:51.

In this study, 100 treated periodontal patients were taken and evaluated for 5 years, and 39 of these patients were followed for 8 years to determine the accuracy of assigned prognosis based on commonly taught clinical criteria. Prognosis was evaluated for all the patients. The ultimate fate of teeth initially labeled as hopeless varied substantially, and even though the average prognosis of the teeth studied at each interval remained relatively stable over time, individual prognosis categories and individual tooth prognosis changed frequently. In conclusion, it was found that projections were ineffective in predicting any prognosis other than good, and that prognosis tended to be more accurate for single rooted teeth than for multirooted teeth.

BIBLIOGRAPHY

1. Eley BM, Manson JD. Diagnosis, prognosis and treatment plan. In, Periodontics 5th ed Wright 2004;149-60.
2. Grant DA, Stern IB, Listgarten MA. Prognosis. In, Periodontics. 6th ed CV Mosby Company 1988;573-91.
3. Goodman SF, Novak KF. Determination of prognosis. In, Newman, Takei, Carranza. Clinical Periodontology 9th ed WB Saunders 2003; 475-86.
4. McGuire MK. Prognosis versus actual outcome: a long-term survey of 100 treated periodontal patients under maintenance care. J Periodontol 1991;62:51.
5. Thomas MV, Mealey BL. Formulating a periodontal diagnosis and prognosis. In, Rose LF, Mealey BL, Genco RJ, Cohen DW. Periodontics, Medicine, Surgery and Implants. Elsevier Mosby 2004;172-99.

MCQs

1. Which of the following statement regarding periodontal prognosis is true?
   A. Maxillary molar's distal furcation involvement has poor prognosis because access for cleaning is poor
   B. If the cause of periodontal diseases is directly related to plaque, then prognosis is much more favorable, than it is in cases where etiological agent is not obvious.
   C. Prognosis depends heavily upon proper diagnosis and therapist's clinical experience.
   D. All of the above.
2. Which of the following does not affect periodontal prognosis:
   A. Enamel pearl
   B. Enamel projection
   C. Bifurcation ridge
   D. Talon's cusp
3. Provided inflammation is controlled, the prognosis for moderate periodontitis is generally:
   A. Good
   B. Fair
   C. Poor
   D. Questionable
4. Prognosis is favorable for:
   A. Two walled intrabony defects
   B. Three walled intrabony defects
   C. One walled intrabony defects
   D. Aggressive periodontitis

Answers

1. D   2. D   3. A   4. B

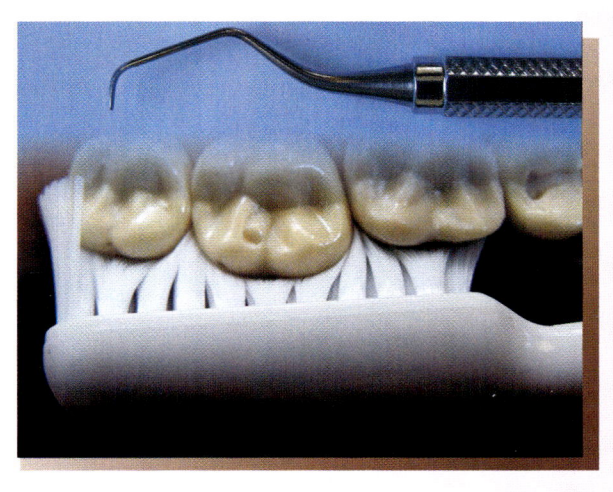

SECTION SIX

A. NON-SURGICAL THERAPY

TREATMENT

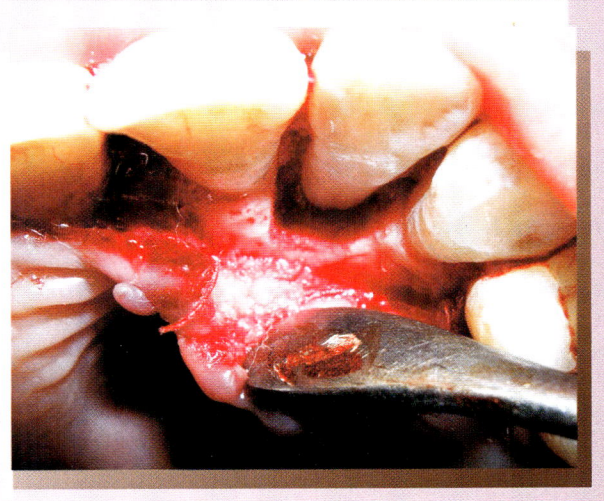

B. SURGICAL THERAPY

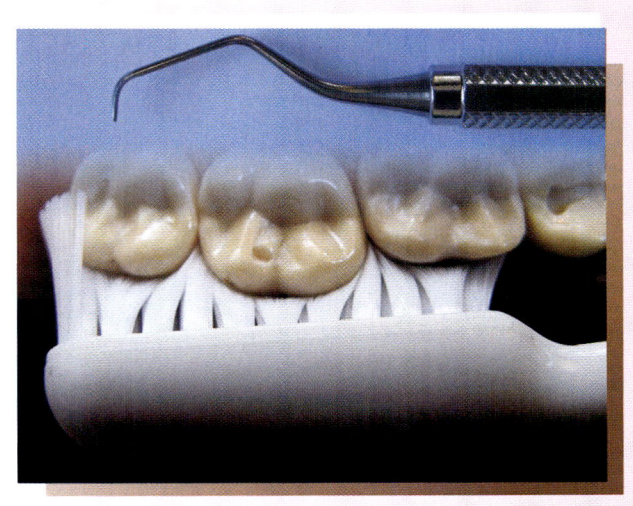

A. NON-SURGICAL THERAPY

Treatment Plan

Shalu Bathla

INTRODUCTION

Treatment plan is the sequential outline of the essential services and procedures that must be carried to eliminate disease and to restore the oral cavity to health and normal function. It is as individualistic as are the patient and the disease. Each patient presents an individual problem, one cannot adhere to a rigid pattern of treatment always. Thus, treatment plan should be tailored to, both physical and psychological needs of the patient. Treatment plan is the blueprint for care management. The aim of the treatment plan is total treatment that is, the coordination of all treatment procedures for the purpose of creating a well – functioning dentition in a healthy periodontal environment. At all times during the course of treatment, the primary focus is on the patient's welfare.

The treatment plan depends on the following major factors:
- Patient's degree of interest and compliance, as well as the ability to participate in therapy
- Findings of the examination
- Nature and extent of the disease diagnosed
- The prognosis of individual teeth segments and arches

PHASES OF PERIODONTAL THERAPY

- Emergency phase
- Etiotropic phase/Phase I
- Surgical phase/Phase II
- Restorative phase/Phase III
- Maintenance phase/Phase IV.

Emergency phase: When the patient has pain, swelling and infection, the emergency condition must be resolved before phase I therapy, just after the history and examination of the area involved in the chief complaint. These emergencies take priority over other treatment scheduling.
- Alleviate pain: The control of pain comes before any other treatment.
- Swelling, even without pain, requires immediate attention.
- Acute infections such as periapical abscess, periodontal abscess, NUG and pericoronitis. Endodontics may be necessary as an emergency measure where there is a pulpitis, apical abscess or a combined periapical - periodontal abscess.

- Traumatic lesions.
- Extraction of hopeless teeth - Extremely mobile teeth which seriously interfere with function should be extracted.
- Repairing of defective prosthesis.

Etiotropic Phase: Phase I

It is etiotropic treatment phase, because its goal is to eliminate the etiologic factor of periodontal disease. The terms Phase I, Initial phase and Hygienic phase are commonly used to refer to this stage of therapy.

The objectives of phase I therapy are:

a. To reduce or to eliminate gingival inflammation.

b. To eliminate periodontal pocket produced by the edematous enlargement of inflamed gingiva.

c. To achieve surgical manageability of the gingiva (i.e. firm consistency and minimal bleeding).

d. To improve healing after periodontal surgery.

Thus, the primary goal of phase I is the elimination of inflammation and plaque control and it includes:

- Patient education and motivation.
- Mechanical plaque control – scaling and root planing.
- Correction of restorative and prosthetic irritational factors- Overhanging margins of dental restorations can be removed using a flame – shaped or flat diamond stone mounted on a handpiece.
- Excavation of caries and temporary restoration - Caries control or temporary fillings can be performed in phase I therapy. Amalgam and composite restorations may be performed to close contacts, to correct food impaction and to remove overhangs.
- Topical and systemic antimicrobial medication- Chemical control of plaque can be achieved by mouth rinses, irrigation or antibiotics.
- Occlusal therapy - Occlusal adjustment should follow scaling and root planing. If a tooth is extremely mobile, gross occlusal adjustment may be done before scaling to reduce mobility.
- Minor orthodontic movement - Orthodontic tooth movement may precede or follow any surgical interventions. Minor orthodontic tooth movement is performed in phase I, when there is inflammation or bony deformities due to tooth malalignment. But major orthodontic tooth movement done for purposes of reconstruction or esthetics, may follow surgery. Orthodontic therapy is now becoming a more integral part of the treatment of patients undergoing periodontal therapy.
- Provisional splinting and prosthesis- Wire ligation and composite acid-etch splinting are generally performed during phase I therapy. Temporary splinting, short-term stabilization for short periods upto six months, or provisional splinting long – term stabilization for up to two years, may be employed to control secondary occlusal trauma during the period before decisions are made about surgery.
- Diet changes/modifications.
- Additional preventive measures such as fluorides can be advised to caries prone patient.

Evaluation of response to etiotropic phase: Thorough, recorded evaluations of the appearance of tissue, the depth of pocket and of level of attachment, mobility, and plaque control should be done. The patient's response should be evaluated to determine whether surgical procedures are indicated and would be beneficial. The frequency of recall visits depends upon the response of the patient.

Surgical Phase: Phase II

Necessary surgery should be carried out in as few stages as possible over short possible time and it includes:

- Periodontal surgery
- Implant surgery - Surgery for first phase insertion of osseointegrated dental implants
- Endodontic therapy.

Evaluation of response to surgical procedures should be done before phase III.

Restorative Phase: Phase III

Restorative phase should follow periodontal surgery and it includes:

- Final restorations
- Fixed/Removable prosthesis are fabricated if needed.

Evaluation of response to restorative procedures should be done.

Maintenance Phase: Phase IV

Patients require recall for inspection, oral hygiene monitoring and scaling at 3, 6, 9 or 12 months intervals, depending upon the previous disease experience and susceptibility.

Periodic rechecking of plaque and calculus, gingival condition, occlusion, tooth mobility and other pathological changes should be done.

SEQUENCE

It is the scheduled sequence of therapeutic measures used to cure or arrest the patient's periodontal disease. It is divided into following 4 phases for each patient according to his needs. **(Fig. 36.1)**

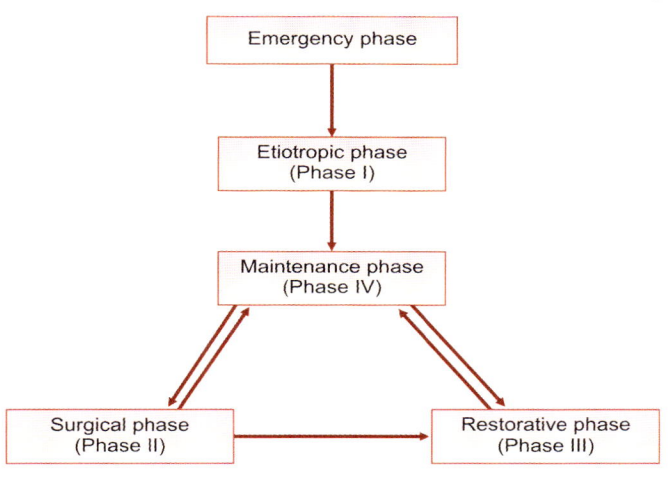

Fig.36.1: Sequence of periodontal therapy

PALLIATIVE TREATMENT

Following are the candidates for palliative treatment:
1. Patients with short life expectancy either due to advanced age/systemic diseases with poor survival prognosis such as poorly controlled diabetes or valvular heart defects.
2. Patients with severe mental and physical disabilities.
3. Patients with severe furcation involvement.
4. Patients with limited financial ability.
5. Noncoopertive patients for existing procedures.

REFERRAL

There are 3 basic reasons for referral:

A. Professional referrals may be medical or dental: Medical referral is indicated when the patient's medical history discloses significant information that may contribute to or influence the course of the treatment. Dental referral is indicated when the general dentist cannot provide the entire periodontal therapy. If clinically observable signs of inflammation and/ or ongoing attachment loss are present after treatment, the general dentist should consider other treatment modalities. If advanced periodontal therapy is among those choices, the general dentist has to consider a possible referral. Other forms of gingivitis and aggressive forms of periodontitis should be referred to the periodontist.

B. Moral and ethical: The specialists or consulting dentists upon completion of their therapy shall return the patient, to the referring dentist.

C. Legal: Dentists are obligated by laws to keep their diagnostic and treatment capabilities up to the standards. Dentists must exercise reasonable judgement in deciding whether to treat or refer their patients.

Other reasons for referral are patient relocation, dentist's preference and dentist-patient personality conflict.

Referral process: Once the general dentist decides to refer, the process should proceed with equal concern for the same communication and quality care that is expected of the periodontist. During the referral consultation, the patient should be informed of the benefits of treatment to be presented by the specialist. The timing of a referral may be fundamental to treatment success. Delay in a referral could change a treatable situation into a hopeless one. The termination of a referral relationship should always be accompanied by an explanation. Lastly, both the periodontist and the referring dentist should be willing to work together at moderate fees and therapy with those patients who are highly motivated but may not be financially competent.

BIBLIOGRAPHY

1. Carranza FA, Takei HH. The treatment plan. In, Newman, Takei, Carranza. Clinical Periodontology 9th ed WB Saunders 2003;503-06.
2. Eley BM, Manson JD. Diagnosis, prognosis and treatment plan. In, Periodontics 5th ed Wright 2004;149-60.
3. Grant DA, Stern IB, Listgarten MA. Treatment plan. In, Periodontics. 6th ed CV Mosby Company 1988;592-10.
4. Wilson RD. Referrals to Specialists. In, Wilson TG, Kornman KS. Fundamentals of Periodontics.Quintessence Publishing Co.1996;457-60.

MCQs

1. Which of all the following come under Phase I therapy:
   A. Excavation of caries
   B. Chemical plaque control
   C. Removal of calculus
   D. All of the above
2. Implant surgery is done in:
   A. Phase I   B. Phase II
   C. Phase III   D. Phase IV
3. Extraction of hopeless teeth is done in:
   A. Emergency Phase   B. Phase I
   C. Phase II   D. Phase III

Answers

   1. D   2. B   3. A

PERIODONTICS REVISITED

Mechanical Plaque Control

Shalu Bathla

INTRODUCTION

Plaque control is the prevention of the accumulation of dental plaque and other deposits on the teeth and adjacent gingival surfaces. The regular use of oral hygiene practices is a requisite for proper supragingival plaque elimination. The conventional toothbrush is the cleaning device most frequently used to remove dental plaque. The effectiveness of a self-care mechanical plaque control depends on motivation, knowledge, provision of oral hygiene instructions, type of oral hygiene aids used and manual dexterity. Motivation is defined as readiness to act or the driving force behind a person's actions. The first condition for success in attempting to establish needs - related toothcleaning habits is a well motivated, well-informed, and well-instructed patient.

TRADITIONAL ORAL HYGIENE METHODS

Traditional methods of oral hygiene have been an integral part of religious and/or traditional beliefs, and because of this and other reasons, such as their availability and low cost, these traditions have been practiced by these cultures for decades. For instance, in certain countries in Asia and Africa, chewing sticks prepared from certain plants have been used as oral hygiene tools. Normally, a stick is cut from the twigs, stems or roots of the plant, then chewed or tapered at one end until it becomes frayed into a brush-like tool. This is then used to brush the facial aspects of teeth and gingiva and the tongue. Some individuals may also leave this tool in the mouth for an extended period of time after brushing, thereby stimulating salivation and enhancing their cleansing effects. In addition, extracts which normally leach out of these sticks into the user's mouth are believed to have biological properties including potential antibacterial effects. It has been suggested that these plants contain antimicrobial substances that naturally protect them against invading microorganisms or other parasites, and that these substances may then exert their effect in protecting the host against cariogenic and periodontopathic bacteria.

Earlier toothbrush bristles were obtained from the hair of the hog or wild boar. Toothbrushes with natural bristles are not recommended now because they wear more rapidly and are hollow which allow microorganisms and debris to collect inside and are water absorbent also. Moreover, their physical qualifications cannot be standardized. Current toothbrushes have nylon bristles or polyester filaments which are durable and resistant to bacteria accumulation than natural bristles.

HISTORICAL PERSPECTIVE OF TOOTHBRUSH

1600 - Bristle toothbrush appear in China
1728 - Pierre Fauchard in his book *'The Surgeon Dentist'* advocated wet sponges and specially prepared herb roots
1780 - William Addis of England made the first toothbrush
1840 - England, France and Germany started producing bristle toothbrush
1857 - HN Wadsworth patented the first American toothbrush
1900 - Celluloid handles were used
1919 - AAP defined specifications
1938 - Nylon was first applied to toothbrush construction
1939 - Synthetic were substituted for natural materials

VARIOUS DESIGNS OF TOOTHBRUSHES

Manual Toothbrushes

Toothbrushes vary in size, design, and bristle hardness, length and arrangement. The choice is a matter of individual preference rather than a demonstrated superiority of any one type. Parts of toothbrush are shown in **Figure 37.1.**

Handle: It is the part that is grasped in the hand during toothbrushing. Handles are usually made of plastic which is sufficiently rigid and durable. The dimension of the handle of an adult is 6 inches, junior - 1/6th smaller than adult size and child is 1/3rd smaller than adult size. The handle should be thick enough to allow firm grip and good control.

Shank: It is the section that connects the head and handle. There may be twist, curve or angle in the shank with or without thumb rests **(Figs 37.2 and 37.3).**

Head: It is the working end which consists of tufts of bristles. The length of head is approximately 1 to 1¼ inch and the width - 5/16 to 3/8 inch. Bristle length / height - 7/16 inches. Brushing plane refers as the trim which is characteristic arrangement of the tips of the filaments at the brushing surface. It may range from filaments of equal length i.e flat planes to those with variable lengths such as bi-level, dome shaped. Bristles in adult toothbrush are usually 10-11 mm long. But the entire

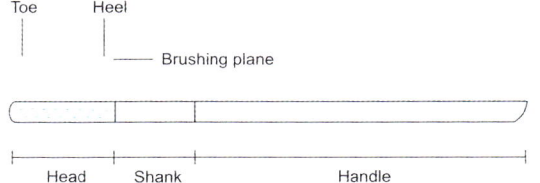

Fig. 37.1: Parts of toothbrush

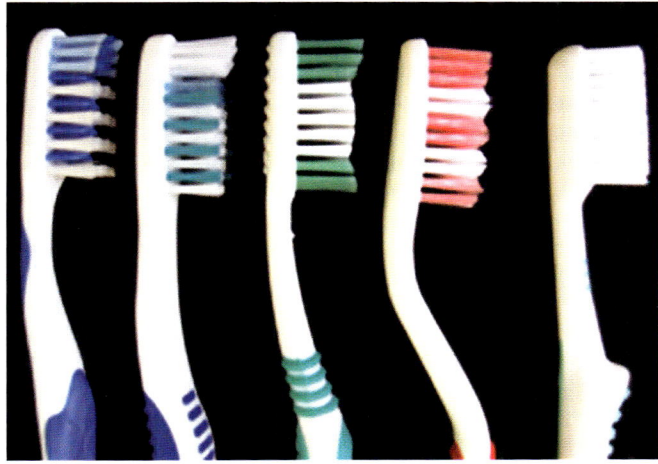

Fig. 37.2: Manual toothbrushes

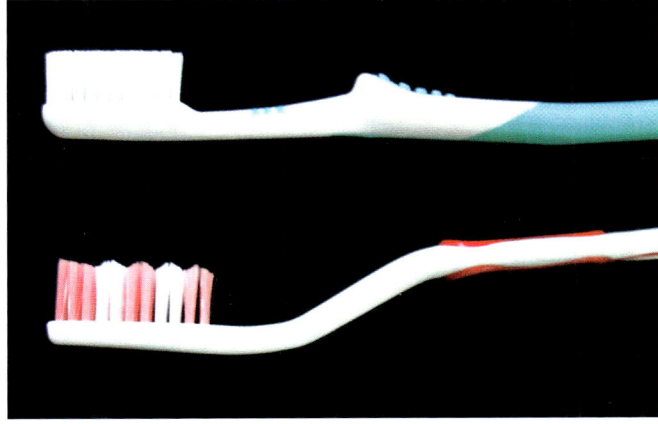

Fig. 37.3: Straight and angled shank toothbrushes

filament should have rounded end because it causes least trauma to the tissues.

ADA specifications of toothbrush
Length - 1 to 1.25 inches
Width - 5/16 to 3/8 inches
Rows - 2 to 4 rows of bristles
Tufts - 5 to 12 per row

PERIODONTICS REVISITED

The filament diameter ranges from soft to hard
- Soft   - 0.2 mm/ 0.007 inches
- Medium - 0.3 mm/ 0.012 inches
- Hard   - 0.4 mm/ 0.014 inches

Filament stiffness α diameter^2/length^2

Care of toothbrushes:
- *Cleaning toothbrushes*: Hold the brush head under strong stream of warm water to remove dentifrices and bacteria present between filaments and then tap the brush handle on edge of sink to remove excess water. Use another toothbrush to clean one tooth brush to remove resistant debris.
- *Brush storage*: It should be kept in open air with head in an upright position, apart from contact with other brushes. Keep the brushes in portable brush container having sufficient holes after being dried completely.
- *Brush replacement*: Toothbrush should be replaced before filaments frayed, at least every 2 to 3 months. But patients who are debilitated, have a known infection or are about to undergo surgery should be advised to disinfect their brush or use disposable brush.

Powered Toothbrushes

Electrically powered toothbrushes were invented in 1939. There are number of designs available with different forms of movements: arcuating, reciprocating and vibrating. The most recent electric toothbrushes have reciprocating, rotating circular head which are designed to clean each tooth surface separately, e.g. Phillips Sonicare, Braun/Oral and Colgate Actibrush. They are also called as mechanical, automatic/ electric brushes. Speed varies from low to high among different models. The thick handles of power assisted brushes have been shown to be easily handled and manipulated by patients with disability. The action is in-built in powered toothbrush. The only muscle training required is turning the handle to apply the brush to each surface of each tooth and holding it on each surface for a reasonable time period in a correct position **(Figs 37.4 and 37.5)**.

Indications:
  i. Those who wear orthodontic appliances
  ii. Children and adolescents
  iii. Those undergoing complex restorative and prostho-dontic treatment
  iv. Those with dental implants
  v. Patients with physical or mental disabilities
  vi. Hospitalized patients, elder ones who need to have their teeth cleaned by caregivers
  vii. Poorly compliant periodontal maintenance patient

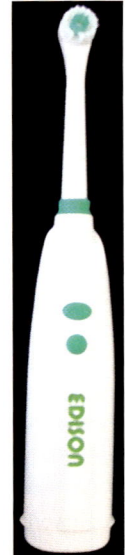

Fig. 37.4: Powered toothbrush

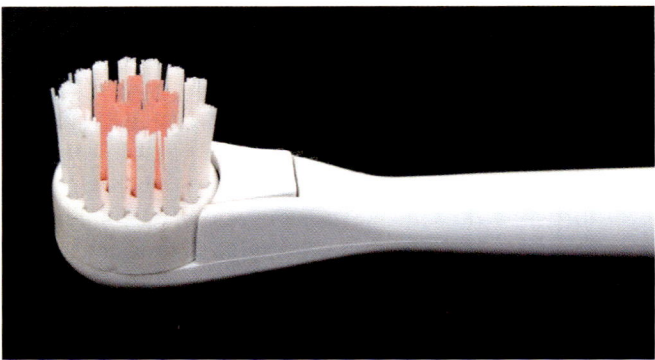

Fig. 37.5: Head of powered toothbrush

Orthodontic Toothbrushes

The head of the brush features soft bristles that are shorter down the center, with hedges of taller bristles on either side, allowing the brush to pass over the appliance without causing abrasion to the teeth. It is also called as bi-level toothbrush **(Figs 37.6 and 37.7)**.

Novel Toothbrushes

These designs are based on the assumption that the majority of the individuals use a simple horizontal brushing action and regular flat-headed brush, which is ineffective to reach the approximal surfaces in the dentition. Therefore, the design of the brush head has been changed and multiple tufts of bristles are angled in different directions **(Fig. 37.8)**. Thus, when the head is located horizontal to the tooth surface, there are bristles angled in the direction of the approximal tooth surfaces.

VARIOUS TOOTHBRUSHING METHODS

i. Roll:
- a. Roll method
- b. Modified Stillman

ii. Vibratory:
- a. Stillman
- b. Charter
- c. Bass

iii. Sulcular: Bass

iv. Simultaneous Sulcular: Collis

v. Circular: Fones

vi. Vertical: Leonard

vii. Horizontal: Scrub

viii. Physiologic: Smith

Bass Method

It is also called as intrasulcular method. This toothbrushing techniques was introduced by Charles Cassedy Bass in 1948, utilizes a soft multitufted brush with bristles 0. 007″ in diameter.

Indications:

a. For open interproximal areas, cervical areas beneath the height of contour of the enamel and exposed root surfaces.

b. Recommended for any patient with or without periodontal involvement.

Technique: Beginning at the most distal tooth in the arch, place the head of a soft brush parallel with the occlusal plane, with the brush head covering three to four teeth. Place the brush with the filament tips directed straight into gingival sulcus and interproximal embrasures **(Figs 37.9 and 37.10)**. The filaments will be directed at approximately 45° to long axis of the tooth **(Fig. 37.11)**. Correct application of brush should produce perceptible blanching of gingiva. Vibrate the brush back and forth with very short strokes without disengaging the tips of the filaments from the sulci.Complete approximately 20 strokes in the same position. Apply the brush to the next group of 2 or 3 teeth with overlap placement. Insert the brush vertically to reach the lingual surface of anterior teeth. Press the heel of the brush into the gingival sulcus area and proximal surfaces at a 45⁰ angle to the long axis of the teeth and brush with multiple short vibratory strokes. On the occlusal surfaces press the bristles firmly into the pits and fissures and brush with about 20 short back-and-forth strokes. Entire stroke is repeated at each position around the maxillary and mandibular arches, both facially and lingually.

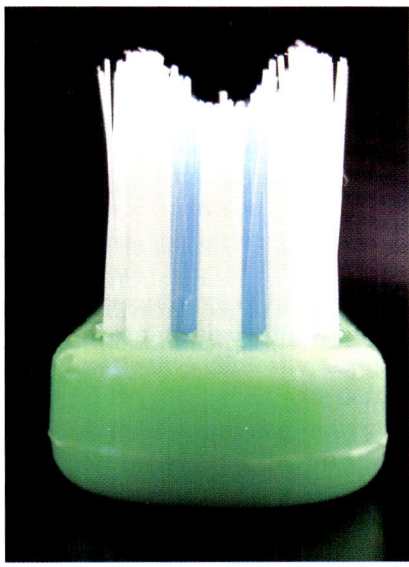

Fig. 37.6: Orthodontic brush

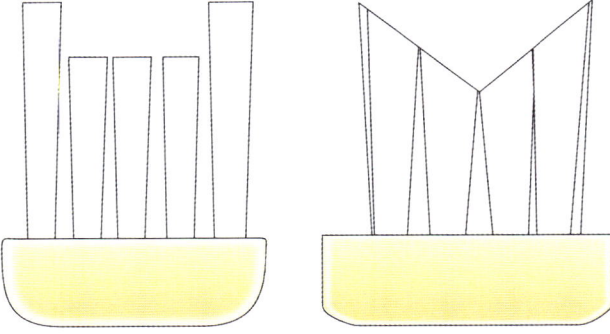

Fig. 37.7: Bi-level orthodontic brush

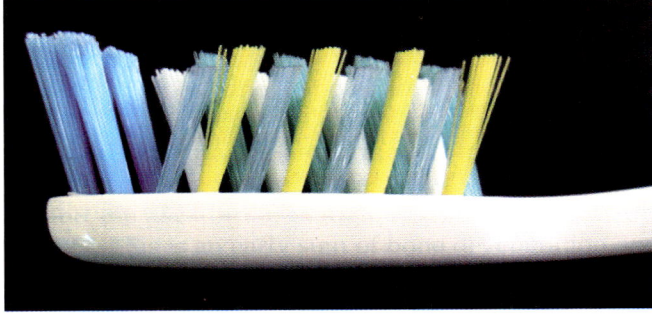

Fig. 37.8: Novel design toothbrush

PERIODONTICS REVISITED

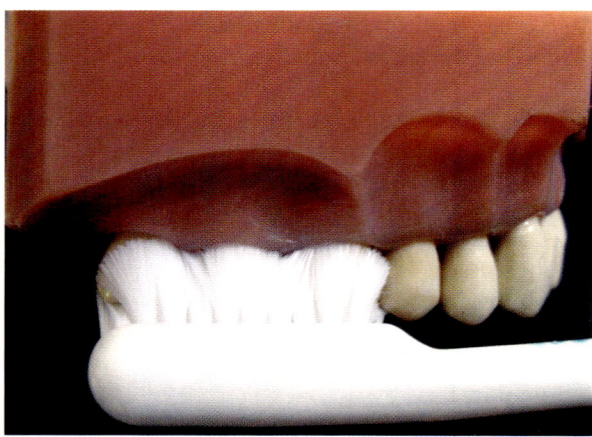

Fig. 37.9: Bass method (Facial view)

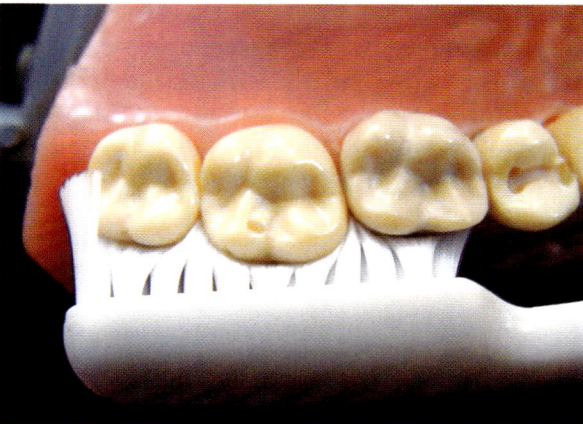

Fig. 37.10: Bass method (Occlusal view)

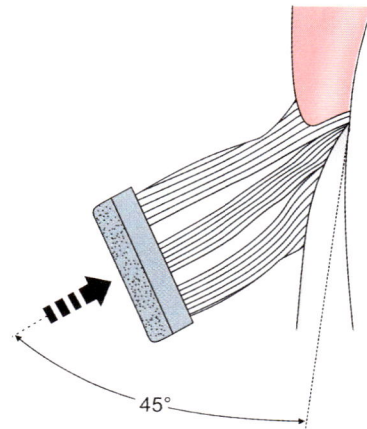

45°

Fig. 37.11: Bass method: Bristle tips are in sulcus and position of the brush is at 45° to long axis of tooth

Advantages:
- It cleans the gingival sulcus.
- It also cleans the interproximal and cervical portion of teeth.

In modified Bass method, bristles are swept towards the occlusal surface after completing the vibratory motion in the gingival sulcus.

Modified Stillman Method

This method was described by Paul R Stillman in 1932.

Indications: In areas with progressing gingival recession and root exposure to minimize abrasive tissue destruction.

Technique: The brush should be placed with the bristle ends resting partly on the cervical portion of the teeth and partly on the adjacent gingiva, pointing in an apical direction and at an oblique angle to the long axis of the teeth. Sides of the bristles are placed against the teeth and gingiva while moving the brush with short, back-and-forth strokes in a coronal direction. The occlusal surfaces of molars and premolars are cleaned with the bristles placed perpendicular to the occlusal plane and penetrating into the grooves and interproximal embrasures **(Figs 37.12 and 37.13)**.

Charters Method

This technique was first described by Leonard Koecker in 1819. However, it was William J Charters, in 1932 who endorsed and documented this technique.

Indications:
a. Cleaning in areas of healing wounds after periodontal surgery.
b. Cleaning in orthodontic appliances patient.
c. Remove bacterial plaque from abutment teeth and under the gingival border of a fixed partial denture(bridge) or from the undersurface of sanitary bridge.

Technique: Hold brush with filaments towards the occlusal or incisal plane of the teeth to be brushed, angle the filaments at 45° to the long axis of teeth **(Fig. 37.14)**. The sides of the bristles should be flexed against the gingiva, and a back-and forth vibratory motion used to brush. The technique was designed to gently massage the gingiva, so the bristle tips should not drag across the gingiva.

Horizontal Method

Place bristle tips at right angle on facial/lingual surfaces of teeth. Draw bristles across adjacent teeth and interdental papillae in horizontal direction.

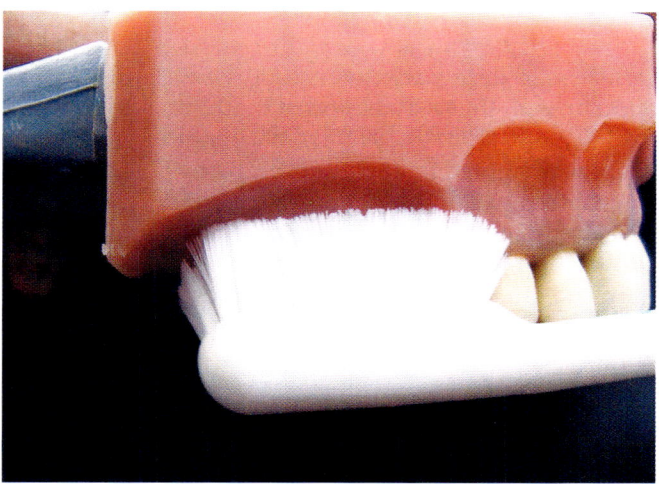

Fig. 37.12: Stillman method – Side of the bristles are placed against the teeth and gingiva

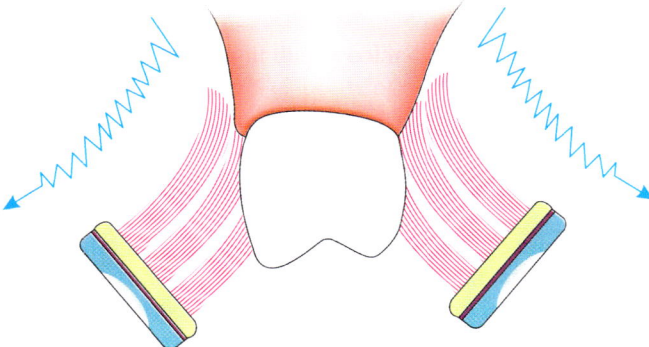

Fig. 37.13: Modified Stillman method – Brush is moved with short back and forth strokes in coronal direction

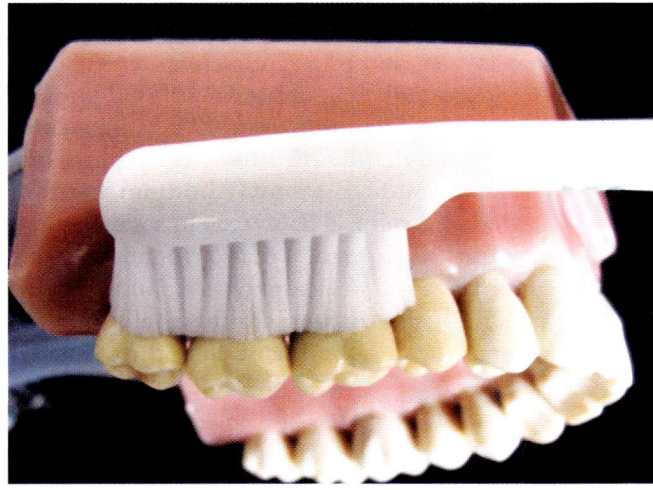

Fig. 37.14: Charters method

Disadvantages:
- This method does not clean the teeth adequately especially the proximal surfaces.
- Injures free gingiva, if performed forcefully can cause gingival recession.
- Can abrade cementum and dentin leading to tooth abrasion.

Physiologic Method

This method was described by T. Sidney Smith in 1940 and advocated later by Bell in 1948. It was based on the principle that the toothbrush should follow the same physiologic pathway that food follows when it traverses over the tissues in a natural masticating act. With soft brush, brush the gingival tissues towards apices of teeth in a gentle sweeping motion. Brushing strokes are directed down over the lower teeth onto the gingiva and upward over the teeth for the maxillary.

Disadvantages:
- Causes injury to soft tissues.
- Does not clean the teeth adequately.

Vertical Method

Leonard described and advocated vertical method of tooth brushing.

Hold teeth in edge to edge position. Direct bristles at right angle to the long axis of teeth. Vigorously move brush up and down on tooth surfaces. Use enough pressure to force the filaments into the embrasures.

Disadvantages:
- Does not clean teeth adequately
- May push debris towards gingival sulci
- May cause McCall's festoons.

Fones Method

Indications: School children/young children because of simplicity.

Dr Fones advocated this circular method. Occlude the teeth and lightly press bristles of toothbrush against posterior teeth and gingiva. Revolve brush head in a fast circular motion, using a large diameter circles. Continue circular motion. Hold maxillary and mandibular teeth apart and use same circular motion on maxillary lingual surfaces and then on mandibular lingual surfaces.

Disadvantages:
- May traumatize soft tissues
- Does not clean teeth adequately especially interproximal areas.

PERIODONTICS REVISITED

Scrub Method

Indications: Very young child to get feeling of brushing his teeth.

It consists of vigorously combined horizontal, vertical and circular strokes with some vibratory motions for certain areas.

Sequence of Toothbrushing

i.   Maxillary teeth first, then mandibular to avoid the deposition of loosened debris from maxillary teeth on brushed mandibular teeth.
ii.   Start brushing from a molar region of one arch around to the opposite side, then back around the lingual/ facial. Repeat in the opposing arch.
iii. Each brush placement must overlap the previous one for thorough coverage.
iv.   Encourage the patient to begin brushing the area that are most frequently missed or most difficult for brush placement.
v.   Sequence is varied at least once each day.

The deleterious effects of overzealous horizontal brushing are gingival recession, bacteremia, abrasion - wedge shaped defects in the cervical area of root surfaces and painful ulceration of the gingiva.

DENTIFRICES

Dentifrices date back over 2000 years and became popular with the re-invention of toothbrush by William Addis about 1770. In 1892, Dr Washington Wentworth Sheffield invented toothpaste tube. Bibby (1942) did first clinical trial of fluoride toothpaste.

Dentifrices are a substance used with a toothbrush or other applicator to remove bacterial plaque and debris from the gingiva and teeth. Thus, they aid in cleaning and polishing tooth surfaces. They are used in the form of pastes, powders and gels.

Different abrasives differ not only with regards to their chemical composition but also in particle size and shape (round, angular). These differences determine the polishing effect of product and abrasiveness of the dentifrices on dentin (measured in vitro as Radioactive/ relative dentin abrasion - RDA value). Therapeutic dentifrice has chemical agent added for a specific preventive/treatment action, e.g. fluoride, desensitizing agent, tartar control agents containing dentifrices. Colgate® Total™ is the first and only toothpaste to be approved by the FDA. For children a pea-sized amount of toothpaste should be used to avoid fluorosis. For adults enough toothpaste to cover the whole length of the toothbrush bristles should be used.

TABEL 37.1: Constituents of dentifrices				
Constituent	Purpose		Powder	Paste/ Gel
Abrasives	Cleaning/stain removal	Calcium Carbonate Calcium Phosphate Hydrated Alumina Hydrated Silica	90-98%	20-25%
Binder	Hold ingredients together	Carrageenan	0	3%
Detergent	Surfactant/foam builder	Sodium lauryl sulphate	1-6%	1-2%
Humectants	Provide creamy texture Moisturizing agent	Sorbitol Glycerin	0	20-35%
Flavoring	Improves taste	Spearmint Wintergreen Cinnamon	1-2%	1-2%
Fluorides	Anticariogenic reduces caries	NaF SnF$_2$	0	0-1%
Tartar control agents	Inhibit calculus formation	Triclosan Disodium pyrophosphate Tetrasodium pyrophosphate Tetrapotassium pyrophosphate	0	0-1%
Water	Solvent		0	15-25%
Desensitizing agent	Reduce hypersensitivity	Potassium nitrate Strontium chloride	0	0-5%
Colorants	Make opaque/ transparent	Food colorants Titanium dioxide	1-2%	1-2%

PERIODONTICS REVISITED

Therapeutic Ingredients:

a. *Fluoride agents*: Fluorides currently used in dentifrices are sodium fluoride, sodium monofluorophosphate, and stabilized stannous fluoride.

b. *Plaque-inhibiting agents*: Sanguinaria, chlorhexidine, lactoperoxidase, triclosan, zinc and stabilized stannous fluoride are the plaque - inhibiting agents used in dentifrices.

c. *Desensitizing agents*: Fluorides agents have been claimed to have desensitizing properties and are contained in specialized dentifrices (e.g. stannous fluoride); nonfluoride agents commonly used in desensitizing agents include strontium chloride, potassium nitrate, and sodium citrate.

d. *Tartar control agents*: Interfere with the calcium phosphate bond in the calculus matrix, thus allowing easier removal of soft calculus during toothbrushing; effective only on formation of supragingival calculus on enamel surfaces.

   1. *Pyrophosphate system*: Pyrophosphate has a negative charge, attracts positively charged calcium ions, and interferes with calculus formation.

   2. *Zinc system*: Zinc has a positive charge, attracts negatively charged phosphate ions, and interferes with calculus formation.

Whitening agents: Several dentifrices are marketed for their ability to remove stains; several whitening dentifrices have low abrasive levels; may be effective for maintenance of cosmetic restorations.

Baking soda: Manufacturers claim benefits from addition of baking soda or baking soda and peroxide to dentifrices; therapeutic benefits have not been demonstrated in controlled clinical trials.

INTERDENTAL CLEANING AIDS

Interdental cleaning aids are interdental brushes, dental floss, interdental tips, wooden tips, rubber tips, plastic tips and dental tape.

The various factors, which should be taken into consideration while recommending an interdental cleaning methods are type and size of the interproximal embrassure **(Fig. 37.15)**, e.g. in type 1 embrassures –no gingival recession, dental floss is been used; type 2 embrassures where there is moderate papillary recession, interdental brush is used; and in type 3 embrassures there is complete loss of papillae, there unitufted brush is used. Other factors are contour and consistency of gingival tissues, tooth position and alignment, ability and

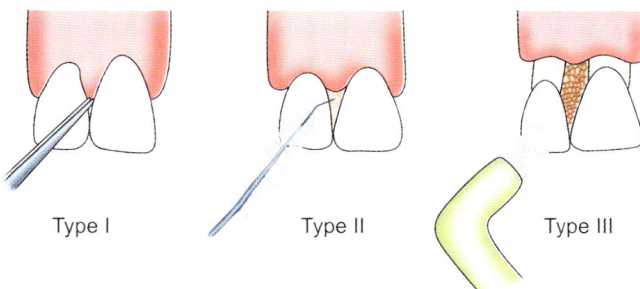

Type I   Type II   Type III

Fig. 37.15: Interproximal embrasure spaces

motivation of patient, presence of orthodontic appliance or fixed prostheses and presence of furcation lesion.

Interproximal brush: Interdental area is the most common site of plaque retention and the most inaccessible area to the toothbrush. Thus, special methods of cleaning is required. The diameter of interproximal brush should be slightly larger than the gingival embrasures to be cleaned, so that bristles can exert pressure on both proximal surfaces as well as root concavities. These brushes are inserted through interproximal spaces and moved back and forth between teeth with short strokes **(Figs 37.16 and 37.17)**.

The types of interdental brushes are:

a. Small insert brushes with reusable handles

b. Brush with wire handle. They are recommended in exposed root surfaces having concavities or grooves, through and through furcation.

The advantages of interdental brushes over dental floss are that: Interdental brushes clean concave root surface and furcations more efficiently than dental floss and are much easier to use than dental floss **(Fig. 37.18)**. When floss is placed over a concave surface in furcation region, contact is not possible and thus supplementary interdental devices are needed to completely remove plaque and deposits. When dentifrices are used, dental tape may be better than floss in retaining the dentifrices against the tooth.

In single tufted brush, there is present a group of small tufts 3 to 6 mm in diameter which may be flat or tapered **(Fig. 37.19)**. These are recommended in furcation areas, distal surfaces of the most posterior molars. These brushes are adaptable around and under fixed partial dentures, pontic and implant abutment easily. The end of tuft is directed into interproximal area and along the gingival margin.

Dental floss and tape: The floss can be waxed or unwaxed. The wax covering waxed dental floss facilitates the movement of floss, prevents excessive absorption of moisture and helps to prevent shredding. Now, powered

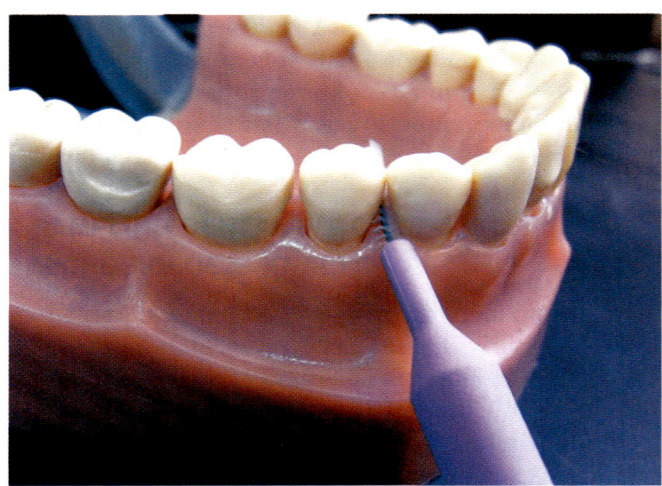

Fig. 37.16: Interdental brush

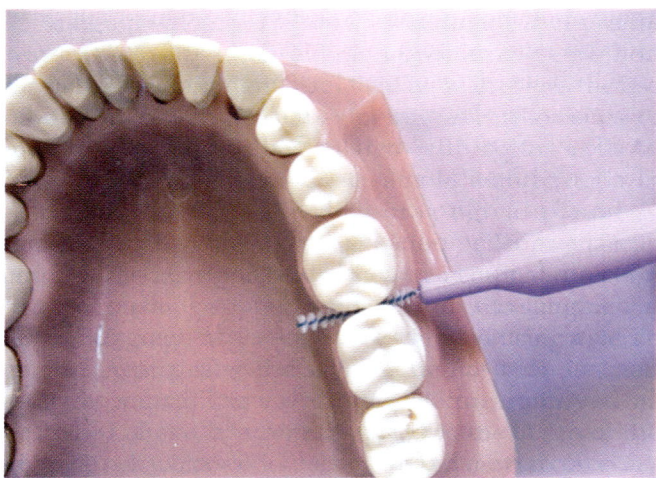

Fig. 37.17: Interdental brush (Occlusal view)

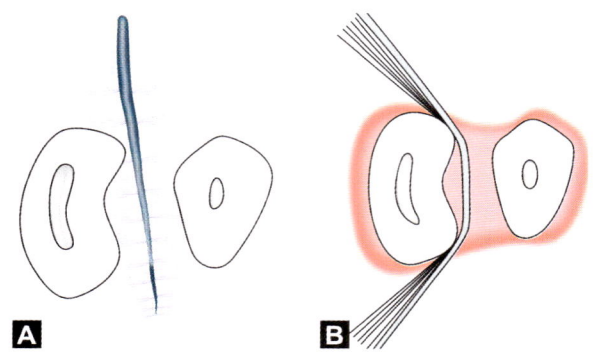

Figs 37.18A and B: Effective cleaning of concave proximal tooth surface with interdental brush (A) as compared to dental floss (B)

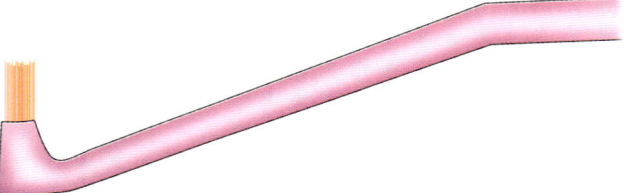

Fig. 37.19: Unituft brush

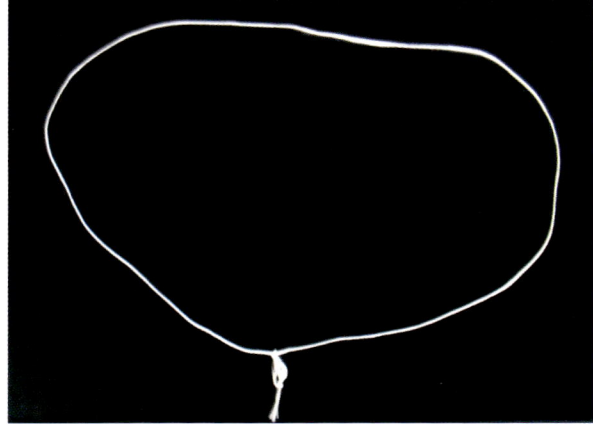

Fig. 37.20: Dental floss in loop

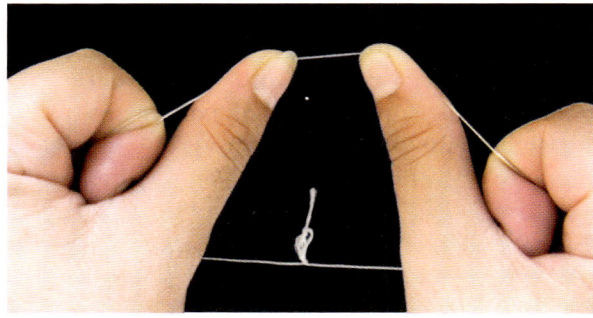

Fig. 37.21: Holding of floss between thumbs for use in maxillary teeth

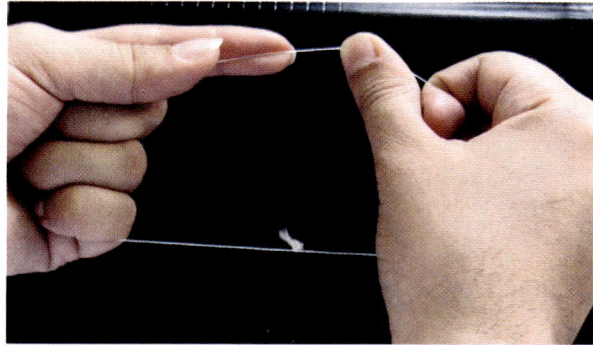

Fig. 37.22: Holding of floss between thumb and index finger for use in maxillary teeth

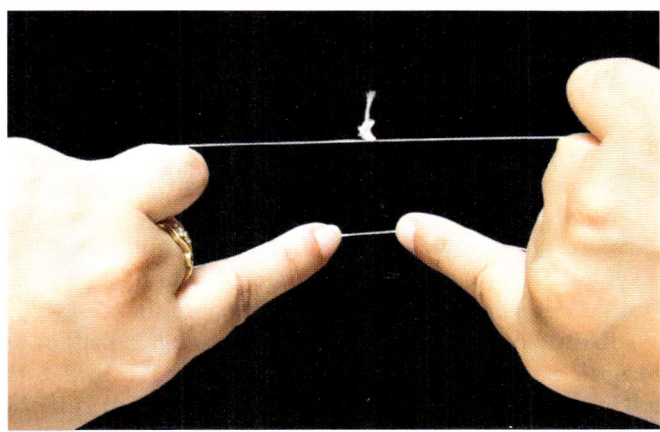

Fig. 37.23: Holding of floss for use in mandibular teeth

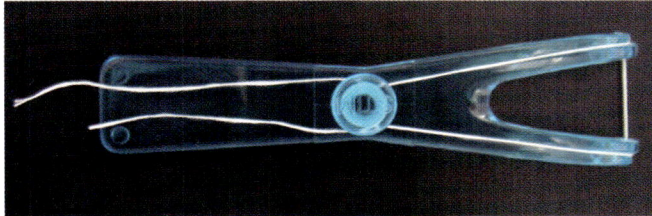

Fig. 37.24: Reusable floss holder

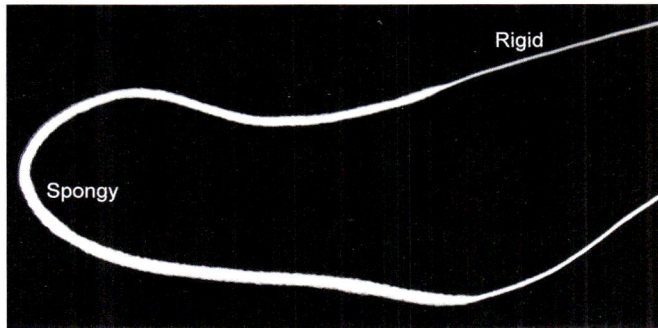

Fig. 37.25: Superfloss

An alternative to the floss threader is Superfloss, a type of floss that incorporates rigid plastic portion that can be introduced under fixed bridges. Distal to the rigid plastic portion is a spongy region that is ideal for plaque removal **(Fig. 37.25)**. The terminal portion of Superfloss is similar to standard dental floss. Superfloss is generally easier to use than floss threaders. The rigid portion is passed into the embrasure space between the retainer and the pontic and pulled through the lingual aspect. The spongy region is then used in an apicocoronal stroke along the intaglio surface of the pontic.

Dental tape: It is used with fluoride dentifrice which is recommended for cleaning the approximal surfaces of molars and premolars in children and adults with a rubbing motion, holding the tape by the hand/in a special holder.

Toothpick: They are usually 2 inch long made of soft wood (basswood/birchwood) and are triangular in shape. They are recommended in patients with open interdental spaces. In fluoridated wooden toothpick, wood can store sodium fluoride crystals both on the surface and in porosites. Sodium fluoride crystal dissolves readily in contact with liquids such as water/saliva. The toothpicks should be moistened in the saliva for a few seconds just before use to accelerate the release of fluoride. Toothpick is contraindicated in children and young adults because interdental space is filled by a normal papilla.

flossing devices are also been introduced. Technique- 12 to 18 inches of dental floss is taken and is wrapped around fingers or ends may be tied together in a loop. **(Fig. 37.20)**. The floss is stretched tightly between thumb and forefinger or between both forefingers and is passed through each contact area with a firm back and forth motion **(Figs 37.21 to 37.23)**. Wrap the floss around the proximal surface of one tooth, once it is placed apical to contact area between the teeth. The floss is then moved firmly along the line angle of tooth upto the contact area and gently down into sulcus, with repeated up and down strokes several times. Then move floss across the interdental gingiva and repeat the procedure on the proximal surface of the adjacent tooth. They are recommended in patients where interdental papillae completely fill the embrasure space.

Floss holders are commercially available to assist patients who have difficulty in flossing. These are primarily plastic handles that hold the floss in such a way as to serve as "substitute fingers" **(Fig. 37.24)**. Some patients benefit from these devices, especially those who have difficulty with manual dexterity, but they can be difficult to use initially.

Other Aids

Tongue scraper: It may be made of plastic, stainless steel or other flexible metal. It is indicated in high caries risk, periodontal risk patients and patients suffering from halitosis. Rationale behind tongue cleaning is that periodontal pathogens produce Volatile Sulphur compounds (VSC) which is responsible for halitosis and accumulates mostly within the filiform papillae and on

PERIODONTICS REVISITED

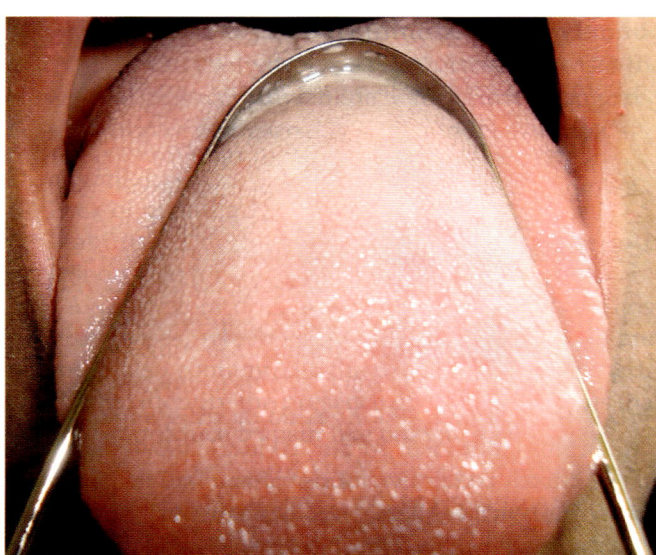

Fig. 37.26: Tongue scraper facilitate removal of microorganism accumulations from the dorsum of tongue, which is the main cause of halitosis

the back of the tongue. The tongue brush/scrapers are placed as far back on the tongue as possible **(Fig. 37.26)**. Once the scraper is in position, gently drag it forward and repeat 2 or 3 times or until tongue is clean.

ASSESSMENT OF HOME CARE

Assessment of the effectiveness of patient plaque control is an ongoing process, beginning at the initial evaluation and continuing throughout therapy, including maintenance. Home care can be assessed using a variety of methods. First, the teeth can simply be inspected visually for the presence or absence of plaque. This is the least effective method, because plaque can be difficult to see. Second, plaque can be made visible through the use of a disclosing solution.

Various indexes have been developed for this purpose. One widely used index is O'Leary plaque index. Such indexes can serve two purposes:

1. For use in monitoring patient's progress (e.g. for assessing whether home care is sufficient to permit surgical intervention), or
2. As a patient motivation tool.

Disclosing agents: Disclosing solution contains a dye or other coloring substance, which imparts its color to calculus, plaque and films on the surface of teeth, tongue and gingiva. It is a excellent oral hygiene aids because they can provide the patient with additional motivational

tool to improve the efficiency of plaque control procedures. It also conserve operating time by making inconspicuous deposits more evident.

Factors to be considered in the selection of a disclosing solution are:

i. Intensity of color
ii. Taste
iii. Non-irritating to mucous membrane
iv. Diffusibility - neither too thin nor too thick
v. Astringent and antiseptic

The various disclosing agents are **(Fig. 37.27)**: Skinner Iodine, Iodine disclosing solution, Diluted Tincture of Iodine, Berwick's solution, Buckley's solution, Talbot Iodoglycerol, Metaphen, Basic fuchsin, Bismarck Brown, Easlick's solution, Bender's solution, Mercurochrome solution, Erythrosin (FDC Red No. 3), DC yellow no. 8 fluorescein, Two tone dye (FDC red no. 3 and FDC green no.3). Two - tone dye test uses FDC red no. 3 and FDC green no. 3 solution which stains thick accumulation of plaque as blue and thin deposits are stained red/pink.

Limitations:

i. Do not selectively disclose bacteria plaque, but rather stain all soft debris and pellicle.
ii. Exposed cementum in particular can stain vividly although it is free of bacterial plaque.
iii. Disclosing solution may stain silicate cement or resin restoration.
iv. Disclosing solutions containing alcohol should not be kept for more than 2-3 months since the alcohol will evaporate and render the solution too highly concentrated.

Strategies for improving home care performance: The first step in addressing insufficient home care is to determine

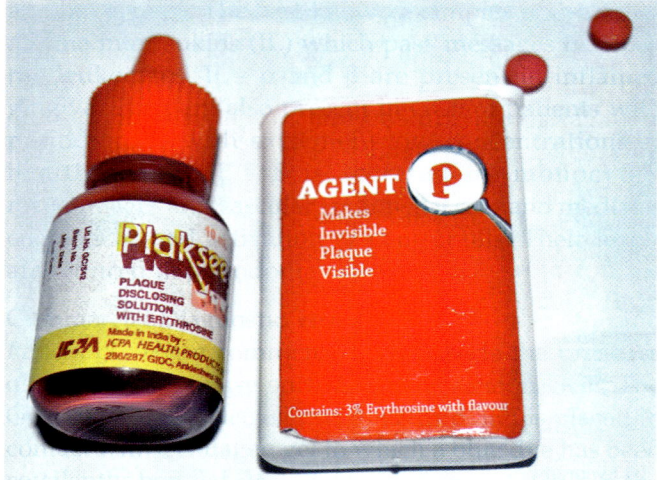

Fig 37.27: Disclosing agents- liquid and tablet form

the cause of the problem. There are, essentially three possibilities:

1. The patient does not know what to do (lacks knowledge).
2. The patient knows what to do, but is unable to perform (lacks dexterity).
3. The patient knows what to do, is able to do it, but simply does not comply with the regimen (lacks motivation).

Toothbrushing techniques can be demonstrated both on a model and in patient's mouth. Ideally, brushing should be performed before a mirror with a good light so that the patient can check the placement of brush and bristles. The patient should brush at night before going to bed. Thus, during the hours of sleep, the mouth will be as clean as possible, and plaque will not be left *in situ* for 12 or more hours.

LANDMARK STUDIES RELATED

Lang NP, Cumming BR, Loe H. Toothbrushing frequency as it relates to plaque development and gingival health. Journal of Periodontology 1973;44:396-405.

Thirty two dental students with clean teeth and healthy gingiva were randomized to four groups and assessed weekly for 6 weeks. The four groups removed plaque respectively every 12 hrs, every 48 hrs, every 72 hrs and every 96 hrs. The 12 hrs group maintained a plaque index of around 0.5 – 0.8, whereas the other three groups eventually reached a plateau of around 1.5. However, the gingival index for both the 12 hrs and 48 hrs group reached a plateau of around 0.1 – 0.2 and stayed there from 4 weeks onwards, whereas the 72 hrs group steadily climbed to 0.5 at 6 weeks and the 96 hrs group reached 0.9 at the same point. Thus, the result showed that the increased plaque of the 48 hrs group did not have the same consequences as the similar quantities in the 72 hrs and 96 hrs groups; this points to factors other than quantity having a role in plaque pathogenicity.

POINTS TO PONDER

✓ Adjunctive aids used for cleansing oral cavity are irrigators, tongue scrapers and dentifrices.
✓ Tooth powders contain about 95% abrasives and five times more abrasive than pastes. Detergents found in dentifrices denature lectin adhesins.
✓ Approximal areas are the visible spaces between teeth that are not under the contact area and interproximal areas refer to the area under and related to the contact point.
✓ "Hawthorne effect", which occurs when research subjects behave differently because they realize that they are being observed.

BIBLIOGRAPHY

1. Axelsson P, Albandar JM, Rams TE. Prevention and control of periodontal diseases in developing and industrialized nations. Periodontol 2000 2002;29:235-46.
2. Echeverria JJ, Sanz M. Mechanical Supragingival Plaque Control. In, Lindhe J, Karring T, Lang NP. Clinical Periodontology and Implant dentistry. 4th ed Blackwell Munksgaard 2003;449-63.
3. Eley BM, Manson JD. Prevention of periodontal disease. In, Periodontics 5th ed Wright 2004;133-43.
4. Grant DA, Stern IB, Listgarten MA. Plaque control (oral hygiene, chemical plaque control), root sensitivity and halitosis. In, Periodontics. 6th ed CV Mosby Company 1988;611-49.
5. Oral infection control: Toothbrushes and toothbrushing. In, Wilkins EM. Clinical practice of the Dental hygienist. 8th ed Lippincott Williams and Wilkins; 350-69.
6. Perry DA. Plaque control for the periodontal patient. In, Newman, Takei, Carranza. Clinical Periodontology 9th ed WB Saunders 2003;651-74.
7. Thomas MV. Oral Physiotherapy. In, Rose LF, Mealey BL, Genco RJ, Cohen DW. Periodontics, Medicine, Surgery and Implants. Elsevier Mosby 2004;214-36.
8. Wilkins EM. Interdental care and chemotherapy. In, Clinical practice of the Dental hygienist. 8th ed Lippincott Williams and Wilkins; 370-93.
9. Woodall IR. Preventing periodontal disease. In, Genco RJ, Goldman HM and Cohen DW. Contemporary Periodontics. CV Mosby Company 1990;361-70.

MCQs

1. Portion of the brush that assists in removal of plaque:
   A. Tip of the brush
   B. Tip of bristle
   C. Sides of bristle
   D. Whole brush
2. The stiffness of the bristles of a nylon toothbrush is dependent on the:
   A. Diameter and length of filament
   B. Amount of polish of filament
   C. Color of filament
   D. Consistency of shape of the filament
3. Humectant in a dentifrice serves:
   A. As an abrasive
   B. Retains moisture
   C. Flavoring agent
   D. Foaming agent

PERIODONTICS REVISITED

4. Which of the following is not found in commercially available toothpaste:
   A. Humectants   B. Sweetening agents
   C. Detergents   D. Astringent

5. The active ingredient present in tartar control toothpaste is:
   A. Pyrophosphate
   B. Metaphosphate
   C. Carboxy methyl
   D. Bicarbonate

6. Which of the following wax is present on dental floss?
   A. Bees wax
   B. Spermaceti wax
   C. Japan wax
   D. Carnauba wax

7. Recommended aid for plaque removal in type II embrasures:
   A. Proxabrush
   B. Floss
   C. Unitufted brush
   D. Stim-U-dent

8. Which one of the following does not provide significant therapeutic value when incorporated in a toothpaste:
   A. Fluorides
   B. Pyrophosphates
   C. Chlorhexidine
   D. All of the above

9. The cleansing property of a dentifrice/ tooth brush is primarily a function of its:
   A. Fluoride content
   B. Physical form viz. Paste/ Powder
   C. Abrasiveness
   D. Binding agents

10. Disclosing agent that differentiates mature and immature plaque:
    A. Two – tone solution
    B. Bismarck Brown
    C. Bender's solution
    D. Mercurochrome solution

11. Natural bristles used in toothbrushes are extracted from:
    A. Hogs   B. Dogs
    C. Hares   D. Horses

12. The angle that should be established between long axis of tooth and toothbrush bristles in bass method:
    A. 55°
    B. 75°
    C. 45°
    D. 65°

13. The brushing technique which is recommended after periodontal surgery is:
    A. Bass technique
    B. Modified stillman method
    C. Charters method
    D. None of the above

14. Adverse effect of oral hygiene aids may be:
    A. Tooth abrasion
    B. Gingival recession
    C. Bacteremia
    D. All of the above

15. Disclosing solution is a useful adjunct for teaching individuals their strengths and weakness in bacterial plaque removal. It is especially important for assessing subgingival plaque removal techniques:
    A. Both statements are TRUE
    B. Both statements are FALSE
    C. The first statement is TRUE, the second statement is FALSE
    D. The first statement is FALSE, the second statement is TRUE

16. The Bass, or sulcular, toothbrushing technique:
    A. Requires a high level of dexterity to perform
    B. Disrupts plaque at and under the gingival margin
    C. Uses a circular vibratory stroke
    D. Directs the toothbrush bristles occlusally at a 45° angle

17. Oral irrigating devices have been shown to:
    A. Reduce the incidence of refractory periodontitis
    B. Initiate keratinization of sulcular epithelium
    C. Promote the healing following periodontal surgery
    D. None of the above

Answers

1. B	2. A	3. B	4. D	5. A
6. B	7. A	8. C	9. C	10. A
11. A	12. C	13. C	14. D	15. C
16. B	17. D			

PERIODONTICS REVISITED

CHAPTER 38

Chemotherapeutic Agents

Shalu Bathla

TERMINOLOGY

Chemotherapeutic agent: Chemotherapeutic agent is a general term for a chemical substance that provides a clinical therapeutic benefit. Chemotherapeutic agents can be administered locally, orally, or parenterally.

Antimicrobial agent: An antimicrobial agent is a chemotherapeutic agent that works by reducing the number of bacteria present. Antibiotics are a naturally occurring, semisynthetic or synthetic type of antimicrobial agents that destroy or inhibit the growth of selective microorganisms, generally at low concentrations.

Antiseptic: An antiseptic is a chemical antimicrobial agent that is applied to living tissues to prevent or arrest the growth or action of microorganisms. In dentistry, antiseptics are widely used as the active ingredient in antiplaque and antigingivitis mouthrinses and dentifrices.

Disinfectant: It is antimicrobial agent, that is generally applied to inanimate surfaces to destroy microorganisms.

COMMONLY USED CHEMOTHERAPEUTIC AGENTS IN PERIODONTICS

i. Antibiotics
ii. Analgesics
iii. Sedatives
iv. Muscle relaxants
v. Postoperative periodontal dressings
vi. Desensitizing agents
vii. Chemical antiplaque agents
viii. Dentifrices
ix. Anticalculus agents
x. Corticosteroids
xi. Hemostatics and Vasoconstrictors
xii. Anesthestics

In this chapter, only chemical antiplaque agents, anticalculus agents and antibiotics will be discussed in detail.

CHEMICAL ANTIPLAQUE AGENTS

Subgingival plaque is derived from supragingival plaque and intimately associated with the advancing lesions of chronic periodontal diseases. On the basis that plaque-induced gingivitis usually precedes the occurrence and re-occurrence of periodontitis, the mainstay of primary and secondary prevention of periodontal diseases is the control of supragingival plaque. Mechanical tooth cleaning through toothbrushing with dentifrice is arguably the most common and potentially effective form of oral hygiene. The chemical preventive agents should be used as adjuncts and not as the replacements for the more conventional and accepted effective mechanical methods. The advantage of chemical approach of antiplaque agent is that zone of diffusion achieved with chemical agent is greater than the limited radius of effect of a mechanical agent.

The action of chemical antiplaque agent can be categorized into **(Fig. 38.1)**:

i. Antiadhesive: Prevents bacterial attachment to the tooth e.g. Chlorhexidine, Delmopinol, Amine alcohol.
ii Antimicrobial: Stop/slow bacterial proliferation, e.g. Chlorhexidine, Antibiotics.
iii. Established plaque removal/Chemical toothbrush e.g. Amine alcohol, Enzymes.
iv. Antipathogenic: Alter the pathogenicity of plaque.

The antiplaque agents accepted by FDA for treatment of gingivitis are: Chlorhexidine (Prescription drug) and Listerine (Over the Counter/Non-prescription drug). In September 1987, Listerine antiseptic mouthwash was the first non-prescription product to be awarded the ADA

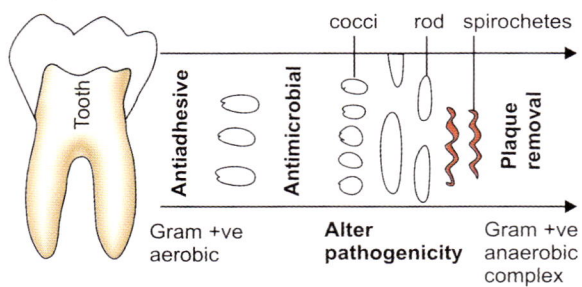

Fig. 38.1: Actions of chemical antiplaque agents

Council on Dental therapeutic seal of acceptance as an aid in controlling supragingival dental plaque.

Chlorhexidine (CHX)

Chlorhexidine was developed by Imperial Chemical Industries, England in 1940s and marketed in 1954 as an antiseptic for skin wound. Plaque inhibition by chlorhexidine was first investigated by Schroeder in 1969, but the definitive study was performed by Loe and Schiott in 1970. Chlorhexidine is available in three forms, the digluconate, acetate and hydrochloride salts. It is the front-runner and bench mark against which most of the other topical supragingival antiplaque agents have been compared.

Structure

It is symmetrical molecule consisting of:

i. Two 4 chlorophenyl rings
ii. Two biguanide groups
iii. A central hexamethylene bridge connecting chlorophenyl and biguanide group

Various chemical antiplaque agents are:

Antibiotics	Penicillin, Vancomycin, Kanamycin
Bisbiguanide antiseptics	Chlorhexidine, Alexidine, Octenidine
Phenols and essential oils	Thymol, Triclosan, Hexylresorinol
Natural products	Sanguinarine
Quartenary ammonium compounds	Cetylpyridinium chloride
Oxygenating agents	Hydrogen peroxide, Sodium peroxyborate, Sodium peroxycarbonate
Detergents	Sodium lauryl sulfate
Enzymes	Protease, Lipase, Nuclease, Dextranase, Mutanase-Glucose oxidase, Amyloglucosidase
Amine alcohol	Octapinol, Delmopinol
Metal salts	Tin, Zinc, Copper
Fluorides	Sodium fluoride, Stannous fluoride, Amine fluoride.

Mechanism of Action

I. *Antibacterial activity:* Cationic chlorhexidine is rapidly attracted to the negatively charged bacterial cell surface, with specific and strong adsorption to phosphate containing compounds.

II. *Antiplaque activity*:
    i. It blocks the acidic groups on the salivary glycoproteins thus, inhibit pellicle formation.
    ii. It directly binds to the bacterial surface in sublethal amounts and thus, prevents the adsorption of bacteria onto tooth surface.
    iii. It inhibits acid production in established plaque.

The peculiar features of chlorhexidine are:

- *Substantivity property*: The quality of prolonged contact time between a substance and substrate is known as substantivity. It is influenced by the concentration of the medication, its pH and temperature and length of contact of the solution with oral surfaces. Substantivity property for chlorhexidine was first described in 1976 by Bonesvoll et al. The substantivity period for chlorhexidine is around 12 hours. The substantivity of plaque – inhibitory substance depends upon pharmacokinetics, concentration and dose, effectiveness over time and site of application.
- Chlorhexidine can be more suitable for repeated use, as it does not suffer from the potential drawback of inducing bacterial resistance. Studies have shown that chlorhexidine is less effective in changing the bacterial flora as compared to tetracycline and metronidazole.

Clinical uses of chlorhexidine are:
    i. Presurgical preparation of periodontal patients
    ii. Postoral surgery including periodontal surgery/root planing
    iii. In patients with jaw fixation
    iv. Medically compromised patients predisposed to oral infections
    v. Mentally and physically handicapped patients
    vi. High caries risk patients
    vii. Recurrent oral ulceration
    viii. Removable and fixed orthodontic appliance wearers
    ix. In the denture stomatitis patients
    x. Preoperative rinsing during ultrasonic scaling and polishing with high speed instruments

Adverse effects:
    i. Staining: Brown discoloration of teeth, restoration and dorsum of tongue. The various proposed mechanism of chlorhexidine staining are:

- Degradation of chlorhexidine molecule to release parachloraniline
- Precipitation of anionic dietary chromogens
- Protein denaturation with metal sulfide formation
- Catalysis of Maillard reactions

    ii. Taste alteration—Interference with taste sensation is probably caused by denaturation of surface proteins on the taste buds.
    iii. Oral mucosal erosion- It is due to precipitation of the mucin layer thus, reducing its lubricating effect.
    iv. Increased calculus formation-The dead microbes due to the use of chlorhexidine may act as an initiator for calculus formation, which is based on the seeding mechanism of calculus formation.
    v. Unilateral or bilateral parotid swelling-Stenosis of the parotid duct has also been reported.

The instructions given to patient after prescribing chlorhexidine mouthwash are that the patient is asked to brush with dentifrice at least after half an hour because of the binding of cationic chlorhexidine to anionic components of the dentifrice. There is reduction in the activity by decreasing the number of active cationic sites. The patients are advised to avoid the intake of tea, coffee and red wine for the duration of use. The Corosdyl available in UK contains 0.2% chlorhexidine and 10 ml volume/rinse is recommended and chlorhexidine mouthwash available in USA is Peridex and in India PerioGard which contains 0.12% chlorhexidine and 15 ml volume/rinse is recommended.

Quarternary Ammonium Compounds

Cetylpyridinium chloride has been widely used as mouthrinses at a concentration of 0.05%, mainly as an antimicrobial agent. Cetylpyridinium chloride molecule has both hydrophilic and hydrophobic interactions. Interaction with bacteria is assumed to be similar to that achieved by chlorhexidine, i.e. via cationic binding. Initial retention of Cetylpyridinium chloride is higher than that of chlorhexidine but clearance of the former is more rapid. The substantivity of Cetylpyridinium chloride appears to be only 3-5 hours due to either loss of activity once adsorbed or rapid desorption.

Listerine

It is phenol related essential oils consisting of thymol (0.064%), eucalyptol (0.092%), methanol (0.042%), methyl salicylate (0.060%) in hydrochloride solution and benzoic acid (0.15%).

The advantages of listerine are that there is no taste alteration or staining as seen with chlorhexidine usage. It is less expensive and is easier to obtain than chlorhexidine, as it is sold over the counter.

The disadvantage of Listerine is its high alcohol concentration (ranging from 21.6 to 26.9%) which, may exacerbate xerostomia. It is contraindicated in patients under the treatment of alcoholism who take antabuse drugs (Disulfiram).

The alcohol is added in mouthrinses to solubilize antimicrobial compound in order to make them bio-available and to improve the shelf-life of the mouthrinse and to some extent improve the pleasurable characteristic of mouthrinsing.

Triclosan

It is off white, odorless, tasteless, crystalline powder with molecular weight of 289.5 and melting point of $57 \pm 1°$ C. It is nonionic antimicrobial which has been widely used over many years in antiperspirants and soaps. Now, it has been formulated into toothpaste and mouthrinses. Triclosan act on the microbial cytoplasmic membrane causing leakage of cellular constitutents and thereby, causing bacteriolysis. Presumably, the hydrophobic portion of the triclosan molecule adsorbs to the lipid portion of the bacterial cell membrane functions. It is bacteriostatic at low concentration and bacteriocidal at high concentration. It has broad spectrum of antimicrobial activity against yeasts, gram-positive and gram-negative bacteria. Triclosan has the substantivity period of approximately 5 hours. Activity of triclosan is enhanced by addition of zinc citrate and polyvinylmethyl ether maleic acid.

Advantages:
- No staining
- Can inhibit several important mediators of gingival inflammation
- It has dual effect both as an antibacterial and anti-inflammatory
- Triclosan is not significantly impaired by the presence of Sodium lauryl sulphate (SLS) as chlorhexidine do.

Povidone Iodine

It was introduced into Anglo-American countries in late 1960s. It is iodophor, a compound that consists of iodine plus a solubilizing agent, i.e. polyvinylpyrrolidone (povidone) from which iodine is continually delivered. Available iodine equivalents can be calculated by dividing the PVP-1 concentration by 10. For example,

povidone-iodine (10%) actually contains 1% iodine. PVP-1 is microbiocidal for gram-positive and gram negative bacteria, fungi, mycobacteria, viruses and protozoans. Its bacterial activity is due to oxidation of amino, thiol and hydroxyl groups. PVP-1 reacts strongly with double bonds of unsaturated fatty acids in cell walls and organelle membranes. Thus, causing transient or permanent pore formation which results in loss of cytoplasmic material and deactivation of enzymes due to direct contact with iodine. The substantivity of povidone iodine is around 60 minutes.

PVP-1 is contraindicated in pregnant women, nursing mothers and in those who are allergic to iodine. Side effects of povidone iodine are staining of teeth and surrounding tissues and interfere with thyroid function due to excessive incorporation of iodine.

Peroxide

Hydrogen peroxide (H_2O_2) is an antiseptic agent that is toxic to many bacteria because of its strongly oxidizing properties. The critical factor in peroxide activity is the fact that H_2O_2 and other reduction products of O_2 (superoxide anions) can generate the more toxic hydroxyl radicals. These reactive O_2 species damage cell membranes, inactivate bacterial enzymes via oxidation of sulfahydryl group and, disrupts bacterial chromosome and destroys the bactericidal action of myeloperoxidase enzyme. The disadvantage of peroxide is that it is toxic to the host, causing peroxidation of lipids in cell membrane and certain chromosomal changes.

Natural Products

- Sanguinarine is a benzophenathridine alkaloids derived from alcoholic extraction of powered rhizosomes of bloodroot plant *Sanguinaria Canadensis*, grown in USA and Canada. After precipitation and putrefaction of alcohol extract an orange powder containing 30-35% of Sanguinarine is obtained. The trade name of Sanguinarine prouct is *Viadent*. It is antimicrobial agent effective against gram-positive and gram-negative bacteria. The exact mode of action is not clear; it seems to interfere with essential steps in the synthesis of bacterial cell wall. It suppresses the activity of several enzymes, possibly through oxidation of thiol group. Sanguinarine containing mouthrinses have been shown to increase the chances of oral precancerous lesion.
- Propolis is a naturally occurring bee product which is used by bees to seal openings in their hives. It

consists of wax and plant extracts. It is used as plaque inhibitory mouthwash because of its antiseptic, anti-inflammatory and bacteriostatic property.

- Viokase is a dehydrated pancreas preparation, which contains trypsin, chymotrypsin, carboxypeptidase, amylase, lipase and nucleases.

ANTICALCULUS AGENTS

I. **1st generation anticalculus agents:**
   a. Dissolution via:
      - Acid: One of the earliest techniques utilized a wooden stick which was moistened with aromatic sulphuric acid before being introduced into a periodontal pocket to dissolve calculus. Other acids included 20% trichloroacetic acid and 10% sulfuric acid. These are caustic to soft tissues and decalcify tooth structure. Thus, the use of acids as anticalculus agents was discontinued.
      - Sodium ricinoleate is the salt of fatty acids produced from castor oil and interferes with the attachment of microorganisms to teeth. Unfortunately, sodium ricinoleate had a particularly unacceptable taste and needed to be applied at high concentrations.
   b. Plaque attachment via:
      - Silicone
      - Ion exchange resins: The resin was a sulphonated polystyrene containing negatively charged ions that would repel the positively charged calcium ions and reduce the degree of mineralization of the calcium.
   c. Plaque inhibition via:
      - Antibiotics (Niddamycin) Penicillin was tested for its anticalculus efficacy due to its known effects on gram-positive cocci.
      - Antiseptics (Chloramine T)
   d. Matrix disruption via:
      - Enzymes: The mode of action of enzyme formulations is to break down plaque matrix or to affect the binding of the calculus to the tooth. The first enzyme to be tested was mucinase, a preparation with proteolytic and amylolytic activity. The theoretical mechanism of action was to breakdown the mucins which were supposed to bind calculus to the tooth.
      - Ascoxal
      - 30% Urea—The anticalculus effect of urea was attributed to its ability to dissolve the mucoproteinaceous material within which the calcium salts are deposited and/or by increasing the solubility of calcium salts in saliva.

II. **2nd generation anticalculus agents:**
   Inhibition of crystal growth via:
   a. *Victamine C (Chlomethyl analog):* Victamine C is a surface active organophosphorus. Victamine C inhibits crystal growth by a crystal poisoning mechanism and has characteristic taste which might have promoted saliva flow, thus reducing calculus levels.
   b. *Pyrophosphates:* The pyrophosphate prevents calcification by interrupting the conversion of amorphous calcium phosphate to hydroxyapatite.
   c. *Diphosphonates:* They are group of synthetic pyrophosphate analog which interact strongly with minerals, and are thought to prevent calculus deposition by inhibiting crystal growth.
   d. *Metal salts (Zinc salts):* They potentially have two mechanisms by which they can affect calculus formation. Firstly, they inhibit plaque growth examples are stannous and stannic salts. The mechanism by which inhibition occurs is probably via the uptake of the metal salt by bacteria, with a consequent disruption of intracellular metabolic processes, or due to extracellular binding of the metal ion, with a consequent change in the bacterial cell wall. This may lead to changes in the adhesive and cohesive nature of the plaque and cause problems with bacterial accretion and binding. Secondly, metal salts are potent inhibitors of mineralization. The metal ion adsorbs to the surface of the growing crystal, and prevents the attachment of lattice ions. Consequently, crystal growth is slowed or inhibited. Metal ions can also bind to hydroxyapatite. This binding is reversible and is itself inhibited by raising the local concentration of calcium. This implies that calcium can compete for binding sites in the crystal lattice and displace other metal ions from that lattice.
   e. *Pyrophosphates, Sodium fluoride, Gantrez copolymer:* Gantrez A has been shown to inhibit the hydrolysis of pyrophosphate by alkaline phosphatase. The proposed mechanism of action is that the copolymer binds tightly with magnesium ions which are a necessary substrate for alkaline phosphatase activity.
   f. Citroxain and Sodium citrate
   g. Calcium lactate

ANTIMICROBIALS/ANTIBIOTICS

In the general category of systemic chemotherapeutic agents, antimicrobials constitute the majority of agents.

Rationale of Using Antimicrobial Agents

- Mechanical therapy alone may not effectively control infection, particularly in deep pockets.
- Poor plaque control increases the rate of reinfection of the pocket.
- Root surface, tongue, tonsils and within other niches in the oral mucosa harbor pathogenic bacteria that recolonize the periodontal pocket and can act as sources for reinfection.
- *Aggregatibacter actinomycetemcomitans* and other tissue-invasive organisms are not easily eradicated without concomitant antibiotic therapy.
- As an adjunct in the treatment of specific disease profiles (refractory disease, severe disease) with periodontitis that could require more aggressive treatment.
- To prevent postsurgical complications including infection.
- In periodontal surgery aiming for regeneration by controlling the subgingival microflora in the early healing phase.

Indications for Use of Antibiotics in Periodontal Therapy

i. *Therapeutic therapy* are those used to treat established clinical infection such as chronic/aggressive periodontitis.
ii. *Prophylactic therapy* involves administration of antimicrobial agents to the individuals susceptible to a clinical disease. Prevention of infective endocarditis is a prime example of prophylactic antibiotic therapy.
iii. *Pre-emptive therapy* involves antimicrobial therapy to individuals prior to the onset of clinical disease based on clinical, epidemiological or laboratory indications of disease risk. Pre-emptive therapy may include *Aggregatibacter actinomycetemcomitans* from younger siblings of adolescents having localized aggressive periodontitis/from children of parents with localized aggressive periodontitis.

Parameters that determine the dosage of an antimicrobial agent include:
- Susceptibility of the pathogen(s)
- Severity of the infection
- Body mass (standard dose should be adjusted for under- and overweight patients);
- Other medications

Combination and Serial Antimicrobial Therapy

A bactericidal antibiotic (e.g., amoxicillin) should not be used simultaneously with a bacteriostatic agent (e.g., tetracycline) because the bactericidal agent exerts activity during cell division that is impaired by the bacteriostatic drugs. When both types of drugs are required, they are best given serially, not in combination.

Combined and serial antimicrobial therapy may help:
- To prevent the emergence of bacterial resistance by using agents with overlapping antimicrobial spectra.
- To lower the dose of individual antibiotics by exploiting possible synergy between two drugs against targeted organisms.
- To broaden the antimicrobial range of the therapeutic regimen beyond that attained by any single antibiotic. For example Metronidazole and Ciprofloxacin combination has both therapeutic as well as prophylactic benefit. Therapeutic benefit as Metronidazole targets obligate anaerobes and Ciprofloxacin acts against facultative anaerobes. Prophylactic benefit as Ciprofloxacin has minimal effect on Streptococcus species, which is responsible for periodontal health.

Generations of Antimicrobials

i. *First generation agents*: Reduces plaque score by 20-50%. Poor substantivity and thus used 4-6 times daily, e.g. Sanguinarine, Quaternary ammonium compounds, Antibiotics.
ii. *Second generation agents*: Reduces plaque score by 70-90%. Used twice daily, e.g. Chlorhexidine, Triclosan.
iii. *Third generation agents*: Effective against specific periodontal pathogens, e.g. Delmopinol.

Various Antibiotics

Amoxicillin

It is semisynthetic penicillin with extended antimicrobial spectrum which inhibit bacterial cell wall. The major side effects associated with Amoxicillin is hypersensitivity. Dosage is 500 mg tid for 8 days.

Tetracyclines

They are broad spectrum antibiotics with activity against gram-negative and gram-positive bacteria as well as mycoplasma infections. Tetracycline hydrochloride, doxycycline and minocycline are all semisynthetic tetracyclines, with tetracycline HCl being derived from oxytetracycline. It consists of 4 fused cyclic rings. The 4th carbon ring has a dimethyl amino group which is responsible for its antimicrobial action. It inhibit bacterial protein synthesis, bind to 30S ribosomes. It has antimicrobial, anticollagenase, anti-inflammatory, anti-proteolytic and fibroblast stimulating activity. Apart from the significant anti-matrixmetalloproteinase effects tetracyclines are also potent inhibitors of osteoclast function, i.e. antiresorptive by altering intracellular calcium concentration and interacting with putative calcium receptor, decreasing ruffled border area, diminishing acid production, diminishing the secretion of cathepsins, inhibiting osteoclast gelatinase activity and inducing apoptosis or programmed cell death of osteoclasts.

Interactions-

- Antacid and iron preparation:Tetracycline HCl is a chelating agent and will chelate Ca^{+2}, Mg^{+2} and Al^{+3} in GIT. These ions especially calcium are present in variety of food substances. Thus, it is advisable to take tetracycline either half an hour before or after food.
- Phenytoin: It decreases concentration of doxycycline.
- Oral contraceptives: Tetracycline causes failure of oral contraceptives.
- Warfarin: Tetracycline increases anticoagulant activity of warfarin.
- Insulin: Tetracycline with insulin increases hypoglycemia.

GIT intolerance, candidiasis, renal diseases, diarrhea, vomiting, nausea, esophageal ulceration, skin rashes, vestibular disturbances, photosensitivity and increased intracranial pressure are few side effects of tetracycline. Hepatic diseases, renal diseases, insulin dependent diabetes, pregnancy, lactating mothers, females taking oral contraceptives, children below 8 years of age and systemic lupus erythematosus (SLE) patients are few contraindications of using tetracycline. Dosage—250 mg qid.

Doxycycline: Dosage—100 mg twice daily the first day, then 100 mg once daily. The advantages of Doxycycline over other tetracyclines are that calcium, antacids, and milk do not alter absorption and has to be given once daily thus show better compliance.

Minocycline: Minocycline are given twice daily, thus facilitating compliance when compared with tetracycline. It shows less phototoxicity and renal toxicity than tetracyclines.

Ciprofloxacin

It is a bactericidal drug which is effective against gram-negative rod and anaerobic bacteria. Advantages of Ciprofloxacin over other antibiotics for combating Aggressive periodontitis are that it has minimal effect on Streptococcus species, which is associated with periodontal health and all strains of *A. actinomyce-temcomitans* are susceptible to Ciprofloxacin.

Clindamycin

It is a chloroderivative of lincomycin. It blocks protein synthesis by binding to 50S bacterial ribosomes and interfering with peptidyl transfer. It is effective against anaerobic bacteria. The major side effects associated with Clindamycin is pseudomembranous ulcerative collitis (due to the result of an overgrowth of toxin producing *Clostridium difficile*) and hepatitis.

Erythromycin

It is a macrolide antibiotic that interferes with protein synthesis at the 50S ribosome site in gram-positive and gram negative bacteria. It is used in patients allergic to pencillin.

Metronidazole

It is a nitroimidazole compound which is bactericidal to anaerobic microorganisms (*P. gingivalis* and *P. intermedia*). It disrupts bacterial DNA synthesis by its hydroxymetabolite. It was originally used in trichomoniasis and amoebiasis. Dosage is 250 mg tid for 7 days. It is used to treat NUG, Aggressive Periodontitis alongwith Amoxicillin and Ciprofloxacin.

Disulfiram like reaction or antabuse effect of alcohol: Disulfiram or Metronidazole irreversibly inhibits ALDH enzyme, which leads to accumulation of toxic levels of acetaldehyde in liver and systemic circulation causing

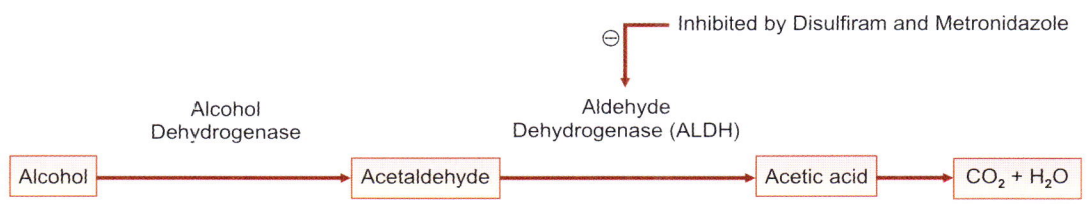

PERIODONTICS REVISITED

vomiting, visual disturbances, postural fainting and circulatory collapse. So, alcohol and products containing alcohol should be avoided during Metronidazole therapy and for at least 1 day after drug is discontinued.

The major side effects associated with Metronidazole are antabuse effect when alcohol is ingested, metallic taste, and GIT intolerance.

Azithromycin

It is a member of azalide class of macrolides which is effective against anaerobes and gram-negative bacilli. Azithromycin penetrates fibroblasts and phagocytes in concentrations 100-200 times greater than extracellular compartment, thus transported and released directly into site of inflammation through phagocytes. Therapeutic dose—Initial loading dose of 500 mg followed by 250 mg/day for 5 days. It is thought to reduce the severity of cyclosporine induced gingival enlargement.

◼ LOCAL DRUG DELIVERY (LDD) SYSTEM

Success of any drug delivery system designed to target periodontal infections depends upon its ability to deliver the antimicrobial agents to the base of the pocket, at a bacteriostatic or bacteriocidal concentration. The rationale behind LDD is the same to disinfect pathogen reservoirs by delivering high concentration of antibiotic or antimicrobial directly to the site of periodontal infection and facilitating the retention of the medicament long enough to ensure efficacious results. LDD system was pioneered by Goodson of the Forsyth Dental Research Center.

LDD system should meet the following criteria to be effective in treating disease:
- Inhibit or kill the putative pathogen
- It should be able to reach the site
- It should be in adequate concentration
- It should be there long enough
- It should not harm

Classification **(Fig. 38.2)**: Subgingival delivery devices are hollow cellulose fiber, dialysis tubing, gels, acrylic strips, and ethylcellulose strips.

Subgingivally applied chemotherapeutic agents are:

i. *Actisite*: It consists of a polymer ethylene vinyl acetate containing 25% of saturated tetracycline HCl. It is marketed in the length of 23 cms and 0.5 mm diameter containing 2.7 mg of tetracycline HCl of flexible yellow fibers.

Technique: Tetracycline fibers have a slight amount of memory and thus can be bent easily. The optimal site for the use of fibers are the periodontal pocket of 5mm or more in the depth that bleeds on probing and does not respond to mechanical therapy. Take 2-3 inches fibers in a forcep and place it in the opening of pocket. This fibre should be folded on itself and packed into the pocket until the pocket is filled to slightly below the gingival margin because gingival shrinkage is known to occur **(Fig. 38.3)**. Interproximal pockets should be packed from both facial and lingual sides. Once the fiber placement is complete, the dentist isolates the area with an air syringe and applies a drop of tissue adhesive at each interdental as well as facial and lingual area. Patient is instructed not to brush, floss in the treated area

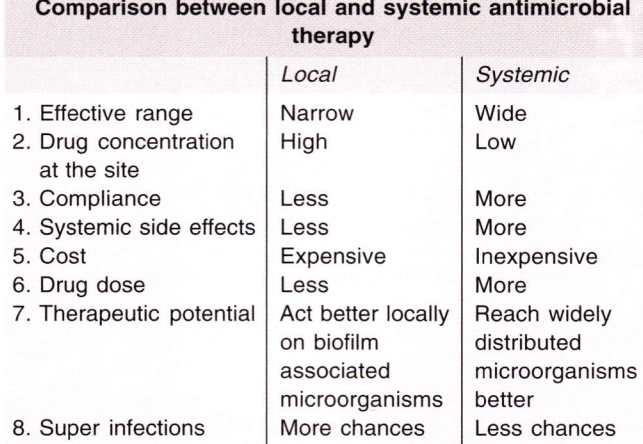

Comparison between local and systemic antimicrobial therapy

	Local	Systemic
1. Effective range	Narrow	Wide
2. Drug concentration at the site	High	Low
3. Compliance	Less	More
4. Systemic side effects	Less	More
5. Cost	Expensive	Inexpensive
6. Drug dose	Less	More
7. Therapeutic potential	Act better locally on biofilm associated microorganisms	Reach widely distributed microorganisms better
8. Super infections	More chances	Less chances

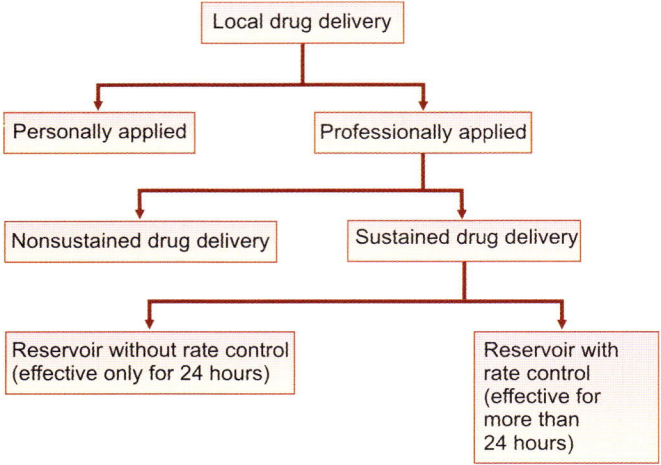

Fig. 38.2: Classification of local drug delivery

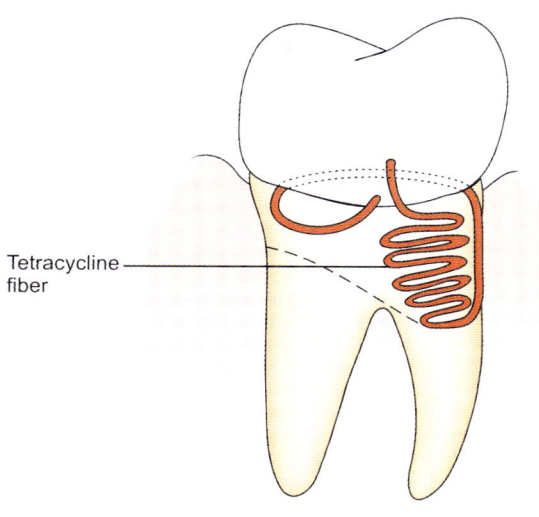

Fig. 38.3: Tetracycline fibers are packed till the base of the pocket

until fibers are removed and chlorhexidine mouthwash is prescribed twice daily.

Disadvantages:

- More length of twice is required for placement.
- Need for a second appointment for the removal of fibers
- Sometimes results in oral candidiasis.

ii. *Atridox*: It is a gel system containing 10% of doxycycline in a syringe. Atridox comes in two syringes that are coupled together before use and mixed by moving the contents of the syringes back and forth for 100 cycles. The delivery syringe is attached to a 23-gauge blunt cannula and the material is injected into the periodontal pocket. This product is also available premixed in a single syringe. Overflow of the material is gently packed in the pocket with a cord packing instrument or the back of a curet. Periodontal dressing or adhesive may aid in retaining the material. Patient is advised to avoid brushing, flossing, or eating in the treated area for a minimum of 7 days. Because the material is biodegradable, no additional appointments for removal are required and the patient is instructed to remove any residual material with their toothbrush and dental floss at the end of 1 week.

iii. *Arestin*: Minocycline microspheres consist of the antibiotic minocycline hydrochloride microencapsulated in a bioabsorbable polymer of polyglycolide-co-dl lactide. The microspheres are dispensed subgingivally using a disposable plastic cartridge (containing 1 mg of minocycline) on a stainless steel handle by inserting the tip to the base of the periodontal pocket and applying the material while withdrawing the tip. The material is bioadhesive on contact with moisture and does not require additional adhesives or periodontal dressings to hold it in place subgingivally. The patient should be instructed to avoid brushing for 12 hours, with no interproximal cleaning for 10 days. No additional appointments are needed for removal of the material because it is bioabsorbable. The minocycline microspheres maintain therapeutic drug concentrations for 14 days.

iv. *Dentamycin/Periocline*: Minocycline ointment contains 2% minocycline hydrochloride and is applied using a syringe with blunt cannula.

v. *Elyzol*: Metronidazole gel contains 25% metronidazole in a glyceryl mono-oleate and sesame oil base and is applied into the pocket by means of a syringe and blunt cannula.

vi. *Periochip*: It is a degradable baby's thumbnail size of 4 × 5 × 0.35 mm orange color chip composed of hydrolyzed gelatin matrix, cross-linked with glutaraldehyde and also contains glycerin and water into which 2.5 mg chlorhexidine gluconate is incorporated. The chip is easily placed into periodontal pockets that are 5 mm or more **(Fig. 38.4)**. Chlorhexidine concentration is 800 -1000 ppm in GCF in the first 48 hours after the placement of Periochip.

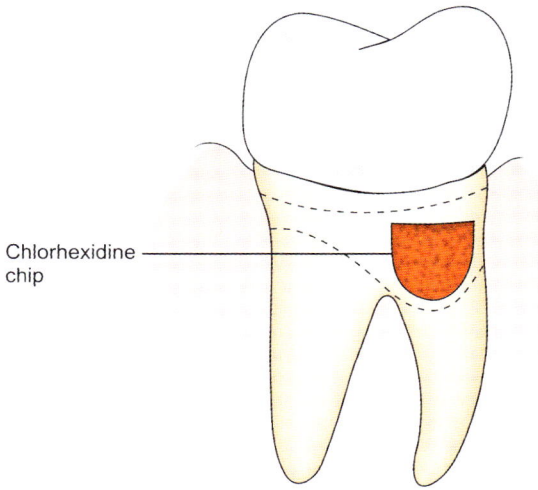

Fig. 38.4: Chlorhexidine chip inserted at the base of the pocket

Later on, 100-500 ppm concentration of chlorhexidine is present over the next 6 days.

vii. *Atrigel*: A biodegradable drug delivery system incorporates 5% Sanguinarine. This delivery system consists of poly (DL- lactide) in a N-methyl-2-pyrrolidone carrier in syringe.

The complicating issues related to LDD is the cost effectiveness—cost includes the price of the local delivery agents, cost associated with clinician's time and the patient's perspective i.e number of trips to the clinician.

Drugs that concentrate in GCF, and thus effective against periodontal pathogens

	Dose (mg)	Crevicular fluid (mg/ml)	Serum conc (mg/ml)
Doxycycline	200	2-8	2-3
Tetracycline	500	5-12	3-4
Metronidazole	500	8-10	6-12
Amoxicillin	500	3-4	8
Chlorhexidine	Periochip	100	-
Actisite	-	1300	5-12
Clindamycin	-	-	1-2

POINTS TO PONDER

✓ Chemotherapeutic agents used as premedication in periodontal surgery are anxiolytics, antibiotics, antiseptics and NSAIDs.

✓ Three groups of antimicrobials which interfere with food absorption are tetracyclines, quinolones and azithromycin.

✓ Chlorhexidine is free from systemic toxicity in oral use.

✓ Chlosite is a gel with 1.5% Chlorhexidine. It is a combination of chlorhexidine gluconate-slow release (0.5%) and chlorhexidine dihydrochloric-rapid release (1.0%).

✓ Antiseptic is applied topically or subgingivally on living surfaces whereas disinfectant is applied to inanimate surfaces to destroy microorganisms.

BIBLIOGRAPHY

1. Addy M. The Use of Antiseptics in Periodontal Therapy. In, Lindhe J, Karring T, Lang NP. Clinical Periodontology and Implant dentistry. 4th ed Blackwell Munksgaard 2003;464-93.
2. Drisko CH. Nonsurgical periodontal therapy. Periodontol 2000 2001;25:77-88.
3. Eley BM, Manson JD. The possible use of antibiotics as adjuncts in the treatment of chronic periodontitis. In, Periodontics 5th ed Wright 2004;223-50.
4. Greenstein G. Povidone Iodine's effects and role in the management of periodontal diseases. A Review. J Periodontol 1999;70:1397-1405.
5. Hammond BF, Genco RJ. Sensitivity of periodontal organisms to antibiotics and other antimicrobial agents.In, Genco RJ, Goldman HM and Cohen DW. Contemporary Periodontics. CV Mosby Company 1990;161-69.
6. Hill M, Moore RL. Locally Acting Oral Chemotherapeutic Agents. In, Rose LF, Mealey BL, Genco RJ, Cohen DW. Periodontics, Medicine, Surgery and Implants. Elsevier Mosby 2004;277-87.
7. Jolkovsky DL, Ciancio SG. Chemotherapeutic agents in the treatment of periodontal diseases. In, Newman, Takei, Carranza. Clinical Periodontology 9th ed WB Saunders 2003;675-87.
8. Killoy WJ, Polson AM. Controlled local delivery of antimicrobial in the treatment of periodontitis. Dent Clin North Am 1998;42(2):263-83.
9. Kinane DF. Systemic Chemotherapeutic Agents. In, Rose LF, Mealey BL, Genco RJ, Cohen DW. Periodontics, Medicine, Surgery and Implants. Elsevier Mosby 2004;289-96.
10. Mombelli A. The Use of Antibiotics in Periodontal Therapy. In, Lindhe J, Karring T, Lang NP. Clinical Periodontology and Implant dentistry. 4th ed Blackwell Munksgaard 2003;494-511.
11. Seymour RA, Heasman PA. Tetracyclines in the management of periodontal diseases: A review. J Clin Periodontol 1995;22:22-35.
12. Walker C, Karpinia K. Rationale for use of antibiotics in periodontics. J Periodontol 2002;73:1188-96.
13. Winkelhoff AJV, Rams TE, Slots J. Systemic antibiotics therapy in periodontics. Periodontol 2000 1996;10:45-78.

MCQs

1. Periostat is:
   A. 20 mg capsule of doxycycline hyclate
   B. 40 mg capsule of doxycycline hyclate
   C. 100 mg capsule of doxycycline hyclate
   D. 200 mg capsule of doxycycline hyclate

2. The active ingredient in periochip is:
   A. Tetracycline
   B. Minocycline
   C. Metronidazole
   D. Chlorhexidine

3. The antibiotic to which all strains of Actinobacillus are susceptible is:
   A. Tetracycline
   B. Ciprofloxacin
   C. Amoxicillin
   D. Metronidazole

4. Which of the following antibiotics can concentrate at sites of periodontal inflammation:
   A. Amoxycillin
   B. Azithromycin
   C. Metronidazole
   D. Clindamycin

5. Metronidazole:
   A. penetrates stagnation areas well
   B. is mainly active against gram-positive aerobes
   C. is effective in the management of necrotizing ulcerative gingivitis.
   D. is mainly concentrated in saliva

6. If periodontal procedures have to be carried out more than once, the minimum gap between two prophylactic antibiotic regimes in case of prophylaxis against SABE, should be:
   A. 2 days
   B. 7 days
   C. 20 days
   D. 42 days

7. Which of the following chemotherapeutic agents has been shown to have a side effect of tooth staining?
   A. Sanguinarine
   B. Chlorhexidine
   C. Hydrogen Peroxide
   D. Phenolic compound
   E. Sodium benzoate

Answers

1. A   2. D   3. B   4. B   5. C
6. B   7. B

C H A P T E R
39

Host Modulatory Therapy

Shalu Bathla

INTRODUCTION

Plaque bacteria are capable of causing direct damage to the periodontal tissues (e.g, by release of hydrogen sulphide, butyric acid and other enzymes and mediators), but now it is recognized that the majority of the destructive events occurring in the periodontal tissues result from the activation of the destructive processes that occur as a part of the host immune - inflammatory response to plaque bacteria. The host response is essentially protective by intent but paradoxically can result in tissue damage, including breakdown of connective tissue fibers in the periodontal ligament and resorption of alveolar bone.

Host modulatory therapy (HMT) do not "switch off" normal defense mechanisms or inflammation; instead they ameliorate excessive or pathologically elevated inflammatory processes to enhance the opportunities for wound healing and periodontal stability.

Host modulatory therapy is a treatment concept that aims to reduce tissue destruction and stabilize or even regenerate the periodontium by modifying or down regulating destructive aspects of the host response and upregulating protective or regenerative responses.

HOST MODULATORY AGENTS

Various HMT have been developed or proposed to block pathways responsible for periodontal tissue breakdown **(Fig. 39.1)**.

A. Inhibition of Matrix metalloproteinases (MMPs): Through Chemically Modified Tetracyclines (CMTs)
B. Inhibition of Arachidonic acid metabolites: Through NSAIDs
   a. COX – 1 inhibitors: Indomethacin, Naproxen, Flurbiprofen
   b. COX – 2 inhibitors: Rofecoxib
   c. COX and LOX inhibitors: Triclosan, Topical Ketoprofen
   d. LOX inhibitors: Lipoxins
C. Modulation of bone metabolism:
   a. Bisphosphonates
   b. Hormone replacement therapy (HRT)
   c. Calcium supplementation
D. Regulation of immune and inflammatory responses:
   a. Suppressing proinflammatory cytokines (IL – 1 and TNF – α receptor antagonists)
   b. Nitric Oxide inhibition

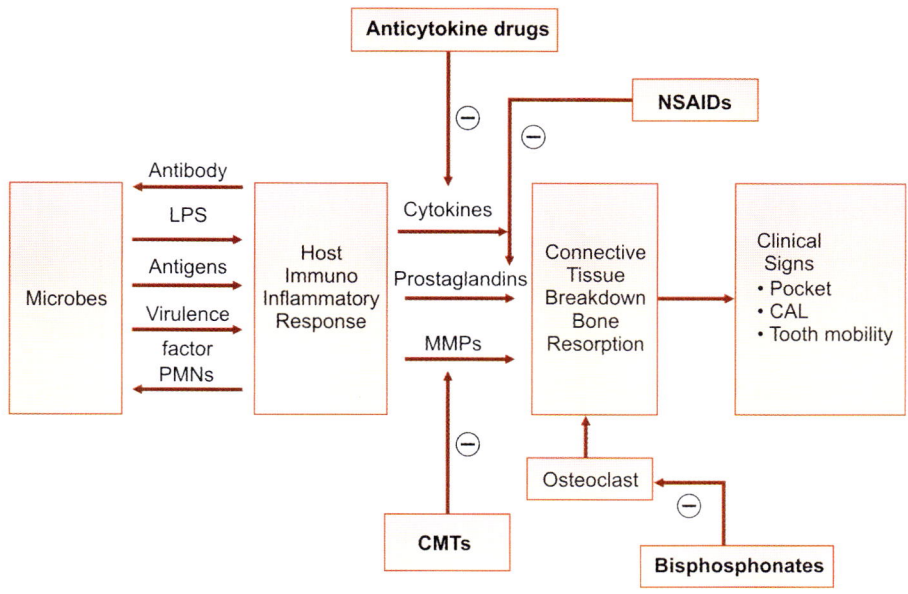

Fig. 39.1: Host modulatory therapies. LPS—Lipopolysaccharide; MMPs—Matrix metalloproteinases; CAL—Clinical attachment loss; CMTs—Chemically modified tetracyclines.

c. Generation of protective antibodies through vaccines
d. Infusion/supplementary anti-inflammatory cytokines IL – 4 and IL – 10.

Inhibition of Matrix Metalloproteinases (MMPs)

Chemically Modified Tetracyclines (CMTs)

Chemically modified Tetracyclines are those which lack dimethylamino group on the 4th carbon atom.

Doxycycline

4-Dedimethylaminosancycline
CMT 3

Mechanism of action of chemically modified tetracyclines **(Fig. 39.2)**:
i. Inhibits or chelates the calcium atoms that Matrix metalloproteinase (MMPs) requires for their action
ii. Inhibit already active MMPs
iii. Down – regulate MMPs expression
iv. Scavenges reactive oxygen species
v. Modulates the osteoclast functions

Periostat: It is subantimicrobial dose of Doxycycline hyclate capsule of 20 mg prescribed for patients with chronic periodontitis twice daily. Indications for periostat are patients who have not responded to nonsurgical therapy, patients with generalized recurrent sites of

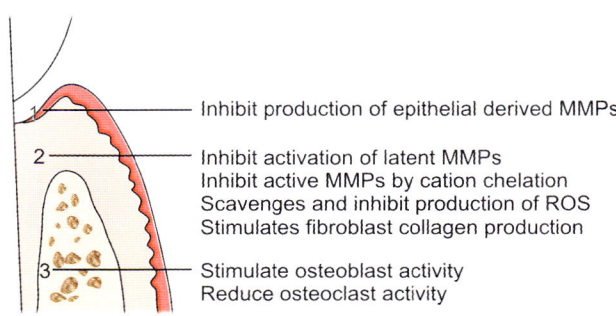

Inhibit production of epithelial derived MMPs
Inhibit activation of latent MMPs
Inhibit active MMPs by cation chelation
Scavenges and inhibit production of ROS
Stimulates fibroblast collagen production
Stimulate osteoblast activity
Reduce osteoclast activity

Action of chemically modified tetracyclines on:
1. Epithelium
2. Connective tissue
3. Alveolar bone

Fig. 39.2: Modes of action of CMTs

PERIODONTICS REVISITED

5 mm or greater pocket depth that bleed on probing, patients with mild to moderate chronic periodontitis and a high susceptibility to rapid periodontal disease progression. The only contraindication for Periostat is the allergy to tetracycline.

Inhibition of Arachidonic Acid Metabolism

In periodontal diseases, prostaglandins and other arachidonic acid (AA) metabolites are synthesized and released within periodontal tissues. AA can be metabolized via the cyclooxygenase (COX) or lipoxygenase (LOX) pathways. One proposed approach to modulate the host response is inhibition of enzymes responsible for the release of these destructive products.

Systemically administered agents NSAIDs: These drugs are propionic acid derivatives, which act by inhibiting the COX pathway of arachidonic acid metabolism; thereby reducing prostaglandin formation. Prostaglandins, including prostaglandin E_2 (PGE_2), is produced by neutrophils, macrophages, fibroblast and gingival epithelial cells in response to the presence of lipopolysaccharide (LPS), a component of the cell wall of gram – negative bacteria. PGE_2 induces bone loss thus, NSAIDs control the alveolar bone loss. Mechanism of action of NSAIDs is explained in **Figure 39.3**.

Locally administered agents NSAIDs: The topical administration of NSAIDs is an alternative method to deliver these agents. In general, topical application of NSAIDs is possible because these drugs are lipophilic and

are absorbed into gingival tissues. NSAIDs that have been evaluated for topical administration includes ketorolac tromethamine rinse and S – ketoprofen dentifrice.

Triclosan: A compound which has received interest as both an antibacterial and anti – inflammatory agent is triclosan. Triclosan (2, 4, 4^1 – trichloro – 2- hydroxyl – diphenyl ether) is an non – ionic antibacterial agent. Triclosan also inhibits COX and LOX and thus, may interfere with the production of AA metabolites.

Modulation of Bone Metabolism (Fig. 39.4)

Bisphosphonates: These are non-biodegradable analogs of pyrophosphate that have a high affinity for calcium phosphate crystals and that inhibit osteoclast activity. These compounds also appear to inhibit MMP activity through a mechanism that involves chelation of cations. Alkyl side chains (e.g. etidronate) characterize first – generation bisphosphonates. Second – generation bisphosphonates include aminobiphosphonates with an amino – terminal group (e.g. alendronate and pamidronate). Third – generation bisphosphonates have cyclic side chains (e.g. risedronate). The antiresorptive properties of bisphosphonates increases approximately ten fold between drug generations.

Modes of action of Bisphosphonates are: 1. inhibition of the development of osteoclasts, 2. induction of osteoclastic apoptosis, 3. reduction of activity of osteoclast 4. prevention of the development of osteoclasts from hematopoietic precursors and 5. stimulation of production of an osteoclast inhibitory factor.

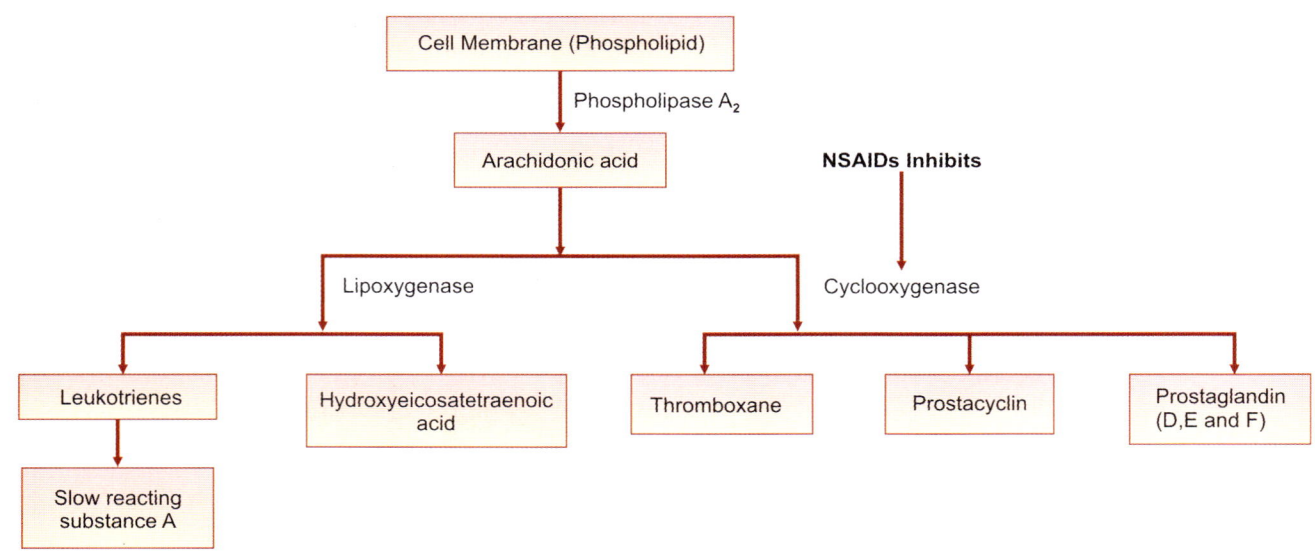

Fig. 39.3: Mechanism of action of NSAIDs

PERIODONTICS REVISITED

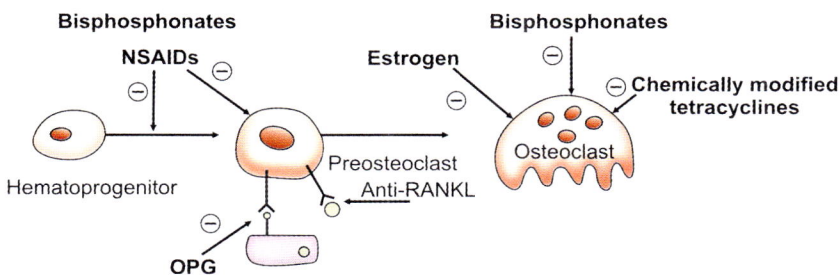

Fig. 39.4: Therapeutic strategies to treat bone resorption

The contraindications for biphosphonates use are the sensitivity to phosphonates and gastrointestinal upset.

Osteoprotegerin (OPG): The discovery of a novel receptor called osteoprotegerin (OPG) revealed a key regulatory mechanism in osteoclast differentiation and activity. OPG and receptor activator of NF-κ B ligand (RANKL) are two molecules that regulate osteoclast formation and bone resorption. RANKL induces osteoclast differentiation and activation, whereas OPG blocks this process by acting as a decoy receptor for RANKL.

Regulation of Immune and Inflammatory Responses

Modulation of Nitric oxide activity: Nitric oxide (NO) is a short lived molecule implicated in a wide range of biological processes. NO is a highly reactive free radical reacting with metal and thiol residues leading to lipid peroxidation, protein and DNA damages and stimulation of cytokine release. Nuclear Poly ADP – ribose polymerase (PARP) enzyme downstream NO toxicity.

Suppressing proinflammatory cytokines: Cytokines are defined as regulatory proteins controlling the survival, growth, differentiation and functions of cells. Cytokines function as a network and are produced by different cell types and share overlapping features. This phenomenon is called biological redundancy. To counteract tissue destruction and maintain homeostasis, cytokine antagonists such as IL – 1 receptor antagonist (IL – 1Ra) or soluble TNF receptors can competitively inhibit receptor mediated signal transduction.

Other Locally administered agents: A number of local host modulation agents i.e enamel matrix proteins, growth factors and bone morphogenetic proteins have been investigated for potential use as adjuncts to surgical procedures, not only to improve wound healing but also to stimulate regeneration of lost bone, periodontal ligament and cementum and thus ,restoring the complete periodontal attachment apparatus. The only local host modulation agent currently approved by the FDA for adjunctive use during surgery is Emdogain.

BIBLIOGRAPHY

1. Choi DH, Moon IS, Paik JW, Kim YS, Choi SH , Kim CK. Effects of sub – antimicrobial dose doxycycline therapy on crevicular fluid MMP – 8, and gingival tissue MMP – 9, TIMP – 1 and IL – 6 levels in chronic periodontitis. J Periodontol Res 2004;39:20-26.
2. Golub LM, McNamara TF, Angelo GD, Greenwald RA, Ramamurthy NS. A Non – antibacterial Chemically – modified Tetracycline Inhibits Mammalian Collagenase Activity. J Den Res 1987;66(8):1310-14.
3. Greenstein G, Lamster I. Efficacy of subantimicrobial dosing with doxycycline. JADA 2001;132 (4):457-66.
4. Modulation of the Host Response in Periodontal Therapy. J Periodontol 2002;73:460-70.
5. Preshaw PM, Ryan ME, Giannobile WV. Host Modulation Agents. In, Newman, Takei, Klokkevold, Carranza. Textbook of Periodontology. 10th ed St Louis Elsevier 2006; 813-27.
6. Preshaw PM, Hefti AF, Jepen S, Etienne D, Walker C, Bradshaw MH. Subantimicrobial dose doxycycline as adjunctive treatment for periodontitis: A review. J Clin Periodontol 2004;31:697-707.
7. Ryan ME, Kinney J, Kim Amy S, Giannobile WV. The Host Modulatory Approach. Dent Clin North Am 2005;49:624-35.
8. Salve GE, Lang NP. Host response modulation in the management of periodontal diseases. J Clin Periodontol 2005;32 (suppl. 6):108-29.
9. Tenenbaum HC, Shelemay A, Girard B, Zohar R, Fritz PC. Biphosphonates and Periodontics: Potential Application for Regulation of Bone Mass in the Periodontium and Other Therapeutic/Diagnostic Uses. J Periodontol 2002;73:813-22.
10. Wang Y, Morlandt AB, Xu X, Carnes DL, Chen Z, Steffenson B. Tetracycline At Subcytotoxic Levels Inhibits Matrix Metalloproteinase – 2 and – 9 But Does Not Remove The Smear Layer. J Periodontol 2005;76:1129-39.

CHAPTER 40

Periodontal Instruments

Suresh DK, Shalu Bathla

1. Common Characteristics of all Periodontal Instruments	3. Nonsurgical Instruments
2. Classification of Periodontal Instruments	4. Surgical Instruments

COMMON CHARACTERISTICS OF ALL PERIODONTAL INSTRUMENTS

A large variety of periodontal instruments are available. Each group of instruments has characteristic features; individual therapists often develop variations with which they operate most effectively. The parts of periodontal instruments are handle, shank and working end **(Fig. 40.1)**. Stainless steel and high carbon steel are used in instrument manufacture. Periodontal instruments are available in single ended and double ended. Each double ended periodontal instrument is identified by the design name and number—When the design name and number are stamped along the length of the handle, each working end is identified by the number closest to it **(Fig. 40.2A)** and when the design name and number are stamped across the instrument handle, the first number (on the left) identifies the working end at the top and the second number identifies the working end at the bottom of the handle **(Fig. 40.2B)**. Balanced instrument: When the working ends are centered on a line running through the long axis of the handle, it is called as balanced instrument.

Instrument Handles

Instrument handles may be designed in various size and shapes and the design of handle depends upon features like:

i. *Weight*: Hollow handle increase tactile transfer and minimize fatigue.

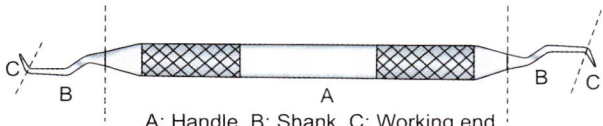

A: Handle, B: Shank, C: Working end

Fig. 40.1: Parts of periodontal instrument

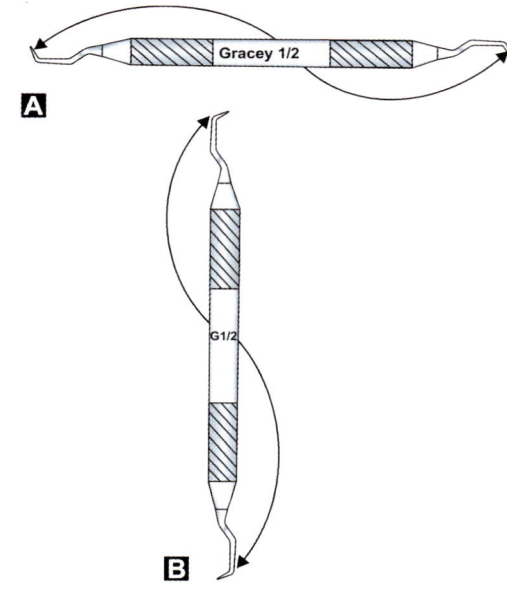

Figs 40.2A and B: (A) Name and number marked along the handle

ii. *Diameter*: Small diameter handle decreases control and increases muscle fatigue. Large diameter handle maximize control and reduces muscle cramps but restrict movement in areas where access is limited (e.g. posterior areas).

iii. *Textures*: Knurled handles maximize control and decreases hand fatigue. Smooth handles decrease control and increase muscle fatigue **(Fig. 40.3)**.

Shank

Design features of Shank—The functional shank length extends from the working end to the shank bend closest to the instrument handles **(Fig. 40.4A)**. Terminal or lower shank is the portion of shank nearest to the working end **(Fig. 40.4B)**. The functional shank length may be short, long or intermediate. Long functional shanks are needed to reach the tooth surfaces of posterior teeth or the root surfaces of teeth within periodontal pockets. Short functional shanks are found on instruments used to remove supragingival calculus deposits or to reach the surfaces of anterior teeth. An instrument shank is curved if it has bends that deviate from the long axis of the shank. Instruments with curved shanks can usually be used on both posterior and anterior teeth and are referred to as universal instruments. Instruments with straight shanks are limited to use on anterior sextants and thus are referred to as anterior instruments. Instruments shank may be flexible, moderately flexible, or rigid in design. Shank flexibility is related to instrument use.

Shank types	Uses	Examples
Rigid	• Removal of heavy or firmly adherent calculus and deposits • Rigid shank limits tactile conduction so that calculus detection is difficult	Sickle scalers, Periodontal files
Moderately flexible	• Removal of moderate or loosely attached calculus • Moderately flexible shank provides better level of tactile transfer, allowing detection and removal of moderate subgingival deposits.	Universal curettes
Flexible	• Detection of subgingival calculus and deposits. • Removal of fine calculus. • Flexible shank provides the best tactile information to the operator's finger pads through the shank and handle.	Explorers Gracey curettes

Working End

An instrument's function is determined primarily by the design of its working end. The design characteristics of working end are face, back, lateral surfaces and cutting edge **(Fig. 40.5)**. The face of the instrument is the surface between the two cutting edges. The surface opposite the face is the instrument back. The surface on either side of the face are called lateral surfaces. Cutting edge is a sharp edge formed where face and lateral surfaces meet.

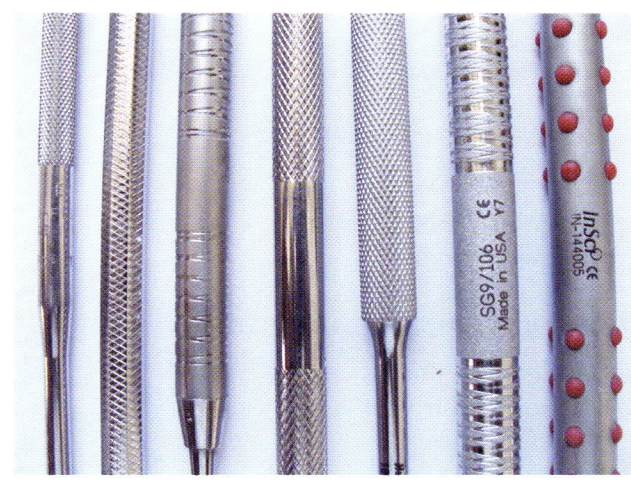

Fig. 40.3: Handle textures

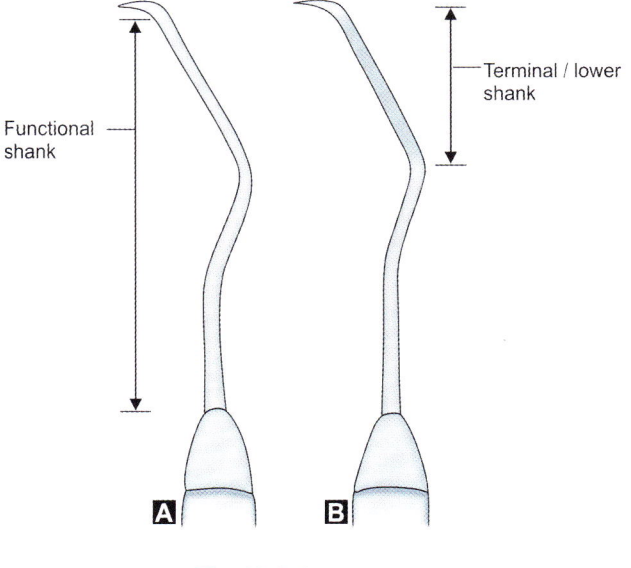

Fig. 40.4: Shank design

PERIODONTICS REVISITED

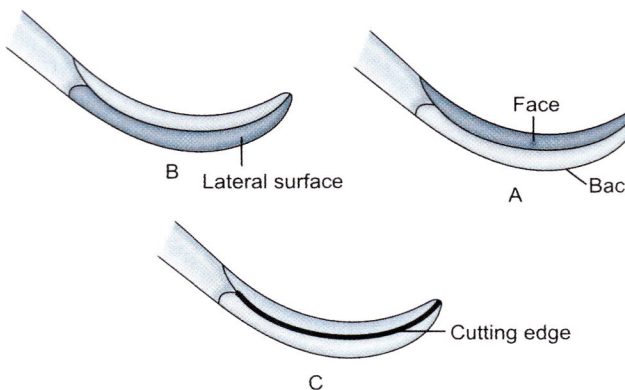

Fig. 40.5: Curette blade: working end design

CLASSIFICATION OF PERIODONTAL INSTRUMENTS

I.   Nonsurgical instruments
II. Surgical instruments

NONSURGICAL INSTRUMENTS

According to the purpose they serve:
1. Diagnostic instruments
   • Dental Mirrors
   • Explorers
   • Tweezers
   • Periodontal probes
2. Scaling and root planing instruments
   i. Hand instruments
      a. Scalers
         • Sickle scalers
         • File scalers
         • Chisel
         • Hoe
      b. Curettes
   ii. Ultrasonic and sonic instruments
   iii. Rotating instruments
   iv. Reciprocating instruments
   v. LASERS
3. Periodontal endoscope
4. Cleaning and polishing instruments

Dental Mirrors

The uses of dental mirrors are indirect vision, indirect illumination, retraction and transillumination. The various types of dental mirror surfaces are:
i. *Plane/Flat surface mirror*: The reflecting surface is at the back of the mirror lens which produces double image.

ii. *Concave surface mirror*: It produces magnified image that may be distorted.
iii. *Front surface mirror*: The reflecting surface is on the front of the lens that eliminates double image, producing actual image. Front surface mirror is the mirror of choice for dental procedures.

Explorers

Types of Explorers

i. *17 – Orbans Explorer*: It is an ideal instrument for calculus detection interproximally and in deep periodontal pocket. Its long, thin shank with fine tip less than 2 mm which curves at right angle to the lower shank facing upwards do not injure soft tissue when placed subgingivally **(Fig. 40.6A)**.

ii. *23 – Shepherd's hook Explorer*: Single ended/paired with 17. It has thicker shank and working end than other explorer which makes it more rigid. Rigidity enhances the role in caries detection, but limits its role in subgingival calculus detection **(Fig. 40.6B)**.

iii. *Pigtail/Cowhorn/3CH Explorer no.21 and 22*: Double ended instrument that is easily adapted throughout the mouth. Working end is curved and shank is thin for calculus detection. Because shank is curved and relatively short, instrument is best used in children/adults with minimal periodontal pocket depth less than 1 mm. It can also be used for detecting calculus in areas of furcation involvement (similar instrument

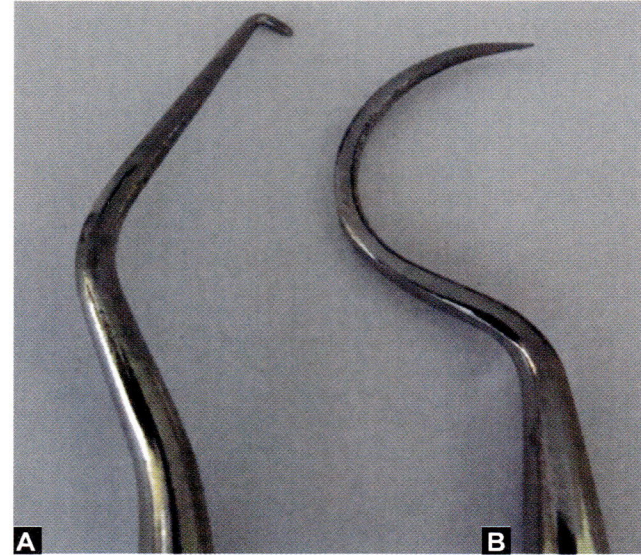

Figs 40.6A and B: 17 and 23 end explorer
(A) 17 Orban explorer (B) 23 Shepherd's hook explorer

design to Naber's probe), detecting proximal and cervical caries. Ineffective in evaluating occlusal caries because the instrument's design limits the force needed to determine occlusal caries.

iv. *3A explorer*: It has a long, fine, arc like tip. It adapts well in deep pocket and furcation areas. Its fine tip allows for good tactile sensitivity, especially for calculus detection.

v. *Old Dominion University (ODU) 11/12 Gracey Type Explorer or EXD 11-12*: Shank design of ODU is similar to that of Gracey 11/12 curette. It was developed by faculty of Old Dominion University, thus named as ODU 11/12. Double ended, paired instrument for calculus detection.

General design features:
- Fine, wire like working end
- Sharp point
- Circular in cross-section

Tweezers

These instruments have serrated handle for secure grip. Tweezers have angled beak which are available in different sizes. They are used to place and remove small items, cotton rolls and gauze from the mouth.

Periodontal Probe

Periodontal probe is a tapered rod like instrument with blunt rounded working end caliberated in mm and color coding. The markings varies from 1 to 15 mm, depending on the type of the probe, which makes it easy in reading and to determine the probing pocket depth. An angled shank places the working end at about a 45° angle in relation to the handle. The thin narrow working end is inserted gently to the depth of the periodontal pocket **(Fig. 40.7)**.

General design features:
- Rod-shaped working ends
- Smooth, rounded tip
- Rounded or rectangular in cross – section
- Caliberated with color coding and millimeter graduations.

Uses of periodontal probe:
i. To locate, mark and measure pocket depth
ii. To determine pocket course and topography
iii. To measure width of attached gingiva
iv. To determine and measure clinical attachment loss
v. To measure gingival recession
vi. To check the bleeding on probing
vii. To evaluate bone support in the furcation areas
viii. To determine amount of bone level that is present
ix. To evaluate the completeness of treatment and its success.

Higher grading should be cosidered as final reading when the gingival margin appears at a level between two markings of the probe.

Various periodontal probes are:
i. University of Michigan 'O' probe with Williams marking at 1, 2, 3, 5, 7, 8, 9, and 10 mm **(Fig. 40.7A)**.
ii. *WHO probe*: 0.5 mm ball at the tip and mm markings at 3.5, 8.5 and 11.5 and color coding from 3.5 to 5.5 **(Fig. 40.7B)**.
iii. *UNC-15 probe*: 15 mm long probe with markings at each mm and color at 5th, 10th and 15th mm **(Fig. 40.7C)**.
iv. *Marquis color coded probe*: Calibrations are in 3 mm sections. The colored band on the periodontal probe is designed to make periodontal examination readings more objective and faster **(Fig. 40.7D)**.
v. Michigan 'O' probe with marking at 3, 6 and 8 mm.
vi. *Goldman fox probe*: Flat, rectangular probe with markings at 1, 2, 3, 5, 7, 8, 9, and 10 mm.
vii. *Nabers probe*: Curved probe used for furcation areas. When periodontal disease causes sufficient loss of attachment around multirooted teeth, the inter-radicular bone (furcation area) may become involved. The presence of gingiva and neighboring teeth frequently prevent accurate probing of the furcation area with the standard periodontal probe. The furcation probe shown in **Figure 40.8** is a double-ended instrument designed to help and determine the extent of the inter-radicular bone loss.

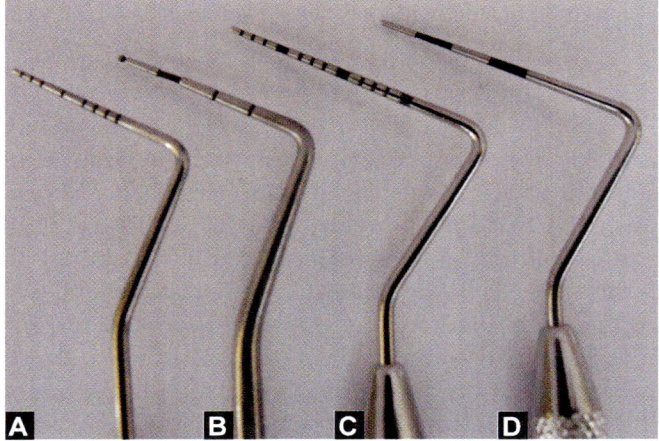

Figs 40.7A to D: Various periodontal probes: (A) Williams probe, (B) WHO probe, (C) UNC-15, (D) Marquis color coded probe

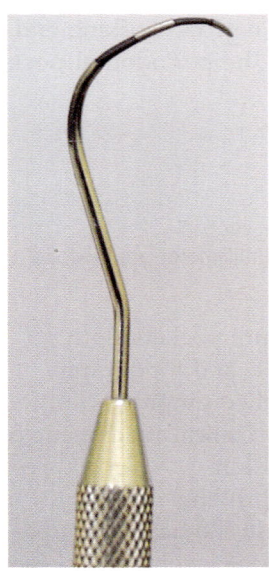

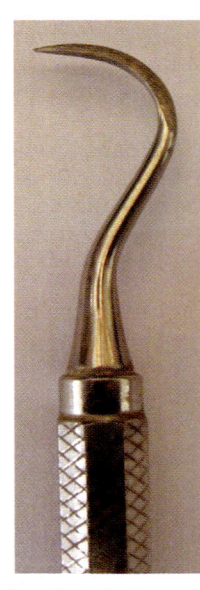

Fig. 40.8: Nabers probe for detection of furcation lesion

Fig. 40.9: Sickle scaler

viii. *Moffitt/Maryland probe*: WHO design with Williams marking.

ix. *NIDR probe*: It is a color coded and is graduated in 2 mm increments at 2, 4, 6, 8, 10 and 12 mm with alternating increments colored in yellow.

x. *Florida probe*: The criteria given by NIDR were met by Florida research group. Gibbs et al in the year 1988 developed the Florida probe system. This incorporates constant probing force, precise electrical measurement, computer storage of data. The parts are Probe hand piece, Digital readout, Switch, Computer interface and Computer. Two models have been developed which differ in their fixed reference point:

   a. *Stent model*: The probe has 1 mm metal collar that rests on a prepared ledge on a prefabricated vacuoform stent.

   b. *Disk model*: Has a 11 mm disk which rests on the occlusal surface or incisal edge of the tooth.

xi. *Toronto automated probe*: Developed by researchers at the University of Toronto. Like the Florida probe, it uses the occlusal – incisal surface to measure clinical attachment levels. The sulcus is probed with 0.5 mm nickel-titanium wire that is extended under air pressure. It controls angular discrepancies by means of a mercury tilt sensor that limits angulation within ± 30°, but it requires reproducible positioning of the patients head and can't easily measure third and second molars.

xii. *Interprobe*: It is also known as Perioprobe, is a third generation probe. Developed by Goodson and Kondon in 1988. This has an optical encoder transduction element with a flexible probe tip, which curves with the tooth as probes enter the pocket area. The probe optical encoder handpieces uses constant probing pressure which provides repeatable measurement of pocket depth and attachment loss.

xiii. *The Jeffcoat probe (or Foster Miller probe)*: Developed by Jeffcoat in 1986. It is capable of coupling pocket depth measurement with detection of the CEJ. The probe extends a thin metal fiber along the tooth surface into the sulcus and detects a slight acceleration rise when encountering the CEJ and then undergoes final extension, under constant force, on reaching the base of the pocket.

Generations of periodontal probe:

First generation; Conventional probes; Manual probes: The usual clinical instrument with a thin tapering line marked to be read in mm.

Second generation; Constant force probes; Pressure sensitive probes: As above, but with a spring or electronic cut-off when the appropriate force is reached. Force 30 g probe tip remains in CEJ and force of 50 g are necessary to diagnose osseous defects, e. g. Vine valley, True Pressure Sensitive TPS.

Third generation; Automated and computerized probes: When probe is in place with specified force, a device is activated that reads the measurement digitally and accurately. e.g. Florida, Foster miller, Toronto automated probes, Inter probe.

Fourth generation—Three-dimensional probes: Currently under development, these are aimed at recording sequential probe positions along gingival sulcus.

Fifth generation—Non-invasive 3 - dimensional probes: These will add ultrasound or another device to a fourth generation probe. These probe aim to identify the attachment level without penetrating it.

Sickle Scaler

A sickle scaler is primarily designed for removal of supragingival calculus. Sickles with straight shanks are designed to adapt to anterior teeth, and those with contra-angled shanks (called Jacquettes) adapt to posterior teeth. Sickle scalers have a flat surface and two cutting edges that converge in a sharply pointed tip. The shape of the instrument makes the tip strong so that it will not break off during use. Because of the design of this instrument, it is difficult to insert a large sickle blade under the gingiva without damaging the surrounding gingival tissues. **(Fig. 40.9).**

Examples of sickle scalers are:
- Anterior sickle scaler: OD-1, Jacquette- 30, Jacquette- 33, Goldman- H6, Goldman- H7
- Posterior sickle scaler: Jacquette- 34/35, Jacquette- 14/15, Jacquette- 31/32.

General design features:
- Two cutting edges
- Cutting edges meet in pointed tip
- Triangular in cross-section

Periodontal File

Periodontal files are strong instruments used to crush large calculus deposits and to smoothen the tooth surface **(Fig. 40.10)**.

General design features:
- Many cutting edges
- Cutting edges at 90 to 105° angle to the shank
- Have strong, rigid shank

Chisel

Use of the periodontal chisel scaler is extremely limited. It is used solely for the removal of heavy supragingival calculus deposits that bridge open interproximal spaces of anterior teeth **(Fig. 40.10)**. The instrument is activated with a push motion while the side of the blade is held firmly against the root.

General design features:
- One straight cutting edge
- Heavy, straight shank

Hoe

Hoe scalers are used for scaling of ledges or rings of calculus. The blade is bent at a 99° angle. The cutting edge is formed by the junction of the flattened terminal surface with the inner aspect of the blade. The cutting edge is beveled at 45°. The blade is slightly bowed so that it can maintain contact at two points on a convex surface. This stabilizes the instrument and prevents nicking of the root. The instrument is activated with a firm pull stroke towards the crown, with every effort being made to preserve the two-point contact with the tooth **(Figs 40.11 and 40.12)**.

General design features:
- One straight cutting edge
- Working end at 99° to 100° angle to the shank
- Strong, rigid shank

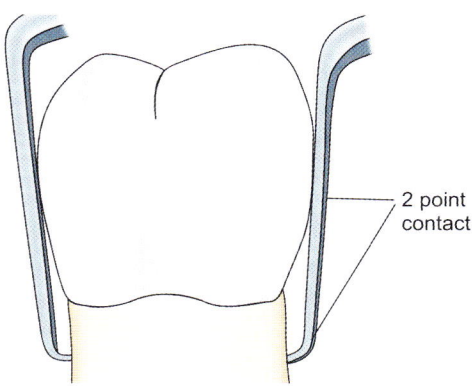

Fig. 40.11: Hoe scaler showing two point contact

2 point contact

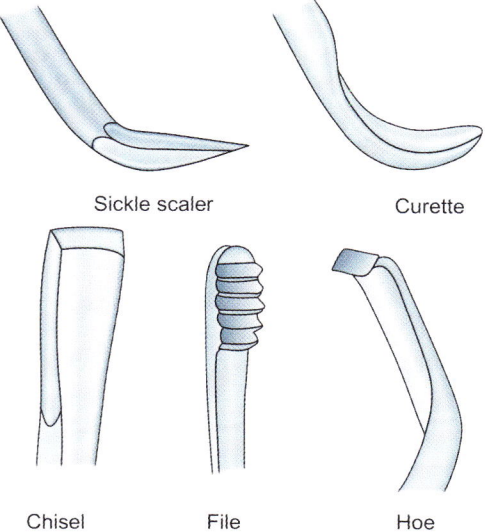

Sickle scaler   Curette

Chisel   File   Hoe

Fig. 40.10: Scaling and root planing instruments

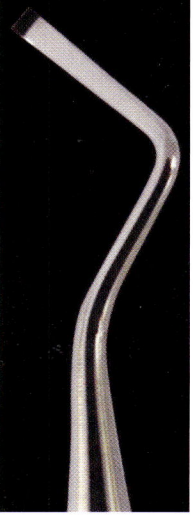

Fig. 40.12: Hoe scaler

Curette

The curette is the instrument of choice for subgingival calculus removal, root planing, and removing soft tissue from the periodontal pocket. The working ends of curettes form a spoon-shaped face and a rounded back. In a cross-section, the curette blade appears semicircular rather than triangular (shape of the sickle scaler) **(Fig. 40.13)**. Two basic types of curettes are the universal and the area specific.

General design features:
- Two cutting edges
- Spoon-shaped working end
- Cutting edges meet in a rounded toe
- Rounded back
- Semicircular in cross-section

Universal curette: The universal curette is a paired instrument designed to adapt to most areas of the dentition by altering and adapting the finger rest, fulcrum, and hand position. Two parallel cutting edges are formed, one on either side of the face. Either cutting edge can be used. Universal instruments come in a variety of sizes and shank lengths **(Figs 40.14 and 40.15)**. Some commonly used instruments are the Columbia 2R-2L and 4R-4L.

Area-specific curettes (Gracey): Area specific curettes differ from the universal curettes in several ways. First, they are a set of several instruments designed and angled to adapt to a specific anatomic area of the dentition. Second, these curettes are designed with only one cutting edge. Area specific curettes are the best choice for subgingival scaling and root planing because they provide the best adaptation to the complex root anatomy.

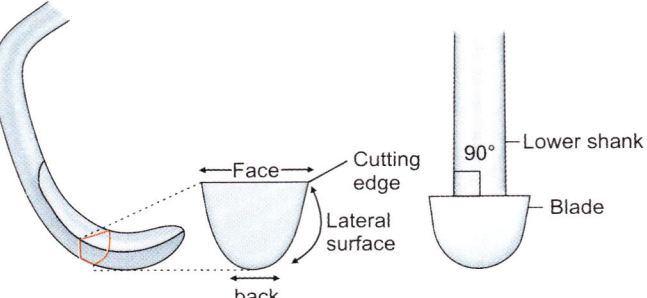

Fig. 40.14: Universal curette blade

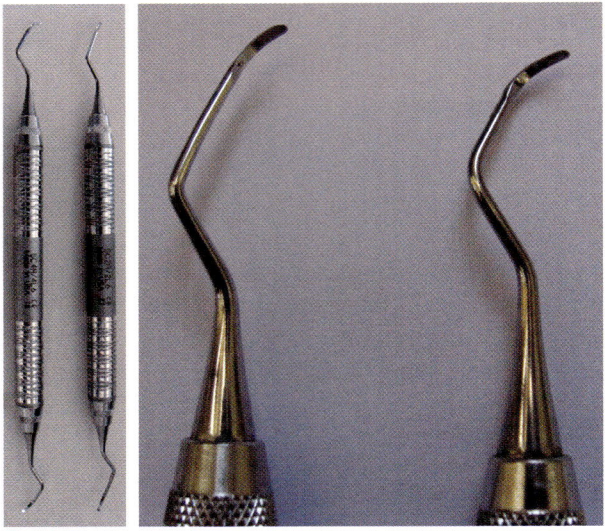

Fig. 40.15: Universal curettes

The Gracey curettes are paired, area-specific instruments that have similar blades with different angulations and contra-angulations of the shank. **(Figs 40.16 and 40.17)** Examples of area-specific curettes are Gracey curettes, Kramer-Nevins series, Turgeon series, Hu-friedy after five series, Hu-friedy Mini five series, Hu-friedy Curvette series and Furcation curettes.

Instrument	Area of use
Gracey 1-2 and 3-4	Anterior teeth
Gracey 5-6	Anterior teeth and premolars
Gracey 7-8 and 9-10	Posterior teeth; facial and lingual surfaces
Gracey 11-12	Posterior teeth; mesial surfaces
Gracey 13-14	Posterior teeth; distal surfaces
Gracey 15-16	Posterior teeth; mesial surfaces
Gracey 17-18	Posterior teeth; distal surfaces

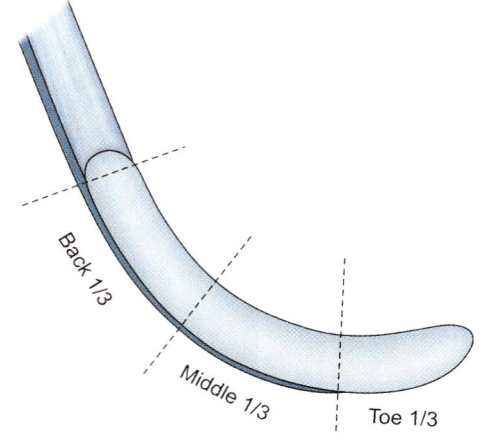

Fig. 40.13: Curette blade- spoon shaped blade and rounded tip

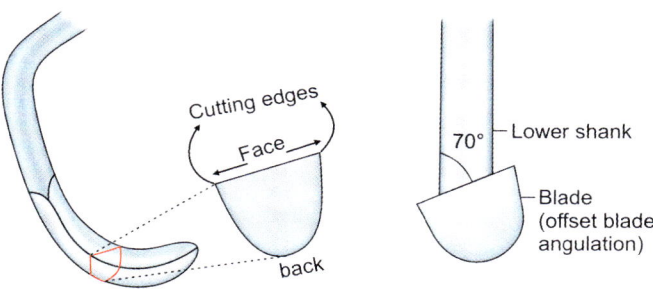

Fig. 40.16: Area specific curette

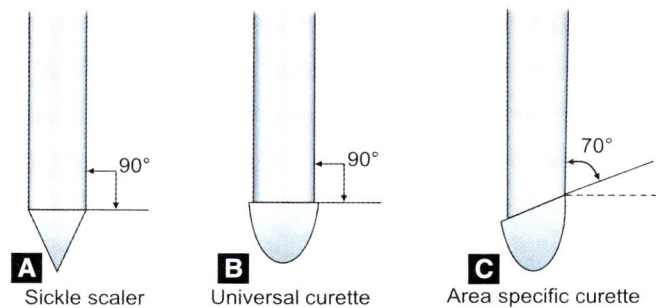

Fig. 40.18: Relation of face to the lower shank

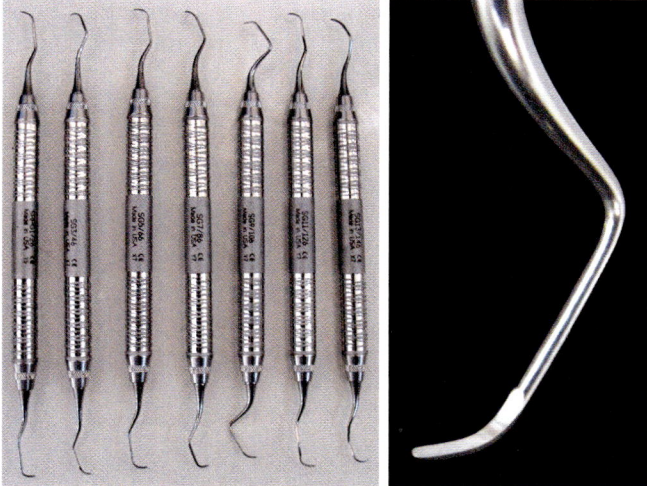

Fig. 40.17: Gracey curettes

Mini-bladed curettes: The blade is half the length of the After Five or standard Gracey curettes **(Fig. 40.19A)**. The shorter blade allows easier insertion and adaptation in deep, narrow pockets; furcations; developmental grooves; line angles; and deep, facial, lingual, or palatal pockets.

After five curettes: These are modifications of the standard Gracey curette design. The terminal shank is 3 mm longer, allowing extension into deeper periodontal pockets of 5 mm or more **(Fig. 40.19B)**. The thinned blade is for smoother subgingival insertion and reduced tissue distention. All standard Gracey numbers except for the #9-10 (i.e #1-2, 3-4, 5-6, 7-8, 11-12, 13-14) are available in the After Five series. These are available in finishing or rigid designs.

TABLE. 40.1: Differences between area specific and universal curettes

	Area specific curettes	Universal curettes
1. Area of use	These are designed for specific areas and surfaces.	Designed for all areas and surfaces.
2. Cutting edge used	One cutting edge, i.e. outer edge	Both cutting edges are used
3. Curvature	Curved in two planes, blade curves up and to the side.	Curved in one plane
4. Blade angle	Offset blade: face of blade beveled at 60-70° to shank **(Fig. 40.18C)**	Not offset: face of blade beveled at 90° to shank **(Fig. 40.18B)**
5. Examples	• Gracey series • Kramer-Nevin series • Turgeon series • After five series • Mini five series • Curvette series	• Columbia 2R/2L • Columbia 4R/4L • Columbia 13-14 • Barnhart 1/2 • Barnhart 5/6

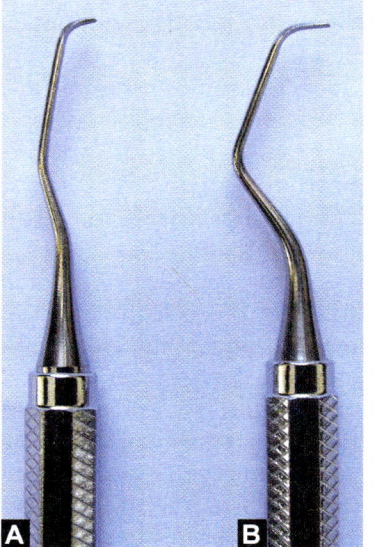

Figs 40.19A and B: (A) Mini bladed curette (B) After five curette

Langer Curettes: The design characteristics of Langer curettes differ from Universal curettes in following manner:

- More than one Langer curette is needed to instrument the entire dentition.
- These curettes combines the shank design of standard Gracey 5-6,11-12 and 13-14 curettes with Universal blade honed at 90°, thus called as the marriage of Gracey and Universal curette design.

Instrument	Area of use
Langer 1/2	Mandilar posterior teeth
Langer 3/4	Maxillary posterior teeth
Langer 5/6	Mandibular and maxillary anterior teeth
Langer 17/18	Mandibular and maxillary second and third molars.

Curvette Area Specific Curettes: The design characteristics of curvette curettes differ from those of standard Gracey curettes in following manner:

- 50% shorter working end
- Increased curvature of the working end
- Straighter shank on anterior instruments
- Extended lower shank on posterior instrument

Instrument	Area of use
Curvette Sub-zero	Anterior teeth and premolars (facial and lingual surfaces)
Curvette 1/2	Anterior teeth and premolars (interproxmial surfaces)
Curvette 11/12	Mesial surface of molars
Curvette 13/14	Distal surface of molars

Ultrasonic and Sonic Instruments

Powered instruments used for periodontal debridement can be classified into two groups on the basis of their operating frequencies: sonic and ultrasonic.

Sonic scalers operate at a relatively low frequency of 3000 to 8000 cycles per second and are driven by compressed air from the dental unit. The stroke pattern of sonic scalers is elliptical to orbital and all the surfaces of the tip can be adapted to root surfaces.

Ultrasonic scalers can be further categorized into magnetostrictive and piezoelectric, on the basis of the mechanism used to convert the electrical current used for energy to activate the tips.

Magnetostrictive ultrasonics operate inaudibly and transfer electrical energy to metal stacks made of nickel-iron alloy or to a ferrous rod. Electrical energy applied to the magnetostrictive insert changes its shape resulting in vibrations. The tip vibrates in an elliptical to orbital motion at 18,000 to 42,000 kHz (cycles per second). The

instrument is comprised of an electronic generator, a handpiece assembly containing a coil to energize the insert, and a variety of interchangeable inserts. The generator produces an alternating low voltage electric current in the handpiece. This current produces a magnetic field in the handpiece that causes the insert to expand and contract along its length and inturn, causes the insert tip to vibrate.

Piezoelectric scalers **(Figs 40.20A and B)** also are inaudible, operating within a range of 24,000 to 45,000 kHz. This type of powered scaler uses electrical energy to activate crystals within the handpiece to vibrate the tip. In contrast to the magnetostrictive scalers, the motion of the tip is linear in nature resulting in activation of mainly the lateral surfaces of the tip. This system is

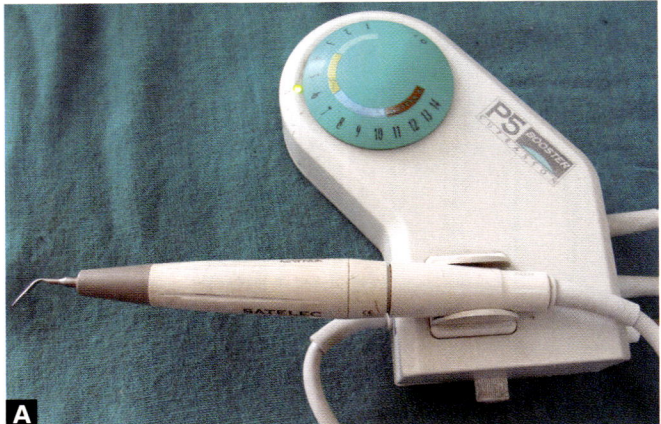

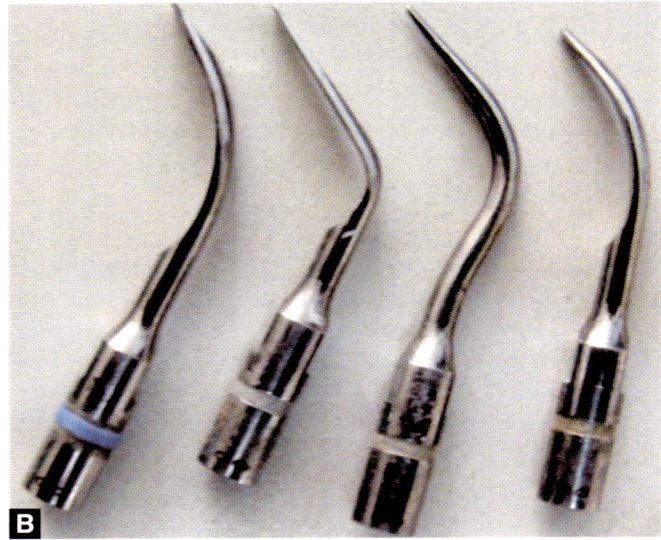

Figs 40.20A and B: (A) Piezoelectric ultrasonic unit (B) Ultrasonic tips

comprised of an electronic generator, a handpiece assembly containinig piezo (ceramic) crystals to energize a scaling tip, and a variety of interchangeable screw-on tips. The generator produces an alternating, high voltage in the handpiece. This voltage produces an electric field in the handpiece that causes the piezo crystals to expand and contract along their diameter and, inturn, causes the scaling tip to vibrate.

Acoustic streaming- The pressure produced by the continuous stream of fluid flowing into the confined space of the periodontal pocket is known as acoustic streaming or turbulence. Bacteria and gram-negative motile rods, in particular, are sensitive to acoustic energy.

Cavitation—The vibratory motion of the tip and the continuous stream of water cause tremendous pressure, creating powerful bursts of collapsing bubbles. This is referred to as cavitation. It is a combination of the vibrating instrument's tip against the deposit, high frequency sound waves, and exploding bubbles that allow for calculus removal.

Pre-procedural antiseptic mouthrinse and use of high volume evacuators can reduce hazards of aerosols production by ultrasonic instrumentation.

Comparison between Ultrasonic and Manual instrumentation.

Ultrasonic instrument	Hand instrument
1. Mechanism of action: Vibration, acoustic streaming and cavitation.	Mechanical removal of deposit
2. Used on heavy tenacious deposits and stains	Used on all amounts of deposits
3. Instrument tip is dull and bulky	Sharp and thin
4. Less tactile sensitivity	Good tactile sensitivity
5. Digital motion activation is used with light pressure	Hand motion activation is used with firm pressure
6. Inaccessible to some areas because of tip design	Greater accessibility
7. Less time required	More time required
8. Less clinician fatigue	More clinician fatigue
9. Water spray cause patient discomfort	No water spray no discomfort
10. Possibility of damage to tooth from heat build up	No heat build up
11. Aerosols are produced	No aerosols are produced
12. Contraindicated in patients with pacemaker and having contagious diseases.	No such contraindications
13. Sharpening not needed frequently	Frequently required
14. Smaller tip size 0.3 - 0.55 mm	Larger tip size 0.76-1 mm

Contraindications:
i. Patients with contagious diseases
ii. Patients with a pacemaker especially to magnetostrictive
iii. Composite resin restorations
iv. Porcelain inlays or crown

Periodontal Endoscope

It consists of a 0.99 mm-diameter reusable fiberoptic endoscope over which is fitted a disposable, sterile sheath. The fiberoptic endoscope fits onto periodontal probes and ultrasonic instruments that have been designed to accept it. The sheath delivers water irrigation that flushes the pocket while the endoscope is in use and keeps the field clear. The fiberoptic endoscope attaches to a medical grade charged coupled device (CCD) video camera and light source that produces an image on a flat panel video monitor for viewing during subgingival exploration and instrumentation. This device allows clear visualization of deep subgingival pockets and furcations. It enables the operator to detect the presence and location of subgingival deposits and guides the operator in their thorough removal.

Cleaning and Polishing Instruments

The primary objective of polishing is the removal of extrinsic stain and supragingival plaque. The rationale for this procedure includes improving the appearance of the dentition, demonstrating a standard of oral cleanliness for the patient to attain on a daily basis, and motivating the patient to improve plaque control, as well as the belief that the outcome of a quality periodontal service should be a plaque-free mouth.

Rubber cups consist of a rubber shell with or without webbed configurations in the hollow interior. They are used in the handpiece with a special prophylaxis angle. A good cleansing and polishing paste that contain fluoride should be used and kept moist to minimize frictional heat as the cup revolves. Polishing pastes are available in fine, medium, or coarse grits and are packaged in small, convenient and single-use containers.

Bristle brushes are available in wheel and cup shapes. The brush is used in the handpiece with a polishing paste. Because the bristles are stiff, use of the brush should be confined to the crown to avoid injuring the cementum and the gingiva.

Air-powered polishing—Prophy-jet contains an air-powered slurry of warm water and sodium bicarbonate.

This system is effective for the removal of extrinsic stains and soft deposits. The slurry removes stains rapidly and efficiently by mechanical abrasion and provides warm water for rinsing and lavage.

Contraindications of polishing:

i. Patients who have communicable disease that could be spread by aerosols.

ii. Patients who are susceptible for bacteremia.

iii. Areas of thin or deficient enamel, cementum or dentin surfaces; areas of hypersensitivity.

iv. Caries susceptible teeth; areas of white spot demineralized mottled teeth.

v. Gold restorations

vi. A restricted sodium diet, including patient with controlled hypertension

vii. Composite restorations.

Dental implant instruments: Plastic probes are available for probing around the implant **(Fig. 40.21).** Special scalers made of plastic or nonmetallic material are designed for cleaning the abutments of dental implants. The special material enables optimum cleaning without damaging the abutment surface. Implacare implant instruments have autoclavable stainless steel handles with different plastic tip designs **(Figs 40.22A and B)**. Metal scalers curettes and ultrasonic tips should never be used because they may damage the surface topography of the implant.

SURGICAL INSTRUMENTS

1. Excisional and incisional instruments
2. Surgical curettes and sickle scaler
3. Periosteal elevators
4. Surgical chisels
5. Surgical files
6. Scissors and Nippers
7. Needle holders

Excisional and Incisional Instruments

Periodontal knives (Gingivectomy knives): The Kirkland knife is kidney-shaped knife with cutting edge all round its periphery **(Fig. 40. 23A)**. Interdental knife is spear-shaped knife having cutting edges on both sides of the blade. Examples are Orban's knife **(Fig. 40.23B)**, Merrifield and Waerhaug knife.

Surgical blades: The most commonly scalpel blades used in periodontal surgery are 11, 12, 15, and 15C. **(Fig. 40.24)**. The 12 no. blade is a beak-shaped blade with cutting edges on both sides, allowing the operator to engage narrow, restricted areas with both pushing and pulling cutting motions. The 15 no. blade is used for thinning flaps and for all-around use. The 15C no. blade, is useful for making the initial, scalloping type incision. When mounted in ordinary handles such as Bard-Parker, they are used for releasing incisions and

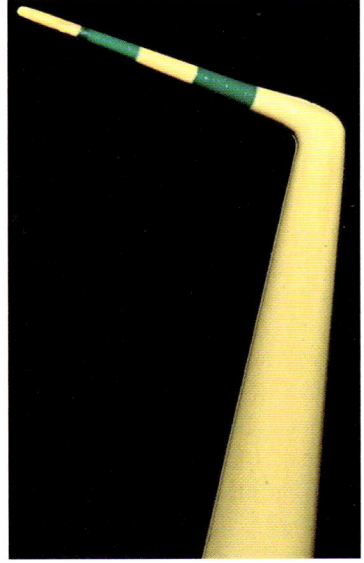

Fig. 40.21: Polymeric color coded plastic probe

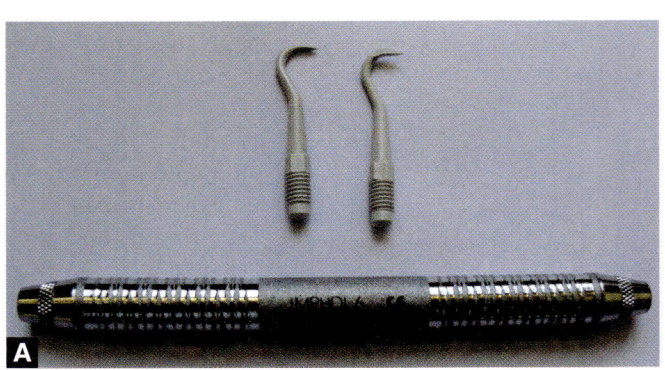

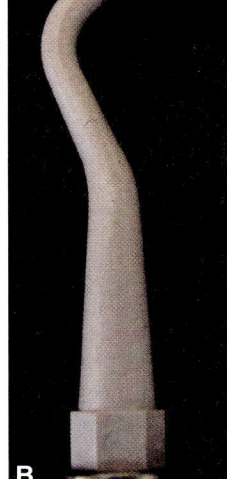

Figs 40.22A and B: (A) Implacare implant maintenance instrument (B) Plastic tip

PERIODONTICS REVISITED

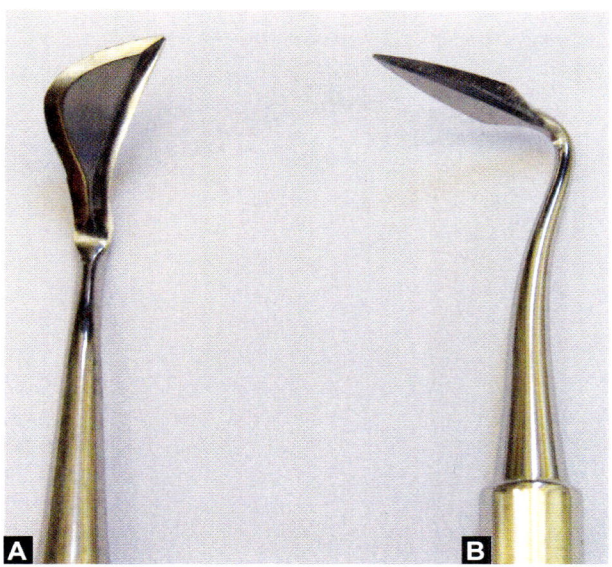

Fig. 40.23: Gingivectomy knives (A) Kirkland knife (B) Orban interdental knife

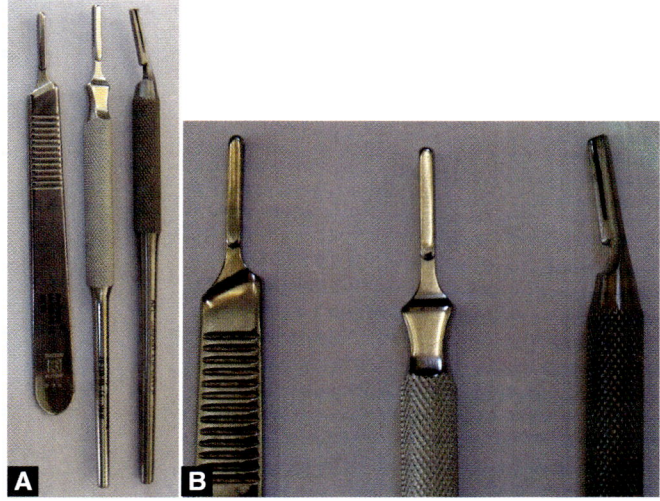

Figs 40.25A and B: Scalpel handle-Bard-Parker handles

facilitates the use of such knives for both gingivectomy excisions and reverse bevel incisions.

Surgical Curettes and Sickles

Surgical curettes and sickles are larger and heavier, often needed during surgical procedure for debridement of granulation tissue, fibrous interdental tissue and tenacious subgingival deposits. The examples are Kramer curettes 1, 2, and 3, Kirkland curettes and Ball scaler B2-B3.

Periosteal Elevators

These instruments are used to reflect full thickness flap and move or to displace the flap after the incision has been made for flap surgery. Example of periosteal elevators are Goldman-Fox 14, Glickman 24G **(Fig. 40.26)**.

Surgical Chisels and Hoes

Chisels and hoes are used for removing and reshaping bone during periodontal osseous surgery. The Ochsenbein 1-2 is a useful chisel with a semicircular indentation on both sides of the shank that allows the instrument to engage around the tooth and into the interdental area **(Fig. 40.27)**.

Surgical Files

Periodontal surgical files are used for removing and reshaping bone primarily to smooth rough bony ledges in all areas of bone. The examples are Schluger **(Fig. 40. 28)** and Sugarman files.

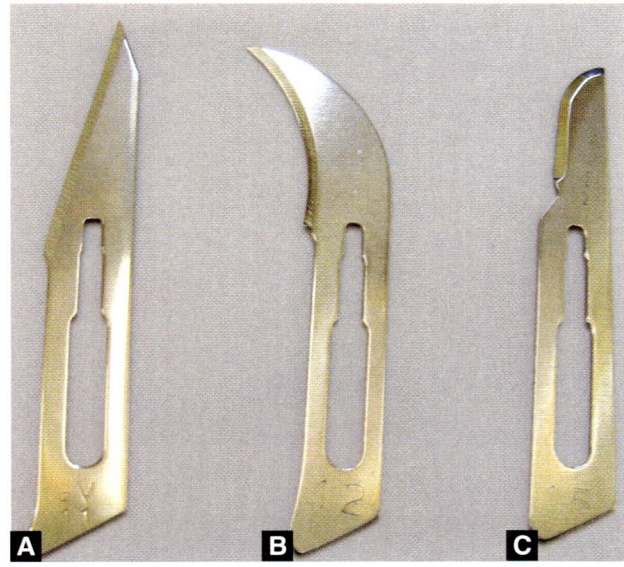

Fig. 40.24: Surgical blades (A) No 11, (B) No 12, (C) No 15

reverse bevel incisions in flap procedures and periodontal plastic surgeries. Bard- Parker scalpel handle has the real advantage of using disposable blade so that sharpening is unnecessary **(Fig. 40.25)**. All of these blades and disposable BP handles are discarded after single use.

Special handles such as Blakes handle make it possible to mount blades in angulated positions, which

PERIODONTICS REVISITED

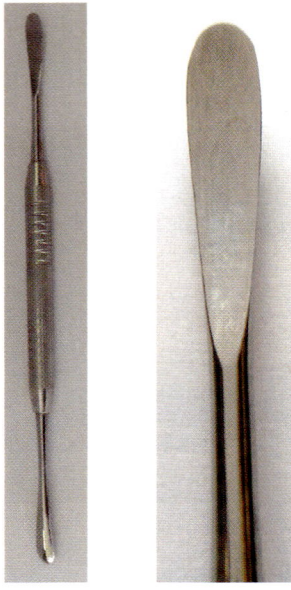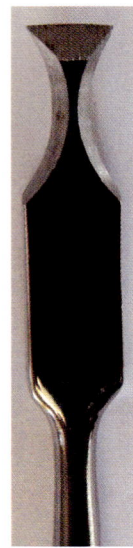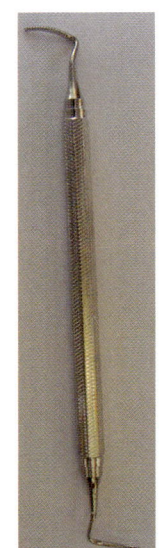

Fig. 40.26: Periosteal elevator (Glickman 24G)

Fig. 40.27: Surgical chisel (Ochsenbein chisel)

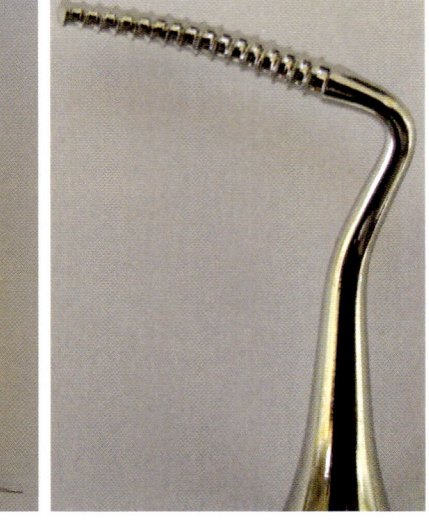

Fig. 40.28: Schluger surgical file

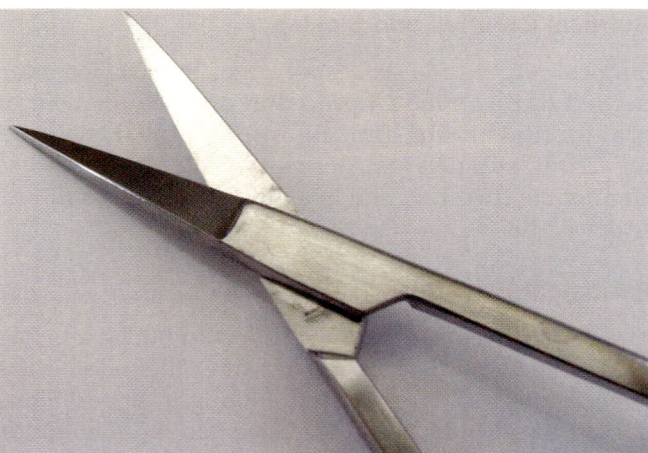

Fig. 40.29: Scissors

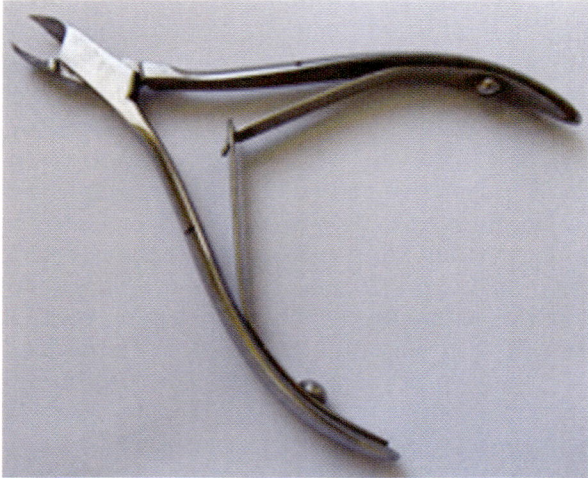

Fig. 40.30: Tissue nipper

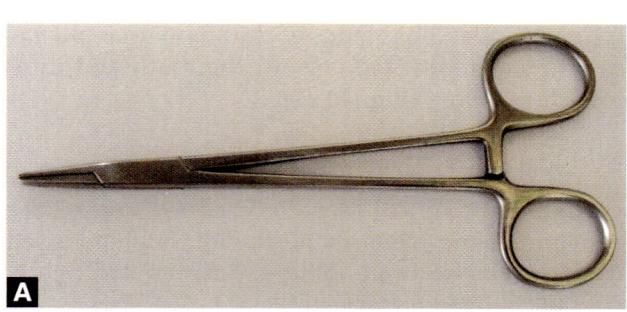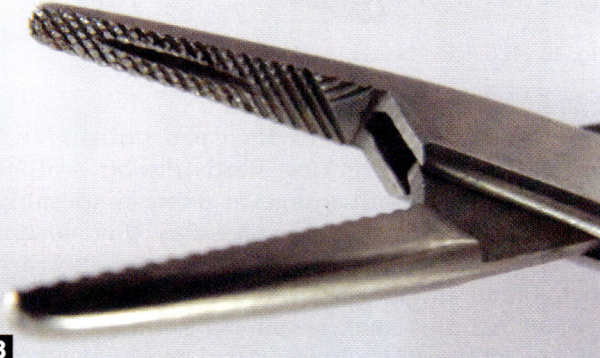

A

B

Figs 40.31A and B: Conventional needle holder

Scissors and Nippers

Scissors and nippers are used in periodontal surgery for removing tissue tabs in gingivectomy procedure, trimming the flap margins, widening the incision in periodontal abscess and removing tissue or muscle attachment in periodontal plastic surgery **(Figs 40.29 and 40.30).**

Needleholders

These are with short or long beak, inner surface of beak serrated criss- crossly with a groove which gives better grip for holding the suture needle **(Figs 40.31A and B)**.

POINTS TO PONDER

✓ *Novatech probes*: These are the probes with unique right angle design for improved adaptability in posterior.
✓ Expros are double end instrument with an explorer on one end and probe on other, e.g. 17/Williams, 23/0 Michigan, 23/Williams.
✓ Merritt and Gilmore periodontal probes are not calibrated probe.
✓ The aerosol which are produced by ultrasonic scaling remains in the air for minimum of 30 minutes.

BIBLIOGRAPHY

1. Grant DA, Stern IB, Listgarten MA. Scaling and root planing. In, Periodontics. 6th ed CV Mosby Company 1988;650-718.
2. Mc Kechnie LB. Instrumentation selection and care. In, Genco RJ, Goldman HM and Cohen DW. Contemporary Periodontics. CV Mosby Company 1990;525-39.
3. Pattison AM, Pattison GL, Takei HH. The Periodontal Instrumentarium. In, Newman, Takei, Carranza. Clinical Periodontology 9th ed WB Saunders 2003;567-93.
4. Plemons J, Eden BD. Non surgical therapy. In, Rose LF, Mealey BL, Genco RJ, Cohen DW. Periodontics, Medicine, Surgery and Implants. Elsevier Mosby 2004;236-62.
5. Scaramucci MK. Instrument Design and Principles of Instrumentation. In, Daniel SJ, Harfst SA. Dental Hygiene - Concepts, Cases and Competencies. Mosby's 2004;137-57.
6. Wennstrom JL, Heijl L, Lindhe J. Periodontal Surgery: Access Therapy. In, Lindhe J, Karring T, Lang NP. Clinical Periodontology and Implant Dentistry. 4th ed Blackwell Munksgaard 2003;519-60.
7. Wilkins EM. Instruments and Principles for Instrumentation. In, Clinical Practice of the Dental Hygienist 8th ed Lippincott Williams and Wilkins 1994;525-39.

MCQs

1. Furcation is best detected by which probe:
   A. WHO probe
   B. University of Michigan 'O' probe
   C. Marquis color coded probe
   D. Naber's probe
2. Which of the following instrument has a two-point contact with the tooth:
   A. Hoe
   B. Sickle
   C. Currette
   D. Cumin scaler
3. Dental instrument used with a "push" motion is:
   A. Hoe
   B. Chisel
   C. Currette
   D. Sickle scaler
4. Gracey Curette No. 11 – 12 are used for:
   A. Anterior teeth
   B. Posterior teeth mesial surfaces
   C. Posterior teeth distal surfaces
   D. Posterior teeth facial and lingual surfaces
5. Cross-section of sickle scaler is:
   A. Triangular
   B. Half circular
   C. Circular
   D. Oval
6. Kirkland and Orban knives are used for:
   A. Curettage
   B. Gingivectomy
   C. Root planing
   D. Scaling
7. Which of the following is a magnetized instrument?
   A. Schwartz periotrievers
   B. Hu-friedy after five curette
   C. Morse sickle scaler
   D. Modified Gracey curette
8. The diameter of dental endoscope is:
   A. 0.66 mm   B. 0.77 mm
   C. 0.88 mm   D. 0.99 mm
9. Instrument for visualization of deposits present in deep periodontal pockets and furcation:
   A. Periotran
   B. Periochip
   C. Perioscope
   D. Prism loupe

10. The millimeter markings that are missing in Williams probe:
    A. 1 and 3
    B. 4 and 6
    C. 7 and 9
    D. 10 and 12
11. Which of the following Gracey Curettes is meant for facial and lingual surface of posterior teeth:
    A. # 9-10
    B. # 11-12
    C. # 13-14
    D. # 15-16
12. Periotriever is used for:
    A. Periosteal elevation
    B. Removal of broken tips of curettes
    C. Measuring crevicular fluid
    D. Local drug delivery
13. The blade of a Hoe is bent at an angle of:
    A. 45°   B. 66°
    C. 90°   D. 99°
14. Linear action of the tip is a feature of:
    A. Sonic scaler
    B. Piezo scaler
    C. Magnetostrictive
    D. All of the above
15. The furcation entrance is narrower than standard curette in first molar in approximately:
    A. 20% cases
    B. 39% cases
    C. 48% cases
    D. 58% cases

16. Which of the following powered instruments use an insert with a stack?
    A. Sonic
    B. Magnetostrictive
    C. Piezoelectric
    D. Manual instrument
17. Which of the following powered instruments function at the highest cycles per second?
    A. Magnetostrictive
    B. Sonic
    C. Piezoelectric
    D. Manual
18. Which of the following health concern contraindicates use of air-powered polishing?
    A. Diabetes
    B. Tuberculosis
    C. Chronic migraine
    D. All of the above
19. Which of the following factors affect the abrasiveness of a polishing agent?
    A. Particle size and shape
    B. Particle hardness and concentration
    C. Amount of water and fluoride
    D. A and B
    E. A and C

Answers

1. D	2. A	3. B	4. B	5. A
6. B	7. A	8. D	9. C	10. B
11. A	12. B	13. D	14. B	15. D
16. B	17. C	18 B.	19. D	

PERIODONTICS REVISITED

CHAPTER 41

General Principles of Instrumentation

Suresh DK, Shalu Bathla

INTRODUCTION

Effective instrumentation is governed by a number of general principles that are common to all periodontal instruments. Proper position of the patient and the operator, illumination and retraction for optimal visibility, and sharp instruments are fundamental prerequisites. The clinician should follow the following principles closely until clinical experience provides the judgment and confidence to modify them for personal preferences or special circumstances, or to achieve a particular outcome.

ACCESSIBILITY

Position of the Operator

The position of the patient and operator should provide maximal accessibility to the operating site and accessibility facilitates thoroughness of instrumentation. The clinician should be seated on a comfortable operating stool that has been positioned so that:

• Head is relatively erect. Head in the least strained position vertically and horizontally.
• Eyes are directed downward in a manner that prevents neck and eye strain.
• Distance from the patient's mouth to the eyes of the clinician should be 14-16 inches.
• Shoulders are relaxed.
• Forearm and wrist are kept in a straight line, wrist is neither flexed nor extended.
• Body weight is completely supported by the chair.
• Back is straight and erect.
• Thighs parallel with the floor.
• Feet are flat on the floor.

Patient/operator positioning is commonly identified by the position of the small hand on a clock in relation to the face of the clock. The patient is represented by the face of the clock. The operator is represented by the small hand of the clock. The patient's chin is at 6 o'clock **(Fig. 41.1)**. The right handed clinician sits between 9 and 12 o'clock. The left-handed clinician sits on the opposite side between 12 to 3 o'clock.

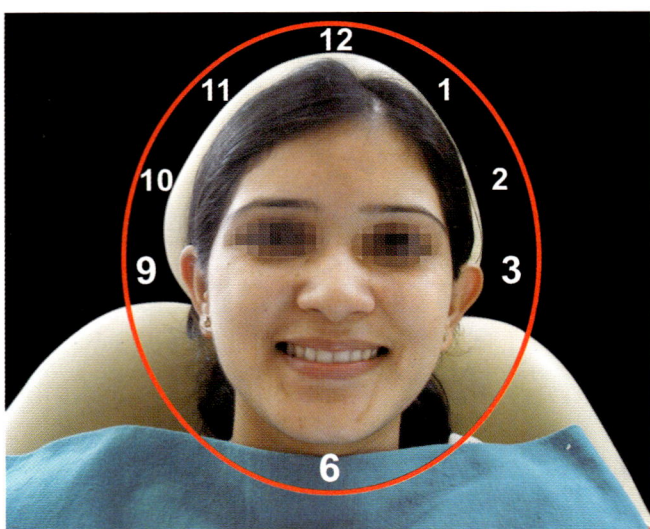

Fig. 41.1: Operator positioning relative to the patient

Position of the Patient

For instrumentation of the maxillary arch, the patient should be asked to raise his or her chin slightly to provide optimal visibility and accessibility. For instrumentation on the mandibular arch, it may be necessary to raise the back of the chair slightly and request that the patient lower his or her chin until the mandible is parallel to the floor. This will especially facilitate work on the lingual surfaces of the mandibular anterior teeth. The distance from the patient's mouth to the eyes of the clinician should be approx. 14 to 16 inches. Assistant is seated with eye level 4 to 6 inches above the clinician's eye level and facing towards the head of dental chair. Following are the various positions of the patient on the dental chair:

- *Upright*: Initial position from which chair adjustments are made.
- *Semi-upright*: Respiratory and Cardiovascular patient should be in a semi-upright position during treatment.
- *Supine*: Flat position with head and feet on the same level.
- *Trendelenburg*: Modified supine position when the head is lower than the heart. The brain is lower than heart and feet slightly elevated.

VISIBILITY, ILLUMINATION AND RETRACTION

Direct vision with direct illumination from the dental light is most desirable. If this is not possible, indirect vision may be obtained by using the mouth mirror. Indirect illumination may also be obtained by using the mirror to reflect light to where it is needed. Indirect vision and indirect illumination are often used simultaneously. Retraction provides visibility, accessibility, and illumination. Depending on the location of the area of operation, the fingers and/or the mirror are used for retraction. The mirror may be used for retraction of the cheeks **(Fig. 41.2)** or the tongue**(Fig. 41.3)**, the index finger is used for retraction of the lips or cheeks. When retracting the lips and cheeks, avoid placing pressure on the labial commissures by pulling the cheeks away from the

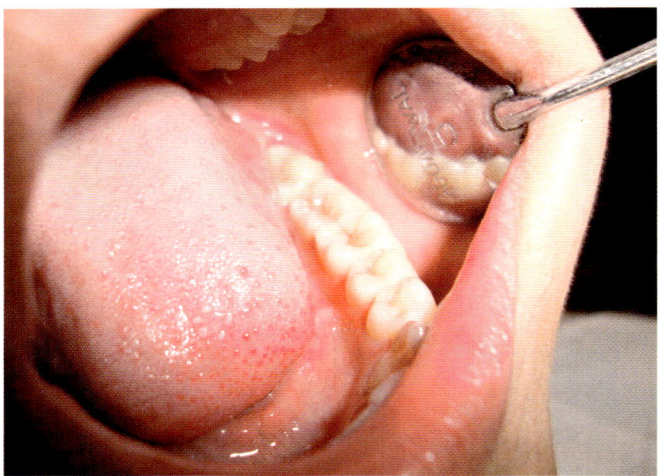

Fig. 41.2: Retraction of cheek by mirror

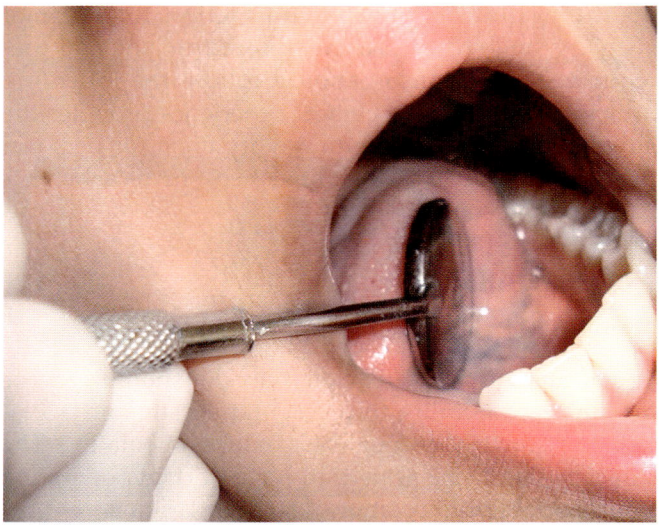

Fig. 41.3: Retraction of tongue by mirror

dentition. Fogging of mirror can be avoided by warming it to body temperature by placing it against the buccal mucosa. Apply petroleum jelly on the angle of mouth and lips before instrumentation is begun which is helpful precaution against cracking and bleeding. Careful retraction is especially important for patients with a history of recurrent herpes labialis, because these patients may easily develop herpetic lesions after instrumentation.

CONDITION OF THE INSTRUMENTS

Steps in the effective care of instruments:
- Instruments are cleaned after each use by removing blood and debris under running water.
- The instruments are sharpen regularly and sharpness is checked thereafter.
- Instruments are sterilized thoroughly.

Sharpness

Instruments are sharpened to produce a functionally sharp edge, to preserve the shape and contour of the instrument. Sharp instruments improves tactile sensations thus, increases efficiency of deposit removal. Using sharp instruments also requires less pressure for calculus and deposit removal.

The various equipments used during sharpening are sharpening stones mounted and unmounted Arkansas and diamond coated stone, lubricating fluids, light mineral oil, water, acrylic test stick and gauge.

The principles of sharpening are:
- Sharpen instrument at the first sign of dullness.
- Choose a suitable sterilized sharpening stone of appropriate shape and abrasiveness for the instrument sharpening.
- Establish the proper angle between sharpening stone and the surface of the instrument.
- Maintain a stable firm grasp of both instrument and sharpening stone.
- Avoid excessive pressure.
- Make the sharpening stroke by moving the instrument towards and not away from you this will minimize the formation of a wire edge.
- Do not overheat the instrument during sharpening. Lubricate the stone well during sharpening.

The methods of testing for sharpness of the instruments are:
- *Effectiveness during use*: A blunt instrument will not bite on root surface and operator will need to apply increased pressure for it to be effective.

- *Visual or Glaze test*: When dull instrument is held under a light, the rounded surface of its cutting edge reflects light back to the observer, appearing bright line running the length of the cutting edge. When sharp instrument is held under light, no bright line can be observed. The cutting edge when examined under magnifying viewer (x5 magnification) should not show any reflection.
- *Acrylic stick test*: Tactile evaluation of sharpness is performed by drawing the instrument lightly across an acrylic rod and evaluating the bite. A dull instrument will slide smoothly, but sharp instrument will bite into the surface, raising a light shaving.

Undesirable edges formed during sharpening are wire edges and beveled edges. Wire edges are undesirable, saw tooth like projections of metal fragments extending beyond the cutting edge from the lateral side or face of the blade. It is formed when a coarse stone is used and instrument is oversharpened. Beveled edges are cutting edges created beneath the original cutting edge by improper stone to instrument placement.

Sterilization of instruments are explained in Section XI Miscellaneous .

MAINTAINING A CLEAN FIELD

Operative field is obscured by saliva, blood and debris. The pooling of saliva interferes with visibility during instrumentation and impedes control because a firm finger rest cannot be established on wet, slippery tooth surfaces. Adequate suction is essential and can be achieved with a saliva ejector, or, if working with an assistant, an aspirator. Blood and debris can be removed from the operative field with suction and by wiping or blotting with gauze squares. Compressed air and gauze squares can be used to facilitate visual inspection of tooth surfaces just below the gingival margin during instrumentation. A jet of air directed into the pocket deflects a retractable gingival margin. Retractable tissue can also be deflected away from the tooth by gently packing the edge of a gauze square into the pocket with the back of a curette. Immediately after the gauze is removed, the subgingival area could be clean, dry and clearly visible for a brief interval.

INSTRUMENT STABILIZATION

Stability of the instrument and the hand is the primary requisite for controlled instrumentation. The two factors of major importance in providing stability are the instrument grasp and the finger rest.

Instrument Grasps

The various instrument grasps are:
1. Standard pen grasp
2. Modified pen grasp
3. Palm and thumb grasp

Standard pen grasp: The thumb, index finger and middle finger are used to hold the instrument as a pen is held and the side of the middle finger rests on the shank **(Fig. 41.4)**.

Modified pen grasp: Modified pen grasp is the most effective and stable grasp for periodontal instruments. Thumb, index finger and middle finger are used to hold the instrument. The pad of the middle finger rests on the shank. The pad of the finger should touch the instrument because this region has the maximum nerve receptors. The index finger is bent at the second joint from the finger tip and is positioned well above the middle finger on the same side of the handle. The pad of the thumb is placed midway between the middle and index fingers on the opposite side of the handle **(Fig. 41.5)**.

Palm and thumb grasp: The handle of the instrument is held in the palm by cupped index, middle, ring and little fingers. The thumb is free to serve as the fulcrum. The palm grasp limits operation in that there is less tactile sensitivity and less flexibility of movement. Palm and thumb grasp is used for stabilizing instruments during sharpening, for manipulating air and water syringes and for manipulating porte polisher **(Fig. 41.6)**.

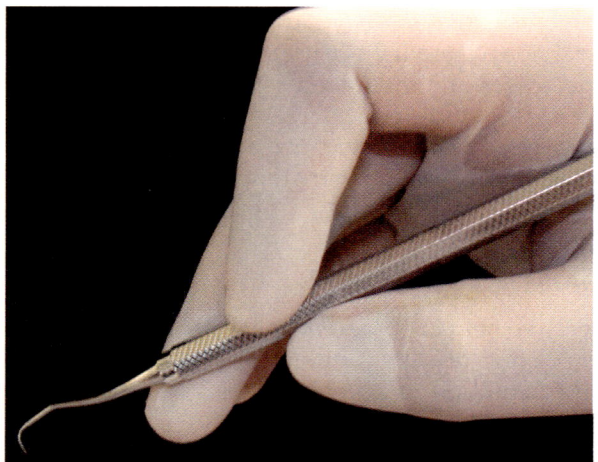

Fig. 41.4: Standard pen grasp (The side of middle finger rests on the shank)

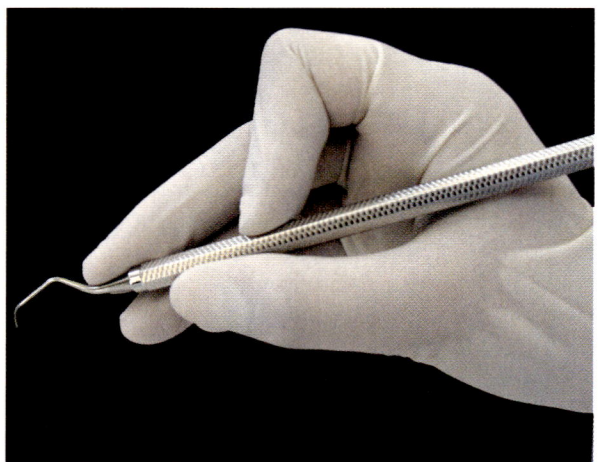

Fig. 41.5: Modified pen grasp (The pad of middle finger rests on the shank)

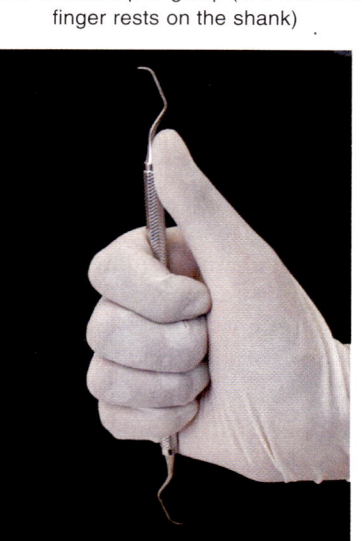

Fig. 41.6: Palm and thumb grasp

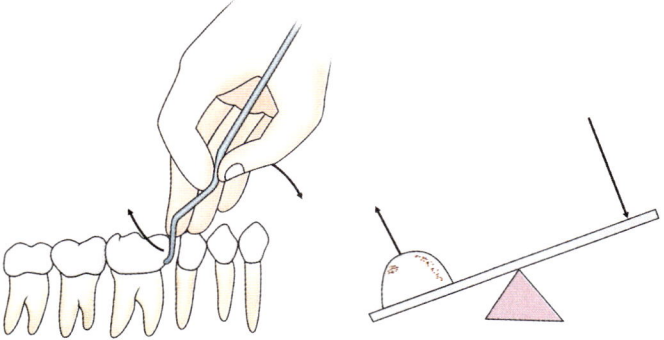

Fig. 41.7: Fulcrum is a stabilizing and pivotal point from which scaling and root planing is done

PERIODONTICS REVISITED

Finger Rests

A scaling instrument operates as a lever, with the third finger (ring finger), serving as a fulcrum and as a stabilizing point for the hand. A fulcrum is the point on which the lever pivots. The fulcrum allows the instrument to function and provides stability and control of the instrument to prevent injury to the surrounding tissues **(Fig. 41.7)**. A proper finger rest provides stable fulcrum, optimal angulation of the blade and enable the use of wrist – forearm motion.

Various Types of Finger Rests

1. *Intraoral finger rests*: Intraoral fulcrum is stabilization of the clinician's dominant hand by placing the pad of the ring finger on a tooth near to the tooth being instrumented in the oral cavity.

   i. *Conventional*: Finger rest is established on the immediately adjacent tooth **(Fig. 41.8)**.

   ii. *Cross-arch*: Finger rest is established on tooth surface on the other side of same arch **(Fig. 41.9)**.

   iii. *Opposite arch*: Finger rest is grasp established on tooth surface on the opposite arch **(Fig. 41.10)**.

   iv. *Finger on finger*: Finger rest is established on the thumb or index finger of the non-operating hand **(Fig. 41.11)**.

2. *Extraoral fulcrums*: Extraoral fulcrum is stabilization of the clinician's hand outside the patient's mouth usually on the chin or cheek. They are essential for

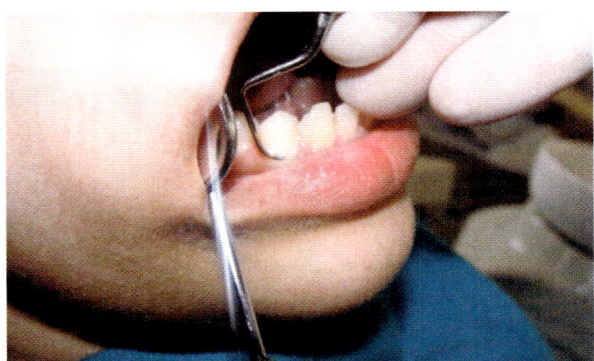

Fig. 41.8: Intraoral Conventional finger rest- 4th finger rests on occlusal surfaces of adjacent teeth

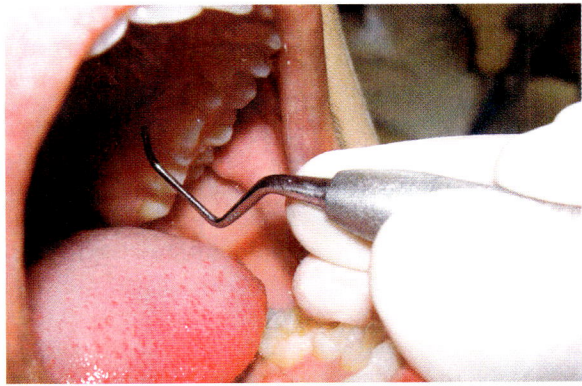

Fig. 41.10: Opposite arch- 4th finger rests on the mandibular teeth while the maxillary posterior teeth are instrumented

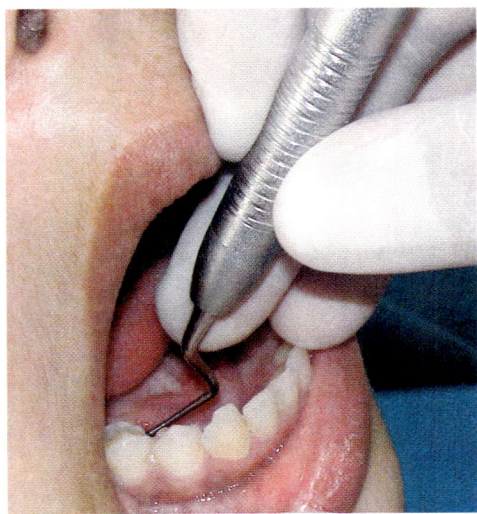

Fig. 41.9: Cross- arch- 4th finger rests on the incisal surface of teeth on the opposite side of the same arch

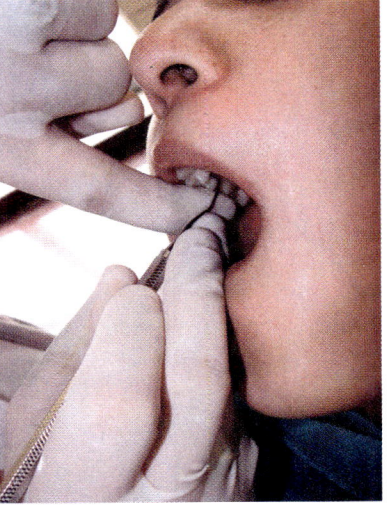

Fig. 41.11: Finger on finger - 4th finger rests on the index finger of non-operating hand

PERIODONTICS REVISITED

effective instrumentation of some aspects of maxillary posterior teeth.

i. *Knuckle rest technique/palm up*: The clinician rests his or her knuckles against the patient's chin or cheek. The back surfaces of the middle and fourth finger is placed on the skin overlying the lateral aspect of the mandible on the right side of the face **(Fig. 41.12)**.

ii. *Chin-cup technique/palm down*: Clinician cups the patient's chin in the palm of his or her hand. The front surfaces of middle and fourth finger is placed on the skin overlying the lateral aspect of the mandible on the left side of the face **(Fig. 41.13)**.

INSTRUMENT ACTIVATION

Adaptation

It refers to the manner in which the working end of a periodontal instrument is placed against the surface of a tooth. The primary goal of adaptation is to keep the instrument tip in continuous contact with the tooth surface during each successive instrument stroke. To accomplish this, the tip must be adapted to the varying contours of each surface, as well as to periodontal structures, by rolling the handle between the index finger and thumb. The instrument tip must be in continual contact with the tooth surface around the circumference of the tooth. Each stroke overlaps the previous one to ensure complete coverage of the surface.

Angulation

It refers to the angle between the face of a bladed instrument and the tooth surface. It is also called as tooth-blade relationship **(Figs 41.14 and 41.15)**.

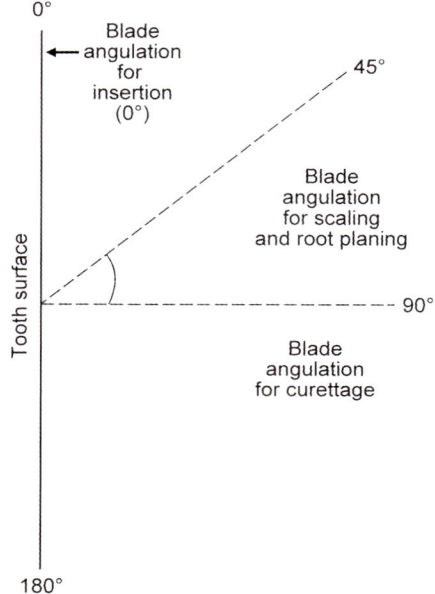

Fig. 41.14: Geometric representation of blade angulation

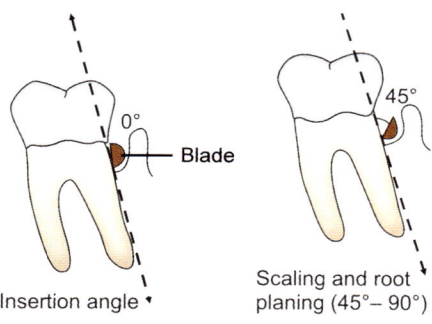

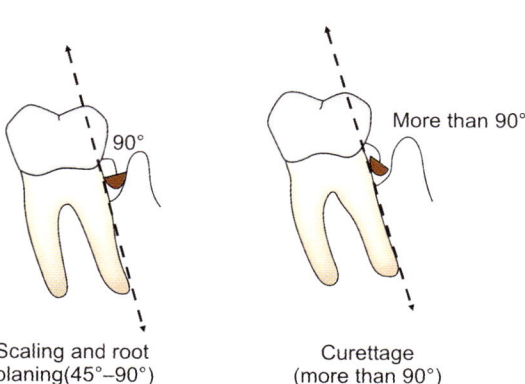

Fig. 41.15: Tooth-blade relationship

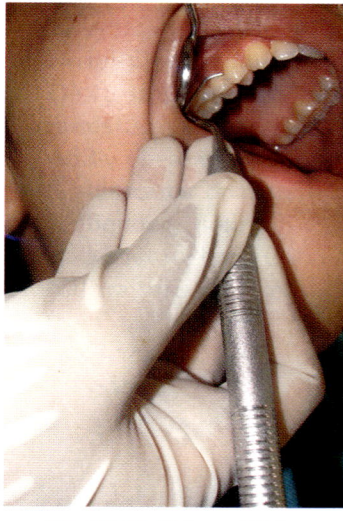

Fig. 41.12: Extraoral Palm up fulcrum

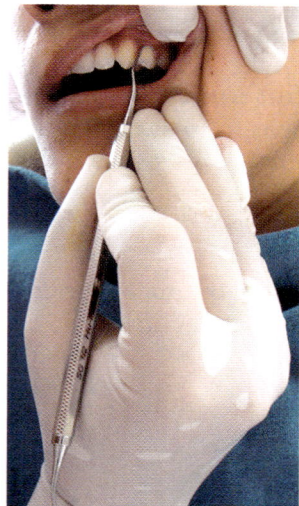

Fig. 41.13: Extraoral Palm down fulcrum

Face to tooth surface angulation for
Insertion beneath the gingival margin is 0°
Scaling and root planing—45° to 90°
Gingival curettage—more than 90°

For successful instrumentation, correct angulation of the working end must be maintained throughout the instrumentation stroke. Lateral pressure refers to the pressure created when force is applied against the surface of a tooth with the cutting edge of a bladed instrument. Lateral pressure may be firm, moderate/light. Lateral pressure is the act of applying equal pressure with the index finger and thumb inward against the instrument handle to press the working end against calculus deposit/tooth surface before and throughout an instrumentation stroke.

INSTRUMENTATION STROKES

Stroke Directions

There are three basic stroke directions **(Fig. 41.16)**.
- *Vertical*: They are used on the facial, lingual and proximal surfaces of anterior teeth. On posterior teeth, vertical strokes are used on the mesial and distal surfaces.
- *Horizontal*: These are made in a perpendicular direction to long axis of the tooth. Horizontal stroke is used at the line angle of posterior teeth, facial and lingual surfaces of anterior teeth, furcation areas and in the areas that are too narrow to allow vertical or oblique stokes.
- *Oblique*: These are used most commonly on the facial and lingual surfaces of anterior and posterior teeth.
Following three basic strokes may be activated by pull or push motion in a vertical, oblique/horizontal direction.
A. *Exploratory stroke/Assessment stroke*: These are light feeling stroke which are used to assess tooth anatomy,

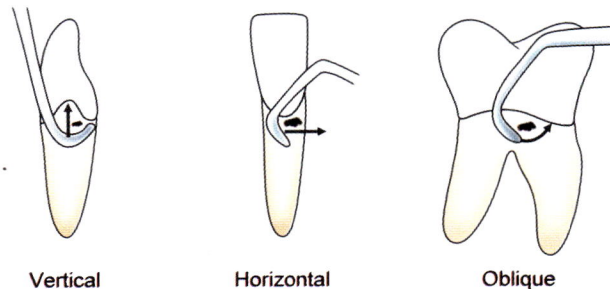

| Vertical | Horizontal | Oblique |

Fig. 41.16: Stroke directions

level of attachment, detect calculus and other plaque retentive factors. Exploratory strokes are used with explorers to locate calculus deposits and with periodontal probes to determine periodontal pocket depths and clinical attachment level.
B. *Scaling stroke*: These are short, powerful pull stroke used to remove supragingival and subgingival calculus with the help of bladed instruments.
C. *Root planing stroke*: These are long, moderate to light pull stroke used for final smoothing and planing of the root surfaces with the help of curettes, hoes, files and ultrasonic instruments.
The walking stroke is the movement of a calibrated probe around the perimeter of the base of a sulcus or pocket. Walking strokes are used to cover the entire circumference of the sulcus or pocket base.
Production of the walking stroke:
1. Walking strokes are a series of bobbing strokes that are made within the sulcus or pocket. The stroke begins when the probe is inserted into the sulcus while keeping the probe tip against the tooth surface.
2. The probe is inserted until the tip encounters the resistance of the junctional epithelium that forms the base of the sulcus. The junctional epithelium feels soft and resilient when touched by probe.
3. Create the walking stroke by moving the probe up and down in short bobbing strokes and forward in 1-mm increments (↔). With each down stroke, the probe returns to touch the junctional epithelium.
4. The probe is not removed from the sulcus with each upward stroke. Repeatedly removing and reinserting the probe can traumatize the tissue at the gingival margin.
5. The pressure exerted with the probe tip against the junctional epithelium should be between 10 and 20 grams.

PRINCIPLES OF SCALING AND ROOT PLANING

Scaling and root planing strokes is confined to the portion of the tooth where calculus or altered cementum is found, this zone is called as instrumentation zone. General principles for use of the curettes for scaling and root planing are as follows:
1. The correct cutting edge should be determined by visually inspecting the blade. With the toe pointed in the direction to be scaled, only the back of the blade can be seen if the correct cutting edge has been selected **(Fig. 41.17)**. If the wrong cutting edge has been adapted, the flat, shiny face of the blade will be seen instead **(Fig. 41.18)**.

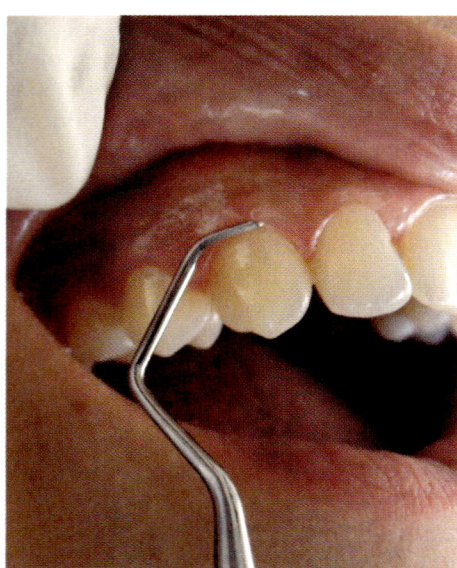

Fig. 41.17: Correct cutting edge of Gracey curette adapted to the tooth

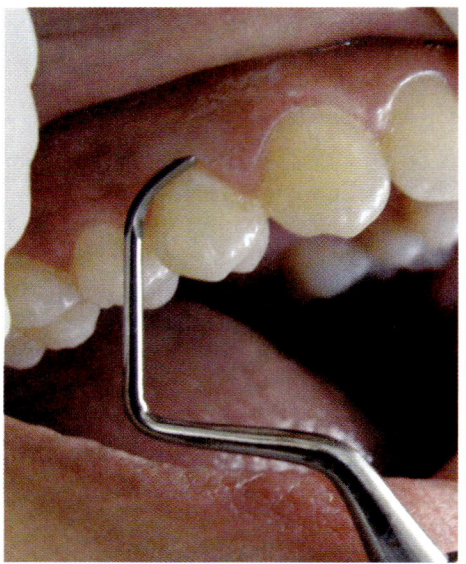

Fig. 41.18: Incorrect cutting edge of Gracey curette

2. The lower shank should be parallel to the surface to be instrumented.
3. When intraoral finger rests are used, the fourth and middle fingers together built-up fulcrum for maximum control and wrist-arm action.
4. For working on the maxillary posterior teeth extraoral fulcrums or mandibular finger rests are used.
5. Concentrate on using the lower third of the cutting edge of instrument for calculus removal, especially on line angles or when attempting to remove a calculus ledge by breaking it away in sections, beginning at the lateral edge.
6. The wrist and forearm should carry the burden of the stroke, rather than flexing the fingers. The clinician activates an instrument with wrist arm motions that roll from the fulcrum finger. Wrist flexion is movement of the hand at the wrist as done in waving or painting with brush. Fingers alone are not used to activate the instrument stroke because finger movements are smaller, has less powerful muscles, produce a limited range of motion, and do not engage the fulcrum.

POINTS TO PONDER

✓ Major difference between standard pen grasp and modified pen grasp: In standard pen grasp, the side of the pad of middle finger rests on the shank while in modified pen grasp, the pad of middle finger rests on the shank.

BIBLIOGRAPHY

1. Grant DA, Stern IB, Listgarten MA. Scaling and root planing. In, Periodontics. 6th ed CV Mosby Company 1988;650-718.
2. Mc Kechnie LB. Instrumentation selection and care. In, Genco RJ, Goldman HM, Cohen DW. Contemporary Periodontics. CV Mosby Company 1990; 525-39.
3. Nield- Gehrig JS. Fundamentals of periodontal instrumentation. 5th ed Lippincott Williams and Wilkins.
4. Pattison GL and Pattison AM. Manual Instrumentation In, Newman, Takei, Carranza. Clinical Periodontology 9th ed WB Saunders 2003; 594-606.
5. Plemons J, Eden BD. Non surgical therapy. In, Rose LF, Mealey BL, Genco RJ, Cohen DW. Periodontics, Medicine, Surgery and Implants. Elsevier Mosby 2004;236-62.
6. Wilkins EM. Instruments and Principles of Instrumentation. In, Clinical practice of the Dental hygienist 8th ed Lippincott Williams and Wilkins 1994; 525-39.

MCQs

1. The most common instrument grasp used is:
   A. Inverted pen grasp
   B. Standard pen grasp
   C. Modified pen grasp
   D. Palm and thumb
2. Correct tooth- blade angulation for curettage is:
   A. 0°
   B. 45°-90°
   C. Less than 45°
   D. More than 90°

PERIODONTICS REVISITED

3. The difference in shank lengths of Gracey and after five curettes is:
   A. 1 mm
   B. 2 mm
   C. 3 mm
   D. 4 mm
4. Aerosols are produced by:
   A. Ultrasonic scaler
   B. Sonic scaler
   C. Both of the above
   D. None of the above
5. The palm and thumb grasp on an instrument:
   A. Is used for removing heavy calculus
   B. Increases maneuverability of the instrument
   C. Is used for stabilizing instrument while sharpening
   D. Enhances sensitivity of the instrument

6. A scaling stroke is a:
   A. Long, powerful pull stroke
   B. Short, moderate to light pull stroke
   C. Long, moderate to light pull stroke
   D. Short, powerful pull stroke
7. In the modified pen grasp, the second finger is positioned with the:
   A. Finger pad on the instrument handle, across from the thumb
   B. Side of the finger resting on a tooth
   C. Finger pad on the instrument shank
   D. Side of the finger against the instrument shank
   E. Finger pad resting on the back of the working end

Answers

1. C 2. D 3. C 4. C 5. C
6. D 7. C

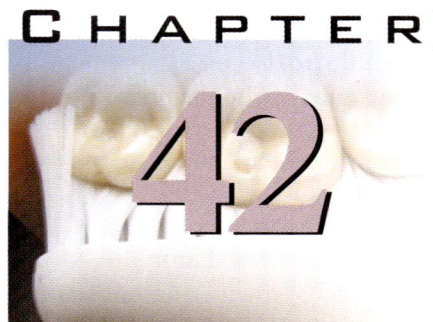

CHAPTER 42

Splinting

Harpreet Singh Grover, Shalu Bathla

HISTORICAL PERSPECTIVE

Early evidence of splinting weakened teeth can be seen in archaeological findings. Etruscans from the 8th century B.C to the first century A.D utilized wire ligation and small gold rings and bands to stabilize loose teeth. Fauchard in 1723 ligated and banded teeth to stabilize them. In the 1900s several authors described splinting techniques that dated back to the 1800s. Hirschfeld (1950) was one of the first modern periodontal author to advocate ligation of periodontally diseased teeth using either stainless steel wire or silk. His technique was extracoronal and involved only the anterior teeth. In 1951, Obin and Arvins advocated the use of self curing internal splint to achieve temporary stabilization. Harrington (1957) modified the splint by incorporating a cemented stainless steel wire. Cross in 1954 suggested the use of a amalgam splint for fixation of mobile posterior teeth.

DEFINITION

A splint is any appliance that joins two or more teeth to provide support. Splintee is the tooth that need support. Splinters are the adjacent teeth that provide support.

RATIONALE FOR SPLINTING

Objectives of splinting are:
1. To provide rest: Occlusal rest provided by splint therapy in one form or another helps to eliminate or neutralize some adverse occlusal factors.
2. For redirection of forces: The forces of occlusion are redirected in a more axial direction over all the teeth included in the splint.
3. For redistribution of forces: Stabilization by splinting increase resistance to applied force. Thus the redistribution of forces ensures that forces do not exceed the adaptive capacity.
4. To preserve arch integrity: Splinting restores proximal contacts and thus reduce food impaction.
5. Restoration of functional stability: Splinting restores functional occlusion, stabilizes mobile abutment teeth and increases masticatory comfort.
6. Psychologic well being: Splinting gives the patient comfort from mobile teeth thereby giving him a sense of well being.
7. To stabilize mobile teeth during surgical, especially regenerative therapy.

8. To protect the tooth supporting tissues during the healing period following surgery or after an accident.
9. To prevent the extrusion of unopposed teeth.
10. To bring into function the teeth that cannot be used to eat efficiently.

Ideal requirements of splints:
- Simple design
- Economical
- Stable and efficient
- Hygienic
- Non – irritating to the soft tissues
- Aesthetically acceptable
- Not provoke iatrogenic disease

INDICATIONS

1. To stabilize moderate to advance tooth mobility that cannot be reduced by occlusal adjustment or periodontal therapy.
2. Stabilize teeth in secondary occlusal trauma.
3. Stabilize teeth with increased tooth mobility which interfere with normal masticatory function.
4. Facilitates scaling and surgical procedures.
5. Stabilize teeth after orthodontic movement.
6. Stabilize teeth after acute dental trauma, i.e. subluxation, avulsion, etc.

CONTRAINDICATIONS

1. Moderate to severe tooth mobility in the presence of periodontal inflammation and/or primary occlusal trauma.
2. Insufficient number of firm teeth to stabilize mobile teeth.
3. Prior occlusal adjustment has not been done on teeth with occlusal trauma or occlusal interferences.
4. Patient not maintaining oral hygiene.
5. When the sole objective of splinting is to decrease tooth mobility following the removal of the splint.

ADVANTAGES OF SPLINTING

1. May establish final stability and comfort for patient with occlusal trauma.
2. Helpful to decrease mobility and accelerate healing following acute trauma to the teeth.
3. Allows remodelling of alveolar bone and periodontal ligament for orthodontically, splinted teeth.

4. Helpful in decreasing mobility favoring regenerative therapy.
5. Distributes occlusal forces over a wide area.

DISADVANTAGES OF SPLINTING

1. *Hygienic*: Accumulation of plaque at the splinted margins can lead to further periodontal breakdown in a patient with already compromised periodontal support.
2. *Mechanical*: The splint being rigid may acts as a lever with uneven distribution of forces. If one tooth of the splint is in traumatic occlusion, it can injure the periodontium of all teeth within the splint.
3. *Biological*: Development of caries is an unavoidable risk and thus, requires excellent maintenance by the patient.

CLASSIFICATION

I. According to the type of material:
   1. A-splints
   2. Braided wire splint
   3. Bonded, composite resin splint
II. According to the location on the tooth:
   1. Intracoronal
      - Composite resin with wire
      - Inlays
      - Nylon wire
   2. Extracoronal
      - Night guard
      - Welded-band
      - Tooth bonded plastic
III. According to the period of stabilization (Schluger et al):
   1. Temporary stabilization—worn for less than 6 months
      - Removable -Occlusal splint with wire, Hawley with splinting arch wire
      - Fixed – Intracoronal, Extracoronal
   2. Provisional stabilization—To be used for 6 months to 12 months, e.g acrylic splints, metal bands.
   3. Permanent splints-Used indefinitely
      - Removable/Fixed
      - Extra/Intracoronal
      - Full/Partial veneer crowns soldered together
      - Inlay/Onlay soldered together
IV. Goldman, Cohen and Chacker classification:
   1. Temporary splints

A. Extracoronal type
   • Wire ligation
   • Orthodontic bands
   • Removable acrylic appliances
   • Removable cast appliances
   • Ultraviolet light polymerizing bonding materials.
B. Intracoronal type
   • Wire and acrylic
   • Wire and amalgam
   • Wire, amalgam and acrylic
   • Cast chrome-cobalt alloy bars with acrylic, or both.
2. Provisional splints
   • All acrylic
   • Adapted metal band and acrylic.
V. Ross, Weisgold and Wright classification:
   1. Temporary stabilization
      • Removable extracoronal splints
      • Fixed extracoronal splints
      • Intracoronal splints
      • Etched metal resin-bonded splints
   2. Provisional stabilization
      • Acrylic splints
      • Metal-band and acrylic splints
   3. Long-term stabilization
      • Removable splints
      • Fixed splints
      • Combination of removable and fixed splints
VI. Permanent splints may be classified as follows:
   1. Removable—external
      • Continuous clasp devices
      • Swing—lock devices
      • Overdenture (full or partial).
   2. Fixed - internal
      • Full coverage, three-fourths coverage crowns and inlays
      • Posts in root canals
      • Horizontal pin splints.
   3. Cast-metal, resin-bonded fixed partial dentures (Maryland splints)
   4. Combined
      • Partial dentures and splinted abutments
      • Removable and fixed splints
      • Full or partial dentures on splinted roots
      • Fixed bridges incorporated in partial dentures, seated on posts or copings
   5. Endodontic posts.

EXTRACORONAL TYPE OF SPLINTS

Extracoronal splints are very simple and are reversible, i.e they do not necessitate any loss of tooth structure. These splints require less chair side time and are economical. The disadvantages of extracoronal splint are that they may interfere plaque removal and maintenance measures. They are cosmetically poor due to bulky contour.

Welded Band Splints

These are useful for temporary stabilization of posterior teeth. Separate the teeth by placing brasswire ligatures interdentally for 24 hours before splinting. Adapt a strip of stainless steel 0.003 to 0.005" thick to a tooth and weld it to form a band. Weld the next strip to the mesial surface of the first band. Seat the two pieces while adapting the second strip to the tooth, then weld the second strip to form a band. Several strips can be added and formed into bands for successive teeth. Bands should not impinge on the gingva. Alternatively, the splint can be fabricated on a model and cemented onto teeth.

Continuous Clasps

These are made of acrylic, gold or cast stainless steel. These splints are seated and removed in the fashion of a partial denture. Sharp edges should be rounded off. Adequate oral hygiene is possible with the continuous clasps.

Night Guards

They are made of heat cured acrylic and completely cover the occlusal surfaces of the teeth. These splints can be made thin enough to be quite comfortable while worn. The splint should cover the occlusal surface of the teeth and extend 1-2 mm over the facial surfaces of the teeth. The occlusal surface must be designed to allow free excursion of the mandible with no greater than 1 mm increase in vertical dimension in the molar regions.

Rochette Splint

An impression of the teeth to be splinted is taken and a chrome - cobalt splint, fitting the lingual surface of these teeth, is constructed. The lingual tooth surfaces are dried and etched and the splint is glued into position with the composite material.

Wire Ligation

These are satisfactory means of stabilizing anterior teeth. Dead-soft stainless steel wire of 0.007 to 0.010" thickness is used. Double a 12 inch length for use as an arch wire and bend it about the 6 anterior teeth. It should be positioned apical to contact points and incisal to the cingula and then loosely twist buccal and lingual strands at one end. Place single, hair-pin bent wires interdentally around the arch wire and below the contact points **(Fig. 42.1)**. Tighten them by twisting clockwise with a needle holder. Tighten the last interdental ligature after all the other interdental ligatures and the arch wire have been tightened. Clip the ends of the wires short 2-3 mm and bend them into the interdental space **(Fig. 42.2)**. Self-cure acrylic or composite-acid etch resin may be placed over the wires.

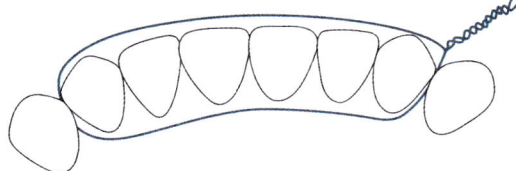

A wire loop is placed around all teeth to be splinted

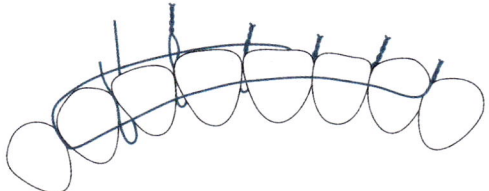

Interdental wires are placed and tightened

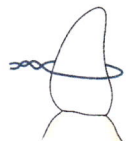

Splint must be placed just apical to contact point

Fig. 42.1: Wire ligation

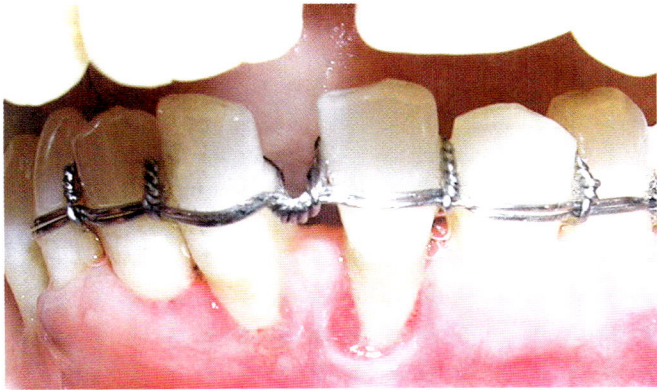

Fig. 42.2: Wire splinting (Interdental ligatures are bent in upward direction instead in interdental spaces, as use of interdental aid was being interfered)

INTRACORONAL TYPE OF SPLINTS

They usually require tooth structure removal and are inconspicuous splints.

Acrylic Splints (A-splint)

Channel/slot is prepared midway between cingulum and incisal edge of approximately 3 mm wide and 2 mm deep on lingual aspect of the tooth **(Fig. 42.3)**. Platinized knurled wire (22 to 16 gauge) or stainless steel wire is placed in the slot. Self cure acrylic is then placed over the wire to seal the slots. It is one of the effective method of stabilizing teeth for prolonged periods of time if proper plaque control is achieved. The main disadvantage associated with this type of splint is the leakage and breakage of acrylic.

Composite Splints

Factors such as position of the opposing teeth, crowding, spacing, rotations and size of embrassures are important in planning such type of splint.

After proper shade selection, rubber dam is placed. Grooves are prepared using a large round carbide bur at high speed with water coolant, a shallow groove is prepared in the enamel layer at a level slightly apical to the contact points. Shallow grooves are prepared in the enamel without reaching the dentin **(Fig. 42.4)**. Prepared surfaces are thoroughly polished with slurry of pumice and water, then it is rinsed and dried with air. Thin layer of hard - setting $Ca(OH)_2$ base is coated over the exposed dentin surfaces to protect pulp. A 0.010 dead, soft single

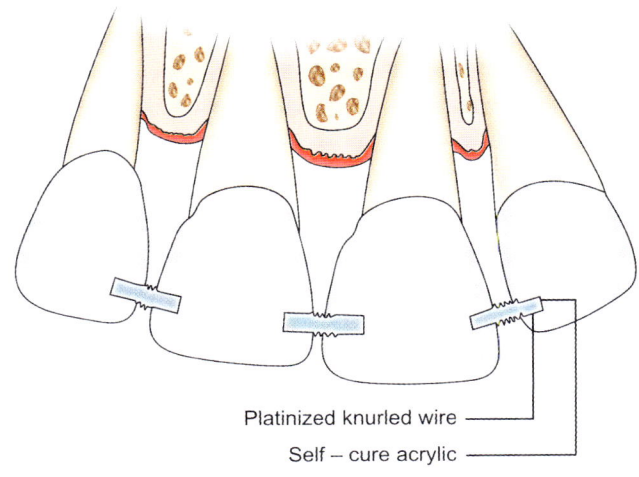

Platinized knurled wire ———

Self – cure acrylic ———

Fig. 42.3: Acrylic-A- splint

PERIODONTICS REVISITED

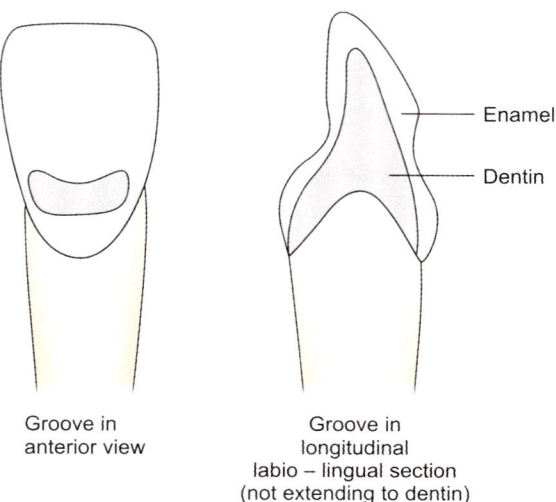

Fig. 42.4: Composite and wire splint

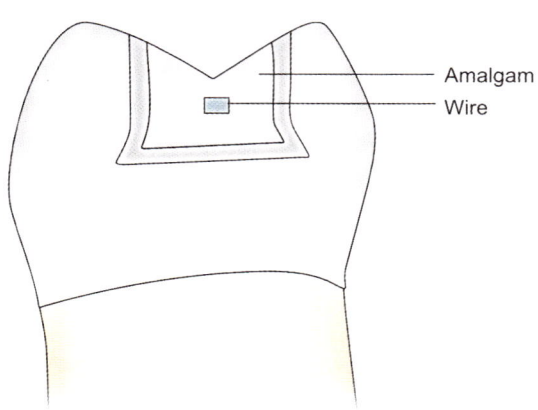

Fig. 42.5: Amalgam and stainless steel wire splint

or double wire is placed in the grooves, ligating the teeth continuous with figure-eight loops. Wood wedges are inserted to all embrasure spaces, so that embrasures are not packed with composite material. 37% phosphoric acid solution is applied to buccal, lingual and interproximal surfaces of the ligated teeth and resin is applied. Finishing of composite is done thereafter.

Amalgam and Stainless Steel Splint

It is similar to the A-splint but used in posterior teeth. A series of mesio-occlusodistal preparations are made and then restored with amalgam that has wire of diameter of 0.050 inches embedded in it at the time of condensation. More amalgam is condensed over the wire in one unit (**Fig. 42.5**). Two or five teeth are splinted together with amalgam splints. The disadvantage associated with it is the frequent fracture of amalgam.

POINTS TO PONDER

✓ The choice of splint should reflect patient needs rather than the artistic aspirations of the operator. When the prognosis is doubtful a simple form of splint is indicated.
✓ Splinting should be undertaken only by patients who prove their willingness and ability to perform plaque control.

BIBLIOGRAPHY

1. Eley BM, Manson JD. Splinting. In, Periodontics 5th ed Wright 2004;366-74.
2. Grant DA, Stern IB, Listgarten MA. Splinting and stabilization. In, Periodontics 6th ed CV Mosby Company 1988;1056-74.
3. Greenfield DS, Nathanson D. Periodontal splinting with wire and composite resin. J Periodontol 1980;51:465-68.
4. Marzouk MA, Simonton AL, Gross RD. Principles for restoration of badly broken down teeth. In, Operative dentistry Modern theory and practice. New Delhi A.I.P.D 2006;435-66.
5. Rosenberg S. A new method for stabilization of periodically involved teeth. J Periodontol 1980;51:469.
6. Simring M, Thaller JL. Temporary splinting for mobile teeth. J Am Dent Assc 1956;53:429.

MCQs

1. Splinting of several teeth together as for a fixed prosthesis is done to:
   A. Distribute occlusal load
   B. Facilitate plaque control
   C. Improve retention of prosthesis
   D. Preserve remaining alveolar bone.
2. Extracoronal splints are:
   A. Continuous clasps   B. Night guards
   C. Both A and B   D. None of the above

Answers

   1. A   2. C

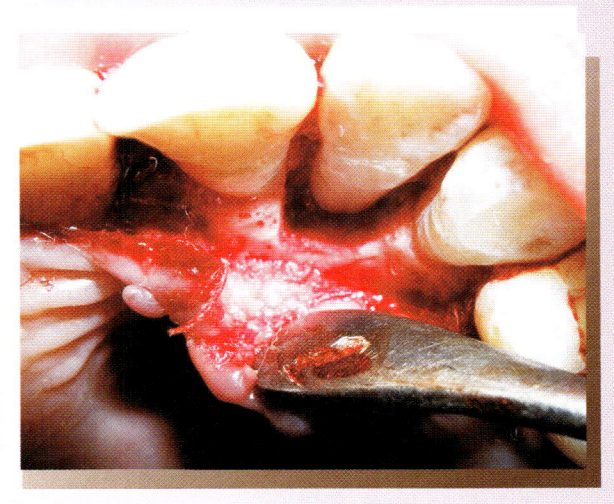

B. SURGICAL THERAPY

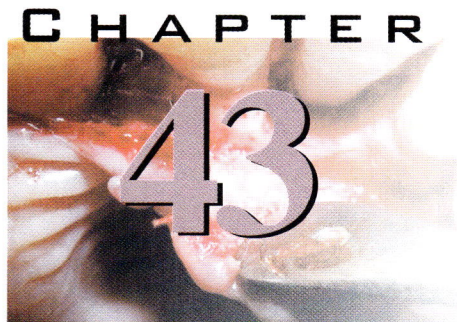

CHAPTER 43

General Principles of Periodontal Surgery

Shalu Bathla

CASE SELECTION

Since, wide range of periodontal surgical therapies are available for the treatment of soft tissue and bony periodontal defects, consideration must be given to the most appropriate surgery for each involved site in each case criteria.

Classification of periodontal surgery:
A. Pocket reduction surgery:
   - Resective: Gingivectomy, apically displaced flap and undisplaced flap with or without osseous resection.
   - Regenerative: Flaps with grafts and membranes.
B. Correction of anatomic/morphologic defects:
   - Plastic surgery techniques to widen attached gingiva:
     - Epithelial grafts
     - Connective tissue grafts
   - Esthetic surgery:
     - Root coverage
     - Recreation of gingival papillae
   - Preprosthetic surgery techniques:
     - Crown lengthening
     - Ridge augmentation
     - Vestibular deepening
   - Placement of dental implants:
     - With GBR
     - Sinus grafts

Objectives of surgical phase of periodontal surgery:
- Regeneration of lost periodontal attachment.
- Improvement of the prognosis of teeth and their replacements.
- Improvement of esthetics.

PREOPERATIVE INFORMATION

Case History

Medical History

The operator should determine if specific preoperative modifications are indicated because of patient's medical history, well before scheduling any surgical procedure. Drug allergy, patient's medication or systemic disease dictate alterations in the type of anesthetic agent, analgesics, prophylactic antibiotic and even surgical procedure.

Indications for Periodontal Surgery

i. Correction of gross gingival aberrations.
ii. Persistent inflammation in areas with moderate to deep pockets.
iii. Areas with irregularly bony contours, deep craters.

iv. When removal of root irritant is not possible due to deep pockets especially in molars and premolars.

v. Furcation lesions.

vi. Infrabony pockets on the distal areas of last molars, complicated by mucogingival problems.

Contraindications for Periodontal Surgery

i. Uncooperative patient

ii. Uncontrolled systemic diseases/hormonal disorders
   a. Uncontrolled diabetes mellitus
   b. Adrenal dysfunction

iii. Blood disorders

iv. Smoking

v. Cardiovascular diseases
   a. Hypertension
   b. Myocardial infarction
   c. Angina pectoris
   d. Anticoagulant therapy
   e. Rheumatic fever

vi. Organ transplantation

vii. Neurological disorders
   a. Multiple sclerosis
   b. Parkinson's disease

Consent

Patient should be fully informed verbally and in writing about the details of the procedure and possible complications. Patient should be given agreement for the procedure both with an oral statement and by signing a consent form.

Premedications

Premedication should be given when indicated. The chemotherapeutic agents used for premedications are:

i. *Anxiolytics*: Apprehensive and neurotic patients are given antianxiety, sedative, hypnotic agents, tranquilizers or barbiturates im or iv prior to surgical therapy.

ii. *Antibiotics*: Given to only medically compromised patients such as infective endocarditis or patients who require prophylactic antibiotics regimen (valvular heart disease). Antibiotics should be given one hour before surgery to attain adequate levels so as to prevent bacteremia.

iii. *Antiseptics*: Oral rinse with 0.12% CHX gluconate mouthwash.

iv. *Nonsteroidal Anti-inflammatory drugs (NSAIDs)*: Ibuprofen can be given as premedication before surgery.

Patients on anticoagulant therapy/aspirin should stop such medicines 7 to 14 days before surgery and 3 to 4 days afterwards with physician's approval.

INTRAOPERATIVE CONSIDERATIONS

Monitoring Presurgical Data

The data necessary to select the surgical procedure includes periapical radiographs, study casts and probing charts.

Anesthesia

Periodontal surgery should be performed painlessly, the entire area of the dentition scheduled for surgery, the teeth as well as periodontal tissues should be anesthetized by proper anesthesia. Local infiltration and block anesthesia are the methods of choice. After the initial administration of local anesthesia, inject a drop of anesthetic solution directly into interdental papilla. It makes the gingiva firmer and easier to incise and has a hemostatic effect because of the vasoconstrictor present in the solution. In general, most periodontal surgical procedures are done under local anesthesia. However, in apprehensive patients or patients suffering from neurological disorders, surgery is done under general anesthesia.

Tissue Management

Flap Preparation

Surgical flap is defined as the separation of a section of tissue from the surrounding tissues except at its base. Flap can be full thickness or partial thickness.

Flap Design

Flap design should be based on the principle of maintaining an optimal blood supply to the tissue. The recommended flap length (height) to base ratio should be no greater than 2:1 **(Fig. 43.1).** The greater the ratio of the flap length to flap base, the greater the vascular compromise at the flap margins.

Flap Reflection

A full thickness flap is elevated using a sharp periosteal elevator directed beneath the periosteum keeping against the bone. Papillae are reflected first, followed by the marginal gingiva, working across the anterior/posterior extent of the incisions until the flap margin has been freed from the teeth or alveolar crest or both. Once the flap

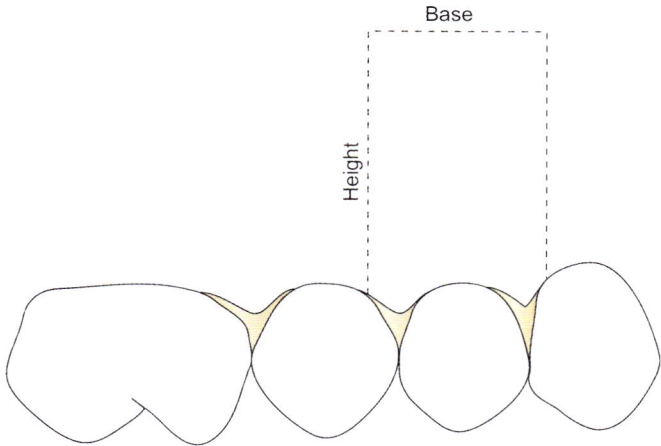

Fig. 43.1: Flap height-to base ratio (Ratio should not exceed 2:1)

margin has been completely released, the periosteal elevator is directed in both horizontal and vertical plane until adequate access is achieved.

Flap Retraction

Surgical retractors are used to hold the flap back from the teeth and bone. Retraction should be passive without any tension. Continuous flap retraction for long period is not advised. When the flap is retracted, the surgical field should be irrigated with the sterile saline to keep the tissues moist, to reduce contamination and to improve visibility.

Flap Repositioning

Surgical flaps may be repositioned, apically positioned, coronally positioned or laterally positioned. The final flap location is determined by the goal of therapy and the specific periodontal surgical technique performed.

Thus in general, tissue should be handled carefully with minimum surgical trauma.

- Use suction during surgery to avoid compression of tissues with dry sponge. Cotton fibers of dry sponge/gauze could be left behind and may be source of future irritation and infection.
- Sterile saline solution should be used.
- Do not blow air into the surgical site as it may induce cervicofacial emphysema which can be fatal.
- Slow-speed sharp surgical bur and adequate cooling should be used for bone removal. Avoid undue drying of the bone and do not heat the bone above 47°C otherwise it will cause necrosis of bone surface.
- Avoid heavy pressure against soft tissues/bone.

Scaling and Root Planing

Scaling and root planing in conjunction with periodontal surgery is done on exposed root surfaces with the help of curettes.

Hemostasis

Steps to minimize postsurgical bleeding:
1. Before approximation of flaps, all areas should be rinsed free of clots and the surgical site should be checked again for bleeding.
2. Pressure should be applied to the flap to encourage minimal clot thickness.
3. Good closure with suturing discourages postsurgical hemorrhage.
4. Distal wedge and edentulous ridge sites should be well approximated carefully with attention because these areas are good source of postoperative bleeding.

Wound Closure

The various techniques of wound closure are sutures, skin clips/staples, skin tapes and wound adhesive [Autologous fibrin glue, fibrin fibronectin sealing system (Tissucol), Cyanoacrylate, Mussel adhesive protein].

The various intraoral anchoring structures useful in securing movable tissues are:
i. *Teeth*: These teeth are easiest and most secure of all intraoral anchors.
ii. *Bound down tissue*: Gingiva affixed to bone via periosteum, is the second most reliable anchor.
iii. *Periosteum*.
iv. *Loose connective tissue*: It is the least secure anchoring structure in the mouth. Connective tissue in the vestibule and fatty tissue in the retromolar area are the examples of loose connective tissue anchor source.

Suture and Suturing Techniques

Selection of the type of suture material and needle is dependent on tissue type and thickness, location in the mouth, ease of handling, cost and the planned time of suture removal.

Parts of Surgical Needle

i. Point – It is the working end of needle.
ii. Body – It refers to the grasping area which forms the majority of length of needle. It starts where the point of needle ends and ends where the contour change, marking the beginning of swage of the needle.

PERIODONTICS REVISITED

iii. Eye/Swage – It is the segment at which needle and suture material are joined.

Types of Needles

A. On the basis of shape:
   i. Straight
   ii. Curved: 1/4, 3/8, 1/2, 5/8 **(Fig. 43.2)**.
B. On the basis of eye:
   i. *Eyed*: Suture material is tied to the needle and is designed to reuse.
   ii. *Eyeless/swaged*: The suture material is inserted into hollow end during manufacturing and metal is compressed around it. Needle is not reusable.
C. On the basis of function:
   i. *Tapered*: Used for closing mesenchymal layers such as muscle/fascia that are soft and easily penetrable.
   ii. *Cutting*: Used for keratinized mucosa and skin.
      a. Conventional cutting **(Fig. 43.3A)**
      b. Reverse cutting **(Fig. 43.3B)**.

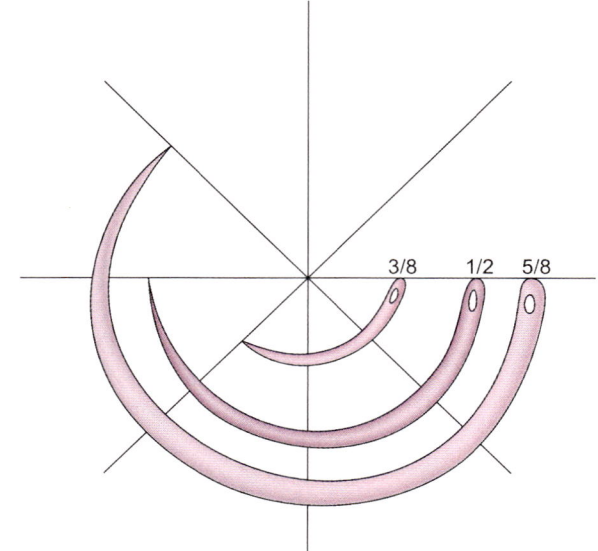

Fig. 43.2: Suture needles: Needles are described by their arc as 3/8, 1/2 or 5/8th of a circle

Types of Suture Materials

A. Based on the number of filaments:
   a. Monofilament, e.g. steel, nylon
   b. Multifilament, e.g. silk, cotton.
B. Based on suture diameter by US Pharmacopoeia in descending order from 5, 4, 3, 2, 1-0 till 11-0 size. 1-0 being the largest diameter and 11-0 the smallest one.
C. Based on resorbability of suture material:
   a. Absorbable
   b. Non absorbable
D. Based on the source:
   a. Natural:
      • *Absorbable*– Plain gut, chromic gut, fast absorbing gut, plain collagen, chromic collagen.
      • *Nonabsorbable*– Silk, cotton, linen.
   b. Synthetic:
      • *Absorbable*– Polyglactin, Polyglyconate, Polyglycolic, Polydioxanone.
      • *Nonabsorbable*– Nylon, Polybutester, Polyester, Decron, Polypropylene, Nurolone.

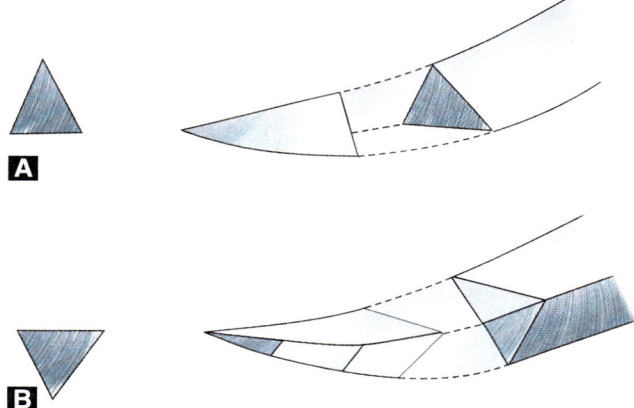

Figs 43.3A and B: A. Conventional cutting needle and B. Reverse cutting needle

Method of Prescription of Suture

It should contain the name of the suture, its size, length and atraumatic, the type of needle, size of the needle and number of foils required, e.g. prolene 2-0, 70 cms with atraumatic reverse cutting needle (3/8 circle 45 mm) – 1 foil.

Objectives of Suturing

   i. To stabilize the tissue
   ii. To secure tissues in the desired locations
   iii. To maintain hemostasis
   iv. To permit healing by primary intention
   v. As a tool to retract flap for photography or to retrieve free gingiva/connective tissue autografts.

Principles of Suturing

   i. Needle holder should grasp the needle approximately ¾th of the distance from point.

ii. Needle should enter the tissue perpendicular to the surface.

iii. Needle should be passed through the tissue following curvature of the needle.

iv. Suture should be placed at an equal distance (2 to 3 mm) from incision on both sides and at an equal depth.

v. Needle should be passed from free to fixed side.

vi. Needle should be passed from thinner to the thicker side.

vii. If one tissue plane is deeper than the other, needle should be passed from deeper to superficial side.

viii. The distance that the needle is passed into tissue should be greater than the distance from the tissue edge.

ix. The tissue should not be closed under tension, it will either tear or necrose.

x. Suture should be tied so that tissue is merely approximated, not blanched.

xi. Suture should not be placed over the incision line.

xii. Suture should be placed approximately 3-4 mm apart.

Various Types of Suturing

A. Interrupted sutures:
   a. Circumferential: Direct/loop
   b. Figure of eight
   c. Mattress: Vertical and horizontal

B. Continuous sutures:
   a. Independent sling suture
   b. Mattress: Vertical and horizontal
   c. Continuous locking

C. Simple sling suture

D. Periosteal sutures

Direct/Loop suture: The needle penetrates the outer surface of the first flap. The undersurface of the opposite flap is engaged and the suture is brought back to the initial side where the knot is tied **(Figs 43.4A to D)**. These

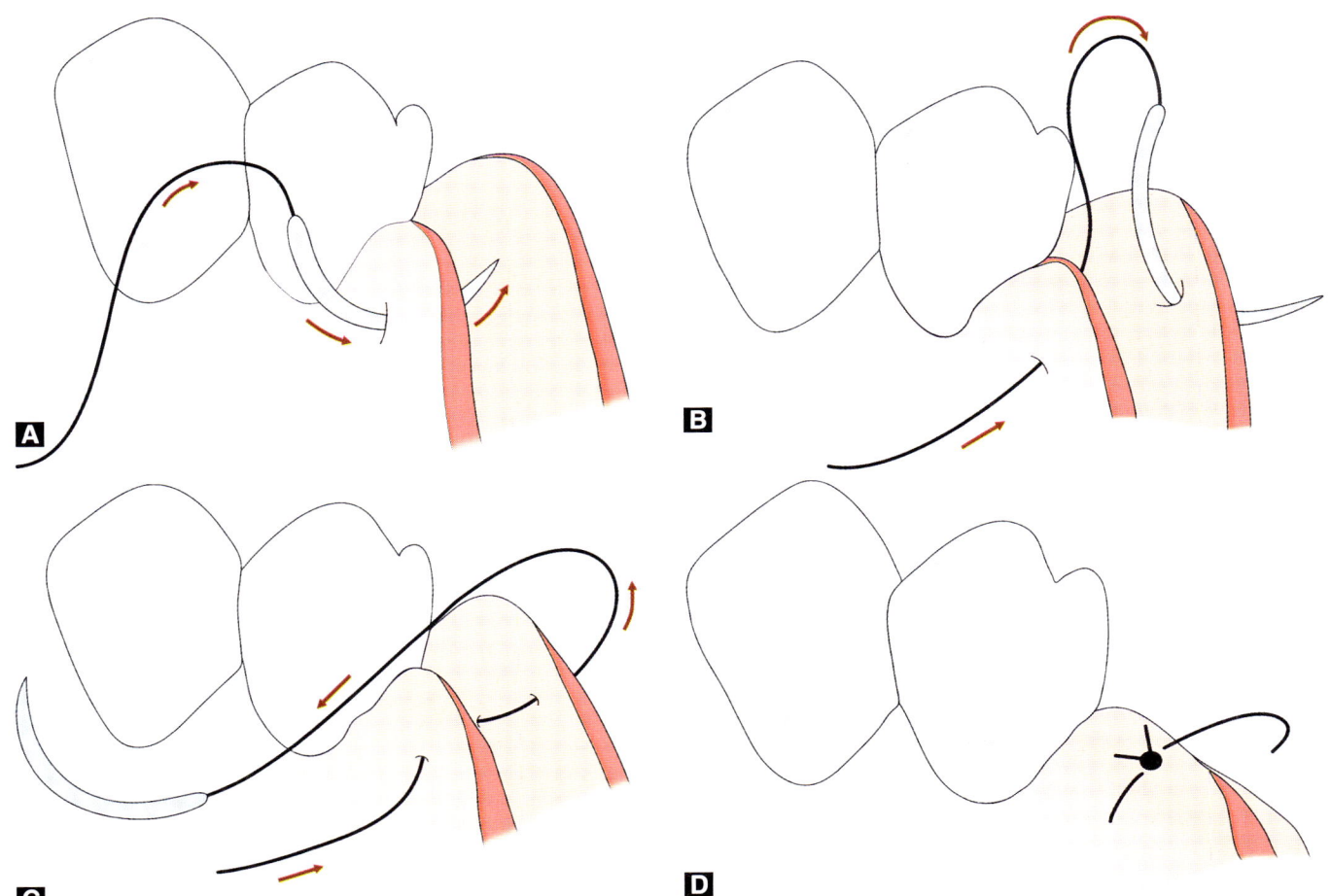

Figs 43.4A to D: Direct loop suture

sutures are used where bone grafts are placed and when closed apposition of scalloped incision is required.

Figure of eight: The needle penetrates the outer surface of the first flap and the outer surface of the opposite flap. The suture is brought back to the first flap and the knot is tied **(Figs 43.5A to D)**. These sutures are placed when flaps are not in close apposition because of apical flap position or nonscalloped incisions.

Simple sling suture: The needle engages the outer surface of the flap and encircles the tooth. The outer surface of the same flap of the adjacent interdental area is engaged. The suture is returned to the initial site and the knot tied **(Figs 43.6A to D)**. It is used primarily with apically positioned flap and in repositioning the flap.

The sling/suspensory suture is used primarily when the surgical procedure is of limited extent and involves only the tissue of the buccal or lingual aspect of the teeth.

It is also the suture of choice when the buccal and lingual flaps are repositioned at different levels and to place barrier membrane onto the tooth surface.

Mattress sutures: Mattress means that the suture passes through the flap twice. The material does not pass under the incision line, thus minimizing wicking.

a. *Vertical mattress*: The needle penetrates the outer/ epithelized surface of the flap 8 to 10 mm apical to the tip of the papilla. It is passed through the under surface of the flap, emerging again from the outer surface of the same flap 2 to 3 mm from the tip of papilla. Thus, a vertical bite of 6 to 7 mm is taken with the needle. The needle is passed through the embrasure, where the technique is again repeated with the opposite/ second flap. The suture is tied on the first flap **(Figs 43.7A to D)**. It is used in areas with long and narrow papillae. It is of two types – everting and inverting.

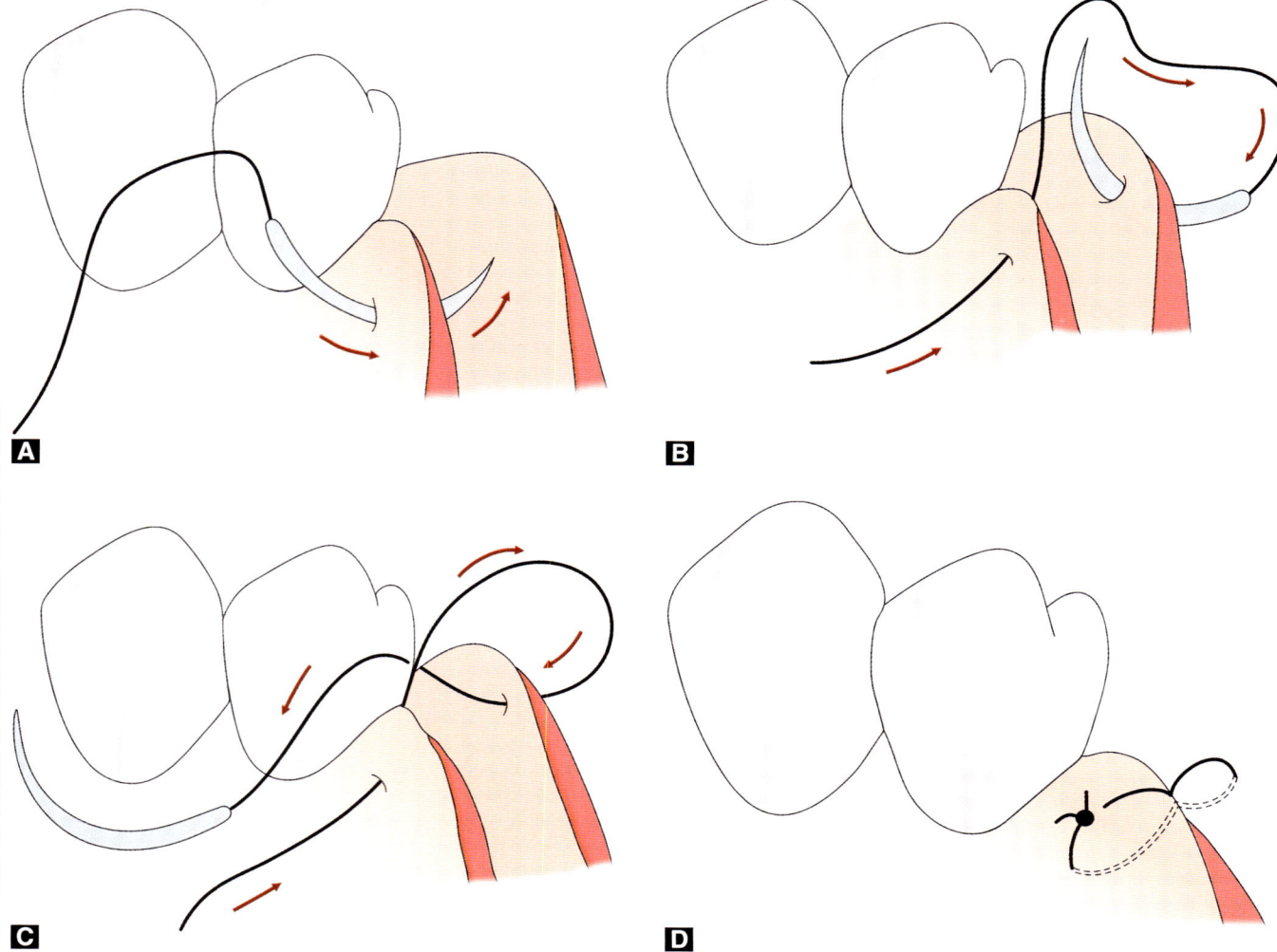

Figs 43.5A to D: Figure of eight suture

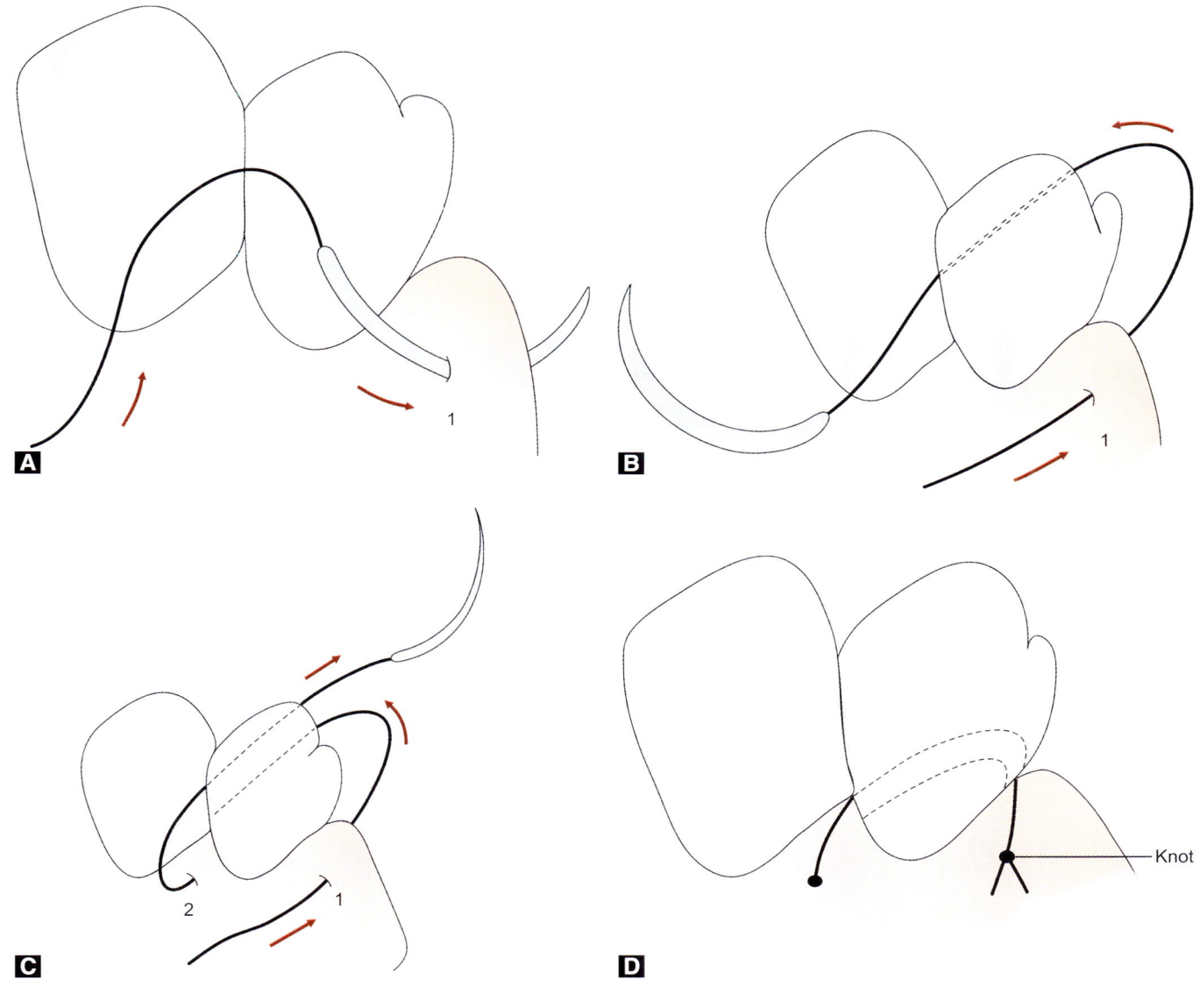

Figs 43.6A to D: Sling suture

b. *Horizontal mattress*: The needle penetrate the outer surfaces of flap 7 to 8 mm apical and to one side of the midline of papilla emerging again 4 to 5 mm through the outer surface on the opposite side of the midline papilla. Thus, horizontal bite of 4 to 5 mm is taken with the needle. The needle is passed the embrasure, where the technique is again repeated with the opposite/second flap. The suture is tied on the first flap **(Figs 43.8 and 43.9)**. It is used in interproximal areas of diastema with short and wide papillae.

Criss Cross suture: The use of a criss- cross as the suture passes through the interproximal areas provides good control of the flap papilla and keeps the suture out of the healing interproximal sulcus area. Thus, criss-cross single horizontal mattress is good for holding osseous grafts in papilla preservation flap **(Fig. 43.10)**.

Circumferential suturing: It is indicated for suturing grafts.

Continuous suture: The suturing procedure is started at the mesial/distal aspect of the buccal flap by passing

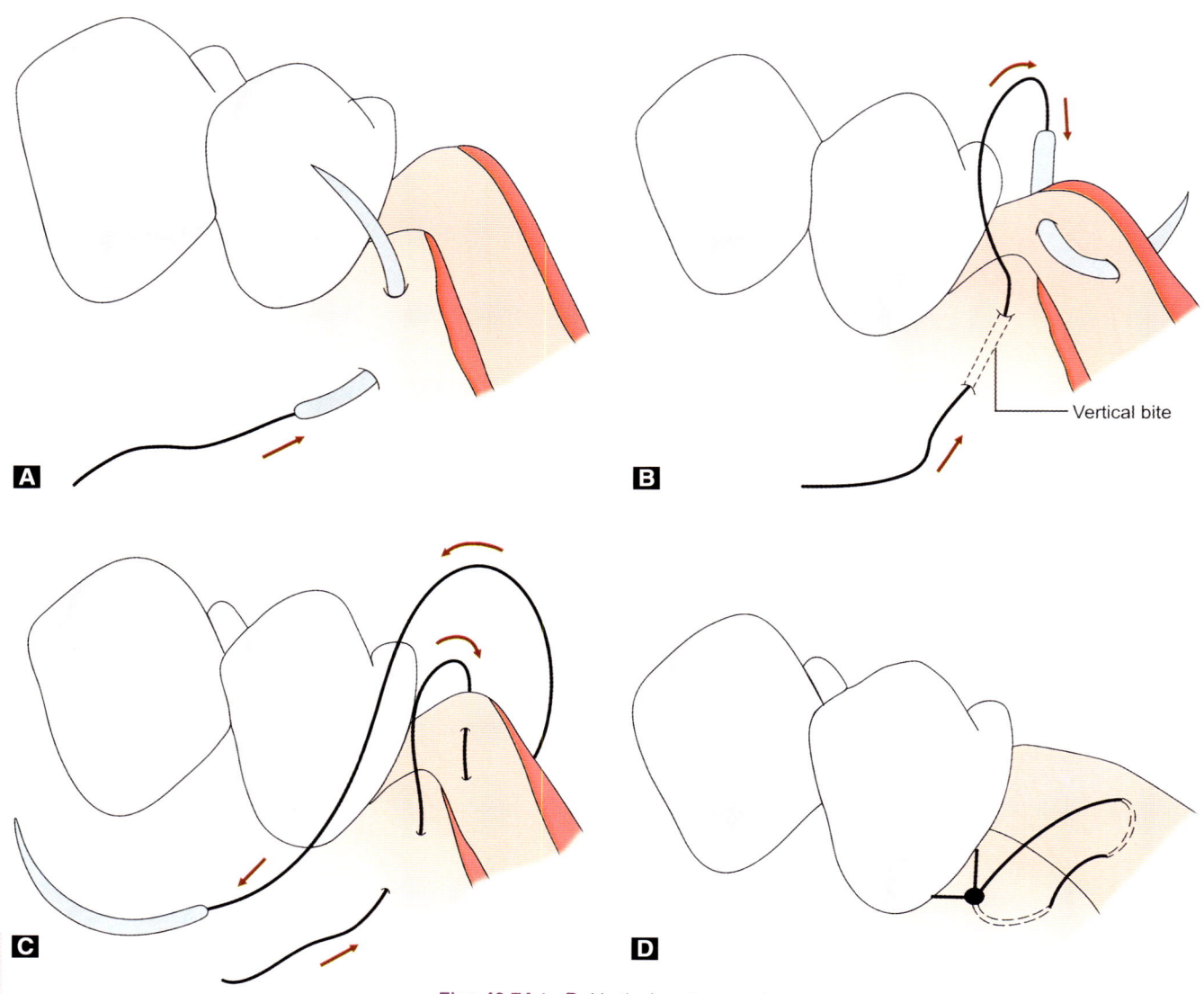

Figs 43.7A to D: Vertical mattress suture

the needle through the flap and across the interdental area. The suture is laid around the lingual surface of the tooth and returned to the buccal side through the next interdental space. The procedure is repeated tooth by tooth until the distal/mesial end of the flap is reached. Thereafter, the needle is passed through the lingual flap, with the suture laid around the buccal aspect of each tooth and through each interproximal space. When the suturing of the lingual flap is completed and the needle has been brought back to the first interdental area, the positions of the flaps are adjusted and secured in their proper positions by closing the suture **(Figs 43.11A and B)**. Thus, only one knot is needed **(Fig. 43.12)**. The continuous suture is

commonly used when flaps involving several teeth are to be apically repositioned. When flaps have been elevated on both sides of the teeth, one flap at a time is secured in its correct position.

Periosteal sutures: It is indicated in apically positioned partial thickness flap **(Fig. 43.13)**.

Sutured Knots

The components of sutured knots are loop, knot and ears. Knot is composed of a number of tight, throws, each throw represents a weave of the two strands and ears that are the cut ends of the suture. Knots should be tied as small as possible. Completed knots should be firm to

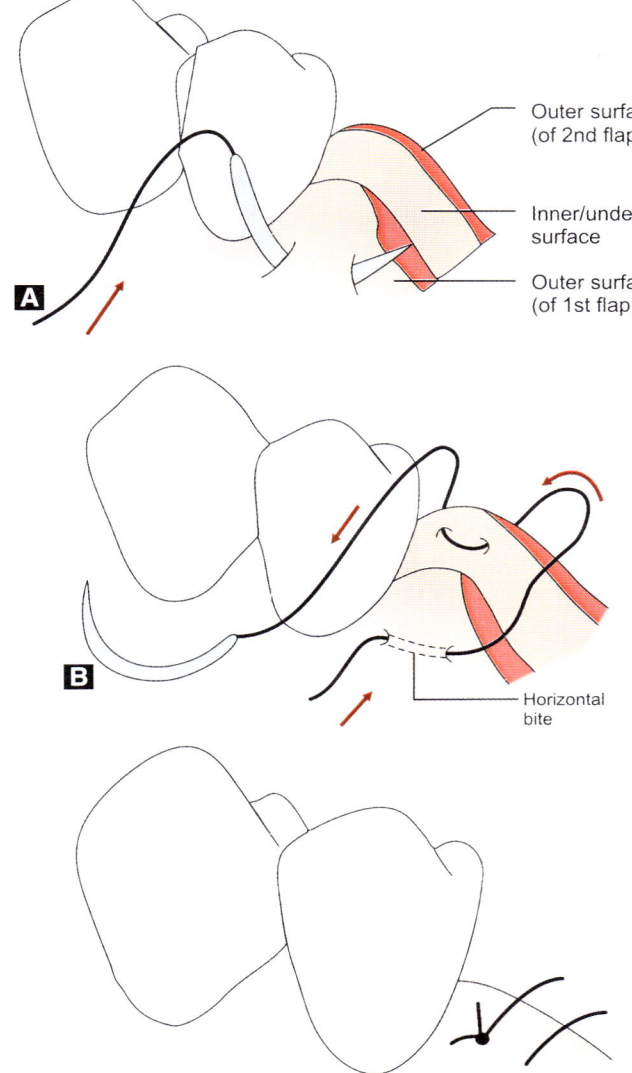

Outer surface (of 2nd flap)

Inner/under surface

Outer surface (of 1st flap)

Horizontal bite

Fig 43.8A to C: Horizontal mattress suture

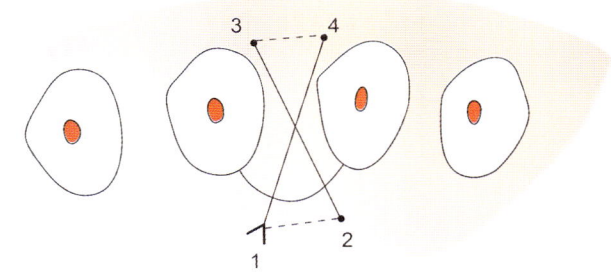

Fig. 43.10: Criss cross horizontal mattress suture

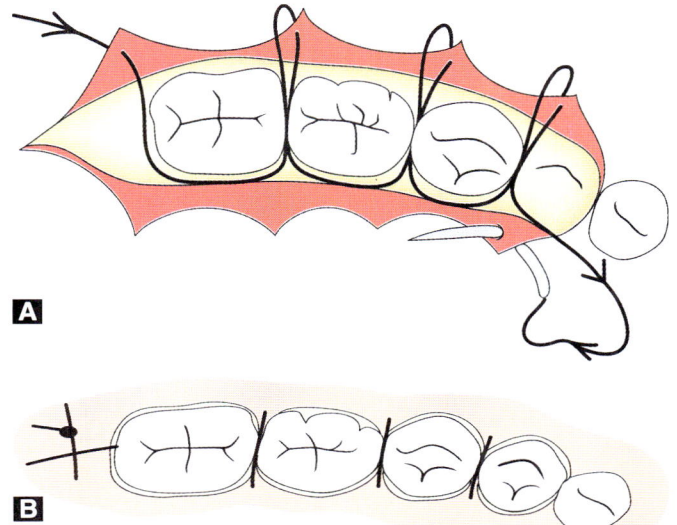

Figs 43.11A and B: Continuous sutures

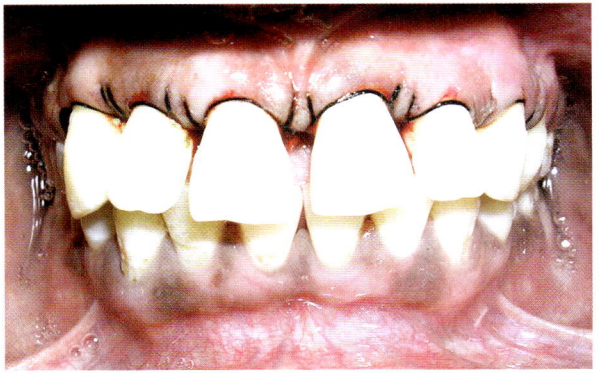

Fig. 43.9: Continuous horizontal mattress sutures

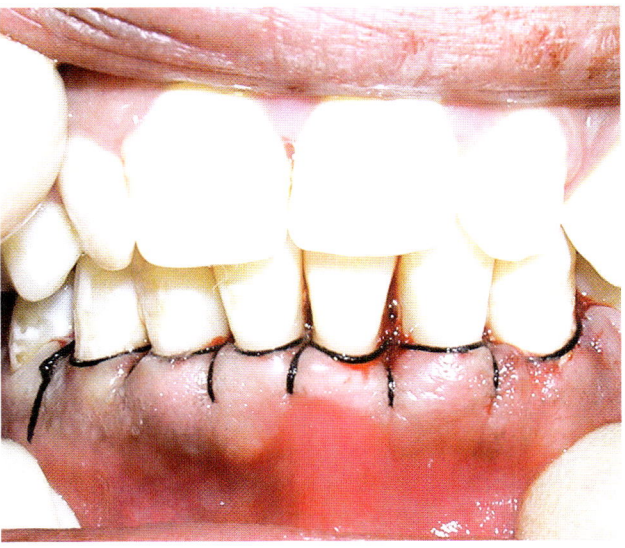

Fig. 43.12: Continuous sutures

PERIODONTICS REVISITED

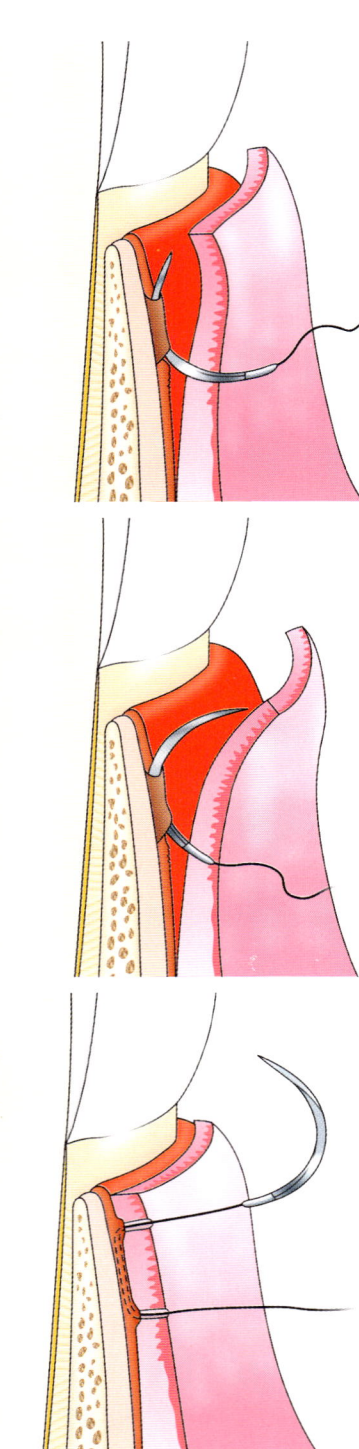

Fig. 43.13: Periosteal suture

reduce slippage. Tie knots on facial aspect for access in removal leaving 2 to 3 mm suture tail.

Types of knots:
  i. *Square knot*: Two single tie in opposite direction.
 ii. *Granny knot*: Two or three tie in same direction.
iii. *Surgeon's knot 2-1*: 1st tie is double and 2nd tie is single in opposite direction.
iv. *Surgeon's knot 2-2*: 1st tie is double and 2nd tie is also double in opposite direction.

Principles of suture removal:
  i. Areas should be swabbed with hydrogen peroxide for removal of encrusted necrotic debris, blood and serum from suture.
 ii. A sharp suture scissor should be used to cut the loops of suture, close to the epithelial surface as possible. In this way, a minimal amount of portion of sutures that was exposed to the outside environment and has become laden with debris and bacteria will be dragged through the tissue.
iii. A cotton plier is then used to remove the sutures. The location of knots should be noted so that they can be removed first, which will prevent unnecessary entrapment of the flap.

Periodontal Dressings

Periodontal dressings were first introduced in 1923 when Dr AW Ward advocated the rules and use of packing material around the teeth following gingival surgery. This material was called Wonder pack, which consisted of zinc oxide eugenol mixed with alcohol, pine oil and asbestos fibers.

Purpose

Periodontal dressings are used for the following reasons:
a. Protect the wound area from irritants such as hot/spicy food.
b. Enhances patient comfort.
c. Helps to maintain the position of repositioned soft tissues and act as a template to prevent formation of excessive granulation tissue.
d. Also protects newly exposed root surfaces from temperature changes, stabilizes mobile teeth and protect sutures.

Properties

a. Dressing should be soft, but with enough plasticity and flexibility.
b. Dressing should set within a reasonable time.
c. Dressing should have sufficient rigidity to prevent fracture and dislocation.

d. Dressing should have a smooth surface after setting to prevent irritation to the cheeks and lips.
e. Dressing should be dimensionally stable to prevent salivary leakage and accumulation of plaque debris.
f. Dressing should preferably have bactericidal properties to prevent excessive plaque formation.
g. Dressing should not induce allergic reactions.
h. Dressing should have an acceptable taste.
i. Dressing must not detrimentally interfere with healing.

Classification of Periodontal Dressing:

i. Zinc oxide eugenol
ii. Zinc oxide noneugenol: Coepak, periocare, periopac, perioputty and vocopac
iii. Others: Photocuring periodontal dressing (Barricaid), collagen dressings, methacrylic gel and cyanoacrylate.

Zinc oxide eugenol dressings:

i. *Powder and liquid form (Kirkland pack)*: Powder is composed of zinc oxide, tannic acid, rosin, kaolin, zinc – steorate, asbestos. Liquid contains eugenol, peanut oil, rosin. When the components of zinc oxide eugenol dressings are mixed, setting occurs as a result of chemical interaction between zinc oxide and eugenol forming zinc eugenolate.
ii. *Paste form* - Tube 1 – Base zinc oxide 87%, fixed vegetable/mineral oil 13%; Tube 2 – Accelerator oil of clove 12%, gum/polymerized rosin.

Zinc oxide non-eugenol dressings:

i. *Coepak*: It is the most common and widely used non – eugenol dressing **(Fig. 43.14)**.

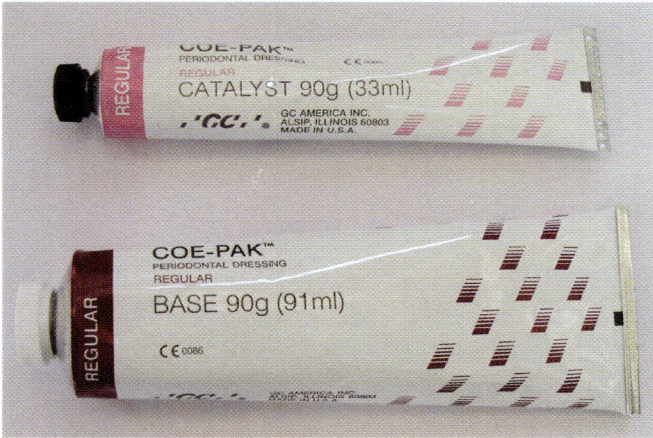

Fig. 43.14: COE PAK: Periodontal dressing

Zinc oxide	:	Main ingredient
Vegetable oil	:	For plasticity
Gum	:	For cohesiveness
Lorothidol	:	Fungicide
Liquid coconut	:	Fatty acids
Chlorothymol	:	Bacteriostatic agent

Colophony resin

ii. *Periocare*: Paste contain zinc oxide, MgO, Ca(OH)$_2$, vegetable oils. Gel contain resins, fatty acids, ethylcellulose, lanolin, Ca(OH)$_2$. The setting of periocare occurs by chemical reaction.
iii. *Periopac*: It is premixed ZnO noneugenol dressing containing Ca$_3$(PO$_4$)$_2$, ZnO, acrylate, organic solvents, flavoring and coloring agents. When this material is exposed to air or moisture, it sets by the loss of organic solvents. After it is set, this dressing becomes quite brittle.
iv. *Vocopac*: It is a new formulated product for use as a periodontal dressing. It contains 90 gm base and 90 gm catalyst. It contains neither eugenol nor coumarin and causes no gingival irritation, it retains its tough elastic qualities throughout its life in the patient's mouth, and does not become brittle. It adheres excellently to the teeth and promotes healing. Mixing time is about 20-30 seconds and its working time is approximately 10-15 minutes.
v. *Perioputty*: It is a noneugenol dressing which contains methyl and propyl-parabens for their effective bacteriocidal and fungicide properties and benzocaine as a topical anesthetic.
vi. *Barricaid visible light cure periodontal dressing*: This single component of periodontal dressing eliminates messy, time consuming mixing of paste. It is available in a syringe for the direct application or dispensing on a mixing pad and placement intraorally. Curing of the material is then accomplished with a visible light curing unit to form a nonbrittle, but firm, protective elastic covering. The principle ingredients of this material are polyether urethane dimethacrylate resin, silica, visible light cure (VLC) photoinitiator, accelerator and stabilizer. It contains polymerisable monomers which may cause skin sensitization (allergic contact dermatitis) in susceptible persons. Eye protection should be worn, while curing with a visible light unit.
vii. *Collagen dressings*: An example of collagen dressing is collocate. Collagen dressing is in the form of collagen sponge which is a type I collagen derived from bovine Achilles tendon. It is completely

resorbable dressing that is used to cover and protect palatal graft sites; the sponge is approximately 3 mm thick and can be cut to fit the graft site. It stops bleeding and can absorb 30-40 times its weight in fluid, without swelling.

viii. *Methacrylate gel dressings*: They have elastic consistency that is soft and resilient and will flow under pressure. They adapt closely to the tissues and are very comfortable with wound site. The major advantage of this material is its ability to carry and release medicaments to the soft tissues.

ix. *Cyanoacrylate*: In 1964 tissue adhesives were introduced to dentistry. Dr SN Bhaskar conceived the idea of their potential use in periodontics and conducted the bulk of the laboratory and clinical research. The basic formula of Cyanoacrylate is CH= C (CN) – COOR. The butyl and isobutyl forms are ideal as periodontal dressings. The use of cyanoacrylate is an alternative to suturing and as a surface adhesive and periodontal dressing. This material has the unique ability to cement together moist, living tissue surfaces. Cyanoacrylate is either applied in drops or sprayed on the tissues. The material is much less bulky than other dressings. Other advantages include lack of apparent side effects, easy adherence to living tissues, immediate hemostasis, lack of evidence of systemic toxicity/sensitivity, precise placement of flaps, decreased suturing time, ease of application and patient preference over bulky dressings. It is most useful in flap control in concave zones such as furcal area fluting. Cyanoacrylate has been used for surface application only; adhesives that become trapped under soft tissue flap will delay wound healing.

Antibacterial properties of packs: Bacitracins, Oxytetracycline (Terramycin), Neomycin and Nitrofuraxone have been tried, but all may produce hypersensitivity reactions. Incorporation of tetracycline powder in Coe – Pak is generally recommended, particularly when long and traumatic surgeries are performed.

Preparation and Application of Periodontal Dressings

Zinc oxide packs are mixed with eugenol or non – eugenol liquids on a wax paper pad with a wooden tongue depressor. The powder is gradually incorporated with the liquid until a thick paste is formed.

Coe-Pak is prepared by mixing equal lengths of paste from tubes containing the accelerator and the base until the resulting paste is of uniform color. The pack is then placed in a cup of water at room temperature, in 2-3 min the paste looses its tackiness and can be molded, and it remains workable for 15-20 min. The pack is then rolled into two strips of approximately the length of the treated area. The end of one strip is bend into a hook shape and fitted around the distal surface of the last tooth, approaching it from the distal surface. The remainder of the strip is brought forward along the facial surface to the midline. The second strip is applied from the lingual surface. It is joined to the pack at the distal surface of the last tooth, and then brought forward along the gingival margin to the midline. The strips are joined interproximally by applying gentle pressure on the facial and lingual surfaces of the pack **(Fig. 43.15)**.

Do Nots

× Periodontal dressing should not extend onto uninvolved mucosa.
× Should not extend over occlusal surfaces of teeth.
× Should not interfere with occlusion.

Placement of Periodontal Dressings

Periodontal dressings are retained mechanically by interlocking in interdental spaces of teeth and joining the lingual and facial portions of the pack. In case of edentulous areas, the periodontal dressing is retained with the help of splints, hawley appliance and stents. In case of isolated teeth, tie dental floss or gauze loosely around the teeth and over which pack is applied.

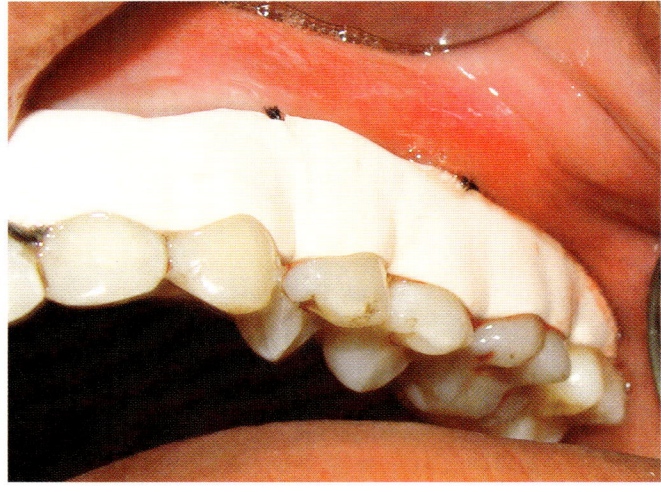

Fig. 43.15: Periodontal pack placement

Periodontal dressing may entrap sutures beneath the dressing and may displace flap.

POSTOPERATIVE INSTRUCTIONS AND CARE

Appropriate postoperative instructions should be given both verbally and in written to the patient including an explanation concerning:
1. Discomfort and potential complications;
2. All medications, especially analgesics and antibiotics;
3. Diet modification

Instructions to the Patient after Surgery

Do's

✓ Take 2 tablets of acetaminophen every 6 hours on first day.
✓ Chew on the nonoperated side
✓ Take semisolid food
✓ Apply ice, intermittently for alternating 20 minutes on and 20 minutes off, on the face over the operated side on the first day
✓ Use chlorhexidine mouthwash
✓ If the bleeding does not stop, take piece of gauge and form it into U-shape and hold it in thumb and index finger, apply it to both sides of the pack, and hold it there under pressure for 20 minutes
✓ Swelling is usual in extensive surgical procedure. It subsides in 3 or 4 days. Apply moist heat if it persists
✓ If any other problem arises do call the doctor.

Do Not's

× Avoid hot food
× Do not smoke or take alcohol
× Avoid citrus, highly spicy food
× Do not brush over the pack
× Avoid exertion
× Do not try to stop bleeding by rinsing.

Postsurgical Care

Day 1: Analgesics, cold packs, moist gauze locally as needed, total avoidance of wound disturbance

After day 1: Pain, swelling, bleeding should diminish or disappear. Begin light activity, warm packs as needed and chemical plaque control are recommended.

After 5 to 10 days: Remove dressing and sutures after 7 days: Professionally de-plaque supragingivally. Begin light oral hygiene.

After 4 to 6 weekly: Biweekly visits for professional de-plaqing and oral hygiene instructions. The dentogingival junction should not be probed or instrumented for 6 to 8 weeks following surgery. Soft toothbrush should be used gently for the first few postoperative weeks. The patient should follow Charter's method avoiding vigorous toothbrushing.

POSTSURGICAL COMPLICATIONS

If postoperative complications occur, they should be managed by prompt and appropriate treatment, which may include control of bleeding, adequate analgesics or antibiotics.

Complications associated with periodontal surgery are:
• Hemorrhage
• Postoperative pain
• Infection
• Swelling
• Reaction to medications
• Other potential risks include root sensitivity, flap sloughing, root resorption or ankylosis, some loss of alveolar crest, flap perforation, abscess formation and irregular gingival contours.

Hemorrhage

Primary postoperative hemorrhage starts at the time of surgery. Intermediate hemorrhage starts soon after the surgery, after having stopped temporarily following surgery. It is usually due to the breakdown of an incomplete clot, such as is associated with loss of the vasoconstrictor effect of anesthesia. Secondary hemorrhage starts from 24 hours to 10 days post-operatively.

Steps to control postsurgical bleeding:
1. First step to control bleeding is to identify the source of bleeding. Suction is done carefully and local pressure with gauze sponges is applied.
2. Judicious injection of vasoconstrictor combined with continuous application of pressure encourages clot formation.
3. Artificial clot may be induced by use of an oxidized cellulose microfibrillar collagen product.
4. Electrocoagulation can be effective for capillary bleeding sites and small arterioles.
5. Large arteriole bleeding sites can be controlled by placing sutures in the soft tissue. Knot is drawn tight to occlude vessel by compression from the surrounding tissue **(Fig. 43.16)**.

PERIODONTICS REVISITED

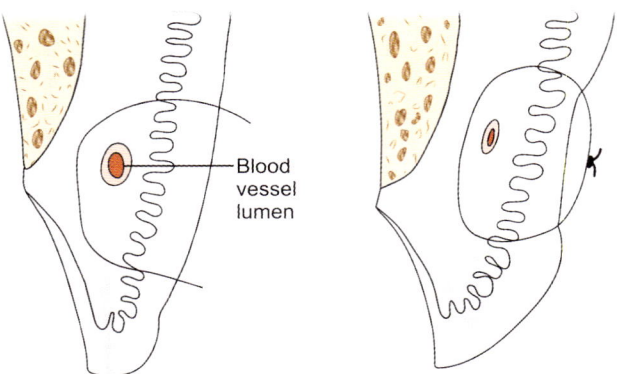

Fig. 43.16: Diagram showing compression suture to control bleeding

6. If bleeding is from intraosseous site then it can be controlled by bone wax (beeswax and salicylic acid) which occlude bony canals.

7. Excessive bleeding from interproximal and infrabony lesions results from inadequate degranulation. Residual granulomatous tissue is a common source of hemorrhage, since it is composed largely of capillaries.

The various topical hemostatic agents are	
Agent	*Main constituent*
Avitene	Collagen
Collacote	Collagen
Collatape	Collagen
Collaplug	Collagen
Thrombinar	Thrombin
Thrombogen	Thrombin
Thrombostat	Thrombin
Gelfoam	Gelatin
Beriplast	Fibrin
Surgicel	Cellulose

Postoperative Pain

The severity of postoperative pain varies depending on the patient threshold level, location, duration, extent of surgery and skill with which the soft and osseous tissue are handled during surgery. Postoperative pain and discomfort for the patient can be minimized by the surgical handling of the soft and osseous tissues atraumatically.

- The bone should be kept moist as dryness of bone induces severe pain. There should be complete soft tissu e coverage of the bone during suturing. Thus bone exposure should not be extensive.
- The periodontal dressing should not over extend beyond the mucogingival junction, or onto frenum and palate.

- Patient should be instructed to avoid chewing from the operated site.
- Two acetoaminophen tablets every 6 hours for the first 24 hours is prescribed for little pain or discomfort. But if pain persists then acetoaminophen plus codeine tablets can be prescribed.
- If the postoperative pain is related to infection which usually start after 4 days following surgery (localized lymphadenopathy and fever), then it should be treated with systemic antibiotics along with analgesics.

Swelling

Swelling after surgery is best prevented by the use of ice packs. After swelling develops, hot moist packs and frequent lavage with warm saline solution are preferred. It generally subsides by the 4th postoperative day. If swelling persists and becomes worse, then amoxicillin (500 mg) should be taken every 8 hours for 1 week. Not all postoperative swelling is caused by inflammation; some may be caused by bleeding into tissues. This may occur after flap operations and are accompanied by discoloration under cheek, chin or eye.

WOUND HEALING

To ensure proper healing, atraumatic surgical principles should be followed including: (1) adequate anesthesia; (2) surface disinfection; (3) sharp instrumentation; (4) minimal, atraumatic tissue handling; (5) short operating time; (6) preventing unnecessary contamination; and (7) proper suturing and dressing, if indicated.

Healing is a phase of the inflammatory response that leads to a new physiological and anatomical relationship among the disrupted body elements. Healing of periodontal tissue can be in the form of repair, new attachment and regeneration. (More is explained in the chapter 48: Regenerative Osseous Surgery)

Healing rates of various periodontal tissues	
Tissue type	*Healing rate (Approximately)*
Junctional epithelium	5 days
Sulcular epithelium	7-10 days
Gingival surface epithelium	10-14 days
Connective tissue	21-28 days
Alveolar bone	4-6 weeks

Gingival wounds heal much more rapidly with much less scar formation when compared to skin. The reason for this reduced scar formation are:

PERIODONTICS REVISITED

a. Gingival fibroblasts unlike the fibroblasts of other connective tissue produce more MMP13 than MMP1. MMP13 has a broad substantivity and is capable of break down/turnover of a number of extracellular matrix proteins. MMP1 on the other hand has a biological activity that is restricted to collagen I. The greater presence of MMP13 in the wound area is thought to produce a greater turnover and thereby, prevent scar formation.

b. There is a greater presence of myofibroblasts in the gingiva when compared to skin. Fibroblasts can differentiate to form the more synthetic myofib-roblasts under the influence of TGF-β. The presence of TGF-β in the wound area enhances the already greater presence of myofibroblasts thereby leading to lesser wound contraction and scarring.

LANDMARK STUDIES RELATED

Lindhe J, Socransky SS, Nyman S, et al. Critical probing depths in periodontal therapy. Journal of Clinical Periodontology 1982;9:323-36.

They reported that scaling and root planing procedures induce loss of attachment if performed in pockets shallower than 2.9 mm, whereas gain of attachment occurs in deeper pockets. The modified Widman flap induces loss of attachment if done in pockets shallower than 4.2 mm but results in a greater gain of attachment than root planing in pockets deeper than 4.2 mm. The critical probing depth at which the attachment level was unchanged after treatment was 2.9 mm for root planing and 4.2 mm for surgery. It was concluded that molars responded better to surgery than to root planing above 4.5 mm. Poor plaque control by patients in the maintenance phase tended to raise the critical probing depth.

POINTS TO PONDER

✓ Causes of excessive bleeding during surgery include laceration of large blood vessels, incomplete removal of granulation tissue, hypertensive patient, bleeding disorder patient and patient on anticoagulant therapy.

✓ If the surrounding tissue blanches, however, the suture is too tight, which may cause necrosis because of poor vascularization.

✓ Hemostasis should be achieved before, and not by, the application of a dressing. The only clear indication for a dressing is to achieve tissue stasis, such as with a free mucosal graft, or to protect a clot over bone in the interdental denudation technique. Application of dressing is a matter of individual preference.

✓ The possible outcomes of surgical periodontal therapy are: Regeneration, new attachment, long junctional epithelium, root resorption/ankylosis and recurrence of pocket.

BIBLIOGRAPHY

1. Eley BM, Manson JD. Surgical periodontal treatment. In, Periodontics, 5th ed Wright 2004;262-75.
2. Genco RJ, Rosenberg ES, Evian C. Periodontal surgery. In, Genco RJ, Goldman HM, Cohen DW. Contemporary Periodontics. CV Mosby Company 1990;554-84.
3. Klokkevold PR, Carranza FM, Takei HH. General principles of periodontal surgery. In, Newman, Takei, Carranza. Clinical Periodontology, 9th ed WB Saunders 2003;725-36.
4. Lindhe J, Socransky SS, Nyman S, et al. Critical probing depths in periodontal therapy. J Clin Periodontol 1982;9:323-36.
5. Mc Donnell HT, Mills MP. Principle and practice of periodontal surgery. In, Rose LF, Mealey BL, Genco RJ, Cohen DW. Periodontics, Medicine, Surgery and Implants. Elsevier Mosby 2004;358-404.
6. Ramfjord SP, Ash MM. Objectives and principles of periodontal surgery. In, Periodontology and Periodontics. Modern Theory and Practice. 1st ed, AITBS Publisher and distributor India, 1996;257-68.
7. Robinson PJ, Goodman CH. General principles of surgical therapy. In, Genco RJ, Goldman HM, Cohen DW. Contemporary Periodontics. CV Mosby Company 1990;543-53.
8. Takei HH, Carranza FM. The surgical phase of therapy. In, Newman, Takei, Carranza. Clinical Periodontology 9th ed WB Saunders 2003;719-24.
9. Wang HL, Greenwell H. Surgical periodontal therapy. Periodontol 2000 2001;25:89-99.

MCQs

1. The purpose of placing sutures after periodontal flap surgery is to:
   A. Hold the soft tissues in place
   B. Protect the wound
   C. Hold the soft tissues in place and maintain the blood clot
   D. All of the above

2. Periosteal sutures in periodontal flaps is usually used in:
   A. Coronally displaced flaps
   B. Apically displaced flaps
   C. Undisplaced flaps
   D. None of the above

PERIODONTICS REVISITED

3. Following statement about suturing is true *except*:
   A. Needle holder should grasp the needle approximately ¾th of the distance from point
   B. Needle should enter the tissue perpendicular to the surface
   C. Needle should be passed through the tissue following curvature of the needle
   D. Needle should be passed from thicker to the thinner side
4. Following statement about periodontal dressings are true *except*:
   A. It protect wound area from irritants such as hot/spicy food
   B. Enhances patient comfort
   C. Eliminate pain
   D. Helps to maintain the position of repositioned soft tissues
5. The most useful periodontal dressing in flap control in concave zones is:
   A. Cyanoacrylate
   B. Collagen dressings
   C. Methacrylic gel
   D. None of the above

6. Which of the following is visible light cure periodontal dressing:
   A. Barricaid
   B. Coepak
   C. Periocare
   D. Periopac
7. The chemotherapeutic agents used for premedications are:
   A. Tranquilizer
   B. Antibiotics
   C. Chlorhexidine gluconate mouthwash
   D. Ibuprofen
   E. All of the above
8. Which of the following is an example of absorbable suture material?
   A. Silk
   B. Propylene
   C. Nylon
   D. Gut

Answers

1. D	2. B	3. D	4. C	5. A
6. A	7. E	8. D		

PERIODONTICS REVISITED

CHAPTER 44

Gingival Curettage

Shalu Bathla

1. Introduction
2. Terminology
3. Indications
4. Contraindications
5. Procedure
   - Basic Technique (With Curette)
   - Excisional New Attachment Procedure (ENAP)
- Ultrasonic curettage
- Chemical curettage
- Laser
6. Present Concepts
7. Healing After Curettage

INTRODUCTION

Gingival curettage consists of the removal of the inflamed soft tissue lateral to the pocket wall. Gingival curettage, as originally conceived, was designed to promote new connective tissue attachment to the tooth, by the removal of pocket lining, junctional epithelium and the subjacent granulation tissue. The actual result obtained with curettage is most often a long junctional epithelium, which is the same result obtained with scaling and root planing alone. Gingival curettage, although surgical in nature, is a closed procedure. It does not afford the improved root surface access and visibility as gained with flap surgery that is needed to achieve complete mechanical removal of plaque, calculus, and biofilm. The major disadvantage of this procedure is limited access especially in deep, tortuous and infrabony pockets.

TERMINOLOGY

- Gingival curettage is a surgical procedure designed to remove the soft tissue lining of the periodontal pocket with a curette, leaving only gingival connective tissue lining.

- Inadvertent curettage is the curettage which is done unintentionally when scaling and root planing procedure is performed.
- Subgingival curettage refers to the procedure that is performed apical to the epithelial attachment, severing the connective tissue attachment down to the osseous crest.

INDICATIONS

1. In patients whom extensive surgery is contra-indicated owing to systemic disease or psychologic problems.
2. Shallow pocket depths with an adequate width and thickness of gingival tissue.
3. It can be performed as a part of new attachment attempts in moderately deep intrabony pockets located in accessible areas.
4. Curettage can be performed on recall visits as a method of maintenance treatment for areas of recurrent inflammation.
5. In suprabony pockets which do not extend beyond the mucogingival junction.

CONTRAINDICATIONS

1. Presence of acute infections such as necrotizing ulcerative gingivitis (NUG).
2. Fibrous enlargement of gingiva such as phenytoin hyperplasia.
3. Extension of the base of the pocket apical to the mucogingival junction.
4. If the patient is medically compromised, the benefits versus the risks of the surgical procedure should be carefully weighed before commiting the patient to the procedure.

PROCEDURE

Curettage can be accomplished as a closed procedure with a sharp curette or as an open procedure with a gingival incision followed by root planing (ENAP).

Basic Technique (With Curette)

Instruments: Gracey curettes, Columbia universal curettes.

- *Isolate and anesthetize*: Local infiltration is given to anesthesize the isolated selected site.
- *Insertion of curette*: Sharp Gracey or Columbia Universal curette is inserted with cutting edge against the tissue so as to engage the inner lining of the pocket wall and junctional epithelium.
- *Curette the soft tissue wall*: Curette is carried along the soft tissue, in a *horizontal stroke* **(Figs 44.1A and B)**. The pocket wall is supported by gentle finger pressure on the external surface. Several overlapping strokes are used to completely remove the epithelium and underlying granulation tissue. In subgingival curettage, the tissues attached between the bottom of the pocket and alveolar crest are removed with a scooping motion of curette to the tooth surface.
- *Irrigation*: Irrigate the area to remove debris and press the tissue to the tooth surface gently which enables the arrest of bleeding and the adaption of soft tissue to the root surface.
- *Suturing*: Suture the tissue if necessary.
- Post operative instructions are given thereafter.

Excisional New Attachment Procedure (ENAP)

It is subgingival curettage performed with a knife. This technique was developed by US Naval Dental Corps. The stated objectives of the procedure are to allow proper soft tissue preparation, to gain better access to the root surface, and to enable soft tissue to adapt intimately to the root surface.

Instruments: Surgical handle (Bard Parker no.3), surgical blades no. 11, 12, 15 and curettes.

Technique:

- *Anesthesia*: Adequate local anesthesia is given to the selected site.
- *Incision*: Internal bevel incision is given with surgical blade no. 15 or 11, from the gingival margin to a point below the bottom of the pocket **(Figs 44.2A and B)**. The intent is to cut the inner portion of the soft tissue wall of the pocket, all around the tooth.
- *Removal of the tissue*: The excised tissue and granulation tissue are removed with curette. Root planing is done after that.
- *Irrigation*: Irrigate the area with saline.
- *Suturing*: Approximate the wound edges and place suitable sutures.
- Postoperative instructions are given.

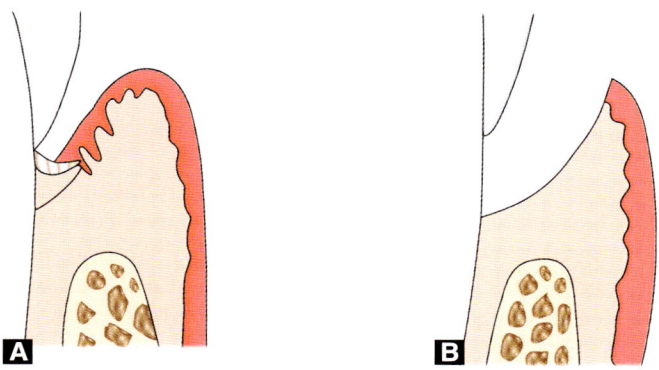

Figs 44.1A and B: Curettage with curette

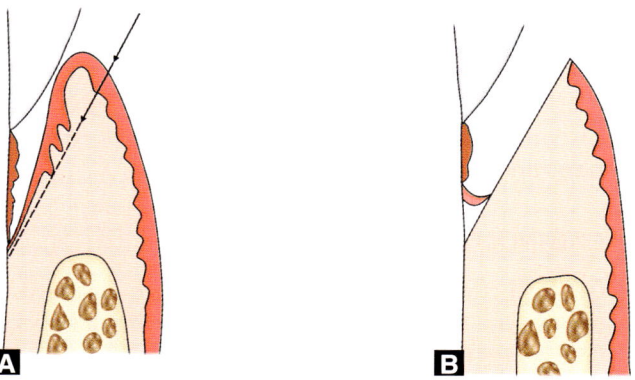

Figs 44.2A and B: Excisional new attachment procedure

Ultrasonic Curettage

Curettage with ultrasonic devices also has been described. Sound energy absorbed at tissue junctions that take the form of heat, results in coagulation. The coagulated epithelium is then removed by mechanical action of the vibrations of ultrasonic instrument.

Chemical Curettage

Sodium sulphide, phenol, camphor, antiformin, and sodium hypochlorite have been used for chemical curettage.

Anesthesia is given to the selected site. After isolating the site with cotton rolls, solution of sodium hypochlorite is placed into the pocket for 1 minute. Then 5% citric acid solution is introduced into the pocket for 1 minute to neutralize the sodium hypochlorite. The coagulated tissue is then removed with a curette and pocket is flushed with saline to remove the remnants of the connective tissue.

The extent of chemical penetration to the tissue cannot be controlled and thus, chemical curettage is discarded.

Laser

Recently, a method of curettage with a dental laser has been proposed. The goals of laser curettage are epithelial removal, as with previous methods, and in addition, bacterial reduction also. A short-term study reported that Nd:YAG laser treatment did not produce statistically significant bacterial reduction.

PRESENT CONCEPTS

Short- and long-term clinical trials have confirmed that gingival curettage provides no additional benefit when compared to scaling and root planing alone in terms of probing depth reduction, attachment gain, or inflammation reduction. After comparing scaling and root planing alone to curettage plus scaling and root planing, it was concluded that curettage "did not serve any additional useful purpose". Following an extensive discussion on the topic in the 1989 World Workshop in Clinical Periodontics, it was concluded that curettage had "no justifiable application during active therapy for chronic adult periodontitis". Since there is no evidence that gingival curettage has any therapeutic benefit in the treatment of chronic periodontitis, the American Dental Association has deleted the code from the fourth edition of *Current Dental Terminology (CDT-4)*. In addition, the American Academy of Periodontology, in its *Guidelines for Periodontal Therapy*, did not include gingival curettage as a method of treatment. This indicates that the dental community as a whole regards gingival curettage as a procedure with no clinical value.

HEALING AFTER CURETTAGE

Gingival sulcus which is totally or partially devoid of epithelial lining is filled by blood clot immediately after curettage. Abundant polymorphonuclear leukocytes occupy the wound site. This is followed by rapid proliferation of granulation tissue.

Epithelium: Sulcular epithelium is restored between 2 to 7 days and junctional epithelium as early as 5 days after curettage.

Connective tissue: Immature collagen fibers appear within 21 days.

POINTS TO PONDER

✓ While performing curettage, Gracey curette No. 11-12 is used for distal surfaces of posteriors and Gracey curette No. 13-14 is used for mesial surfaces of posteriors (which is opposite for scaling and root planing).

✓ For gingival curettage blade face to tooth surface angulation is more than 90°.

BIBLIOGRAPHY

1. Academy report. The American Academy of Periodontology Statement Regarding Gingival Curettage. J Periodontol 2002;73:1229-30.
2. Carranza FM,Takei HH Gingival curettage. In, Newman, Takei, Carranza. Clinical Periodontology, 9th ed WB Saunders 2003;744-48.
3. Genco RJ, Rosenberg ES, Evian C. Periodontal surgery. In, Genco RJ, Goldman HM and Cohen DW. Contemporary Periodontics CV Mosby Company 1990;553-84.
4. Grant DA, Stern IB, Listgarten MA. Gingival and subgingival curettage: Curettage of the pocket wall. In, Periodontics 6th ed CV Mosby Company 1988;740-60.
5. Ramfjord SP, Ash MM. Curettage. In, Periodontology and Periodontics. Modern Theory and Practice. 1st ed AITBS Publisher and Distributor India 1996;269-74.
6. Wang HL, Greenwell H. Surgical periodontal therapy. Periodontol 2000 2001;2589-99.

MCQs

1. Curettage of posterior mesial gingiva is done by:
   A. Gracey curettes 11-12
   B. Gracey curettes 13-14

C. Gracey curettes 1-2

D. Gracey curettes 9-10

2. Which is true about ENAP:

A. Resective osseous surgery

B. Subgingival curettage by knife

C. Bone grafting procedure

D. Gingivectomy procedure

3. Which of the following is true about gingival curettage *except*:

A. Blade face to tooth surface is less than 90°

B. It is removal of soft tissue lining of periodontal pocket

C. Can be done with curette or knife

D. Done in patients in whom extensive surgery is contraindicated

4. After curettage re-epithelization occurs in:

A. Two weeks   B. One week (2-7 days)

C. 1-2 days   D. 2-3 days

Answers

1. B   2. B   3. A   4. B

CHAPTER
45

Gingivectomy

Shalu Bathla

HISTORICAL PERSPECTIVE

History of gingivectomy can be dated back to 1742, when Fauchard describe the procedure to remove excessive tissue. Robicsek in 1884, later on described the so called gingivectomy procedure as straight incision technique in which the tissues were excised and the granulation tissue eliminated. Pickerill's book "Stomatology in General Practice", published in 1912, described the procedure and very reasonably named the operation gingivectomy. Zentler in 1918 gave scalloped incision technique for gingivectomy. Gingivectomy is thought to be introduced as an official periodontal therapy when the idea of periodontal etiology shifts from bone to soft tissue. This is mainly due to Kronfeld in 1935, who emphasized that periodontal disease is not the disease of the bone. Gingivectomy was later defined by Grant et al in 1979 as being the excision of the soft tissue wall of a pathologic periodontal pocket.

DEFINITION

According to the World Workshop in Periodontics (1989), gingivectomy is defined as "an excision of the soft tissue wall of the periodontal pocket".

OBJECTIVES

i. Pocket elimination by gingival resection.
ii. Development of physiologic tissue form for disease prevention.

INDICATIONS

i. Elimination of suprabony pockets.
ii. Elimination of gingival enlargement.
iii. Elimination of suprabony periodontal abscess.
iv. To expose additional clinical crown to gain added retention for restorative purposes and to provide access to subgingival caries.
v. The presence of furcation involvement (without associated bone defects) where there is a wide zone of attached gingiva.
vi. Pericoronal flap.

CONTRAINDICATIONS

i. The need for bone surgery or examination of the bone shape and morphology.
ii. Situations in which the bottom of the pocket is apical to the mucogingival junction, gingivectomy will

excise most of the gingiva and leave an inadequate zone of gingiva.

iii. Esthetic considerations, particularly in anterior maxilla.

iv. If the patient complains of tooth senstivity before surgery. Although it is relative contraindication, as the cause of any complaint should be treated before the surgery and if the sensitivity cannot be controlled, surgery should be contraindicated.

LIMITING CIRCUMSTANCES

1. *Palatal aspects of maxillary posterior teeth*: When the palatal vault is shallow and the depth of periodontal involvement is near or enters the vault area, gingivectomy on the palatal aspect of maxillary posterior teeth may result in elimination of most if not all of the palatal gingiva, placing the gingival margin at or near a level of coincident with that of the roof of the mouth.

2. *Mandibular retromolar lesions*: When an incision is made on movable and delicate mucosa, this tissue often cuts poorly, bleeds profusely and may be difficult to resect and shape. The use of the distal wedge procedure, often simplifies the management of retromolar tissue.

3. *Maxillary tuberosity areas*: When soft tissue is so great, relative to the depth of periodontal involvement on the distal aspect of the last molar, that its level resection would bring about surgical entry into the mucosa of the hamular notch. It may be more appropriate to perform a distal wedge procedure to eliminate diseased tissue immediately adjacent to the distal portion of the molar.

4. *Cases of emotional stress*: With age, diminish patient cooperation and motivation, retarded healing, etc. have a direct bearing upon the desirability of the surgical therapy. Such patient is a poor surgical risk and requires therapeutic modification.

DRAWBACKS

1. Tissue wound heals by secondary intention.
2. Alveolar bone defects are not revealed and therefore cannot be treated adequately.
3. Gingivectomy is a radical procedure in which zone of attached gingiva is compromised/may be eliminated. Thus, attached gingiva is wasted.
4. Clinical crown are lengthened considerably and need to be explained to the patient before surgery.

5. It may lead to dentin hypersensitivity due to root exposure.

GINGIVOPLASTY

Gingivoplasty first described by Goldman in 1950 as a plastic procedure of which the gingival tissue was removed. Sugarman in 1951 describe electrosurgical gingivoplasty in his case report. Gingivoplasty can be defined as recontouring of gingiva that has lost its physiologic form. Gingivoplasty was introduced to facilitate dealing with abnormal form of gingiva and was essentially a surgical procedure designed to reshape gingiva without necessarily reducing sulcular depth.

The purpose of gingivoplasty is different from gingivectomy, as gingivoplasty is just reshaping of gingiva to create physiologic gingival contours, with the sole purpose of recontouring the gingiva in the absence of pockets, while the objective of gingivectomy is to eliminate pocket.

Indications of gingivoplasty:

i. Need for correction of the grossly thickened gingival margin.

ii. Gingival clefts and craters caused by necrotizing ulcerative gingivitis that interfere with normal food excursion, collect plaque and food debris.

iii. Sharply varying levels of gingival margin in adjacent areas.

iv. Saucer shaped deformities, buccolingual in the interproximal regions.

Instruments: Gingivoplasty may be done with a periodontal knife, scalpel, rotary coarse diamond stones or electrode.

Steps in the gingivoplasty procedure are similar and resembles those performed in festooning artificial dentures namely:

i. Tapering the gingival margin.

ii. Creating a scalloped marginal outline.

iii. Thinning the attached gingiva.

iv. Creating vertical interdental grooves and shaping the interdental papillae to provide embrasures for the passage of food.

Scrapping: Use a scalpel as a hoe and pass the instrument tightly but firmly over a firm, tough tissue surface which results in shaving of the surface. The use of rotary abrasives consists essentially of abrading tissue until it has assumed the desired form. The rules governing the application of the rotary abrasive to soft tissue are exactly those that apply to hard tissue. A steam of water on the instrument expediates the procedure immeasurably just as it does on bone, enamel or dentin. Accelerated speed ensures a smooth, rapid operation while the stream of water provides temperature control and prevents clogging of instruments.

TYPES OF GINGIVECTOMY PROCEDURE

Surgical Gingivectomy

Surgical Instruments

- Pocket markers: Goldman-fox, Crane Kaplan **(Fig. 45.1A)**
- Broad-bladed, round scalpels: Goldman-fox no. 7, Kirkland knife **(Fig. 45.1B)**
- Interproximal knife: Goldman-fox no. 8, 9 and 10, Orban's knife **(Fig. 45.1C)**

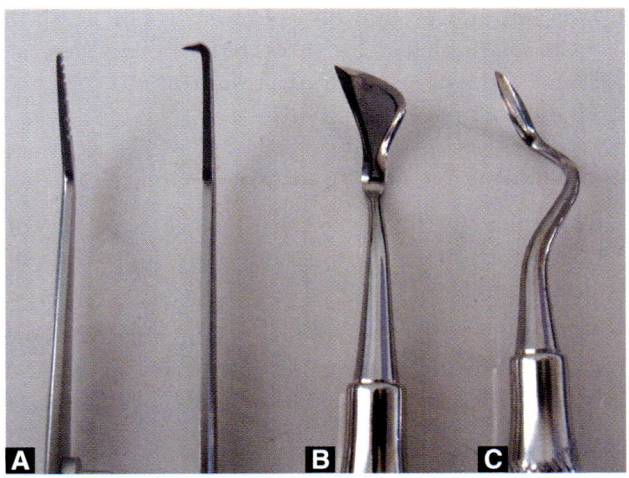

Fig. 45.1: A. Pocket marker. B. Kirkland knife C. Orban's knife.

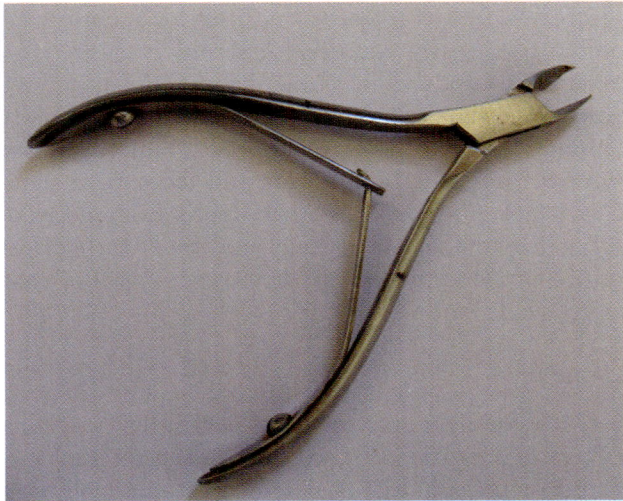

Fig. 45.2: Tissue nipper

- Surgical handle: Bard Parker no.3 or angulated handle (Blake's handle) with blade no 11,12,15
- Curettes
- Tissue nipper **(Fig. 45.2)**, scissors.

Procedure

- *Mark bleeding points*: After LA is given in the selected site, mark bleeding points with the help of pocket marker systematically, beginning on the distal surface of the tooth, then on the facial and mesial surface. The procedure is repeated on the lingual/palatal surface. Beak of pocket marker must be parallel to root surface. Pinpoint perforations individuate pocket depth which is used as a guideline for the incision.
- *Incisions*: Discontinuous/continuous incision is given apical to the bottom of the bleeding point beginning at the most terminal tooth **(Fig. 45.3)**. External bevel incision is given at an angle of 45° apical to the base of the pocket with the help of Kirkland knife or blade no.11 or 15 with BP handle no.3 or angulated Blake's handle. The blade must pass fully through the tissue to the tooth in coronal direction **(Figs 45.4 and 45.5)**. The incision should be as close as possible to the bone without exposing it so as to remove the soft tissue coronal to the bone. The main principle here is to eliminate pocket all the way to the base without exposing the bone. Once the primary incision is completed on the buccal and lingual aspect, Orban's knife or Waerhaug knife is placed at angle of 45° to free the tissue interproximally.
- *Tissue removed*: The incised tissues are carefully removed with the help of curette or scaler. The remaining tissue tabs are removed with scissors. The gingival margins should be thin and beveled and if necessary corrected by means of knives or rotating diamond burs.
- *Scaling and root planing*: The calculus and necrotic cementum on the tooth are removed with the help of scalers and curettes.
- *Periodontal dressing*: Bleeding is controlled and after that periodontal dressing is applied over the treated site primarily for patient comfort. Thereafter, patient is given postoperative instructions.

Laser Gingivectomy

The lasers most commonly used for gingivectomy are the CO_2 having wavelength of 10600 nm and Neodymium:yttrium-Aluminium-garnet (Nd:YAGtr) having wavelength of 1064 nm both in infrared range.

PERIODONTICS REVISITED

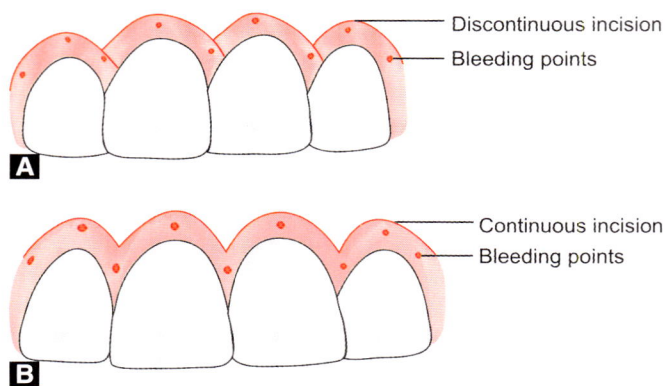

Figs 45.3A and B: Incisions: (A) Discontinuous incision; (B) Continuous incision

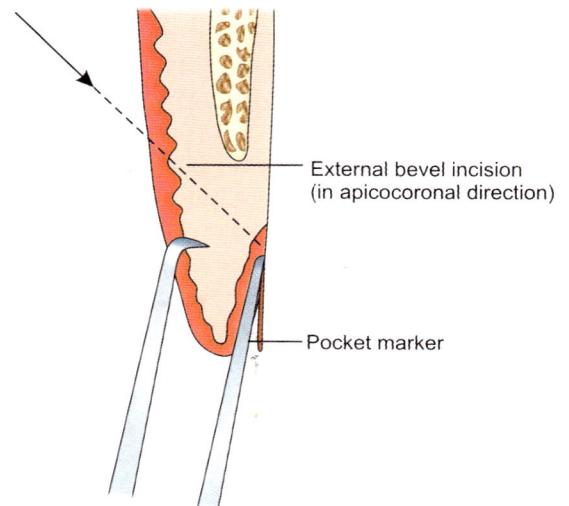

Fig. 45.4: Mark the depth of pocket with pocket marker and give external bevel incision apical to the bleeding point making 45° angle to the long axis of tooth

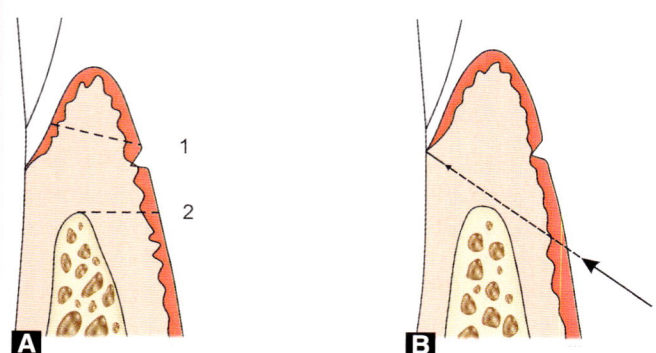

Figs 45.5A and B : (A) Incorrect incisions: 1. Shallow incision (Fail to remove pocket), 2. No bevel incision (Result in bone exposure); (B) Correct incision

PERIODONTICS REVISITED

Advantages

i. Laser offers an almost completely dry, bloodless surgery.
ii. Because of dried field, surgical time may be reduced.
iii. There is instant sterilization of the area, decreasing the chances of bacteremia.
iv. This is noncontact surgery, thus no mechanical trauma to the surgical site.
v. There is prompt healing with minimal postoperative swelling and scarring.
vi. Postoperative pain appears to be greatly reduced.

Disadvantages

i. There is loss of tactile feedback in using the instrument.
ii. It is imperative that all operating room personnel wear safety glasses for protection of their eyes.
iii. There is the necessity for hospitalization.
iv. High cost of the equipment.

Gingivectomy by Electrosurgery

Instruments: Needle electrode (thickness varying from 0.0075 inch to 0.015 inch), small ovoid loop/diamond shaped electrodes.

Procedure: The site must not be too dry otherwise excessive sparking will result. Conversely, if excessive moisture is present, considerable surface coagulation will occur instantly. For the best results, the site should be very slightly moist. The removal of gingival enlargements and gingivoplasty is performed with the needle electrode, supplemented by the small ovoid loop/ diamond shaped electrodes for festooning. A blended cutting and coagulating (fully rectified) current is used. In all reshaping procedures, electrode is activated and moved in a concise shaving motion. Electrode should be kept in constant motion in order to prevent a build-up of heat with appropriate current setting and the patient should be properly grounded. Clean all debris from electrodes with gauze sponges after each movement through soft tissue. The sponge may be dry or moistened with absolute isopropyl alcohol.

Advantages

i. It provide clear operating area with little/no leeding.
ii. Lack of pressure to incise tissue, thus allowing a more precise incision than is obtained by a scalpel.
iii. Minor tissue loss after healing.

iv. Self-sterilization of the tip of the active electrode.
v. Scar-free healing by primary intention, when used properly.
vi. Greater ease for the patient as well as for the operator.

Disadvantages

- It causes an unpleasant odor.
- If the electrosurgery point touches the bone, irreparable damage can occur.
- When electrode touches the root, areas of cementum burns are produced.

Contraindication

One major contraindication to electro-surgery is a cardiac pacemaker. Since an electrosurgical unit generates radiofrequency energy, it should never be used within 15 feet of an individual with a cardiac pacemaker.

Gingivectomy by Chemosurgery

Five percent paraformaldehyde or potassium hydroxide were the chemicals used to perform gingivectomy which is no longer in use because of the following disadvantages associated with it:
- The depth of chemical action cannot be controlled.
- Gingival remodeling cannot be accomplished effectively.
- Epithelialization and reformation of the junctional epithelium, re-establishment of the alveolar crest fiber system are slower in chemically treated gingival wounds than in those produced by scalpel.

HEALING AFTER GINGIVECTOMY

Healing after gingivectomy is by secondary intention. Bernier J and Kaplan H reported the following time sequence for healing following gingivectomy in humans. The initial response after gingivectomy is the formation of a protective surface clot; the underlying tissue becomes acutely inflamed with some necrosis.

The outer epithelium heals by approximately 14 days but sulcular epithelium requires 3 to 5 weeks to heal. Twelve hours after gingivectomy there is slight reduction in cementoblasts and some loss of continuity of the osteoblastic layer on the outer aspect of alveolar crest. New bone formation occurs at the alveolar crest as early as the 4th day after gingivectomy and new cementoid appears after about 10 to 15 days.

Thus, total gingivectomy healing takes place in about 4 to 5 weeks and remodeling of the alveolar bone crest

has been shown to occur during this phase. Gingivoplasty wound often heal faster than gingivectomy wound.

2nd day	Clot formation ↓
4th day	• Clot replaced by granulation tissue • Epithelium without rete pegs extends over part of the surface • Dense inflammatory infiltration ↓
6th day	• Wound is covered by stratified squamous epithelium • Collagen formation starts in the connective tissue ↓
16th day	• Epithelium with rete pegs appear • Dense collagenous connective tissue appears ↓
21st day	• Epithelial rete pegs well developed, with thickening of stratum corneum • Increased Collagen formation in the connective tissue • Gingiva clinically appear normal

The tissue changes that occur in post gingivectomy healing are the same in all individuals, but the time required for complete healing varies, depending upon the local and systemic factors influencing wound healing (interference from local irritation, infection and age).

Gingivectomy may be performed be means of scalpels, lasers, electrode or chemicals.
In gingivectomy, external bevel incision is given at 45° to the tooth surface in apicocoronal direction.
Gingivectomy wound heals by secondary intention.

POINTS TO PONDER

✓ Failure to produce beveled incision leaves a broad plateau which takes more time than ordinarily required to develop the physiologic contour of gingiva, thus the incision should be beveled at approximately 45° to the tooth surface.
✓ The granulomatous tissue is removed first and then thorough scaling is attempted on the tooth, so that hemorrhage from the granulomatous tissue should not obscure the scaling during surgical procedure.

BIBLIOGRAPHY

1. Carranza FM, The gingivectomy technique. In, Newman, Takei, Carranza. Clinical Periodontology, 9th ed Saunders 2003;749-53.
2. Electrosurgical Management of soft tissues and restorative dentistry. Dent Clin North Am 1980;24(2):247-69.
3. Eley BM, Manson JD. Surgical Periodontal treatment. In, Periodontics, 5th ed Wright 2004;262-75.

PERIODONTICS REVISITED

4. Genco RJ, Rosenberg ES, Evian C. Periodontal surgery. In, Genco RJ, Goldman HM, Cohen DW. Contemporary Periodontics. CV Mosby 1999;554-84.
5. Grant DA, Stern IB, Listgarten MA. Gingivectomy and Gingivoplasty. In, Periodontics 6th ed CV Mosby Company 1988;761-85.
6. In, Ramfjord SP, Ash MM. Gingivectomy, wound healing. Periodontology and Periodontics. Modern Theory and Practice. 1st ed AITBS Publisher and Distributor India 1996; 275-84.
7. Pick R, Pecaro B, Silberman C. The Laser Gingivectomy, the use of the CO2 laser for the removal of Phenytoin hyperplasia. J Periodontol 1985;56(8):492-6.
8. Tibbetts LS, Ammons WF. Resective Periodontal Surgery. In, Rose LF, Mealey BL, Genco RJ, Cohen DW. Periodontics, Medicine, Surgery and Implants. Elsevier Mosby 2004;502-52.
9. Wang HL, Greenwell H. Surgical periodontal therapy. Periodontol 2000 2001;25:89-99.
10. Wennstrom JL, Heijl L, Lindhe J. Periodontal Surgery: Access Therapy. In, Lindhe J, Karring T, Lang NP. Clinical Periodontology and Implant dentistry, 4th ed Blackwell Munksgaard 2003;519-60.

MCQs

1. Which of the following about conventional gingivectomy is false?
   A. Eliminate false pockets
   B. Heal by secondary intention
   C. Leads to decrease in the width of attached gingiva
   D. Provides accessibility to alveolar bone

2. Gingivoplasty is more likely to be useful in:
   A. NUG
   B. Juvenile periodontitis
   C. Desquamative gingivitis
   D. All of the above

3. Indication of gingivectomy is:
   A. Pocket depth below mucogingival junction
   B. Infrabony pockets
   C. 5 mm periodontal pocket
   D. A fibrotic area of the free gingiva that covers part of the occlusal surface of tooth

4. External bevel incision is beveled at approximately _____ to the tooth surface:
   A. 15°
   B. 30°
   C. 45°
   D. 90°

5. Gingivectomy wound basically heals by:
   A. Secondary intention
   B. Primary intention
   C. Tertiary intention
   D. None of the above

Answers

1. D   2. A   3. D   4. C   5. A

Periodontal Flap

Shalu Bathla

VARIOUS INCISIONS USED IN PERIODONTAL SURGERY

I. **Horizontal Incisions (Fig. 46.1A):**

A. *Internal bevel incision—First/basic incision.* It starts from a designated area on the gingiva and is directed to an area at or near the crest of the alveolar bone **(Fig. 46.2)**. Given with the help of 11 or 15 no. surgical blade. Morris in 1965 introduced internal bevel incision which separated the pocket wall from the rest of the mucoperiosteal flap and produced a healthy thin and flexible margin. It is also called as reverse bevel incision because its bevel is in reverse direction from that of gingivectomy incision.

Objectives:

It accomplishes three important objectives:

1. It removes the pocket lining.
2. It conserves the relatively uninvolved outer surface of the gingiva.
3. It produces a sharp, thin flap margin for adaptation to the bone–tooth junction.

Indications: Primary incision of flap surgery is given if;

1. There is a sufficient band of attached gingiva.
2. Thick gingiva (such as palatal gingiva).
3. Deep periodontal pockets and bone defect.
4. Desire to lengthen clinical crown.

B. *Crevicular/Sulcular incision—Second incision.* It is made from the base of the pocket to the crest of the alveolar bone **(Fig. 46.1B)**. This incision is carried around the entire tooth with the help of 12 no. surgical blade. Its purpose is to facilitate the removal of the inflammatory granulation tissue surrounding the cervical area (cervical wedge) left after reflecting the primary flap.

Indications:

1. Narrow band of attached gingiva.
2. Thin gingiva and alveolar process.
3. Shallow periodontal pocket.
4. Desire to lessen postoperative gingival recession for esthetic reasons in the maxillary anterior region.
5. As a secondary incision of usual flap surgery.
6. Bone graft or GTR procedure: Desire to preserve as much periodontal tissue (especially interdental papilla) as possible to completely cover grafted bone and membrane by flap.

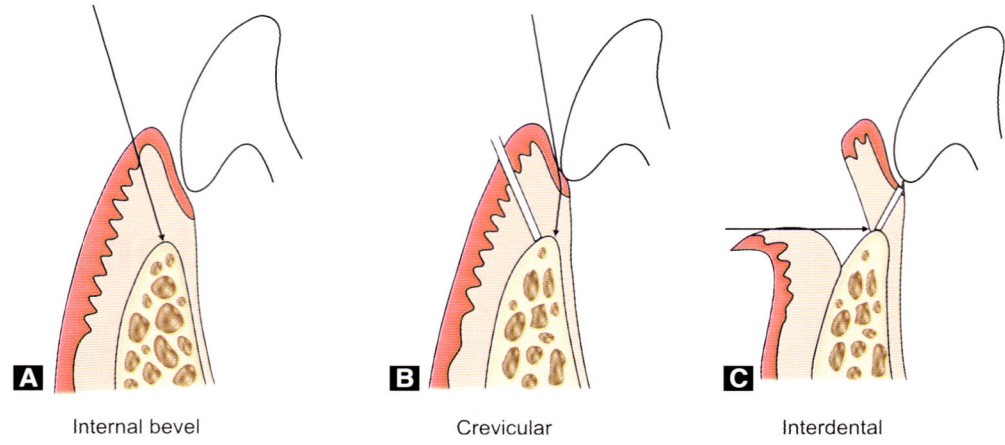

Internal bevel   Crevicular   Interdental

Figs 46.1A to C: Horizontal incisions

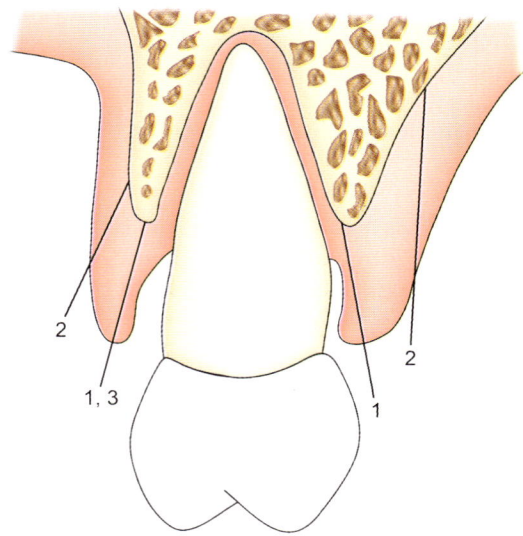

1. Modified widman flap
2. Undisplaced flap
3. Apical displaced flap

Fig. 46.2: Varying locations of internal bevel incision for different flaps (*Courtesy:* Dr SK Salaria)

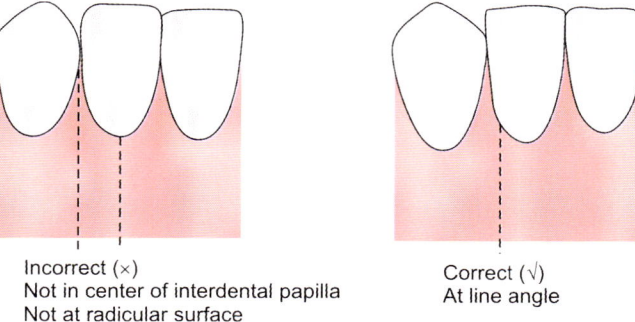

Incorrect (×)
Not in center of interdental papilla
Not at radicular surface

Correct (√)
At line angle

Fig. 46.3: Vertical incision

C. *Interdental incision*: *Third incision*. This incision is made in a horizontal direction and close to the surface of the bone crest, thereby separating the soft tissue collar from the root surfaces and alveolar bone **(Fig. 46.1C)**. Given by Orban's knife. The third incision facilitates secondary flap removal as a single piece.

II. **Vertical Incision/Oblique releasing incision**: Vertical incision must extend beyond the mucogingival line. It should be made at the line angles of a tooth either to include the papilla in the flap or to avoid it completely. Thus, vertical incision should be placed on the tooth surface rather than on interdental gingiva **(Fig. 46.3)**. Vertical incision in lingual and palatal areas are avoided. These should be designed so as to avoid short flap mesiodistally with long apically directed horizontal incision because this could jeopardize the blood supply to the flap. Given with the help of 11 or 15 no. surgical blade.

III. **Thinning incision:** Extends from gingiva towards the base of the flap in palatal flap and distal wedge procedures. Given with the help of 11 or 15 no. surgical blade.

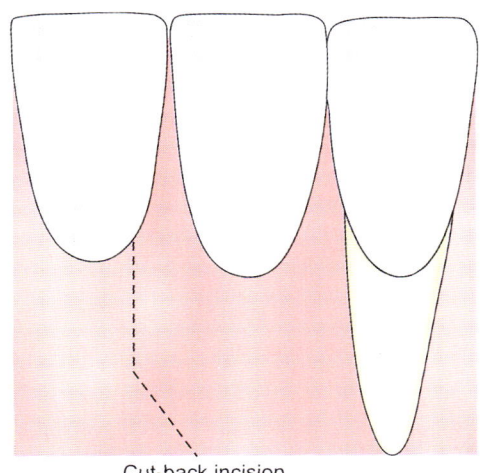

Cut-back incision

Fig. 46.4: Cut-back incision

IV. **Cut-back incision:** Made at apical aspect of releasing incision and directed towards base of the flap in laterally positioned flap **(Fig. 46.4)**. Given with the help of 11 or 15 no. surgical blade.

V. **Periosteal releasing incision:** Made at the base of flap severing the underlying periosteum. Given with the help of 15 or 15C no. surgical blade.

Incisions used in periodontal surgery:

Horizontal Incisions: Internal bevel incision, Crevicular/ Sulcular incision and Interdental incision

Vertical incision

Thinning incision

Cut back incision

Periosteal incision

DEFINITION OF PERIODONTAL FLAP

It is the portion of gingiva and or alveolar mucosa surgically separated from the underlying tissues to provide visibility and access to the bone and root surface.

OBJECTIVES OF PERIODONTAL FLAP

i. Provide access for root surface detoxification.

ii. Reducing probing depth including those that extend to or beyond the mucogingival junction.

iii. Preserve/create an adequate zone of attached gingiva.

iv. Permits access to underlying bone for treatment of osseous defects.

v. Facilitate regenerative procedures.

PRINCIPLES OF FLAP DESIGN

According to Hupp (1993), the following principles should be followed for flap design.

Prevention of flap necrosis:

- The apex of the flap should never be wider than the base
- The flap sides should either run parallel to each other or preferably converge moving from the base of the flap to the apex of the flap
- Length of the flap should be no more than twice the width of the base
- The base of the flaps should not be excessively twisted or stretched
- Whenever possible, an axial blood supply should be included in the base of the flap.

Prevention of flap tearing:

- Vertical releasing incisions should be placed one full tooth anterior to the sites of any anticipated bone removal
- Vertical incision should be started at the line angle of the tooth or in the adjacent interdental papilla and carried obliquely apically into the unattached gingiva.

Basic flap requirements:

- Base of the flap must be wide enough to maintain an adequate blood supply
- Flap must be big enough to expose any underlying bone defects
- No important vessels or nerves should be damaged in raising the flap
- Incisions must allow movement of flap without tension.

CLASSIFICATION OF PERIODONTAL FLAPS

Classification of periodontal flaps

A. According to flap reflection or tissue content:
   a. Full thickness flap
   b. Split-thickness flap

B. According to management of papilla:
   a. Conventional flap
   b. Papilla preservation flap

C. According to flap placement after surgery:
   a. Non displaced flap
   b. Displaced flap:
      - Apical displaced flap
      - Coronal displaced flap
      - Lateral displaced flap

Full-thickness/mucoperiosteal flap: It consists of the complete mucoperiosteum i.e surface epithelium, connective tissue and periosteum which is raised by a periosteal elevator **(Fig. 46.5A)**.

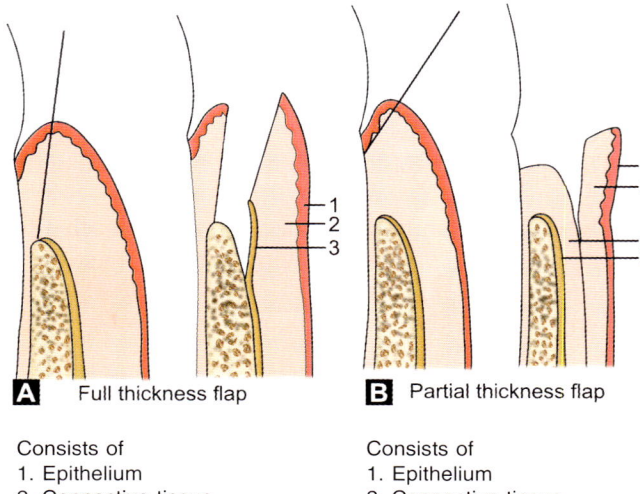

Figs 46.5A and B: A. Full thickness and B. Partial thickness flap

Consists of
1. Epithelium
2. Connective tissue
3. Periosteum
Incision ends on bone

Consists of
1. Epithelium
2. Connective tissue

Incision ends on root surface

Indication: A full-thickness flap is used to expose the bone surface in osseous surgery.

Contraindications:
1. Area where treatment for osseous defect with mucogingival problem is not required.
2. Thin periodontal tissue with probable osseous dehiscence and osseous fenestration.
3. Area where alveolar bone is thin.

Split-thickness/mucosal flap: Gingiva is dissected from the underlying periosteum which is left on the bone and consists of epithelium and thin layer of connective tissue **(Fig. 46.5B)**. Sharp dissection is used to produce a partial thickness flap. Partial-thickness flap is prepared while holding and pulling the flap edge with tissue pliers, turning the blade toward the gingival margin. The flap is dissected slowly from an apico-occlusal direction. To prevent flap penetration, use the side of the blade and hold it parallel to the periosteum to make the incision.

Indications: Partial thickness flaps are especially useful for augmentation of the attached gingiva. This is done by positioning the flap apically or laterally. Partial thickness flap is employed, when exposure of bone is to be avoided as in the case of fenestration/dehiscence.

Advantages: The flap can be attached firmly to the desired position with a periosteal suture if the reflected flap is displaced apically and the thin marginal bone can be protected by the periosteum-connective tissue bed.

Disadvantages: The biggest problem of a partial-thickness flap is with the thickness of the remaining periosteum-connective tissue bed on the bone. If it is less than 0.5 mm, the remaining periosteum-connective tissue may become necrotic, with decreased protective effect for the alveolar bone. However, the partial-thickness flap is a difficult technique and causes much discomfort because of postoperative swelling.

Comparison between full-thickness and partial-thickness flaps		
	Full thickness flap	*Partial thickness flap*
1. Degree of technical difficulty	Moderate	High
2. Osseous surgery	Possible	Difficult
3. Blood supply to flaps	Sufficient	Decrease
4. Periosteal retention	No	Yes
5. Widen zone of keratinized gingiva	No	Yes
6. Bleeding and tissue trauma	Limited	Greater
7. Variability of suture	Low	High
8. Healing	Primary intention	Secondary intention

VARIOUS FLAP PROCEDURES FOR POCKET ELIMINATION

MODIFIED WIDMAN FLAP PROCEDURE

Historical perspective: In 1918, Widman introduced Widman flap surgery. In 1965, Morris revived this technique and called it as unrepositioned mucoperiosteal flap. The same

Differences between Original and Modified Widman flap		
	Original Widman flap	*Modified Widman flap*
1. Given by	Leonard Widman, 1918	Ramfjord and Nissle,1974
2. Purpose	For pocket elimination	Provide access for adequate instrumentation
3. Collar of tissue attached to the teeth torn	With curettes	With Orban's knife
4. Releasing incision	Given	Not given
5. Flap reflection	High flap reflection	Minimal flap reflection
6. Bone contouring	Done	No bone contouring
7. After suturing	Flaps do not cover interproximal bone, remains exposed	Flaps cover interproximal bone

PERIODONTICS REVISITED

procedure was presented in 1974 by Ramfjord and Nissle who called it the modified Widman flap.

The advantages of Modified Widman flap over Original Widman flap procedure are i) close adaptation of soft tissue to root surface, ii) minimum trauma to alveolar bone and iii) access to adequate instrumentation of the root surface.

Objectives: The main purpose of the modified widman technique is to facilitate instrumentation on root surfaces by exposing them and to remove the pocket lining. Resdiual deposits of subgingival calculus left in deep pockets are thus removed.

Surgical Instruments

Blade no. 11, 12, 15, Bard Parker handle no. 3, Periosteal elevator and Curettes.

Procedure

- *Incision and flap reflection*: The internal bevel incision is the initial incision starting 0.5 to 1 mm from the gingival margin to the alveolar crest **(Fig. 46.6A)**. Scalloping follows the gingival margin. Care should be taken to insert the blade in such a way that the papilla is left with a thickness similar to that of the remaining facial flap. The gingiva is reflected with a periosteal elevator. A *crevicular incision* is made from the bottom of the pocket to the alveolar bone, circumscribing the triangular wedge of tissue containing the pocket lining. After the flap is reflected, a *third incision* is made in the interdental space, coronal to the bone, with an interproximal knife **(Fig. 46.6B)**.
- *Cervical wedge*: The gingival collar is removed with the help of curette.
- *Curettage, scaling and root planing*: Tissue tags and granulation tissue are removed with a curette. The root surfaces are checked and are scaled and planed, if necessary. Residual periodontal fibers attached to the tooth surface should not be disturbed.
- Bone architecture is not corrected unless it prevents good tissue adaptation to the neck of the teeth. Every effort is made to adapt the facial and lingual interproximal tissue adjacent to each other in such a way that no interproximal bone remains exposed at the time of suturing. The flaps may be thinned to allow for close adaptation of the gingiva around the entire circumference of the tooth and to each other interproximally.

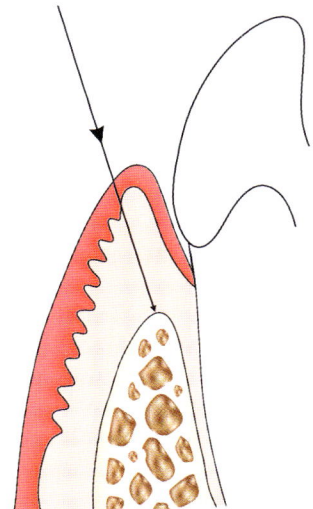

Fig. 46.6A: Internal bevel incision of modified widman flap

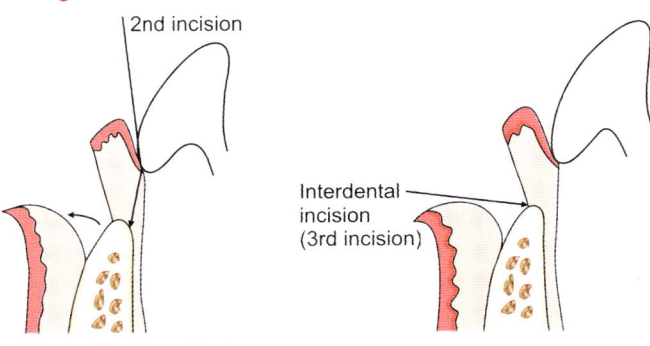

Flap reflected and 2nd incision (crevicular) given

Fig. 46.6B: Crevicular incision and interdental incision of modified widman flap

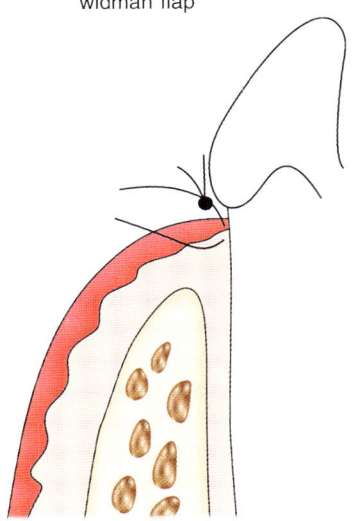

After root surface debridement flap is sutured to its original position

Fig. 46.6C: Modified widman flap sutured

PERIODONTICS REVISITED

- *Suturing*: The flaps are replaced in their original position and secured by interdental suturing **(Fig. 46.6C)**.
- *Postoperative management*: The operated site is covered with periodontal surgical pack and postoperative instructions are given thereafter.

UNDISPLACED FLAP PROCEDURE

It is also called as internal bevel gingivectomy because the soft tissue pocket wall is removed with the initial incision.

Objectives
i. To reduce or eliminate pocket by removing pocket wall.
ii. To improve accessibility for instrumentation.

Surgical Instruments

Pocket marker, Blade no. 11, 12, 15, Bard Parker handle no. 3, Periosteal elevator and Curettes.

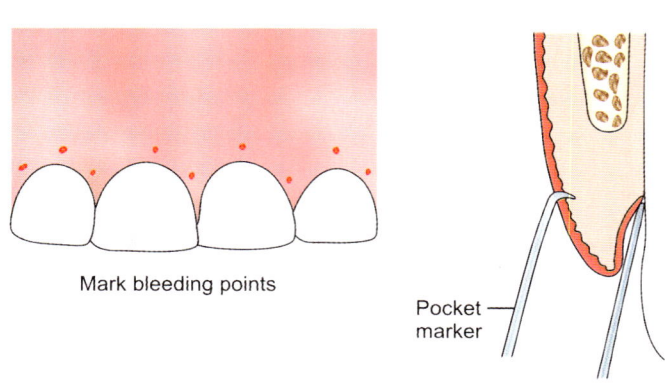

Mark bleeding points

Pocket marker

Mark the depth of pocket with pocket marker

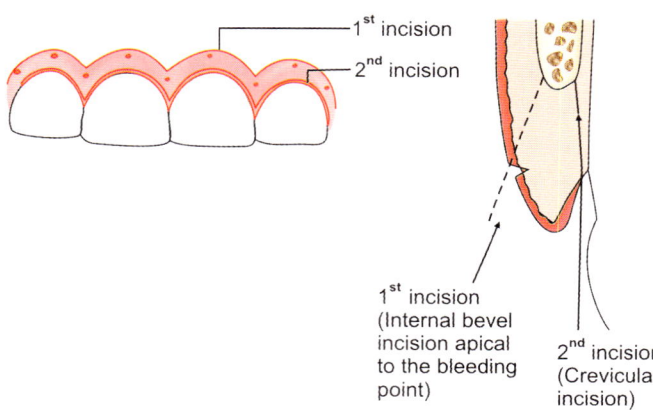

1st incision
2nd incision

1st incision
(Internal bevel incision apical to the bleeding point)

2nd incision
(Crevicular incision)

Fig. 46.7: Undisplaced flap

Procedure *(Fig. 46.7)*

- *Mark bleeding points*: The pockets are measured with a periodontal probe and bleeding points are produced on the outer surface of the gingiva to mark the pocket bottom with the help of pocket marker.
- *Incision and flap reflection*: The initial, internal bevel incision is made following the scalloping of the bleeding marks on the gingiva. The incision is usually carried to a point apical to the alveolar crest, depending on the thickness of the tissue. The thicker the tissue is, the more apical will be the ending point of the incision. Then crevicular incision is made from the bottom of the pocket to the bone to detach the connective tissue from the tooth. Full thickness flap is reflected with a periosteal elevator. The third incision, i.e. interdental incision is made with an interdental knife, separating the connective tissue from the bone. The triangular wedge of tissue created by the three incisions is removed with a curette.
- *Removal of granulation tissue*: The area is debrided, removing all tissue tags and granulation tissue with sharp curettes.
- *Curettage, scaling and root planing*: After the necessary scaling and root planing, the flap edge should rest on the root—bone junction.
- *Suturing*: A continuous sling suture is utilized to secure the facial and the lingual or palatal flaps. This type of suture, which uses the tooth as an anchor, is advantageous to position and hold the flap edges at the root—bone junction. The area is covered with a periodontal pack.
- Postoperative instructions are given thereafter.

APICALLY DISPLACED FLAP PROCEDURE

Historical Perspective

In 1954, Nabers described the repositioning of the attached gingiva. For the first time, a mucoperiosteal flap was apically positioned after treatment. He utilized one vertical releasing incision which is placed mesially to the area of the deepest pocket. Later in 1957, he introduced the inverse bevel incision of which he called the "repositioning incision" which includes the internal incision from the gingival margin to the alveolar crest. This incision, he stated, would permit an easier flap reflection and result in a thinner gingival margin. In that same year, Ariaudo and Tyrrell modified Nabers' technique and recommended two vertical releasing incisions instead of just one to facilitate the mobilization of the flap. At this point, the only difference from the flap design of Widman is the apical positioning. Finally, in 1962, Friedman published the technique in his paper and coined the term "apically repositioned flap". In his paper, he described the use of inverse beveled incision to thin the marginal tissue and the papillae. This thinning incision eliminates thick gingival margin and papillae with large triangular pieces of interdental tissue. A thick tissue would be difficult to be eliminated from the already raised flap and also created problem in approximation of tissue for primary intention healing, resulting in bulbous or ledging tissue upon healing. This flap designed could be referred to as the partial full-thickness flap since the marginal papillae was partially disected with the inverse bevel incision, then this incision continue to include the mucoperiosteum of the full thickness flap. Goldman in 1982 introduced another variation of which he followed the full thickness flap with a partial dissection, allowing the use of periosteal suture to position the flap. This flap design, he called the tertiary flap or the partial-full-partial-thickness flap. Today, the word "reposition" is replaced by the term "position" since reposition means place the flap back to where it was before. The flap can be positioned apically or reposition, depending on each individualized case. The sling suture is recommended for better flap placement. Pocket elimination is achieved only by apically positioning of the flap.

Objectives:

i. To eliminate pocket by apically positioning the soft tissue wall of the pocket.
ii. To preserve/increase the width of attached gingiva.
iii. To improve accessibility.

The position of the flap displacement varies depending on the:

1. Thickness of alveolar margin in operating area.
2. Width of attached gingiva.
3. Clinical crown length necessary for an abutment.

Procedure (Figs 46.8A to D)

- *Incisions and flap reflection*: First incision, internal bevel incision is made 1 mm from the crest of the gingiva and directed towards the crest of the alveolar bone. The beveling incision should be given a scalloped outline to ensure maximal interproximal coverage of the alveolar bone, when the flap subsequently is repositioned. Second incision, crevicular incision is made, followed by the elevation of the full thickness mucoperiosteal flap. Third incision, interdental incision is given and the wedge of the tissue that contains pocket wall is removed. Vertical incision extending out into alveolar mucosa (i.e. past the

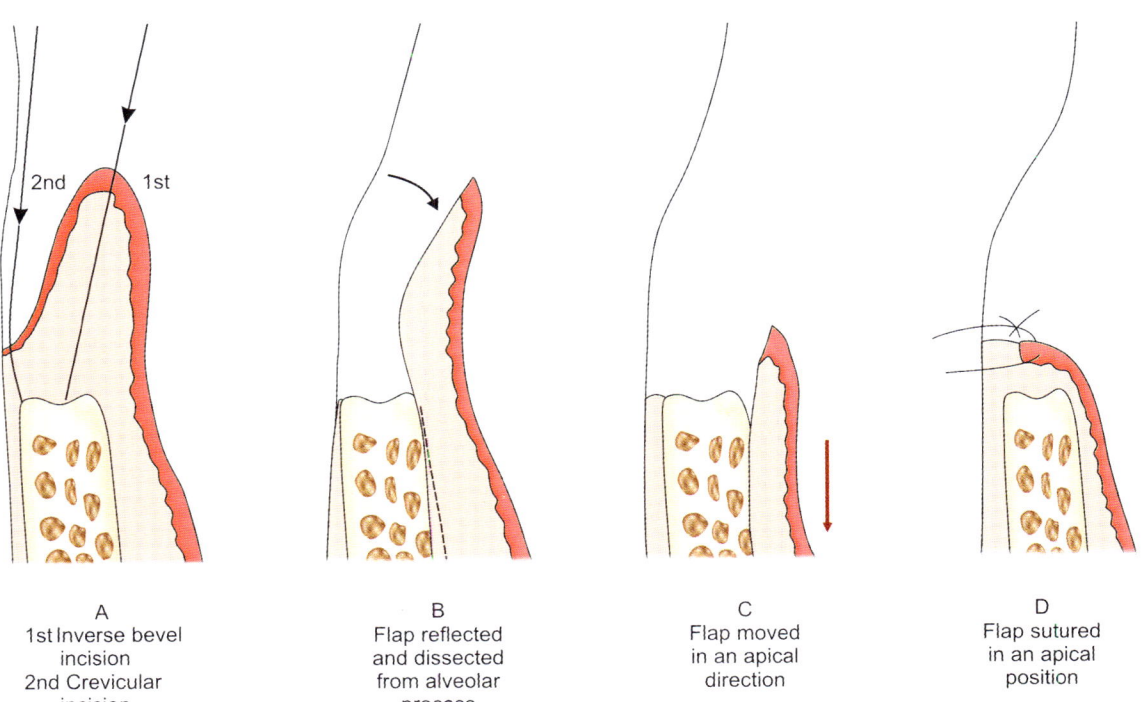

A	B	C	D
1st Inverse bevel incision 2nd Crevicular incision	Flap reflected and dissected from alveolar process	Flap moved in an apical direction	Flap sutured in an apical position

Figs 46.8A to D: Apically positioned flap

mucogingival junction) are made at each end points of the internal bevel incision, making the apical repositioning of the flap. For full thickness flap, periosteal elevator is used to reflect the flap.

- *Removal of granulation tissue:* Marginal collar tissue and granulation tissue are removed with curettes.
- *Scaling and root planing*: Scaling and root planing is done carefully with scalers and curettes.
- *Osseous recontouring*: Alveolar bone crest is recontoured with the help of bur and bone chisels.
- *Apical positioning and suturing:* The flap is reflected to the base of the vestibule. Once released, the flap tends to contract and fold up so that apical positioning takes place. Flap is displaced apically so that edge just covers the newly recontoured alveolar crest. Interrupted sutures should be placed first at the mesial and distal vertical incisions. Full thickness flap is sutured using sling suture while partial thickness flap is secured with direct loop suture or a combination of loop and anchor suture. Periodontal dressing is applied on the operated site over the dry foil.
- Postoperative instructions are given thereafter.

Advantages:
1. Eliminates periodontal pocket- Apically repositioned flap results in pocket elimination and the formation of a normal/physiological length of junctional epithelium whereas the replaced flap results in the formation of a long junctional epithelium which may adhere to the root surface. The long junctional epithelium is inherently less stable than the physiological junctional epithelium and demands much higher frequencies of recall for maintenance than pocket elimination procedures.
2. Preserves attached gingiva and increases its width.
3. Establishes gingival morphology facilitating good hygiene.
4. Ensures healthy root surface necessary for the biologic width on alveolar margin and lengthen clinical crown.

Disadvantages:
1. May cause esthetic problems due to root exposure.
2. May cause attachment loss due to surgery.
3. May cause hypersensitivity.
4. May increase the risk of root caries.
5. Possibility of exposure of furcations and roots, which complicates postoperative supragingival plaque control.

PAPILLA PRESERVATION FLAP

In 1985, Takei et al proposed surgical approach called as Papilla preservation technique. Later, Cortellini et al described modifications of this flap designs. It is the procedure which incorporates the entire papilla in one of the flaps by means of crevicular and interdental incisions to sever the connective tissue attachment and a horizontal incision at the base of the papilla, leaving it connected to one of the flaps.

Indications:
i. Diastema region.
ii. Bone grafting areas.

Contraindication:
i. Narrow embrasures.

Procedure

- *Incisions*: Crevicular incisions are made at the facial and proximal aspects of the teeth without making incisions through the interdental papillae. Subsequently, crevicular incision is made along the lingual/palatal aspect of teeth with a semilunar incision made across each interdental area with the blade perpendicular to the outer surface of gingiva and extending through the periosteum to the alveolar process (**Fig. 46.9A**). Semilunar incision should dip apically atleast 5 mm from the line angles of teeth, which will allow the interdental tissue to be dissected from the lingual/palatal aspect so that it can be elevated intact with the facial flap.
- *Reflection of flap*: A curette or interproximal knife is used to carefully free the interdental papilla from the underlying hard tissue. The detached interdental tissue is pushed through the embrasure with a blunt instrument (**Fig. 46.9B**). A full–thickness flap is reflected with a periosteal elevator on both facial/palatal surfaces. The exposed root surfaces are thoroughly scaled and root planed and bone defects carefully curetted.
- *Removal of granulomatous tissue*: While holding the reflected flap, the margins of the flap and the interdental tissue are scrapped to remove pocket epithelium and excessive granulation tissue. In anterior areas, the trimming of granulation tissue should be limited so as to maintain the thickness of tissue. After reflection of flap, access to the interdental bony defect will be obtained. The bony defect is cleaned out using curette. The bone graft material is placed if required.

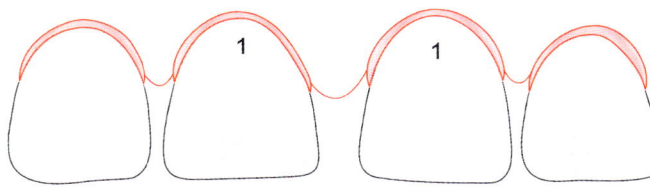

1. Intrasulcular incision
(Facial aspect)

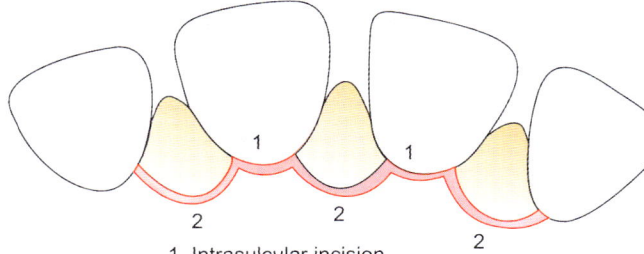

1. Intrasulcular incision
2. Semilunar incision
(Palatal aspect)

Fig. 46.9A: Papilla preservation flap incisions

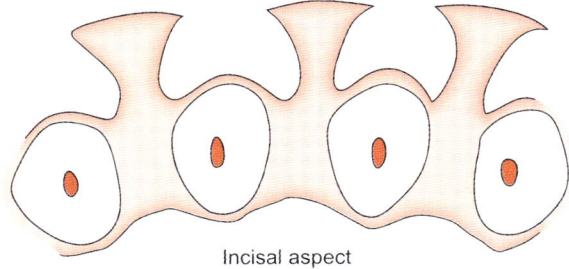

Incisal aspect

Fig. 46.9B: Reflected papilla preservation flap

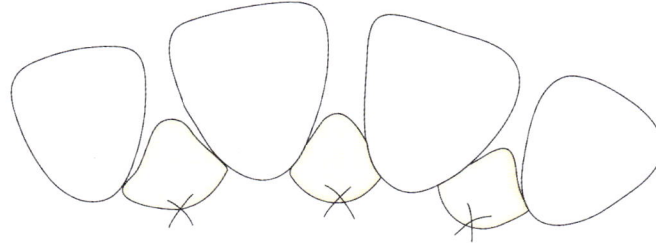

Fig. 46.9C: Papilla preservation flap sutured

- *Suturing*: The flaps are repositioned and sutured using criss cross mattress. The cross mattress suture results in optimal flap closure without having suture material in direct contact with the graft material. Alternatively, a direct suture of the semilunar incisions can be done as the only means of flap closure **(Fig. 46.9C)**. Periodontal dressing may be placed to protect the surgical area.

- Postoperative instructions are given thereafter.

Advantages:
 i. Esthetically pleasing.
 ii. Primary coverage of implant.
iii. Prevents postoperative tissue craters.

Disadvantages:
 i. Technically difficult.
 ii. Time consuming.

PALATAL FLAP

The surgical approach for palatal flap is different from other flaps because of the nature of palatal tissue which is attached and keratinized with no elastic properties. The apical portion of the scalloping should be narrower than the line angle area because of the taper of palatal root apically. Palatal flap cannot be displaced apically nor can a split-thickness palatal flap be accomplished.

Indications:
 i. Areas that require osseous surgery.
 ii. Pocket elimination.
iii. Reduction of enlarged and bulbous tissue.

Contraindication:
It is contraindicated when the palate is broad and shallow.

Special care must be taken performing a palatal flap due to several anatomic structures:
- Greater palatine artery and nerve may be damaged if flap reflection is extensive in molar region.
- Palatal exostoses present in molar region in 1/3rd of the patient. It creates thin tissue in the region and make proper flap margin placement difficult.
- Incisive papilla present in anterior palate.
- Presence of palatal rugae at or near the flap margin create poor gingival margin contours postsurgically.

Procedure

- *Incisions*: The outline of initial incision for palatal flap varies and is determined with consideration for the: i) thickness of palatal soft tissue; ii) depth of periodontal pocket; iii) necessity for osteoplasty; and iv) clinical crown length required for restorative treatment. If the purpose of surgery is debridement then internal bevel incision is given such that palatal flap is adapted at root bone junction, when sutured. If osseous resection is to be done, then palatal incision is planned to compensate for lowered level of bone when the flap is closed.

PERIODONTICS REVISITED

The initial incision may be the usual internal bevel incision, followed by crevicular and interdental incisions. If the tissue is thick, a horizontal gingivectomy incision may be made, followed by an internal bevel incision that starts at the edge of this incision and ends on the lateral surface of the underlying bone. The placement of the internal bevel incision must be done in such a way that the flap fits around the tooth without exposing the bone. The blade should be parallel to the palatal soft tissue to prepare a thin and uniform primary flap (1.5–2.0 mm thickness). Caution must be taken to avoid perforating the flap or making the flap too thin, which will cut off the necessary blood supply.

- *Flap reflection*: Before the flap is reflected to the final position for scaling and management of the osseous lesions, its thickness must be checked. Flaps should be thin to adapt to the underlying osseous tissue and provide a thin, knife like gingival margin.
- *Scaling, root planing*: With the help of scalers and curettes scaling, root planing is performed. Osteoplasty is done only if required.
- *Suturing*: Suture the flap's edge at the level of the bone margin or slightly over the alveolar crest (approximately 1–2 mm above the bone margin).
- Post operative instructions are given thereafter.

Beveled Flap

Friedman developed the beveled flap, a modification of the apically repositioned flap for the periodontal pockets on the palatal aspect of the teeth. As there is no alveolar mucosa present on the palatal aspect of the teeth, it is not possible to reposition the flap in an apical direction.

A primary incision is made intracrevicularly through the bottom of the periodontal pocket and a mucoperiosteal flap is elevated. Scaling, root planing and osseous recontouring is performed in the surgical area. The palatal flap is replaced and a secondary, scalloped, reverse bevel incision is made to adjust the length of the flap to the height of the remaining alveolar bone. The shortened and thinned flap is replaced over the alveolar bone and in close contact with the root surface **(Fig. 46.10)**.

Advantages of palatal approach procedures are esthetics, easier access for osseous surgery, wider palatal embrassure space and less resorption because of thicker bone. The only disadvantage is close root proximity.

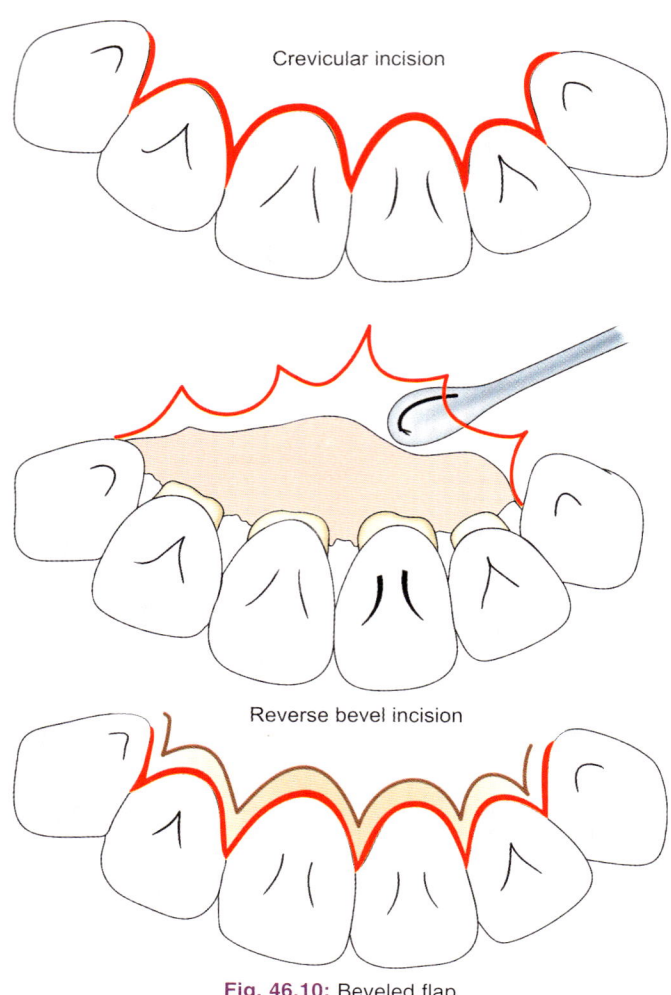

Crevicular incision

Reverse bevel incision

Fig. 46.10: Beveled flap

DISTAL MOLAR SURGERY

Treatment of periodontal pocket on the distal surface of terminal molar is often complicated by the presence of bulbous fibrous tissue over the maxillary tuberosity or prominent retromolar pad in the mandible. Deep vertical defects are also commonly present in conjunction with the redundant fibrous tissue. This procedure enables the removal of thick gingival tissue on the adjacent edentulous site. If there is an osseous defect, it corrects the bone morphology by flattening it and the intrabony defect may be eliminated. The periodontal pocket is eliminated and a shallow gingival sulcus favorable for postoperative maintenance is created.

Objectives of distal wedge procedure
1. To maintain and preserve attached gingiva.
2. To eliminate periodontal pocket.
3. To lengthen clinical crown.
4. To create easily cleansable gingiva-alveolar form.

The various incisions for distal molar surgery **(Fig. 46.11)**:
i. Linear incision
ii. Triangular incision
iii. Pedicle incision
iv. Square, parallel incision

Indications for the square incision:
- Long and large edentulous ridge, maxillary tuberosity and retromolar triangle
- Much tissue to be removed in the wedge area
- Sufficient existing band of attached gingiva
- Deep periodontal pockets and osseous defects on the mesial and distal aspects of the abutment.

Maxillary molars: Two parallel incisions, beginning at the distal portion of the tooth and extending to the mucogingival junction distal to the tuberosity, are made. These incisions are usually interconnected with the incisions for the remainder of the surgery in the quadrant involved. The amount of wedge tissue to be removed (the distance between the two internal bevel incisions) is determined by a number of factors, such as i) depth of periodontal pocket, ii) thickness of the soft tissue wedge, iii) whether osteoplasty or osseous resection is necessary and, iv) clinical crown length required for abutment. A transversal incision is made at the distal end of the two parallel incisions so that a long, rectangular piece of tissue can be removed. The parallel distal incisions should be confined to the attached gingiva because bleeding and flap management becomes problem when the incision is extended into the alveolar mucosa. When the tissue between the two incisions is removed and the flaps are thinned, the two flap edges must approximate each other at a new apical position without overlapping.

Mandibular molars: Incisions for the mandibular arch differ from those used for the tuberosity, owing to differences in the anatomy and histologic features of the areas. The retromolar pad area does not usually present as much fibrous attached gingiva. The two incisions distal to the molar should follow the area with the greatest amount of attached gingiva. Therefore, the incisions could be directed distolingually or distofacially, depending on which area has more attached gingiva. Before the flap is completely reflected, it is thinned with

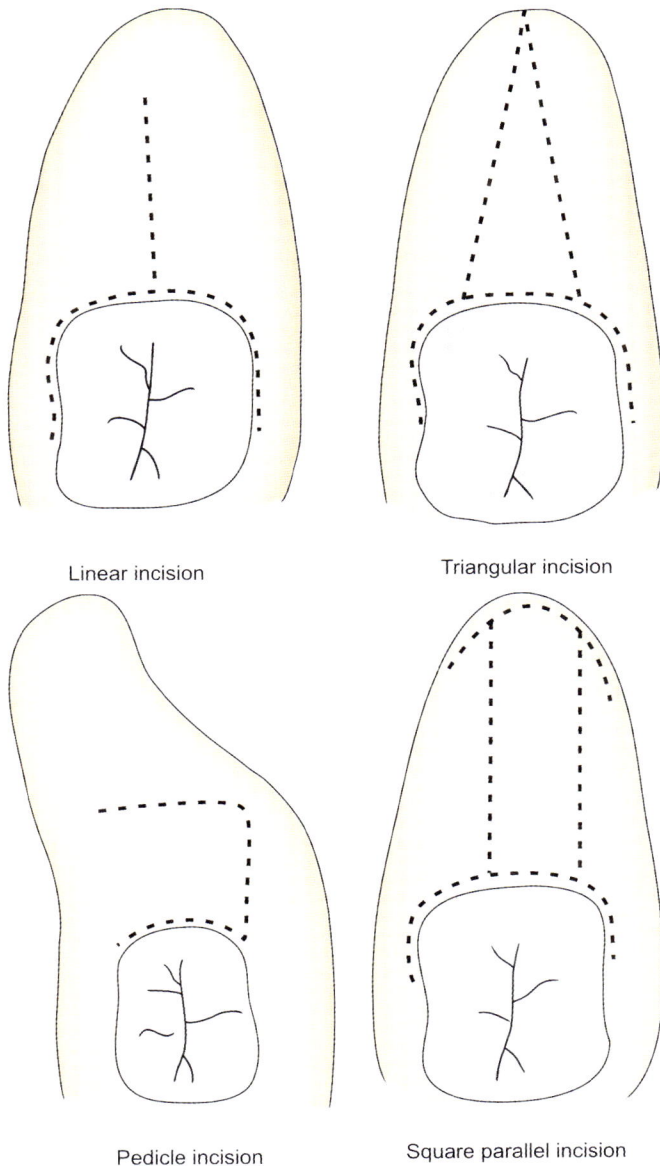

Linear incision   Triangular incision

Pedicle incision   Square parallel incision

Fig. 46.11: Various incisions for distal molar surgery

a 15 no. blade. It is easier to thin the flap before it is completely free and mobile. After the reflection of the flap and the removal of the redundant fibrous tissue, any necessary osseous surgery is performed. The flaps are approximated similarly to those in the maxillary tuberosity area.

Advantages of distal wedge procedure
i. Maintenance of attached tissue.
ii. Accessibility for treatment of both distal furcation and underlying osseous irregularities.

Coronally Displaced Flap

Explained in chapter no. 50 Periodontal Plastic Surgery.

Laterally Positioned Pedicle Flap

It was originally developed by Grupe and Warren in 1956. In this procedure a pedicle graft is taken from a donor site and is placed on the adjoining site by moving the flap towards the recipient site and suture are placed (Rest is described in chapter no. 50 Periodontal Plastic Surgery).

Double Papilla Pedicle Flap

Explained in chapter no. 50 Periodontal Plastic Surgery.

Comparison between Flap Procedure and Gingivectomy

	Flap Procedure	Gingivectomy
1. Reattachment	Possible	No
2. Healing	Primary intention	Secondary intention
3. Bleeding postoperatively	Low	High
4. Preservation of keratinized gingiva	Yes	No
5. Visibility and ability to treat osseous irregularities and defects	Good	Inadequate
6. Time required	Slow	Fast
7. Degree of difficulty	High	Low

POINTS TO PONDER

✓ Incisions are either coronally directed incisions (external bevel incision) or apically directed incisions (Internal bevel, sulcular incision).

✓ Undisplaced flap is considered as Internal bevel gingivectomy. Undisplaced flap and gingivectomy procedures surgically remove the pocket wall.

✓ Apically positioned flap surgery, is one of the most reliable technique for the elimination of periodontal pockets.

✓ The flap without vertical incision is called envelope flap.

✓ The tissue which is left on the surface of tooth when the flap is raised is called as cervical wedge.

✓ Neumann flap: Neumann in 1911, introduced the flap in which the intrasulcular incision was made along with two vertical releasing incision, a full thickness flap raised and the area was curetted thoroughly to eliminate all the granulation tissue to prevent reinfection. Root was planed smooth and bone was superficially removed.

✓ Conventional flap is the flap in which the papilla is split into facial half and lingual/palatal half.

BIBLIOGRAPHY

1. Carranza FM, Takei HH. The flap technique for pocket therapy. In, Newman, Takei, Carranza. Clinical Periodontology. 9th ed Philadelphia WB Saunders 2003;774-85.
2. Eley BM, Manson JD. Surgical Periodontal treatment. In, Periodontics. 5th ed Wright 2004;262-75.
3. Genco RJ, Rosenberg ES, Evian C. Periodontal surgery. In, Genco RJ, Goldman HM, Cohen DW. Contemporary Periodontics C.V Mosby 1999;554-84.
4. Hupp JR. Contemporary Oral and Maxillofacial Surgery. 2nd ed Singapore Harcourt Brace and Company Asia (Pvt.) Ltd. 1993.
5. Mc Donnell HT, Mills MP. Principles and Practice of Periodontal surgery. In, Rose LF, Mealey BL, Genco RJ, Cohen DW. Periodontics, Medicine, Surgery and Implants. Elsevier Mosby. 2004;358-404.
6. Robinson PJ, Goodman CH. General principles of surgical therapy. In, Genco RJ, Goldman HM, Cohen DW. Contemporary Periodontics CV Mosby 1999;543-53.
7. Ramfjord SP, Nissle R. The modified Widman flap. J Periodontol 1974;45:601-18.
8. Takei HH, Caranza FA. The periodontal flap. In, Newman, Takei, Carranza. Clinical Periodontology 9th ed Philadelphia WB Saunders 2003;762-73.
9. Wang HL, Greenwell H. Surgical periodontal therapy. Periodontol 2000 2001;25:89–99.

MCQs

1. An apically repositioned flap:
   A. Is the procedure of choice for palatal pockets
   B. Does not preserve the attached gingiva
   C. Does not increase the length of clinical crown
   D. Is a pocket elimination procedure
2. A split thickness flap is indicated where:
   A. Fenestration and Dehiscence are suspected
   B. Three walled osseous defects are present
   C. Osseous craters are present
   D. Buttressing bone formation is present
3. Which of the following flaps can be considered as "internal bevel" gingivectomy procedure:
   A. Modified widman flap
   B. Undisplaced flap
   C. Apically displaced flap
   D. Coronally displaced flap
4. External bevel incision is:
   A. Apically directed incision
   B. Coronally directed incision
   C. Vertical incision
   D. None of the above
5. Following are the basic flap requirements except:
   A. No important vessels or nerves should be damaged in raising the flap
   B. Incisions must allow movement of flap without tension

C. The apex of the flap should be wider than the base
D. Length of the flap should be no more than twice the width of the base

6. Distal wedge procedure:
A. Maintain and preserve attached gingiva
B. Eliminate periodontal pockets
C. Lengthen clinical crown
D. All of the above

7. Cut-back incision is:
A. Made at apical aspect of releasing incision directing towards base of the flap in laterally positioned flap
B. Made at the base of flap severing the underlying periosteum
C. Extends from gingiva towards the base of the flap in palatal flap and distal wedge procedures
D. None of the above

8. Indication of Papilla preservation flap:
A. Diastema region   B. Bone grafting areas
C. Narrow embrasures   D. Both A and B

Answers

1. D   2. A   3. B   4. B   5. C
6. D   7. A   8. D

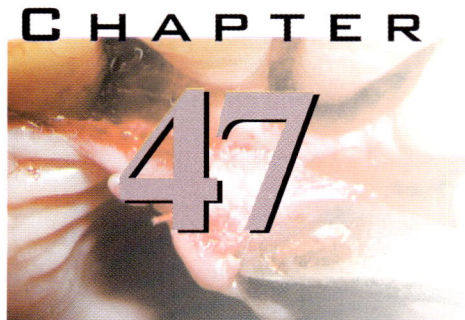
Resective Osseous Surgery

Shalu Bathla

DEFINITION

Schluger is considered to be the father of resective osseous surgery and advocated osseous resective treatment of periodontitis, rather than scaling and root planing or the gingivectomy.

The procedure designed to restore the form of pre-existing alveolar bone to the level existing at the time of surgery or slightly more apical to this level is called as resective osseous surgery.

It is the combined use of both osteoplasty and ostectomy to reestablish the marginal bone morphology around the teeth to resemble normal bone with a positive architecture.

TERMINOLOGY

- *Ideal architecture:* The bone level is more coronal in the interproximal areas, with a gradual slope around and away from the tooth.
- *Positive architecture:* The level of radicular bone is apical to the interdental bone **(Fig. 47.1A)**.
- *Negative architecture:* The level of interdental bone is more apical to radicular bone. It is also called as reversed architecture **(Fig. 47.1B)**.

- *Flat architecture:* The interdental bone is at the same level to that of radicular bone **(Fig. 47.1C)**.
- *Osteoplasty:* It is a procedure to create a physiologic form of alveolar bone without removing any supporting bone.
- *Ostectomy:* It is a procedure in which supporting bone i.e. bone involved in the attachment of tooth is removed to reshape deformities.

The objectives of osseous resection are to remove osseous defects, to correct bone morphology, to create a harmonious relation between the gingiva and alveolar bone by eliminating periodontal pockets, and to create a favourable postoperative gingival morphology.

RATIONALE

To achieve physiologic architecture of marginal alveolar bone conducive to gingival flap adaption with minimal probing depth. The end points of osseous resective surgery are minimal probing depths and a gingival tissue morphology that enhances good self performed oral hygiene and periodontal health.

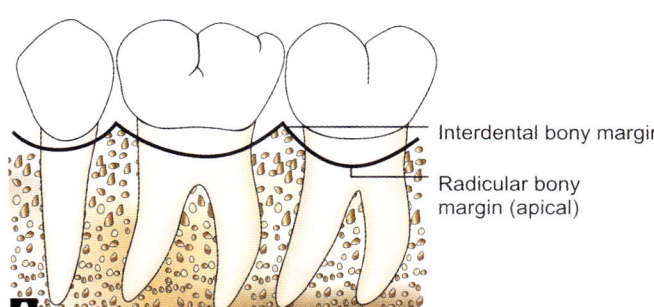

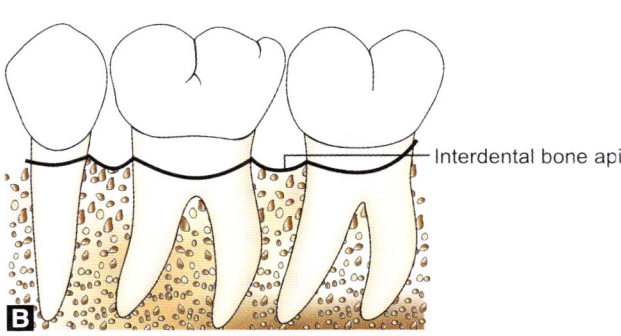

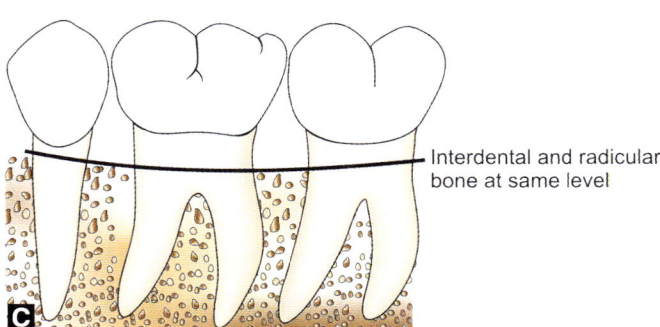

Figs 47.1A to C: Bone architecture A. Positive,
B. Reversed/Negative, C. Flat

INDICATIONS OF OSTEOPLASTY

i. Removing exotoses/ledges
ii. Tori that interferes with plaque control and persistent pocket
iii. Early grade I furcation lesion
iv. To contour alveolar ridge to make room for pontics
v. Open furcation in tunneling procedure.

INDICATIONS OF OSTECTOMY

i. Crown lengthening
ii. Exposure of sound dentin apical to caries/fractures
iii. Opening of interradicular spaces for the treatment of furcation involvement.

EXAMINATION AND TREATMENT PLANNING FOR RESECTIVE OSSEOUS SURGERY

1. Soft tissue palpation.
2. Radiographic examination:
   • Provide information about the interproximal bone loss, the presence of angular or irregular bone loss.
   • Provide the information about the extent of bony defect or the number of bony walls remaining.
3. Probing: It reveals the presence of-
   • Pocket depth greater than that of normal gingival sulcus.
   • The location of the base of pocket relative to the mucogingival junction and attachment level on adjacent teeth.
   • The number of bony walls.
   • The presence of furcation defects.
4. Transgingival probing (sounding):
   • Under local anesthesia confirms the extent and configuration of the intrabony component of the pocket or furcation defects.
   • The probe walks along the tissue-tooth interface to feel the bony topography.
   • The probe may pass horizontally through the tissue to provide three-dimensional information regarding bony contours.

INSTRUMENTS USED IN RESECTIVE OSSEOUS SURGERY

i. Rongeurs - Friedman, Blumenthal **(Figs 47.2A and B)**
ii. Files - Sugarman, Schluger **(Figs 47.3A and B)**
iii. Chisels - Backaction, Ochsenbein **(Fig. 47.4)**
iv. Burs - Carbide, Diamond

PROCEDURE

I. Anesthesia- Appropriate local anesthesia is given in the selected area.
II. Incision and flap reflection- Mucoperiosteal flap is reflected by giving horizontal and vertical incisions

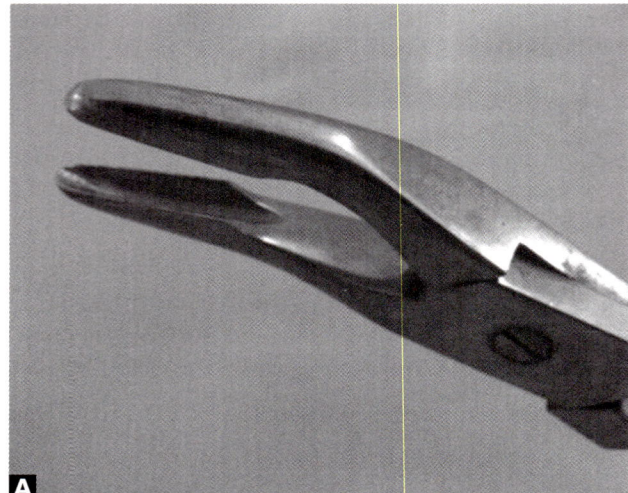

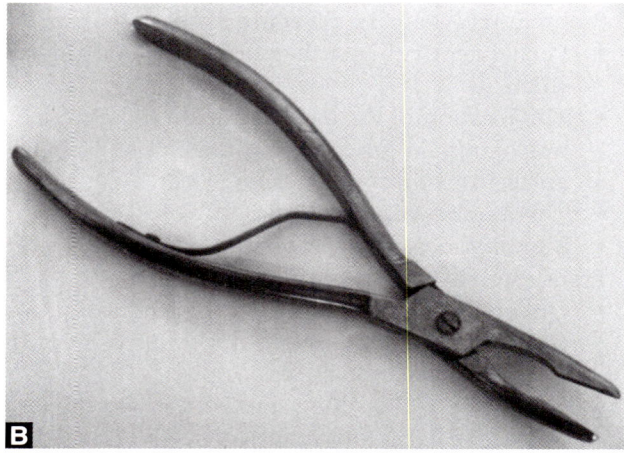

Figs 47.2A and B: Bone rongeur

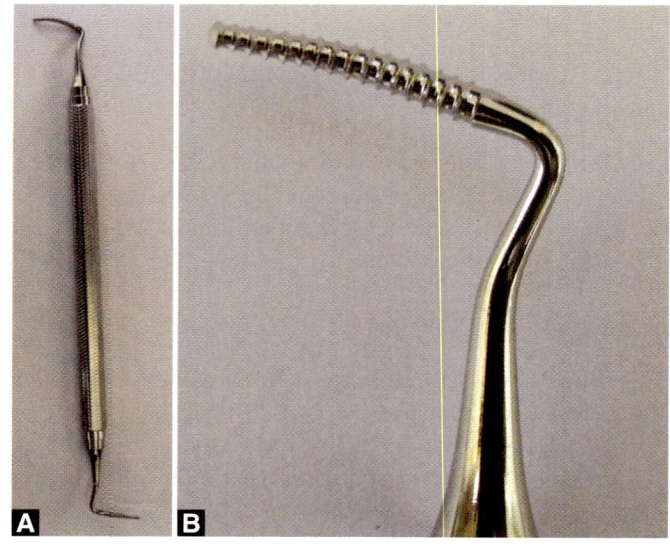

Figs 47.3A and B: Schluger file

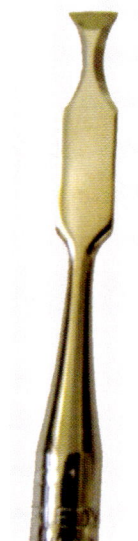

Fig. 47.4: Ochsenbein chisel

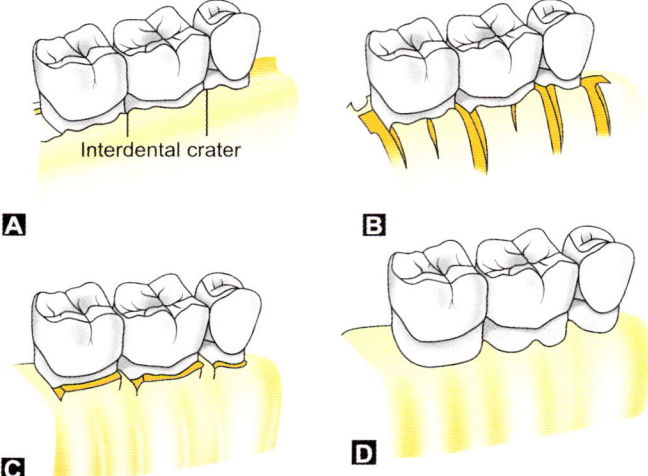

Figs 47.5A to D: A. Bony topography showing interdental craters, B. Vertical grooving, C.Radicular blending and flattening of interproximal bone, and D. Gradualizing the marginal bone (*Courtesy:* Dr SK Salaria)

in the surgical area. (For apically displaced flap vertical incision should be given).

III. Resective osseous technique is carried out in 4 steps: **(Figs 47.5A to D)**

a. Vertical grooving/festooning: It is the first step of the resective osseous surgery designed to reduce the thickness of the alveolar housing and to provide prominence to the radicular aspects of the teeth. Slow speed (2000 rpm) handpiece with a sharp carbide surgical bur is used to perform the vertical grooving. Cooling with a copious spray of sterile saline is necessary so that the temperature of the bone is not raised beyond 47°C. It is contraindicated in close root proximity or thin alveolar housing areas.

It is designed:
  i. To reduce the thickness of the alveolar housing,
  ii. To provide relative prominence to the radicular aspect of the teeth, and
  iii. To provide continuity from interproximal surface onto the radicular surface.

  b. *Radicular blending*: It is the extension of vertical grooving which gradualize the bone over the entire radicular surface to produce smooth and blended surface for good flap adaptation. It is indicated where thick ledges of bone present on the radicular surface, whereas it is contraindicated where thin, fenestrated radicular bone is present.

Both vertical grooving and radicular blending may be used for treatment of:
• Thick osseous ledges of bone on radicular surface.
• Class I and early class II furcation involvement.

  c. *Flattening of interproximal bone*: This is done where interproximal bone levels vary horizontally. There small amount of supporting bone is removed with the help of chisel.
  d. *Gradualizing marginal bone*: It is the minimal bone removal to provide a sound, regular base for gingival tissue to follow. The bone is removed with chisel. Saline irrigation should also be carried out during chiseling, since this generates heat.
IV. *Suturing*: After removal of the osseous tissue, the flap is adapted closely to cover the bone with the flap apically displaced, which is then sutured in place.
 V. *Postoperative instructions*: The patient is followed postoperatively as with other flap procedures.

Specific Osseous Reshaping Situations

Correction of one walled hemiseptal defect

• The bone should be reduce to the level of the most apical portion of the defect. It requires removal of some bone on the side with greatest coronal bony height. This result in significant reduction in attachment on relatively unaffected adjacent teeth to eliminate the defect.

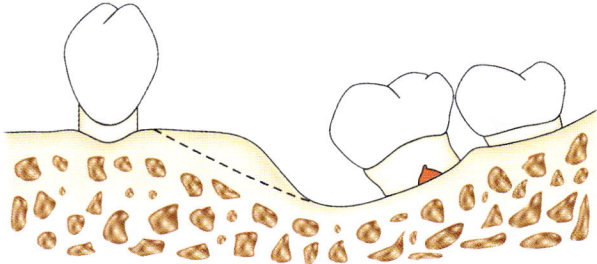

Fig. 47.6: Reduction of one-wall angular defect by ramping

• If the tooth has one wall defect on both its mesial and distal surfaces, the severely affected tooth may be extruded by orthodontics during disease control to minimize the need for resection of bone from the adjacent teeth.
• If one walled defect occurs next to edentulous area, the edentulous ridge is reduced to the level of the osseous defect **(Fig. 47.6)**.

In case of exostoses, malpositioned or supraerupted tooth

• Osteoplasty is done to eliminate the exostoses or reduce the buccal/lingual bulk of bone.
• It is common to incorporate a degree of vertical grooving during reduction of the bony ledges, since it facilitate the process of blending the radicular bone into interproximal areas.
• Follow all the four steps explained above

DISADVANTAGES OF RESECTIVE OSSEOUS SURGERY

• Causes recession, hypersensitivity
• Reduces tooth bone support
• Removes bone that may be needed if implants are desired
• Exposed roots could be at higher risk for caries in patients with poor oral hygiene
• More access for brush but more challenge for patient to maintain

POINTS TO PONDER

✓ Resective osseous surgery is the most predictable pocket reduction technique.
✓ *Spheroiding/Parabolizing:* It is the removal of supporting bone to produce a positive gingival and osseous architecture.

PERIODONTICS REVISITED

✓ *Scribbing:* It is the technique by which high speed rotary instruments are used to outline the radicular bone which is to be removed by hand instrumentation.

✓ *Widow's peaks*: Schluger in 1949 described widow's peaks as the residual pieces of cortical bone left over facial or lingual line angle from the horizontal grooving that form a crater in a mesiodistal direction. They will not be absorbed and will result in immediate postoperative tissue pocketing. Hand instrumentation with Ochsenbein chisel is used to eliminate widow's peak.

BIBLIOGRAPHY

1. Carnevale G, Kaldahl WB. Osseous resective surgery. Periodontol 2000 2000;22:59-87.
2. Genco RJ, Rosenberg ES, Evian C. Periodontal Surgery. In, Genco RJ, Goldman HM and Cohen DW. Contemporary Periodontics. CV Mosby Company 1990;554-84.
3. Grant DA, Stern IB, Listgarten MA. Periodontal osseous resection. In, Periodontics 6th ed CV Mosby Company 1988;838-59.
4. Sims NH , Ammons WF. Resective osseous surgery. In, Newman, Takei, Carranza. Clinical Periodontology 9th ed WB Saunders 2003;786-803.
5. Tibbetts LS, Ammons WF. Resective Periodontal Surgery. In, Rose LF, Mealey BL, Genco RJ, Cohen DW. Periodontics, Medicine, Surgery and Implants. Elsevier Mosby 2004;502-52.

MCQs

1. Radicular blending is a _____ procedure:
   A. Osteoplasty
   B. Ostectomy
   C. A and B
   D. None of the above

2. The level of interdental bone is more apical to radicular bone in:
   A. Negative architecture   B. Positive architecture
   C. Flat architecture   D. Ideal architecture

3. The most predictable pocket reduction technique:
   A. Regenerative osseous surgery
   B. Resective osseous surgery
   C. Gingivectomy
   D. Modified widman flap

4. Sequence of resective osseous surgery is:
   A. Vertical grooving, flattening interproximal bone, radicular blending and gradualizing marginal bone.
   B. Radicular blending, vertical grooving, flattening interproximal bone and gradualizing marginal bone.
   C. Vertical grooving, radicular blending, flattening interproximal bone and gradualizing marginal bone
   D. None of the above

5. Instruments used in resective osseous surgery are *except:*
   A. Friedman and Blumenthal rongeurs
   B. Schluger and sugarman files
   C. Back action and Ochsenbein chisels
   D. Kirkland and Orbans knife

Answers

1. A   2. A   3. B   4. C   5. D

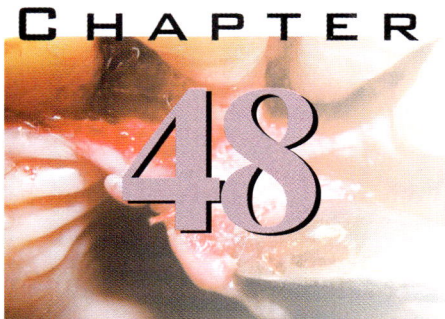

Regenerative Osseous Surgery

Shalu Bathla

INTRODUCTION

New attachment with periodontal regeneration is the ideal outcome of periodontal therapy because it results in obliteration of the pocket and reconstruction of the marginal periodontium. On the cellular level, periodontal regeneration is a complex process requiring coordinated proliferation, differentiation and development of various cell types to form the periodontal attachment apparatus.

TERMINOLOGY

- *Repair:* Healing of a wound by a tissue that does not fully restore the architecture/function of the part.
- *Regeneration:* It refers to the reproduction/reconstruction of a lost/injured tissue.
- *New attachment:* It is defined as the union of connective tissue or epithelium with a root surface that has been deprived of its original attachment apparatus. New attachment can also be defined as the embedding of new periodontal ligament fibers into new cementum and the attachment of the gingival epithelium to a tooth surface previously denuded by disease.

- *Reattachment:* It describes the reunion of epithelial and connective tissue with a root surface.
- *Periodontal regeneration:* It is defined as the restoration of lost periodontium/supporting tissues and includes formation of new alveolar bone, new cementum and new periodontal ligament.

REGENERATIVE SURGICAL MANAGEMENT

Incision: Usually, sulcular incision is given in regenerative surgical procedure. Incision for regenerative surgery is given such as to preserve the maximum amount of gingival tissue.

Flap design: The flap design of choice in regenerative surgery is the papilla preservation flap, which retains the entire papilla covering the lesion. However, to use this flap, there must be adequate interdental space to allow the intact papilla to be reflected with the facial or lingual/palatal flap. When the interdental space is very narrow, making it impossible to perform a papilla preservation flap, a conventional flap with only sulcular incisions is made. Surgical flap design should be such that after sulcular incision, buccal and lingual full thickness flaps are reflected, extending to atleast one to three teeth mesially and distally to the treated tooth. Interdental tissues should be preserved in their entirety so that flap margins cover the graft or membrane completely preventing their exposure during healing. The flap in regenerative surgery is not thinned out as for other surgical procedures.

Regenerative surgical techniques can be subdivided into two major areas:
- Non-graft-associated new attachment
- Graft-associated new attachment

NON-GRAFT-ASSOCIATED NEW ATTACHMENT

Periodontal reconstruction can be attained without the use of grafts in meticulously treated three-wall defects (intrabony defects) and in periodontal abscess.

Removal of junctional and pocket epithelium: The presence of junctional and pocket epithelium has been perceived as a barrier to successful therapy because its presence interferes with the direct apposition of connective tissue and cementum, thus limiting the height to which periodontal fibers can become inserted to the cementum. Several methods to remove junctional and pocket epithelium are curettage, chemical agents, ultrasonic methods and surgical techniques like ENAP.

Prevention of epithelial migration: The epithelium from the excised margin may rapidly proliferate to become interposed between the healing connective tissue and the cementum. Thus, prevention of epithelial migration is required.

Guided Tissue Regeneration (GTR)

Historical Perspective

A technique pioneered by Nyman et al. in 1982, was introduced in periodontal therapy which was later named "Guided Tissue Regeneration" (GTR) by Gottlow in 1986, slowly became acceptable for regenerative therapy. Nyman et al. in 1982 carried out the first human study to test the hypothesis that new attachment may form on a previously periodontitis involved root surface, provided the cells originating from the periodontal ligament were enabled to repopulate the root surface first during healing.

Definition

The 1996 World Workshop in Periodontics defined GTR as "procedures attempting to regenerate lost periodontal

structures through differential tissue responses. Barriers are employed in the hope of excluding epithelium and gingival corium from the root surface in the belief that they interfere with regeneration."

Rationale behind using GTR barrier membranes (Fig. 48.1)
i. Exclusion of epithelium and gingival connective tissue.
ii. Barrier membrane maintain space between the defect and tooth.
iii. Stabilize the clot.

Biologic Requirements

Scantlebury describes the historical development of barrier membranes and proposes five general criteria that must be considered in the design of membranes intended for use in regenerative applications in the oral cavity. In brief, membranes used for dentoalveolar regeneration must exhibit the following characteristics:

i. *Tissue integration:* Tissue may grow into the material without penetrating all the way through. The goal of tissue integration is to prevent rapid epithelial downgrowth on the outer surface of the material or encapsulation of the material and to provide stability to the overlying flap.

ii. *Cell occlusivity:* George Winter, an English researcher had proposed that specific porosities ingrew with connective tissue and stopped or slowed the migration and pocketing of epithelial tissues. He called this phenomenon as contact inhibition. The material should act as a barrier to exclude

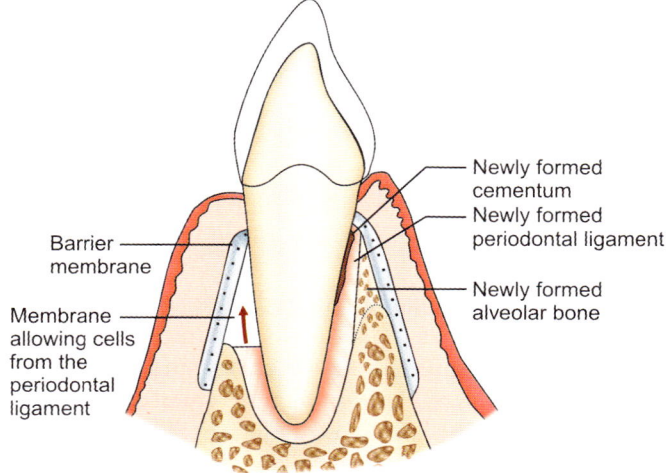

Fig. 48.1: Barrier membrane which prevents epithelium and gingival connective tissue

undesirable cell types from entering the secluded space adjacent to the root surface. It is also considered an advantage that the material would allow the passage of nutrients and gases.

iii. *Clinical manageability:* Barrier should be provided in configurations which are easy to trim and to place.

iv. *Space making:* Barrier material should be capable of creating and maintaining the space, adjacent to the root surface allowing the ingrowth of tissue from the periodontal ligament. Some materials may be so soft and flexible that they collapse into the defect and others are too stiff that they may perforate the overlying tissues.

v. *Biocompatibility:* The material should not elicit an immune response, sensitization or chronic inflammation which may interfere with healing and present a hazard to the patient.

Indications for GTR procedures:
i. Narrow 2 or 3 wall infrabony defects
ii. Circumferential defects
iii. Class II furcation defects
iv. Recession defects

Contraindications for GTR procedures:
i. Any medical condition contraindicating surgery
ii. Infection at defect site
iii. Poor oral hygiene
iv. Smoking (Heavy)
v. Tooth mobility > 1 mm
vi. Defect < 4 mm deep
vii. Width of attached gingiva at defect site ≤ 1 mm
viii. Thickness of attached gingiva at defect site ≤ 0.5 mm
ix. Furcation with short root trunks
x. Generalized horizontal bone loss
xi. Advanced lesions with little remaining support
xii. Multiple defects

Materials used for GTR:

A. *First generation material*: Non-Resorbable: Expanded polytetrafluorethylene (ePTFE), GORE-TEX membrane, dense polytetrafluorethylene (dPTFE), Nucleopore, Millipore filters, Ethyl cellulose and Semipermeable silicone barrier.

Expanded PTFE is one of the most inert materials known. It has an extremely long carbon chain protected by a dense sheath of fluorine atoms and because the body cannot react with it chemically, tissue "accepts" it, while exhibiting a healthy tissue reaction.

B. *Second generation material*: Resorbable membranes:

a. Collagen – Biomend, Biomend – extend, Periogen, Paroguide, Biostite, Biogide, Tissue Guide and Biobar

b. Polylactide and Polyglycolide – Guidor, Vicryl, Atrisorb, Resolut, Epiguide and Biofix

c. Others – Periosteum, Connective tissue graft, Alloderm, Emdogain, Surgicel, Gelform, Gengiflex, Capset, Hapset and Cargile membrane.

C. *Third generation material* -Resorbable bioactive barrier membranes with added growth factors.

Absorbable GTR barrier materials: Several features make these bioresorbable membranes easier to manage clinically: i) they are more tissue compatible than nonresorbable membranes; ii) the timing for resorption can be regulated by the amount of cross-linkage in the synthetic polymer and collagen membrane; iii) a second surgical procedure is not required to retrieve the membrane.

A disadvantage of many resorbable membranes is the relative lack of rigidity, because resorbable membranes, unlike titanium reinforced ePTFE membranes, have no embedded support structures.

i. *Guidor:* It is a hydrophobic barrier material made from Polylactic acid (PLA) combined with a citric acid ester softening agent. It is a bilayered consisting of an external layer having large rectangular perforations (400 to 500/cm^2) and internal layer having smaller circular perforations (4000 to 5000/cm^2).

ii. *Vicryl:* It is made from copolymer of glycolide and lactide. It is available in two forms:

a. *Knitted mesh:* These have large pore size with better handling property **(Fig. 48.2)**.

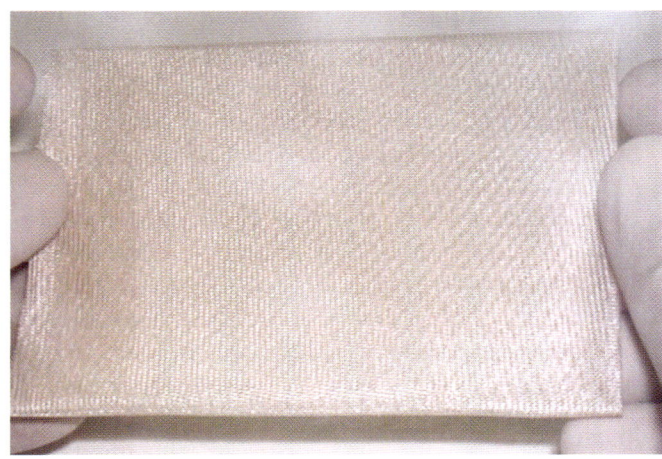

Fig. 48.2: Vicryl knitted mesh - resorbable membrane

b. *Woven mesh:* These have smaller pore size but tends to fray.

These membranes degrade to produce polylactide and polyglycolide, which are converted to lactic acid and pyruvate, respectively, and metabolized by the enzymes of the Krebs cycle and are eliminated as carbon dioxide and water.

iii. *Artisorb:* It is a polymer of lactic acid and poly (D, L – lactic acid), dissolved in N- methyl – 2 pyrrolidone (NMP). It is prepared as a solution that coagulates or sets to a firm consistency on contact with water/other aqueous solution; this principle is used in forming a barrier that is partially coagulated to a semirigid state in a chairside mixing kit, which can be trimmed to the dimensions of defect. Kit contains sufficient material for the fabrication of upto 10 membranes. However, excess material cannot be stored for future use and thus may results in wastage of material.

iv. *Resolut:* It is a copolymer of PGA and PLA which is supplied with a bioresorbable suture.

v. *Epiguide:* It is a hydrophilic membrane formed from PLA (D, L – form). It contains flexible open cell structure and internal void spaces.

vi. *Collagen membrane:* It's antigenicity and rate of degradation can be controlled by varying its cross linkage. Collagen membranes are degraded by collagenases and subsequently by gelatinases and peptidase. The various advantages associated with collagen membranes are: hemostasis, chemotaxis for periodontal ligament fibroblasts and gingival fibroblasts, weak immunogenicity, easy manipulation and ability to augment tissue thickness.

Bio-Gide - The collagen membrane is prepared from pig which involve several technological processing steps. An alkaline treatment is carried out for several hours to eliminate any viral/ bacterial contamination of the material. The structural quality of membrane is controlled by segment analysis. Collagen fibres are obtained without any other organic residues. Collagen membrane should be devoid of antigenicity. For this, terminal peptides/telopeptides are split off and fat and protein residues are also removed by specific purification process for the same reason of reducing antigenicity. The collagen membranes are cross linked to extend absorption time and to reduce antigenicity. Cross linking agents used in collagen barrier membrane are physical agents (Gamma, UV radiation) and chemical agents (Formaldehyde and Diphenylphosphorylazide). The resorption of collagen membranes starts with the action of collagenase which splits the molecule at specific sites. The resultant fragments are denatured at 37°C to gelatin and then gelatinases and other proteinase degrade gelatin to oligopeptides and amino acids.

Advantages of Absorbable GTR barrier materials:
- Elimination of second surgery for barrier removal
- Reduce operatory time
- Increase patient acceptance
- Reduce risk of loss of regenerated attachment owing to re-entry surgery
- More tissue friendly.

Disadvantages of Absorbable GTR barrier materials:
- Instability of barrier against root
- High cost
- Biodegradation rate cannot be controlled
- In case of infection or strong tissue response, if there is a need to remove the membrane, disintegration of the material in its various stages, makes it impossible.

Surgical Procedure

- *Incision:* Intrasulcular incision is made to preserve as much as attached gingiva as possible, including the adjacent interdental papilla. Mucoperiosteal or full thickness flap is raised with vertical incisions, extending a minimum of two teeth anteriorly and one tooth distally to the tooth being treated.
- *Defect preparation and membrane placement:* Debride the osseous defect and thoroughly plane the roots. Appropriate membrane is selected among the several membranes available. Trim the membrane with sharp scissors to the approximate size of the area being treated. The apical border of the material should extend 3 to 4 mm apical to the margin of the defect and laterally 2 to 3 mm beyond the defect; the occlusal border of the membrane should be placed 2 mm apical to the cementoenamel junction **(Fig. 48.3)**.
- *Suturing:* Suture the membrane tightly around the tooth with a sling suture. Suture the flap back in its original position or slightly coronal to it, using independent sutures interdentally and in the vertical incisions. The flap should cover the membrane completely. The use of periodontal dressing is optional and the patient is placed on antibiotic therapy for 1 week.

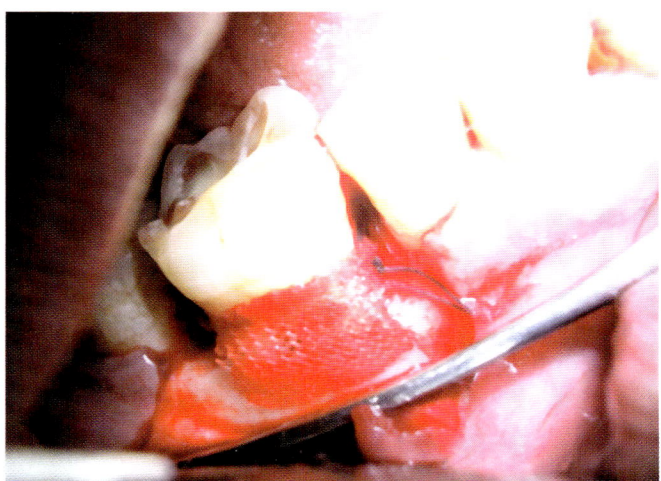

Fig. 48.3: Placement of GTR membrane

- *Removal of membrane:* If the nonresorable membrane is used, then remove it after 4-6 weeks of placement. The material is removed by making a sharp access incision for dissection of the material from the flap. The flap is then dissected from the membrane. Sutures holding the membrane are cut and the membrane is removed.

Root Biomodification

Biologic concept: The biologic concept behind root biomodification is that the acid treatment causes demineralization of the root planed dentin, hereby exposing collagen fibrils of the dentin matrix. It is assumed that this exposure of collagen fibrils may facilitate adhesion of the blood clot to the root surface and favour migration of fibroblasts and that the exposed collagen fibrils of the dentin matrix may interdigitate with newly formed collagen fibrils in the adjacent healing tissues. Root surface conditioning was originally suggested because of the ability of acid to modify the root surface by "detoxifying". Thus, the rationale of root biomodification is to make contaminated root surfaces biologically acceptable.

Various physical and chemical methods that have been tried to enhance new attachment by root conditioning are:
1. Physical methods include root conditioning by lasers.
2. Chemical methods include the use of various chemicals like Citric acid, Tetracycline, Ethylene diamine tetra acetic acid (EDTA), Fibronectin (Tissucol), Laminin, Sodium Deoxycholate, Human Plasma fraction Cohn IV and Growth factors (PDGF, bFGF, IGF, TGF).

Lasers: Lasers are capable of sterilizing the diseased root surface and thus, ultimately promoting cell reattachment. The lasers ability to sterilize, vaporize and ablate appears to offer an effective means of removing or altering adsorbed endotoxin, calculus, plaque and other root surface contaminants. Carbon – dioxide, Nd:YAG (Neodynium:Yttrium; aluminium and garnet) and Er:YAG (Erbium: Yttrium; aluminium and garnet) are commercially available laser systems.

Citric acid: The potential of acid demineralization of root surface as an adjunct to new attachment procedures gained new popularity following studies by Urist (1965). He suggested that dentin following acid demineralization possessed inductive properties.

It has been shown that citric acid demineralization enhances new attachment or reattachment and regeneration by one or more of the following mechanisms:
1. Antibacterial effect
2. Root detoxification
3. Exposure of root collagen and opening of dentinal tubules
4. Removal of smear laser
5. Initial clot stabilization
6. Demineralization prior to cementogenesis
7. Enhanced fibroblasts growth and stability
8. Attachment by direct linkage with or without cementogenesis
9. Prevention of epithelial migration along the denuded roots
10. Accelerated healing and new cementum formation after detachment of the gingival tissues and demineralization of the root surface by means of citric acid.

Technique

The recommended technique of application is as follows:
a. Raise a mucoperiosteal flap.
b. Thoroughly instrument the root surface removing calculus and underlying cementum.
c. Apply cotton pellets soaked in a saturated solution of citric acid (pH1) and leave on for 2–4 minutes. 61 gm of citric acid per 100 ml of distilled water is added to achieve pH of 1.
d. Remove pellets and irrigate root surface profusely with water.
e. Replace the flap and suture.

The use of citric acid has also been recommended in conjunction with coverage of denuded roots using free gingival grafts.

Fibronectin: Fibronectin is a high molecular weight glycoprotein (mol wt = 440,000) that is found in the extracellular tissue and is the main component that holds the clot together. It promotes cell adhesion to both collagen and scaled root surfaces and has a chemotactic effect on fibroblasts and mesenchymal cells.

The use of fibronectin as a supplement to demineralization is, therefore, strongly supported by the following:

1. The initial stage after demineralization and prior to new attachment is fibrin formation and linkage.
2. It is the coronal growth of cells from the periodontal ligament that is responsible for new attachment and fibronectin stimulates this growth.
3. Favours the growth and attachment of fibroblasts over epithelial cells to the root surface.
4. Speeds the linkage process by being chemoattractive for fibroblasts and stabilizing the clot between the exposed root surface collagen and new fibers within the tissue.

Laminin: Laminin is a glycoprotein of high molecular weight. It is capable of adhering to various substrates. Laminin promotes gingival epithelial and fibroblast chemotaxis. It also promotes epithelial cell adhesion and growth to tetracycline and glycoprotein conditioned surfaces.

Sodium-Deoxycholate and Human Plasma fraction Cohn IV as Root conditioners: These agents can dissociate endotoxin into subunits and might thereby detoxify the diseased root surface. The human plasma fraction possibly contains fibronectin.

Growth Factors

Growth factors are polypeptide molecules, released by cells in the inflamed area, which regulate events in wound healing. These factors primarily secreted by macrophages, endothelial cells, fibroblasts and platelets, include platelet – derived growth factor (PDGF), insulin like growth factor (IGF), basic fibroblasts growth factor (bFGF) and transforming growth factor α (TGF- α). Growth factors could be used to control events during periodontal wound healing (e.g. promoting proliferation of fibroblasts from the periodontal ligament and favoring bone formation). A combination of PDGF and IGF-1 would be effective in promoting growth of all the components of the periodontium.

Bone Morphogenetic Protein (BMPs)

The history of the identification and purification of bone morphogenetic proteins began in 1965, when Marshall Urist demonstrated that the cellular events associated with embryonic bone development could be reproduced in heterotrophic sites by implants of demineralized bone segments. In the late 1960's and early 1970's, it was recognized that dentin also contained bone morphogenetic activity. Bone morphogenetic proteins form a subgroup of a larger family of structurally related proteins known as the transforming growth factor-β superfamily.

Types: Atleast 15 BMPs have been identified upto date. Most of them are identified by their capacity to induce bone in vivo or extraskeletal sites in mammals.

- BMP-1 Protease; not osteoinductive
- BMP-2 Osteoinductive; located in bone, spleen, liver, brain, kidney
- BMP-3 Osteogenin osteoinductive, located in lung, kidney, brain
- BMP-4 Osteoinductive, located in apical ectodermal ridge, meninges,lung, kidney, liver
- BMP-5 Osteoinductive, located in lung,kidney, liver
- BMP-6 Not osteoinductive, found in lung, brain, kidney, uterus, muscle, skin
- BMP-7 Osteoinductive, located in adrenal glands, placental, spleen, skeletal muscle
- BMP-8 Osteoinductive
- BMP-9 Osteoinductive; stimulates hepatocyte proliferation; hepatocycte growth and function
- BMP-12 and BMP-13; Inhibition of terminal differentiation of myloblasts.

Tissucol

A fibrin – fibronectin sealing system (FFSS) has been commercially available (Tissucol – Tisseel) in Europe since 1975. It is a human plasma cryoprecipitate, which consists of highly concentrated fibrinogen, fibronectin, factor XIII, platelet – derived growth factor (PDGF), antiplasmins and plasminogen. Aprotinin (bovine antiplasmin), thrombin and calcium chloride are added at the moment of use.

Highly concentrated fibrinogen, fibronectin, PDGF plays a significant role not only in the coagulation process, but also in wound healing. Activated thrombin induces the clotting of cryoprecipitate. Aprotinin in different concentrations can modulate the stability of artificial clot. Fibrinogen is a high molecular weight 340 kda protein, which is transformed into fibrin by thrombin to form bulk of the blood clot, thereby providing hemostasis. It is arranged to form a network, lining collagen and glycosaminoglycans in such a way that tissue adhesion occurs. Fibronectin is found in plasma on the cell surface, in the extracellular matrix and in the basement membrane of epithelium. Fibronectin promotes cell to cell adhesion and cell mobility. Thus, fibronectin promotes migration, adhesion, attachment and synthetic activity of fibroblasts. Factor XIII is a transglutaminase, an enzyme that mediates the links between the clot and the collagen and glycosamino-glycans of the connective tissue. Plasminogen is a glycoprotein (90 kda) that is transformed into plasmin under effect of active thrombin. The protease activity of plasmin causes the lysis of fibrin. The plasminogen – fibrinogen ratio in Tissucol is reduced upto 30 times less than in human plasma. This reduced proportion is more favorable to clot stability. Anti-plasmin are macro-globulin that modulates the rate of coagulum lysis inhibiting plasmin activity. Thrombin is a serinoprotease (40 kda) that activates fibrinogen and factor XIII in the presence of Ca^{+2}, which is provided by calcium chloride($CaCl_2$) in Tissucol. Thrombin stimulates the growth of fibroblasts and synthesis of fibronectin and collagen. Aprotinin is a polypeptide extracted from bovine lungs and it inhibits plasmin activity. PDGF is a major human serum polypeptide growth factor. It is stored in granules of circulating platelets and is released into serum during blood clotting. It is a potent mitogen and chemo-attractant for fibroblasts. Thus, there are several promising areas of research for the use of biologic mediators such as in guided tissue regeneration procedures, coronally positioned flaps for furcations, ridge augmentation and implant surgery.

Emdogain

It is a resorbable, implantable material that consists of enamel matrix proteins extracted from developing embryonic enamel of porcine origin supplied in sterile, lyophilized form.

Emdogain contains a protein preparation that mimics the matrix proteins that induce cementogenesis. During root development, the Hertwig's epithelial sheath deposits enamel matrix proteins on the newly formed root dentin surface. These proteins stimulate the differentiation of surrounding mesenchymal cells into cementoblasts, which form acellular cementum. Once a new cementum layer is formed, collagen fibers form in the adjacent periodontal ligament, attaching into the new cementum.

The major constituents are amelogenins, which are highly hydrophobic proteins that aggregate and serve as a nidus for crystallization. Other proteins identified include ameloblastin and enamelin. This protein preparation uses propylene glycol alginate (PGA) as a carrier. The EMD-containing PGA remains highly viscous when stored in the cold or at room temperature. Once it is applied to the tissue at a neutral pH and at body temperature, the PGA carrier decreases in viscosity and the EMD preparation precipitates. EMD is absorbed into the hydroxyapatite and collagen fibers of the root surface, where it induces cementum formation followed by periodontal regeneration.

Emdogain has two presentation forms: One is in liquid and powder form, in 2 separate bottles containing the vehicle and the protein powder and the other is in the form of gel in syringe. The material is stored in the refrigerator, at 2 - 8°C. It should be used in no more than 2 hours from opening, because it gelifies and hardens.

Emdogain is used in various osseous and recession defects.

Platelet Rich Plasma (PRP)

PRP is an autologous thrombocyte concentrate. The thrombocytes contain various components with hemostatic effects and also factors that stimulate the healing process. It induces neoformation of blood vessels, which are essential in the process of regeneration. Because PRP has an osteostimulant, not osteoinductive effect, in case of using synthetic materials it is recommended to add a small amount of autologous bone. It accelerates the bone maturation and the bone quality. PRP is obtained through direct centrifugation from the patient's blood and should be applied as quickly as possible.

Components:
- Growth factors (PDGFs)
- WBC, phagocytic cells
- Native fibrinogen concentration
- Vasoactive and chemotactic agents
- High concentration of platelets

Platelet count in PRP often ranges from 5 lakh to 1 million. Thus, PRP is a way to accelerate and enhance the body's natural wound healing mechanisms.

PERIODONTICS REVISITED

GRAFT – ASSOCIATED NEW ATTACHMENT

Bone Graft Materials

There are numerous therapeutic grafting modalities for reconstructing periodontal osseous defects. Classification of bone graft materials are:

A. According to the type of graft:
   i.   Autogenous grafts
   ii. Allogenic grafts
   iii. Xenogenic grafts
   iv. Alloplastic materials
B. According to their mode of action:
   i.   Osteogenetic/Osteoproliferative means that new bone is formed by bone forming cells contained in the graft.
   ii. Osteoinductive means that bone formation is induced in the surrounding soft tissues immediately adjacent to the graft.
   iii. Osteoconductive means that the grafted material does not contribute to new bone formation but serves as scaffold for bone formation originating from adjacent host bone.

Autogenous Bone Graft

Grafts transferred from one position to another within the same individual. Autogenous bone, which is certainly the best, since it may have both osteogenetic and osteoinductive potency. Its availability is nevertheless limited, and its use generally results in additional inconvenience for the patient. They are resorbed and replaced by few viable bones. Autogenous bone grafts can be harvested from intraoral or extraoral sites and can be cortical bone or cancellous bone.

The various sites for procuring autogenous bone graft are:

A. *Intra oral sites:* Healing extraction wounds, edentulous ridges, exostoses, lingual ridge on the mandible, bone distal to a terminal tooth, lingual surface of the mandible at least 5 mm from the roots, maxillary tuberosity and mandibular retromolar area **(Figs 48.4A and B)**.

B. *Extra oral sites:* Iliac autografts – Posterior iliac crest. Problems associated with iliac autografts are postoperative infection, exfoliation, sequestration, varying rates of healing, root resorption and rapid recurrence of the defect. Due to the morbidity associated with donor site and root resorption, the iliac crest marrow graft are not used now in regenerative periodontal therapy.

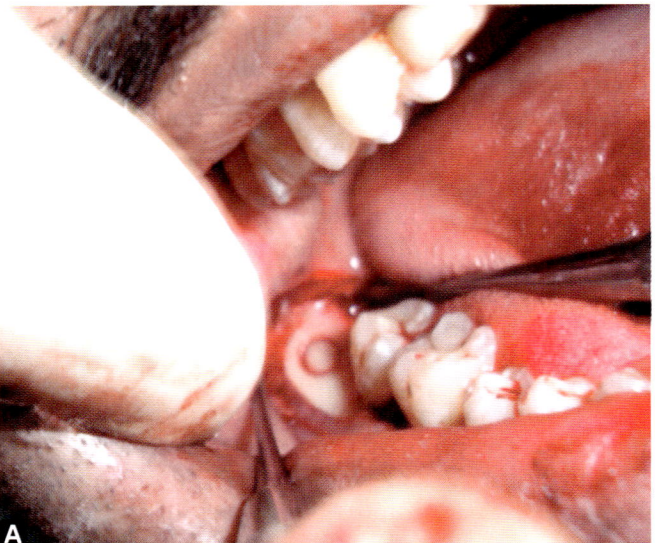

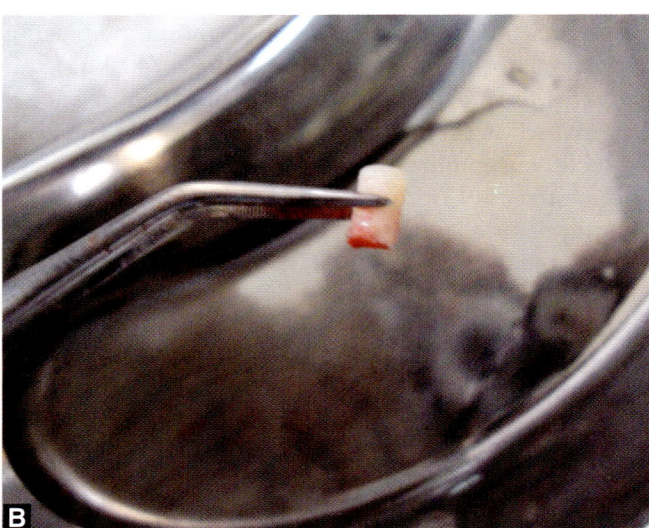

Figs 48.4A and B: Taking autogenous bone graft from mandibular retromolar area by trephine (*Courtesy*: Dr Vikender Yadav)

Osseous coagulum: It is a mixture of bone dust obtained by grounding cortical bone and blood. Round carbide bur revolving at 25,000 to 30,000 rpm is used within the surgical site to reduce donor bone to small particles, which then coated with the patient's blood to make coagulum.

Advantages:
   i. Relatively rapid technique
   ii. Complements osseous resective procedures that may be required at surgical site

iii. Particle size provides additional surface area for the interaction between cellular and vascular elements.

Disadvantages:

i. Cannot be used in larger defects because of inability to procure adequate material
ii. Poor surgical visibility
iii. Relatively low predictability
iv. Inability to use aspiration during accumulation of the coagulum
v. Fluidity of the material makes it difficult to transfer the coagulum to the defect.

Bone Swaging: Piece of bone is incompletely detached from its base by a chisel and swung into a neighboring bone defect with some of its blood supply maintained. It is the technique which requires existence of an edentulous area adjacent to the defect. It represents a contiguous/pedicle bony autograft utilizing the principle of greenstick fracture of long bones.

Bone Blend: It involves removing bone (cortical, cancellous or both) from accessible intraoral donor site by chisel/rongeur forceps, placing it in a sterile plastic amalgam capsule with pestle and then triturating.

Allograft

Allografts are the grafts transferred between genetically dissimilar members of the same species. They can be Undemineralized freeze dried bone allograft or Demineralized freeze dried bone allograft.

Bone allografts are commercially available from tissue banks. They are obtained from cortical bone within 12 hours of the death of the donor, defatted, cut in pieces, washed in absolute alcohol and deep frozen. The material may then be demineralized and subsequently ground and sieved to a particle size 250 to 750 μm, freeze dried and vacuum sealed in glass vials. The various methods to suppress the antigenic potential of allograft and xenograft are:

- *Radiation treatment:* 6 Mega Rads of high intensity of Gamma radiation is adequate.
- *Freezing:* Deep frozen -197°C liquid Nitrogen freezer for a period of atleast 4 weeks.
- *Chemical treatment:* Through keeping in Merthiolate solution.

Demineralization in cold, diluted hydrochloric acid exposes the components of bone matrix, closely associated with collagen fibrils that have been termed bone morphogenetic protein.

Bone allografts does not require additional surgical site for the removal of donor material from the same patient, but can provoke an immune response in the recipient patient.

Comparison between freeze dried bone allograft (FDBA) and demineralized freeze dried bone allograft (DFDBA)	
FDBA	*DFDBA*
1. Not demineralized	Demineralized
2. More radio-opaque	More radiolucent
3. Breakdown by way of foreign body reaction	Rapid resorption
4. Primary indication : Bone augmentation associated with implant treatment	Primary indication : Periodontal disease associated with natural tooth
5. Osteoconductive	Osteoinductive
6. No bone morphogenetic protein expression.	More bone morphogenetic protein.

Xenogenic Graft

These are the grafts taken from a donor of another species. They are referred as anorganic bone. Proprietary processes remove all cells and proteinaceous material and what is left behind is inert, absorbable bone scaffolding. It is on this scaffolding that revascularization, osteoblast migration and woven bone formation supposedly occur. Resorption of xenografts has been reported to occur very slowly.

Sclera as non bone graft material: There are some structural similarities of sclera to the periodontal ligament. Sclera is derived from mesoderm and consists of obliquely arranged collagen fibers of 640 to 700 A^0 axial periodicity. Sclera is easily sterilized and show low levels of antigenicity due to minimal cellularity and poor vascularity. But, sclera has tissue memory and tends to return to its original curvature, this limits its application to wide and shallow defects.

Alloplastic Graft/Inert Biologic Fillers

Synthetic or inorganic implant materials which are used as substitutes for bone graft, functions primarily as defect fillers. Ideally alloplasts bone substitutes should have the following properties - 1. biocompatibility, 2. minimal fibrotic reaction, 3. the ability to undergo remodeling and support new bone formation, 4. similar strength comparable to cortical/cancellous bone, and 5. similar modulus of elasticity comparable to bone to prevent fatigue fracture under cyclic loading.

PERIODONTICS REVISITED

These are namely Polymers, Tricalcium phosphate, Hydroxyapatite and Bioactive glasses.

Biocompatible composite polymer (Bioplant HTR or "hard tissue replacement" material) consists of polymethylmethacrylate- poly-hydroxyl-ethylmethacrylate beads coated by calcium hydroxide. This calcium hydroxide surface forms a calcium carbonate apatite when introduced into the body.

Tricalcium phosphate (TCP): It has a calcium-to-phosphate ratio of 1.5 and are β-whitlockite crystals. TCP is partially bioresorbable.

Hydroxyapatite (HA) has a calcium-to-phosphate ratio of 1.67, similar to that found in bone material. HA is generally nonbioresorbable.

Bioactive glass ceramics: They are made of CaO, Na$_2$O, SiO$_2$, and P$_2$O$_5$ in the same proportions as in bone and teeth and are referred to as 45S5 bioactive glass. This material was initially introduced as an amorphous material (Bioglass). The material has subsequently been produced in a particulate form with a 90 to 710 μm diameter (PerioGlas) and with a 300 to 350 μm (BioGran) diameter. Bioactive glass enhances bone formation by ionic dissolution of the ceramic particles such that a silica gel layer forms over the particles on contact with body fluid. Over this silica gel layer, a calcium phosphate layer forms, which is quickly converted into a hydroxy-carbonate apatite layer. This apatite layer has been shown to be identical to bone mineral and to provide the surface for osteoblast cell attachment and bone deposition. The continuous ionic exchange results in dissolution of the ceramic particles such that after 1 to 3 years, the particles have been shown to be replaced by bone.

Calcium carbonates: Calcium carbonates are processed natural coral skeletons (NCSs) from Porites coral, which can serve as resorbable bone graft substitutes.

Bone Grafting Technique

1. Flap design:
   a. Sulcular incision: Preservation of flap tissue is important for regenerative techniques to ensure coverage and containment of the graft postsurgically. Thus, sulcular incision is given on facial and lingual with interproximal space being conserved by papilla preservation.
   b. Avoid flap perforation or loss of the papilla, due to granulomatous tissue from the lesion that adheres to the inner aspect of the flap. Excessive thinning can compromise blood supply and flap survival.

2. Defect/Root debridement:
   a. Debride the defect of all soft tissue using hand, ultrasonic and rotating instruments.
   b. Meticulously remove all hard and soft accretions on the root surface.
   c. Root biomodification is done by using saturated solution of citric acid (pH 1).
   d. If the bone lesion is more chronic in nature i.e. lined with an intact cortical plate a one-quarter or one-half round bur can be used to perforate the bone and create a bleeding environment. The theory behind cortical/intramarrow penetration is that bone marrow, like the periodontal ligament space, serves as a repository for the pleuripotent progenitor cells essential for regeneration. Intramarrow penetration is intended to enhance rapid revascularization and incorporation of the graft.
   e. Placement of the graft into the osseous defect - Graft is contoured and the graft material is packed firmly, but not too tight, as some space is necessary for the development of granulation tissue.
   f. Suturing: The flaps are closed using a mono - filament suture with an interrupted or vertical mattress suture technique.
   g. Postoperative instructions are given thereafter.

VARIOUS METHODS USED TO QUANTIFY TISSUE CHANGES AFTER REGENERATIVE PERIODONTAL SURGERY

1. *Histological evaluation of biopsy material:* The most reliable outcome variable for evaluating periodontal regeneration, is human histology. However, the morbidity associated with this technique makes it possible only in isolated case studies designed to prove that a drug, device, or technique is capable of regenerating the lost periodontium including bone, cementum, and periodontal ligament. In the absence of this genuine variable, other "surrogate" variables must be used.

2. *Clinical evaluation of hard tissue changes (Bone formation):* Of all the surrogate variables available for use in regenerative clinical trials, new bone formation is the primary alternative, as it directly measures the formation of one of the three components required for successful regeneration. However, new bone formation may sometimes be a "stand alone" phenomenon without an accompanying cementum

and functional periodontal ligament (PDL). There are several alternative methods for measuring new bone formation:

Direct Bone Measurements

Linear measurements: A series of linear measurements using a fixed reference point such as the cemento-enamel junction (CEJ), restorative margins, or tooth notch are performed at baseline and at the final evaluation, the net changes are calculated from these two observations.

Typically three sets of measurements are made: distance from a landmark to the bone crest, distance from a landmark to the base of the defect and distance from the crest to the base of defect.

Volumetric measurements: An elastomeric impression material is placed into the alveolar defect, either *in vivo* or on a plaster model of the teeth and surrounding bone reproduced from an impression of the surgical site. When set, the material in the defect is removed carefully weighed, and weight values translated into volumetric units based on the material's specific gravity. A potential disadvantage of this method is distortion of the impression material which might affect the measurements. Also, this method does not discriminate between defect resolutions which results from bone fill and that which results from crestal resorption, thus it is likely to overestimate positive changes.

Indirect Bone Measurements include sounding bone measurement and radiographic bone measurement.

3. *Clinical evaluation of attachment levels and other soft tissue parameters*-They include clinical attachment level measurements, probing depth measurements, gingival recession, measurements of gingival infection and inflammation and tissue formation.

The nature of the cell population on the inner surface of the barrier membrane was investigated using scanning electron microscopy (SEM). Fibroblast-like cells, together with inflammatory cells, red blood cells and some bacterial cells, were observed on the inner surface of the middle portion of the membrane.

4. *Radiographic evaluation of hard tissue changes:* Radiographic evaluation of bone regeneration requires careful standardized techniques for reproducible positioning of the film and the tube.

5. *Ancillary methods.* Gingival Bone Count Index (GCBI): Dunning JM and Leach DB (1960).

6. *Surgical re-entry:* The surgical re-entry of operated site after a period of healing gives a good view of the state of the bone crest that can be compared with the view taken during the initial surgical intervention and can also be subject to measurements. But the disadvantages associated with surgical re – entry are that it requires unnecessary second operation and does not show the type of attachment. Moreover, it is an unethical issue.

FACTORS INFLUENCING THERAPEUTIC SUCCESS OF REGENERATIVE PROCEDURES

Factors that can adversely affect clinical outcome after regenerative therapy are:

A. Barrier dependent factors:
   1. Inadequate root – barrier adaptation: Absence of barrier effect
   2. Non–sterile technique: Plaque/saliva contamination of barrier
   3. Instability (movement) of barrier against root
   4. Premature exposure of barrier to oral environment and microbes.
   5. Premature loss or degradation of barrier.

B. Barrier independent factors:
   1. Poor plaque control
   2. Smoking
   3. Occlusal trauma: Hyperocclusion
   4. Suboptimal tissue health: Inflammation persists
   5. Mechanical habits: Aggressive tooth – brushing techniques
   6. Overlying gingival tissue:
      a. Inadequate zone of keratinized tissue
      b. Inadequate tissue thickness
   7. Surgical technique:
      a. Improper incision placement: Excessive loss of marginal tissue
      b. Traumatic flap elevation and management
      c. Excessive surgical tissue: Tissue/flap desiccation
      d. Inadequate closure/suturing: Failure to achieve and maintain primary closure.
   8. Postsurgical factor:
      a. Premature tissue challenge
         • Plaque recolonization
         • Mechanical insult
      b. Loss of wound stability – Loose sutures, loss of early fibrin clot.

Factors that can limit regenerative healing after GTR surgery are above and most important among these, are presence of smoking habit, poor plaque control and premature exposure of barrier material.

LANDMARK STUDIES RELATED

Melcher AH. On the repair potential of periodontal tissues. Journal of Periodontology 1976;47:256-60.
In 1976, Melcher in a review paper suggested that the type of cell which repopulates the root surface after periodontal surgery determines the nature of the attachment that will form. After flap surgery the curetted root surface may be repopulated by four different types of cell: 1. Epithelial cells, 2. Cells derived from the gingival connective tissue, 3. Cells derived from the bone, 4. Cells derived from the periodontal ligament. If epithelial cells proliferate along the root surface, a long junctional epithelium will result. If gingival connective tissue populates the root surface, a connective tissue attachment will form and root resorption may occur. If bone cells migrate and adhere to the root surface, root resorption and ankylosis occur. If cells from the periodontal ligament proliferate and colonize the root surface, regeneration occurs **(Figs 48.5A to D)**. Thus, the concept of "compartmentalization" was developed.

POINTS TO PONDER

✓ Various Star healing are:
  − *One – star healing:* Control of inflammation
  − *Two – star healing:* Long junctional epithelium
  − *Three – star healing:* New attachment
  − *Four – star healing:* Partial regeneration
  − *Five – star healing:* Complete regeneration
✓ Root conditioning, now also called as chemically guided tissue regeneration.

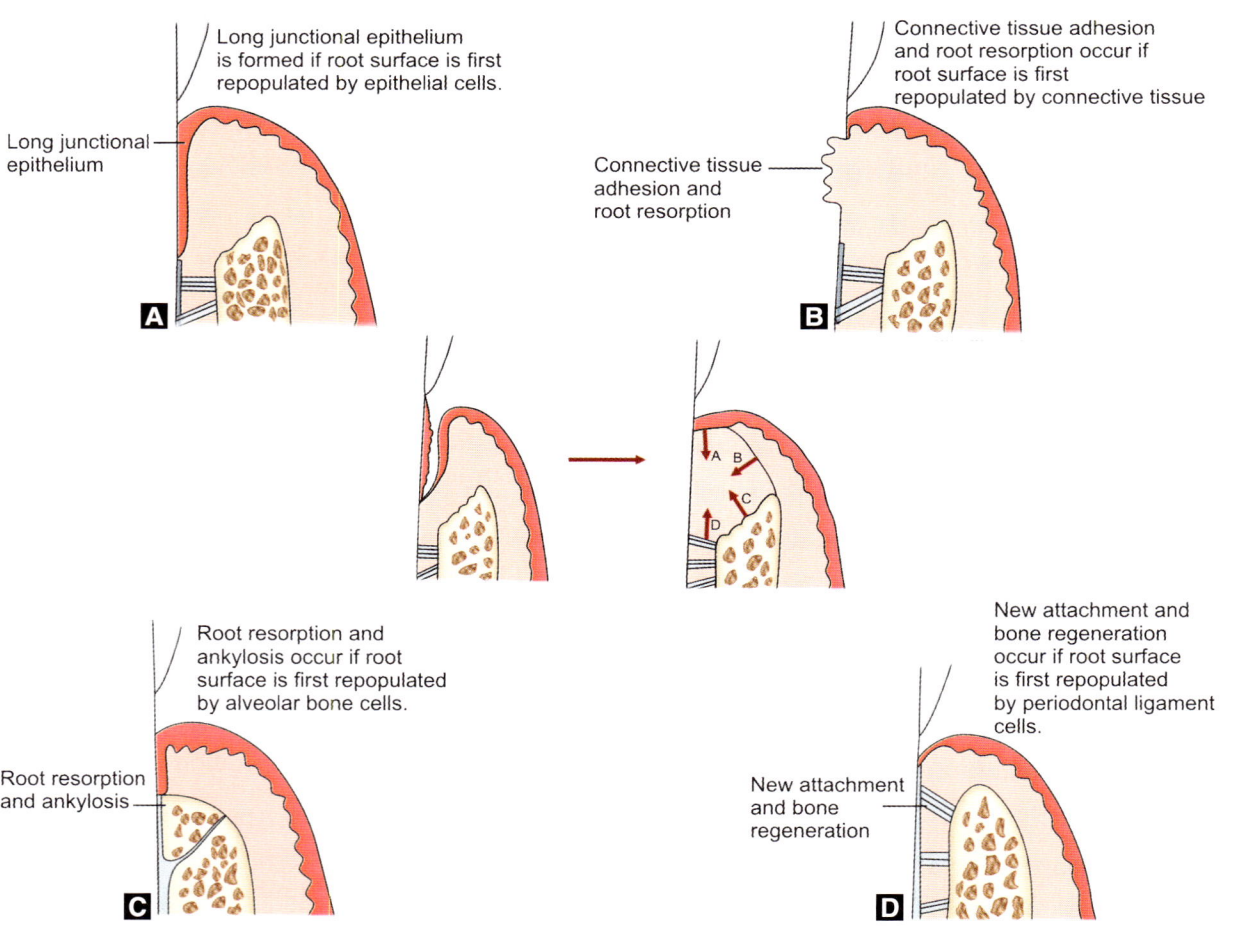

Figs 48.5A to D: Outcomes of periodontal therapy (*Courtesy:* Dr.SK Salaria)

PERIODONTICS REVISITED

✓ The advantage of autogenous grafts over allografts is that there is no problem of disease transmission or histocompatibility.

✓ Radiographically, FDBA appears radiopaque because it is not demineralized.

BIBLIOGRAPHY

1. Aravind B, Koshy C, Bhat GS, Bhat KM. Root conditioning - A review. JISP 2003;6:88-93.
2. Becker W. Guided tissue regeneration for Periodontal Defects. In, Polson AM. Periodontal Regeneration Current status and Directions.Quintessence Publishing Co, Inc 1994;137-50.
3. Bunyaratavej P, Wang HL. Collagen membranes: a review J Periodontol 2001;72:215-29.
4. Caffesse RG, Nasjleti CE. Clinical and Histologic Results of Regenerative Procedures. In, Polson AM. Periodontal Regeneration Current status and Directions.Quintessence Publishing Co, Inc 1994;113-36.
5. Carranza FM, Mclain PK, Schallhorn RG. Regenerative osseous surgery. In, Newman, Takei, Carranza. Clinical Periodontology 9th ed WB Saunders 2003;804-24.
6. Grant DA, Stern IB, Listgarten MA. Bone grafts and transplants. In, Periodontics 6th ed CV Mosby Company 1988;860-82.
7. Greenstein G, Caton JG. Biodegradable barriers and guided tissue regeneration. Periodontol 2000 1993;1:36-45.
8. Greenstein G, Caton JG. Resorbable Barriers and Periodontal Regeneration. In, Polson AM. Periodontal Regeneration Current status and Directions.Quintessence Publishing Co, Inc 1994; 151-66.
9. Hiatt WH, Genco RJ. Regenerative therapy in Periodontics. In, Genco RJ, Goldman HM, Cohen DW. Contemporary Periodontics. CV Mosby 1990;585-604.
10. Kao RT. Periodontal Regeneration and Reconstructive surgery. Rose LF, Mealey BL, Genco RJ, Cohen DW. Periodontics, Medicine, Surgery and Implants. Elsevier Mosby 2004;572-609.
11. Karring T, Jan Lindhe J, Cortellini P. Regenerative Periodontal Therapy. In, Lindhe J, Karring T, Lang NP. Clinical Periodontology and Implant dentistry. 4th ed Blackwell Munksgaard 2003;650-704.
12. Lowenguth RA, Blieden TM. Periodontal Regeneration: root surface demineralization. Periodontol 2000 1993;1:54-68.
13. Lynch SE. The role of Growth Factors in Periodontal Repair. In, Polson AM. Periodontal Regeneration Current status and Directions.Quintessence Publishing Co, Inc 1994;179-98.
14. Mellonig JT. Osseous Grafts and Periodontal Regeneration. In, Polson AM. Periodontal Regeneration Current status and Directions.Quintessence Publishing Co, Inc 1994;71-102.
15. Polson AM, Hanes PJ. Root Surface and Periodontal Regeneration. In, Polson AM. Periodontal Regeneration Current status and Directions.Quintessence Publishing Co, Inc 1994; 21-40.
16. Position Paper. Periodontal Regeneration. J Periodontol 2005;76: 1601-22.
17. Ramfjord SP, Ash MM. Flap surgery for reattachment and adaptation in periodontal pockets. In, Periodontology and Periodontics. Modern Theory and Practice 1st ed AITBS Publisher and distributor India, 1996;297-304.
18. Sanz M, Giovannoli JL. Focus on furcation defects: guided tissue regeneration. Periodontol 2000 2002;22:169-89.
19. Yukna RA. Synthetic Grafts and Regeneration. In, Polson AM. Periodontal Regeneration Current status and Directions. Quintessence Publishing Co, Inc 1994;103-112.

MCQs

1. Resorbable membrane is:
   A. dPTFE
   B. Nucleopore
   C. Vicryl membrane
   D. ePTFE
2. Which of the BMP is not osteoinductive:
   A. BMP-1
   B. BMP-6
   C. BMP-1 and 6
   D. BMP-2
3. Grafts taken from a donor of another species are:
   A. Xenogenic grafts
   B. Alloplastic grafts
   C. Autogenous grafts
   D. Allogenic grafts
4. Which is true about collagen membrane except:
   A. Hemostatic
   B. Chemotaxis for fibroblasts
   C. Rate of degradation can be controlled by varying its cross-linkage
   D. Anticoagulant
5. For regenerative surgery, first incision usually is:
   A. Internal bevel incision
   B. Sulcular incision
   C. External bevel incision
   D. Interdental incision
6. Tissucol consist of:
   A. Fibronectin
   B. Fibrinogen
   C. PDGF
   D. All of the above
7. The purpose of guided tissue regeneration is:
   A. Prevention of epithelial migration
   B. Elimination of junctional and pocket epithelium
   C. Complete removal of all irritants
   D. Careful curettage of the pocket wall surface
8. Transgingival probing is performed to:
   A. Know the bone architecture after the area is anesthetized
   B. Know the level of attachment
   C. Determine the disease activity
   D. Know the functional occlusal relationship

PERIODONTICS REVISITED

9. The best indication for osseous grafts for bone regeneration procedure is:
   A. One - walled intrabony defect
   B. One - walled suprabony pocket
   C. Two - walled intrabony defect
   D. Three - walled intrabony defect

10. Grafts taken from the different individual of the same species:
    A. Alloplast
    B. Xenograft
    C. Autograft
    D. Allograft

11. Which of the following materials has osteoinductive property:
    A. Autogenous graft
    B. Hydroxyapatite
    C. Plastic materials
    D. Cartilage

12. Anorganic bone is an example of:
    A. Autografts
    B. Alloplasts
    C. Xenografts
    D. Allografts

Answers

1. C	2. C	3. A	4. D	5. B
6. D	7. A	8. A	9. D	10. D
11. A	12. C			

CHAPTER 49

Furcation Involvement and Management

Shalu Bathla

INTRODUCTION

The furcation lesion defect represents a serious complication in periodontal therapy due to inaccessibility to adequate instrumentation, presence of root concavities and furrows making proper cleaning of the area difficult. Thus, loss of periodontal attachment in the furcation area is a condition that requires careful evaluation and management in order to achieve stability of dentition.

TERMINOLOGY

• *Furcation* is the area located between individual root cones.
• *Furcation involvement* is the extension of pocket formation into interradicular area of bone of multirooted tooth.
• *Furcation entrance* is the transitional area between the undivided and divided part of the root.
• *Furcation fornix* is the roof of the furcation.
• *Degree of Separation* is the angle of separation between two roots (cones) **(Fig. 49.1)**.
• *Co-efficient of Separation* is the length of root cones in relation to the length of root complex **(Fig. 49.1)**.

• *Root amputation* is the removal of one or more roots from a multirooted tooth leaving the majority of crown intact.
• *Sectioning* is the surgical sectioning of a tooth into segments consisting of the root and overlying crown.

CLASSIFICATION

I. According to Glickman (1953):

Grade I: It is the incipient stage of furcation involvement, but radiographically changes are not usually found.

Grade II: The furcation lesion is a cul-de-sac with a definite horizontal component. Radiographs may or may not depict the furcation involvement **(Fig. 49.2)**.

Grade III: The bone is not attached to the dome of the furcation. Class III furcation display the defect as a radiolucent area in the crotch of the tooth **(Fig. 49.3)**.

Grade IV: The interdental bone is destroyed and soft tissues have receded apically so that the furcation opening is clinically visible.

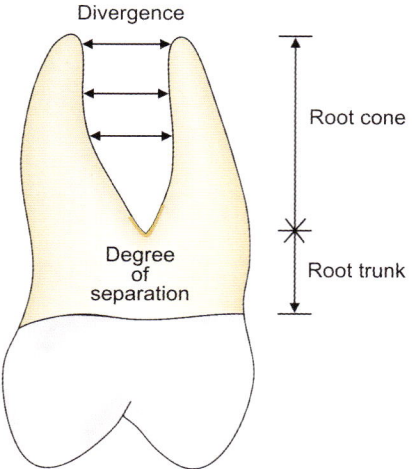

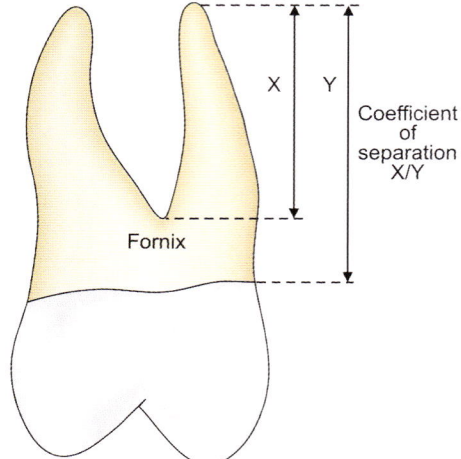

Fig. 49.1: Terminology in relation to furcation

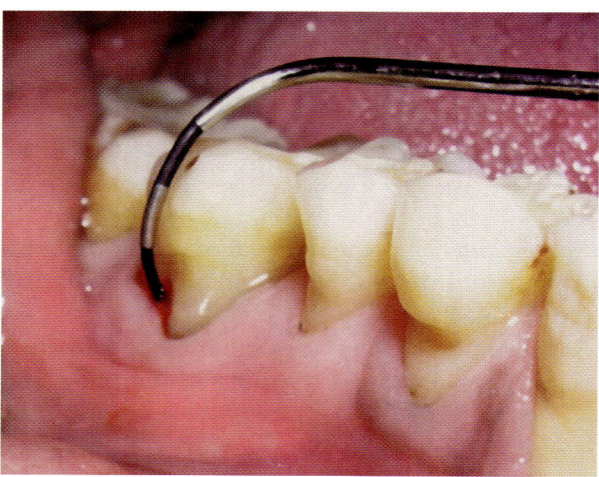

Fig. 49.2: Grade II furcation defect

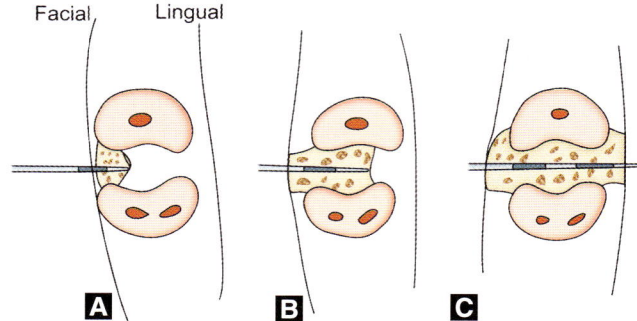

Figs 49.4A to C: (A) Furcation probed up to the depth of 3 mm, (B) Furcation probed more than 3 mm but not through and through, and (C) Furcation probed through and through

II. According to Hamp et al (1975) **(Figs 49.4A to C):**

Degree I: Horizontal loss of periodontal support not exceeding 1/3rd of the width of the tooth (< 3 mm).

Degree II: Horizontal loss of periodontal support exceeding 1/3rd of the width of the tooth (≥ 3 mm).

Degree III: Horizontal through and through destruction of periodontal tissue in the furcation area.

III. According to Tarnow and Fletcher (1984): Based on vertical component of furcation involvement depending on the distance from the base of the defect to the roof of the furcation they are classified into :

Subgroup A: Vertical destruction of bone upto one – third of the inter-radicular height (1– 3 mm).

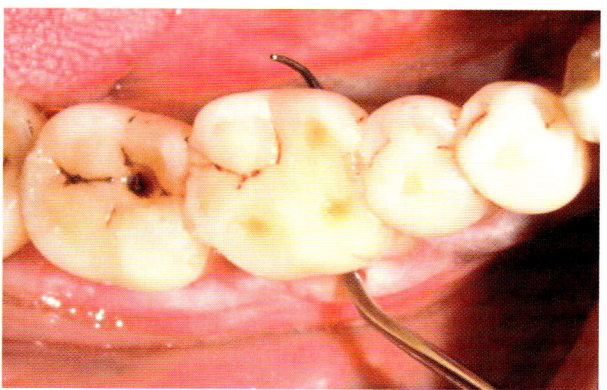

Fig. 49.3: Grade III furcation defect (Occlusal view): Naber's probe passes through and through the furcation lesion

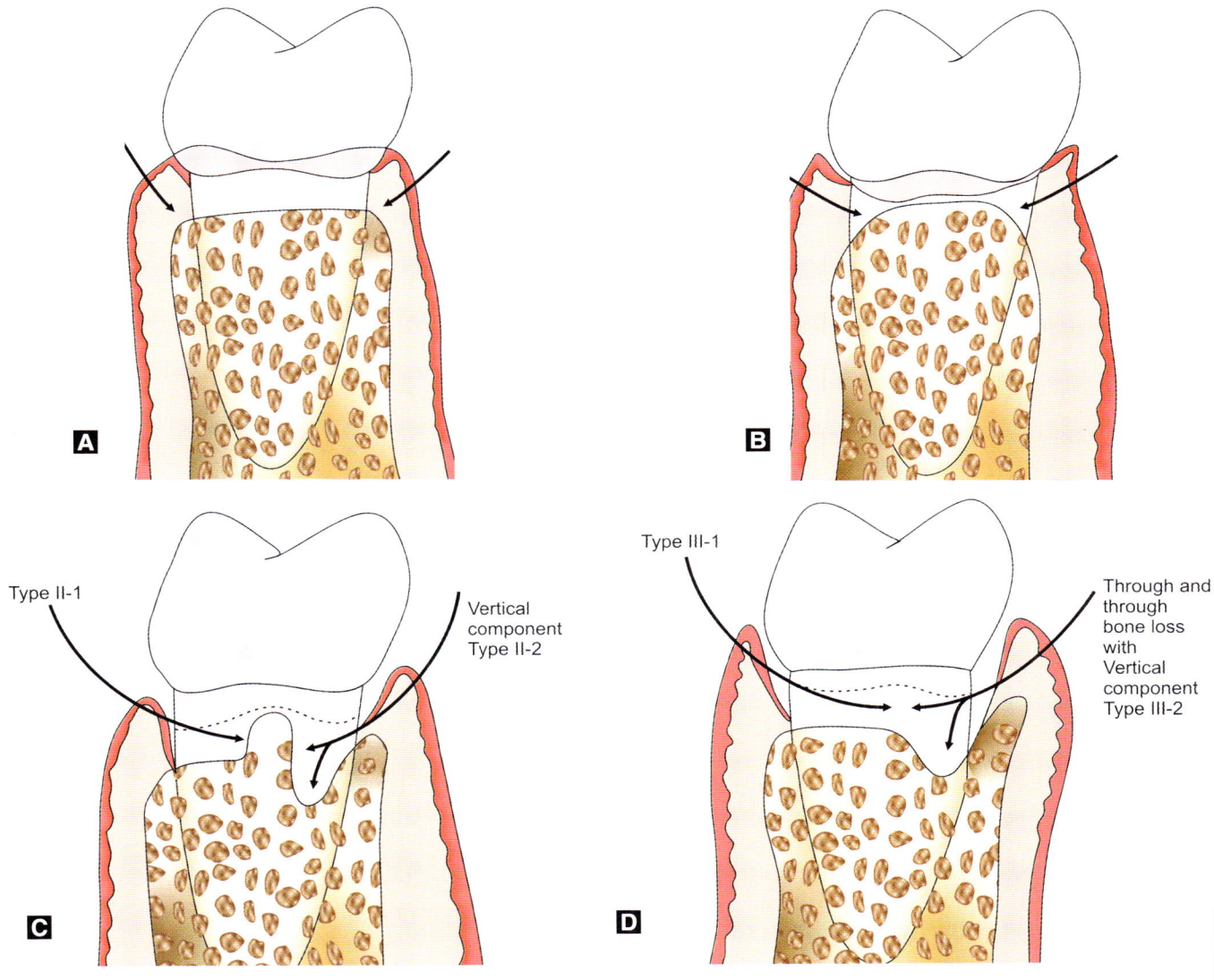

Type II-1

Vertical
component
Type II-2

Type III-1

Through and
through
bone loss
with
Vertical
component
Type III-2

Figs 49.5A to D: Easley and Drennan defect classification: (A) No furcation involvement, (B) Class I- Incipient involvement,
(C) Class II Type-1, Type-2, (D) Class III Type-1, Type-2

Subgroup B: Vertical destruction of bone upto two –
third of the inter-radicular height (4 – 6 mm).
Subgroup C: Vertical destruction beyond the apical –
third (7 mm or more).

IV. According to Goldman and Cohen (1968)
Grade I: Incipient lesion
Grade II: Cul- de-sac lesion
Grade III: Through and through lesion

V. According to Eskow and Kapin: Based on vertical
component of furcation involvement
Subgroup A: Vertical osseous defect up to 1/3rd of root

Subgroup B: Vertical osseous defect up to 2/3rd of root
Subgroup C: Vertical osseous defect > 2/3rd of root

VI. According to Easley and Drennan: **(Figs 49.5A to D)**
Class I: Incipient involvement in which the fluting
coronal to the furcation entrance is affected but there
is no definite horizontal component to the furcation
involvement.

In this classification system, Class II and III
furcations are separated into subtypes 1 and 2 on the
basis of the configuration of the alveolar bone at the
entrance to the furcation. Horizontal resorption into

the furca is subtype 1, whereas subtype 2 indicates a significant vertical component to the defect.

Class II: Type 1—A definite horizontal loss of attachment into the furcation, but the pattern of bone loss is essentially horizontal. There is no definite buccal or lingual ledge of bone. Type 2—There is a buccal or lingual bony ledge and a definite vertical component to the attachment loss.

Class III: A through and through loss of attachment in the furcation. As with Class II furcation defects, the pattern of attachment loss may be horizontal type 1 or there may be a vertical component type 2 of varying depth.

ETIOLOGY

There is no difference in basic etiology and pathology between furcation involvements and other periodontal pockets. However, the anatomical and morphological features of the furcations and their relationship to the adjacent structures pose specific problems in treatment of involved teeth.

i. The primary cause of furcation involvement is the progressive loss of attachment that results from inflammatory periodontal disease. Bacterial plaque is the most common cause of marginal periodontitis, which progressively invades one or more furcation areas to varying degrees, resulting in irreversible bone loss in the inter-radicular area. In most patients, the response to bacterial plaque, in the absence of therapy, is a progressive and site-specific attachment loss. Although the rate of response may vary from individual to individual, local anatomic factors that affect the deposition of plaque or hamper its removal can exert a significant impact on the development of attachment loss.

ii. Predisposing factors:
   • *Cervical enamel projections (CEPs):* Cervical enamel projections that are present on the root surface in the furcation region has been considered to be predisposing etiologic factor for periodontal attachment loss.
   • *Trauma from occlusion:* Trauma from occlusion acting as a predisposing cofactor for rapid formation of furcation involvement is controversial. Glickman (1961) assign a key role to trauma, since furcation areas are most sensitive to injury from excessive occlusal forces. Waerhaug (1979) denied the initiating effect of trauma and considered that inflammation and edema caused by plaque in the furcation area tend to extrude the tooth, which becomes traumatized and sensitive.
   • *Pulpal periodontal disease:* The high percentage of molar teeth with patent accessory canal opening into the furcation suggests that pulpal disease could be an initiating cofactor in the development of furcation involvement.
   • *Iatrogenic cofactors*: Iatrogenic predisposing cofactors, i.e. pin and endodontic perforations and overhanging restorations can lead to the formation of isolated furcation lesion by therapists themselves. Overhanging restorations harbor dental plaque which causes periodontal inflammation and attachment loss.
   • *Root fractures involving furcations:* If these root fractures involve the trunk of a multirooted molar and extend into the furcation, this can result in a rapidly forming isolated furcation defect. The prognosis for these situations is poor and usually results in loss of the tooth.

VARIOUS ANATOMIC FACTORS WHICH INFLUENCE THE TREATMENT OF FURCATION LESION (FIG. 49.6)

i. *Root trunk length:* Root trunk length is a key factor that affects both the development of furcation involvement and the mode of treatment. If root trunk is short, less attachment has to be lost before furcation is involved and when the root trunk is long, furcation will be invaded later but will be difficult to instrument. Short root trunk facilitates surgical procedure and is more accessible to maintenance therapy than long root trunk.

• Maxillary molars - Mesial furcation entrance is located about 3 mm from CEJ while buccal furcation entrance is approx. about 4 mm and distal furcation entrance is located about 5 mm from CEJ.
• Maxillary premolars – Length of root trunk is approx. 8 mm.
• Mandibular molars – The length of root trunk at the lingual entrance is 4 mm and at buccal entrance it is approx. 3 mm.

ii. *Root length:* Root length is directly related to the quantity of attachment supporting the tooth.

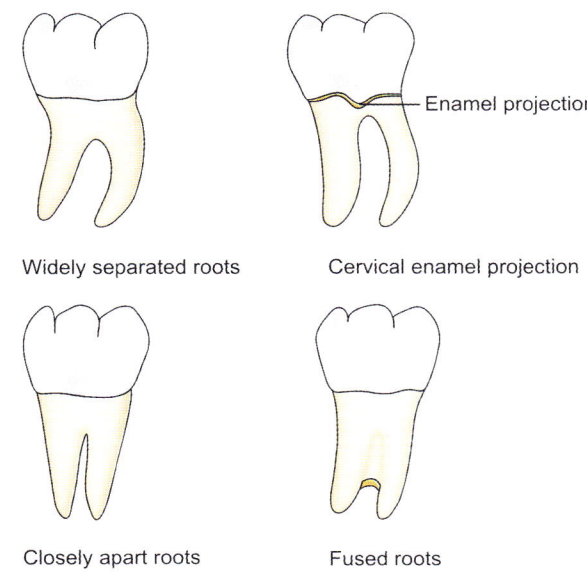

Widely separated roots

Cervical enamel projection — Enamel projection

Closely apart roots

Fused roots

Figs 49.6A to D: Anatomic variation of furcation areas
(*Courtesy:* Dr SK Salaria)

iii. *Root form:* The roots of molars may be fused, partially fused, closely approximated, or widely divergent. Curvature and fluting increases the potential for root perforation during endodontics and vertical root fracture. Marked concavities appear in the mesiobuccal root of the maxillary first molar and both roots of mandibular first molar.

iv. *Inter-radicular dimensions:* Narrow, inter-radicular zone complicate the surgical procedure where as widely separated roots have more treatment options and easily hemisected, readily treated. In divergent rooted tooth adequate instrumentation can be done during scaling, root planing and surgery. The dimensions of furcation entrance should be taken into consideration during the selection of instruments.

- Maxillary premolars – The width of furcation entrance of maxillary premolars is approx. 0.7 mm.
- Maxillary molars – The width of buccal entrance is 0.5 mm, mesial entrance is 0.75 mm and distal entrance is approx 0.5 mm to 0.75 mm.
- Mandibular molars – The buccal entrance is often less than 0.75 mm while the lingual entrance is more than 0.75 mm.

v. *Anatomy of furcation:* An intermediate bifurcation ridges has been described in 73% of mandibular first molars, crossing from the mesial to the distal root at the midroot of the bifurcation. Bifurcational ridges, concavity in the dome and accessory canals complicates scaling, root planing, surgical procedures and maintenance.

vi. *Cervical enamel projections (CEPs):* They favour plaque accumulation and complicate scaling and root planing. Enamel projections act as local factor in the development of gingivitis and periodontitis.

Masters and Hoskins in 1964 classified CEPs into 3 grades:
Grade I – The enamel projection extends from CEJ towards the furcation entrance.
Grade II – Enamel projection approaches the entrance of the furcation without entering the furcation with no horizontal component.
Grade III – Enamel projection extends horizontally into the furcation.
The prevalence of CEPs is highest in mandibular and maxillary second molar teeth.

DIAGNOSIS

The position and morphology of the furcation region complicates the clinician's ability to identify the location and extent of furcation defect. Furcation must be diagnosed at the earliest possible time.

i. *Radiographically:* Radiographs are useful in assessing root morphology and apicocoronal position of the furcation but do not allow the clinician to determine attachment loss in the furcation. Thus, two dimensional radiographic pictures provide meager information about furcation involvement, especially in maxilla. High resolution spiral CT, CADIA and digital radiography will allow cross-section views of interior furcation lesions. It appears that radiographs alone do not detect the furcation lesion with any predictable accuracy and that probing the furcation areas is necessary to confirm the presence and severity of furcation defect.

ii. *Clinically:* Periodontal probes are useful for determining the probing depth in a vertical direction, but less useful for determining the degree of horizontal involvement. For this purpose either curved Cowhorn explorer or *Naber's probe* are very useful. Furcation probes have curved, blunt tip that allows easy access to furcation areas. Example of furcation probes are Nabers 1N and Nabers 2N. The probe is directed beneath the gingival margin. At the base of pocket, rotate the probe tip toward the tooth to fit the tip into the entrance of the furcation. Terminal shank of Nabers

PERIODONTICS REVISITED

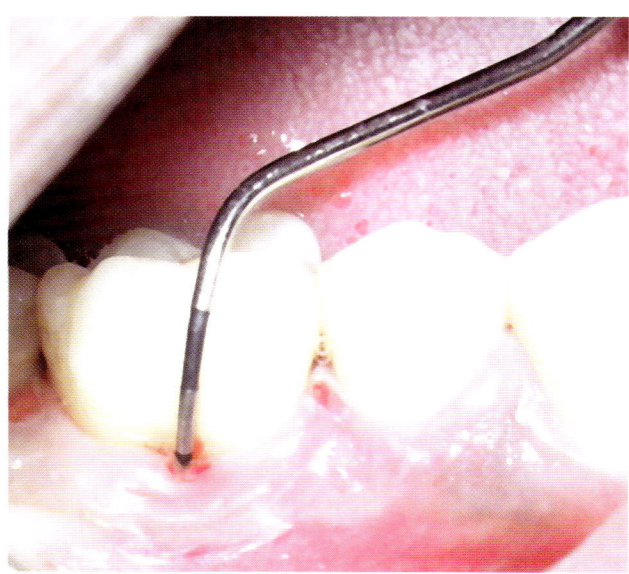

Fig. 49.7: Probing of molar furcation with Naber's probe

probe is positioned parallel to the long axis of tooth surface being examined **(Fig. 49.7)**.

- Probing of mandibular molar furcations is relatively easy because there are only buccal and lingual entrances each of which is located midway mesiodistally.
- Probing of maxillary molar furcations - Buccal entrance is accessible midway mesiodistally. Distal furcation is present midway buccolingually, thus can be probed from either buccal or palatal aspect. Mesial furcation of maxillary molar is easily probed from the palatal aspect because mesial furcation opens about 2/3rd of the way towards the palate, rather than midway buccolingually.

iii. *Transgingival probing/bone sounding*: To determine the bone contours associated with furcation lesions more accurately, transgingival probing can be accomplished through anesthetized soft tissues. (More is explained in chapter no. 30 Clinical Diagnosis)

PROGNOSIS

In general, teeth with furcation involvements have a poor prognosis.

- Prognosis of furcation involvement in maxillary first premolar has poor prognosis.
- Prognosis of maxillary molars is not good whereas prognosis of mandibular first molar is considered good.

The following factors should be considered in projecting a prognosis of tooth with furcation involvement:

a. Extent of involvement
b. Status of bone support
c. Root separation
d. Health of neighbouring teeth

Other factors involved in establishing a treatment prognosis are related to personal, psychologic, sociologic and financial considerations.

MANAGEMENT

Objectives of Furcation Therapy

i. To facilitate maintenance of existing furcation defect through scaling and root planing.
ii. To increase access to the furcation through gingivectomy, apically positioned flap, odontoplasty, ostectomy/osteoplasty and tunnel preparation.
iii. To prevent further attachment loss or eliminate the furcation through root amputation, tooth resection and hemisection.
iv. To obliterate the furcation defect by filling furcation defects with biocompatible material such as polymeric reinforced Zinc oxide eugenol (IRM) and GIC.
v. To regenerate the lost attachment through GTR procedures and bone grafting.

Following are the factors to be considered during treatment of furcation lesion:

A. Tooth related factors:
   i. Degree of furcation involved
   ii. Amount of remaining periodontal support
   iii. Probing depth
   iv. Tooth mobility
   v. Root trunk length
   vi. Root length
   vii. Root form
   viii. Inter-radicular dimensions
   ix. Anatomy of furcation
   x. Cervical enamel projections
   xi. Tooth position and occlusal antagonisms
   xii. Endodontic conditions and root canal anatomy
B. Patient related factors:
   i. Strategic value of the tooth in relation to the overall plan
   ii. Patient's age and health condition
   iii. Oral hygiene capacity

Treatment Modalities for Class I, II, III and IV Furcation Defects

The keys to successful treatment of molar furcation involvement are the same as for any other periodontal problem—that is, early diagnosis, thorough treatment planning, good oral hygiene by the patient, careful technical execution of the therapeutic modality, and a well designed and implemented program of periodontal maintenance. Depending upon the severity of furcation involvement as well as tooth position in either maxilla or mandible, various therapeutic methods are attempted.

Class I Furcation Defects

A. *Furcationplasty:* In 1975, Hamp, Nyman and Lindhe described furcationplasty as raising a mucoperiosteal flap to provide access to the furcation area and combining scaling and root planing, osteoplasty and odontoplasty to remove local irritants and to open the furcation to allow the patient access to clean the area. It is done in Grade I and early Grade II furcation lesions.

B. *Scaling and root planing:* In Grade I, furcation lesions have not lost bone within the furcation, so closed or open scaling and root planing procedures can resolve inflammation. If inflammation is not resolved then gingivectomy or apically positioned flap can be done depending upon the width of attached gingiva.

C. *Odontoplasty:* Odontoplasty is defined as the reshaping of a tooth coronal to the furcation. It widens and shallow the furcation by raising the roof of furcation. The rationale behind this technique is to create improved access for plaque control and maintenance. If CEP is found then it is removed and the area is recontoured. Odontoplasty must be approached with caution due to the potential complications of hypersensitivity, pulpal exposure and increased risk of root caries.

D. *Osteoplasty:* It is done to provide better gingival form by grooving the bone between the roots and then, festooning and beveling the bone over the roots.

E. *Gingivectomy/Apical positioned flap:* Can be used in reducing or eliminating the soft tissue pockets over the furcation region to increase access for plaque control and allows resolution of periodontal inflammation.

Class II Furcation Defects

A. *Open flap debridement:* If sufficient subgingival access is not possible with a closed approach, for furcated molars with deep lesions, then open flap debridement or modified widman flap yields more effective plaque and calculus removal.

B. *Guided tissue regeneration:* Organic or synthetic barrier membranes are used based on the principles of guided tissue regeneration.

C. *Bone grafting:* The strong focus on bone formation as a prerequisite for new attachment formation has led to implantation of bone grafts or different types of bone substitutes into furcation defects. Among these are bone autografts, allografts, xenografts and alloplastic materials designed as either bone substitutes or biologic barriers.

Class III and Class IV Furcation Defects

A. *Tunnel preparation:* Tunneling is the process of deliberately removing bone from the furcation to produce an open tunnel through the furcation. It is a resective technique use to treat advanced class II and class III furcation defects. The objective of this technique is to make the furcal area accessible to home care instruments by the patient.

The factors to be considered while selecting the case of tunnel preparation are

- Tooth should be mandibular molar for clear two way access
- Patient should have low caries index
- Good patient compliance towards plaque control.
- Root trunk should be short with high furcation entrance and long roots
- Root should have wide furcal entrance with the degree of divergence more than 30°
- The floor of the pulp chamber should not be close to the roof of the furcation to allow for possible odontoplasty of the entrance.

Procedure:

Buccal and lingual flaps are reflected and the involved area is widened by the removal of some of the inter-radicular bone. Some of the interfurcal bone is sacrificed vertically and is recontoured to obtain a flat outline of the bone. Following bone resection enough space is established in the furcation area to allow access for cleaning devices to be used by the patient itself. Main advantage associated with tunneling is the avoidance of prosthetic recon-struction and endodontic therapy.

The drawbacks associated with tunnel preparation are threat of root caries, subsequent pulpal pathology, reverse architecture and retained plaque in furcation cavities leading to progressive periodontal breakdown.

B. *Root resection:* It is often the treatment of choice for deep grade II and III furcation lesions when regeneration is unpredictable. Root with the greatest bone loss should be considered for amputation. Indications for root resection include:

- Severe and disproportionate attachment loss around the affected root
- Furcation defects that can be eliminated by root amputation
- Elimination of cracked or deeply fissured roots
- Elimination of an endodontically untreatable root
- Inoperable root caries
- Recession exposing most or all of the root in a multirooted tooth

Factors determining for the root resection are:

- Bone levels in the furcation
- Accessibility for plaque removal
- Root proximity
- Position of the root in the arch
- Root morphology
- Endodontic complications

Technique (Figs 49.8A to D):

Root selection of mandibular molar: The mesial root concavities are less accessible for plaque removal and two narrow pulp canals of the mesial root are more difficult to treat endodontically than distal root. Post and core restoration are easily constructed on the distal root. Thus, mesial root of mandibular molar is preferred over distal root for root resection.

Root selection of maxillary molar: The most commonly performed root resection is the distobuccal root of maxillary first molar. When both the mesial and distal furcation is involved palatal root amputation should be considered if buccal furcation is intact. Palatal root has an unfavourable axial inclination and unfavourable prosthetic relationship with the first bicuspid.

Endodontic Phase

In non vital root resection, the endodontic therapy (root canal therapy) is done prior to root resection and in vital root resection, the root resection is accomplished first and then endodontic therapy.

Resective Phase

- Flap reflection: After LA is given to the selected site, through crevicular incision full thickness mucoperiosteal buccal and lingual flap are reflected.

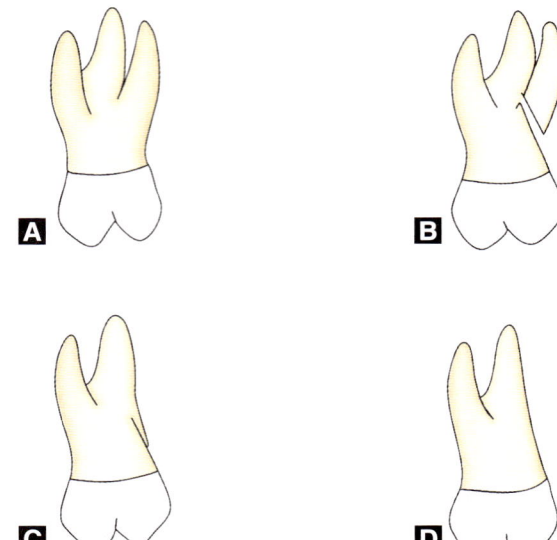

A. Maxillary molar
B. Root resection cut to separate the root from root trunk
C. Extraction of separated root
D. Final recontouring of the root trunk

Figs 49.8A to D: Root resection of maxillary molar

- Cut: Small amount of bone covering the root (which is to be resected) is removed to provide access for elevation and root removal. Cut is made with high speed surgical length fissure or cross cut fissure carbide bur. Cut is then directed from just apical to the contact point of the tooth, through the tooth, to the other orifices of furcation. In vital root resection the cut is made more horizontally, so as to expose less surface area of pulp chamber.
- Root removal: After sectioning, the root is elevated from its socket. Before flap closure it is important to check for any residual root spurs and ledges that can act as subgingival overhangs to retain plaque and cause future periodontal destruction.
- Suturing: Sutures are placed over the approximated flap.

Restorative Phase

The removal of a root alters the direction of occlusal forces on the remaining roots. Occlusion of that tooth is evaluated and adjusted. Crowns should be placed. But before giving permanent restoration the quality of the endodontic filling, residual ledges should be examined radiographically and clinically.

C. *Hemisection:* Hemisection is the splitting of a two rooted tooth into two separate teeth. This process is also called as bicuspidization.

Indications:
- Strategic teeth with Grade III furcation involvement
- Teeth with divergent well supported roots

Contraindications:
- When the remaining periodontal support is inadequate
- Tooth that cannot be treated endodontically
- Where adequate restorations of the remaining tooth including splinting cannot be performed.

Procedure **(Fig. 49.9)**:
- *Cut:* Vertically oriented cut is made faciolingually through the buccal and lingual developmental grooves of the tooth, through the pulp chamber and through the furcation. The metallic portion of the cut should be made before flap elevation which will prevent the contamination of the surgical field with metallic particles.
- *Flap raised:* Buccal and lingual flaps are raised and the area is curetted. Osseous surgery is completed by removing the residual internal osseous crater on the mesial or distal aspect of the remaining root.
- *Tooth reshaping:* Roof of furcation is carefully perforated with dull rounded bur in a slow handpiece. Each half of the tooth is reshaped into a single rooted tooth and will be prepared to receive crown.
- Orthodontic separation of the roots is required to allow restoration with adequate embrasure form.

D. *Tooth resection:* Tooth resection involves removal of one or more roots of tooth as well as corresponding portion of the crown.

Direction of tooth section

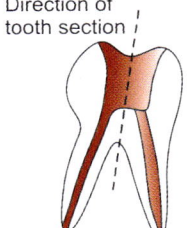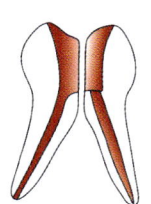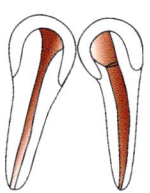

Fig. 49.9: Hemisection of mandibular molar

Advanced Class IV Furcation Defects

Tooth Extraction

Indications for removal of a tooth with a Grade III and IV furcal defects are:
   i. Individuals who do not maintain oral hygiene
   ii. Patients with high level of caries activity
   iii. The existence of an unopposed molar which is the terminal tooth in the arch.
   iv. Financial consideration preclude acceptance of treatment.
   v. If an otherwise heroic effort for a tooth with a questionable prognosis would be better handled by an implant.

Failures in Surgical Furcation Therapy

Failures in surgical furcation therapy are due to the following reasons:
   i. Inadequate plaque control and maintenance
   ii. Poor root resection
   iii. Improper restoration
   iv. Endodontic failures
   v. Cracked roots
   vi. Root caries
   vii. Patients who respond poorly despite best treatment

LANDMARK STUDIES RELATED

Bower RC. Furcation morphology relative to periodontal treatment: Furcation root surface anatomy. Journal of Periodontology 1979;50:366-74.

A random sample of 114 maxillary and 103 first permanent mandibular molar teeth were selected from a collection of extracted teeth at University of Michigan Dental School. Measurement of furcation entrance diameter was performed using a dissecting microscope. Following were the results: Maxillary first molar furcation- in 85% of buccal furcations the diameter was 0.75 mm or less, whereas in 49% of mesiopalatal and 54% of distopalatal furcations the entrance diameter were 0.7 mm or less. Mandibular first molars - in 63% of the cases the buccal furcation entrance diameter and 37% of lingual furcation entrance diameter was 0.75 mm or less. The blade face width of 12 commonly used curette types was measured using a Vernier caliper and recorded. Blade face width of all the curettes was within the range of 0.75 mm to 1.10 mm. Thus, study showed that in 81% of furcation (maxillary and mandibular teeth) the entrance diameter was found to be 1.0 mm or less and in 58% the diameter was 0.75 mm or less. Comparison of the furcation entrance diameters of first molar teeth and blade face width of some of the more commonly used periodontal curettes reveals a size disparity which makes it unlikely that curettes used alone will achieve adequate preparation of furcation area.

Bower RC. Furcation morphology relative to periodontal treatment. Furcation entrance architecture. Journal of Periodontology 1979; 50:23-27.

In this study internal furcation root surface morphology was studied. A sample of 114 maxillary and 103 mandibular first molar teeth were sectioned transversely at a level of 2 mm apical to the most apical root division. Following were the results:

Maxillary First Molar Teeth

a. The furcal aspect of the root was concave in 94% of mesiobuccal roots, 31% of distobuccal roots and 17% of palatal roots.
b. The deepest concavity was in the furcal aspect of the mesiobuccal root (mean concavity 0.3 mm).
c. The furcal aspects of the buccal roots diverge toward the palate in 97% teeth (mean divergence 22^0).

Mandibular First Molar Teeth

a. Concavity of the furcal aspects was found in 100% of mesial roots and 99% of distal roots.
b. Deeper concavity was found in the mesial root (mean concavity 0.7 mm) than the distal root (mean concavity 0.5 mm).

Hirschfeld L, Wasserman B. A long term survey of tooth loss in 600 treated periodontal patients. Journal of Periodontology 1978; 49: 225-237.

After 15-50+ years (mean 22 years) of post treatment maintenance, 600 patients were re-examined. Prognosis was originally described as questionable for teeth with furcation involvement, deep ineradicable pocket, severe bone loss or marked mobility with deep pocket. During maintenance, patients varied greatly and were grouped according to response to treatment: 499 well maintained patients (WM) lost three teeth or fewer; 76 downhill patients (D) lost 4 – 9 teeth; and 25 extreme downhill patients (ED) lost 10 – 23 teeth. Overall 2 out of 3 questionable teeth were kept; 7% of all teeth were lost for periodontal reasons and 1% for other reasons. Thus, treatment outcome was less predictable in the ED and D groups.

POINTS TO PONDER

✓ The dimensions of furcation entrance should be taken into consideration during the selection of instruments.
✓ Furcation defects of maxillary molars are more difficult to interpret on radiographs because of the superimposition of the large palatal root.
✓ In hemisection, two rooted molar tooth is converted into two single rooted teeth.

BIBLIOGRAPHY

1. Ammons WF, Harrington GW Jr. Furcation; The problem and its management. In, Newman, Takei, Carranza. Clinical Periodontology 9th ed Philadelphia WB Saunders 2003;825-39.
2. Bower RC. Furcation morphology relative to periodontal treatment: Furcation root surface anatomy. J Periodontol 1979;50:366-74.
3. Carnevale G, Pontoriero R, Lindhe J. Treatment of furcation - Involved teeth. In, Lindhe J, Karring T, Lang NP. Clinical Periodontology and Implant dentistry. 4th ed Blackwell Munksgaard 2003;705-30.
4. Garette S, Bogle G. Periodontal Regeneration with bone grafts. Curr Opin Periodontol 1994;187-93.
5. Hamp SE, Nyman S, Lindhe J. Periodontal treatment of multirooted teeth: Result after 5 years. J Clin Periodontol 1975;2:126.
6. Kalkwarf KL, Reinhardt RA. The furcation problem. Dent Clin North Am 1988;32(2):243-66.
7. Newell DH. The diagnosis and treatment of molar furcation invasions. Dent Clin North Am 1998;42(2):301-38.
8. Sanctis M, Piniprato GP. Root resection and root amputation. Curr Opin Periodontol 1993;105-10.
9. Sanz M, Giovannoli JL. Focus on furcation defects: guided tissue regeneration. Periodontol 2000 2002;22:169-89.
10. Tarnow D, Fletcher P. Classification of the vertical component of furcation involvement. J Periodontol 1984;55:283.
11. The periodontally diseased furcation. In, Grant DA, Stern IB, Listgarten MA. Periodontics 6th ed CV Mosby Company 1988;921-49.
12. Treatment of intrabony pockets and furcation involvement:bone implants. In, Ramfjord SP and Ash MM. Periodontology and Periodontics Modern Theory and Practice 1st ed A.I.T.B.S Publisher and distributor India, 1996;327-38.
13. Waerhaug J. The furcation problem, etiology, pathogenesis, diagnosis, therapy, and prognosis. J Clin Periodontol 1980;7:73-95.
14. Zappa U, Grosso L, Simona C, Graf H, Case D. Clinical furcation diagnosis and interradicular bone defects. J Periodontol 1993;64:219-27.

MCQs

1. Furcation lesion can be clinically detected by:
   A. Curette   B. Hoe
   C. Naber's probe   D. 17 end explorer

2. Cul de sac lesion is:
   A. Grade I furcation   B. Grade II furcation
   C. Grade III furcation   D. Grade IV furcation
3. Hemisection is commonly done in:
   A. Maxillary molar
   B. Mandibular molar
   C. Maxillary premolar
   D. None of the above
4. Tunnel preparation is usually done in:
   A. Grade I furcation lesion
   B. Grade II furcation lesion
   C. Grade III and IV furcation lesion
   D. None of the above
5. In vital root resection:
   A. Endodontic therapy is done prior to root resection
   B. Root resection is done prior to endodontic therapy
   C. Endodontic therapy is not done at all
   D. None of the above
6. Indication for vital root amputation during periodontal surgery *except*:
   A. Root fracture
   B. External resorption
   C. Root anomalies
   D. Grade I Furcation defect
7. Prognosis is worst for furcation involvement of:
   A. Maxillary 1st premolar
   B. Maxillary 2nd premolar
   C. Mandibular 1st premolar
   D. Mandibular 1st molar
8. Hemisection is:
   A. Removal of one or more roots from a multirooted tooth leaving the majority of crown intact
   B. Removal of one or more roots from a multirooted tooth with the crown
   C. Splitting of a two rooted tooth into two separate teeth
   D. None of the above

Answers

1. C	2. B	3. B	4. C	5. B
6. D	7. A	8. C		

PERIODONTICS REVISITED

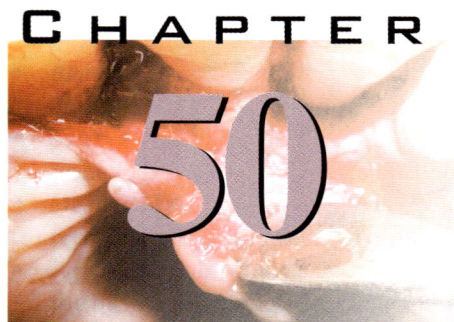

CHAPTER 50

Periodontal Plastic Surgery

Shalu Bathla

INTRODUCTION

Mucogingival therapy was defined as the correction of defects in morphology, position or amount of soft tissue and underlying bone. This is the most comprehensive definition because it includes both nonsurgical and surgical mucogingival therapy of the gingiva, alveolar mucosa and bone such as papilla reconstruction by means of orthodontics or restorative dentistry. The term *mucogingival surgery* was initially used in the literature by Friedman in 1957, he referred to corrective surgery of the alveolar mucosa and the gingiva which included problems with attached gingiva, aberrant frenum and shallow vestibule.

The 1996 World Workshop renamed mucogingival surgery as periodontal plastic surgery, a term originally proposed by Miller in 1993 because the term muco-gingival surgery did not adequately describe all the periodontal procedures that were being performed under this section. The goal is the creation of form and appearance that is acceptable and pleasing to both patient and therapist. The word plastic means to mould or shape, therefore periodontal plastic surgery literally means to mould or shape the tissues around the teeth or implants to create optimal aesthetics.

Periodontal plastic surgery is defined as the surgical procedures performed to correct/ eliminate anatomic, developmental/ traumatic deformities of the gingiva/ alveolar mucosa.

It includes the following:
i. Periodontal prosthetic corrections
ii. Crown lengthening
iii. Ridge augmentation
iv. Aesthetic surgical corrections
v. Coverage of the denuded root surface
vi. Reconstruction of papillae
vii. Aesthetic surgical correction around implants
viii. Surgical exposure of unerupted teeth for orthodontics

OBJECTIVES

The objectives of periodontal plastic surgery is to deal with:
- *The problem associated with attached gingiva*: Widening the attached gingiva enhances plaque removal around the gingival margin, improves esthetics and reduces inflammation around restored teeth.
- *The problems associated with shallow vestibule*: The sulcular brushing technique requires the placement of the toothbrush at the gingival margin, which may

not be possible with reduced vestibular depth. Adequate vestibular depth may also be necessary for proper placement of removable prosthesis.

- *The problems associated with aberrant frenum:* A frenum that encroaches on the margin of the gingiva may interfere with plaque removal and tension on this frenum may tend to open the sulcus.
- *The problems associated with papilla.*
- *The problems associated with resorbed alveolar ridge.*

CRITERIA FOR SELECTION OF TECHNIQUES FOR SOLVING MUCOGINGIVAL PROBLEMS

- *Surgical site free of plaque, calculus and inflammation*: Periodontal plastic surgical procedures should be undertaken in a plaque and inflammation free environment to enable precise incisions on the firm gingival tissue.
- *Adequate blood supply to the donor tissue:* Root coverage procedures present a portion of the recipient site (denuded root surface) without blood supply. A pedicle displaced flap has a better blood supply than a free graft, with the base of the flap intact. If the anatomy is favorable, the pedicle flap is the best procedure for localized root coverage. The subepithelial connective tissue graft and the pouch and tunnel techniques use a split flap with the connective tissue sandwiched in between the flap. This flap design maximizes the blood supply to the donor tissue. If large areas require root coverage, these sandwich-type recipient sites provide the best flap design.
- *Anatomy of the recipient site:* The presence or absence of vestibular depth is an important anatomic criteria at the recipient site for gingival augmentation. If gingival augmentation is indicated apical to the area of recession, there must be adequate vestibular depth apical to the recessed gingival margin to provide space for either a free or pedicle graft. When split thickness, sandwich-type flap e.g subepithelial connective graft are indicated then adequate amount of gingival thickness is required at the recipient site.
- *Anatomy of the donor site:* Pedicle displacement of tissue necessitates the presence of an adjacent donor site that presents gingival thickness and width. Palatal tissue thickness is also necessary for the connective tissue donor autograft.
- *Stability of the grafted tissue to the recipient site.*
- *Minimal trauma to the surgical site:* Poor incisions, flap perforations, tears, traumatic and excessive placement of sutures can lead to tissue necrosis. The selection of

proper instruments, needles, and sutures are mandatory to minimize tissue trauma. Sharp, contoured blades; smaller diameter needles; and resorbable, monofilament sutures should be used for atraumatic surgery.

TECHNIQUES FOR INCREASING ATTACHED GINGIVA

Following are the techniques for increasing attached gingiva:
I.   Gingival augmentation apical to recession:
  1. Free epithelial autograft
  2. Free connective tissue autograft
  3. Apically positioned flap
  4. Fenestration
  5. Vestibular extension
II. Gingival augmentation coronal to recession/root coverage:
  1. Free epithelial autograft
  2. Free connective tissue autograft
  3. Pedicle autografts:
      A   Rotational:
          a. Lateral Pedicle
          b. Double Papilla
      B   Advanced:
          a. Coronally displaced
          b. Semilunar
  4. Subepithelial connective tissue
  5. Subpedicle connective tissue
  6. Pouch and Tunnel technique
  7. Envelope technique
  8. Guided tissue regeneration technique

Epithelial Graft

In a brief report from Sweden, Bjorn (1963) published the first illustrated success of gingival grafting. Free epithelial grafts are used to create a widened zone of attached gingiva.

Procedure

- Adequate anesthesia is injected on to the recipient as well as donor site.
- *Prepare the Recipient Site:* A firm connective tissue bed is prepared to receive the graft. The recipient site can be prepared by incising at the existing mucogingival junction with a 15 no. blade to the desired depth, blending the incision on both ends with the existing mucogingival line. The incision is extended to approximately twice the desired width of the attached

gingiva which allows for 50% contraction of the graft when healing is complete. Insert 15 no. blade along the cut gingival margin and separate a flap consisting of epithelium and underlying connective tissue without disturbing the periosteum. The recipient bed should be smooth and essentially free of muscle attachment tissue. At this point, gauze square is packed between the wound and the lip or cheek to limit bleeding and promote hemostasis in the recipient area while the donor tissue is being obtained.

- *Obtain the Graft from the Donor Site:* Donor site may be gingivectomy tissue, an edentulous ridge or the palate. The amount of donor palatal tissue needed can be accurately determined by using a foil template. Place the template over the donor site and make a shallow incision around it with a 15 no. blade. All palatal incisions are made in such a fashion as to create a butt joint margin at the donor site. Insert the blade to the desired thickness at one edge of the graft. Elevate the edge and hold it with tissue forceps. Continue to separate the graft with the blade, lifting it gently and as separation progresses, visibility increases. A partial thickness graft consisting of epithelium and a thin layer of underlying connective tissue is used. The ideal thickness of the graft is in between 1.0 mm to 1.5 mm. Thinner graft shrivels and exposes the recipient site while thicker graft jeopardizes the circulation and nutrient diffusion.

- *Transfer and Immobilize the Graft:* Pressure is applied on the recipient site to remove the excess clot as thick clot interferes with vascularization of the graft. Suture the graft at the lateral borders and to the periosteum to secure it in position. The graft should be immobilized because any movement interferes with healing. Avoid excessive tension, which can distort the graft from the underlying surface.

- *Protect the Donor Site:* Once the graft is free, firm pressure should be applied to the donor site with a gauze square. Cover the donor site with a periodontal pack for 1 week and repeat if necessary. A modified hawley retainer is useful to cover the pack on the palate.

- *Postoperative Instructions:* Instructions to the patient are most important to the success of the graft. Patient should be advised not to brush at the recipient site for the week. Should not retract the lip or cheek to observe the graft. No postoperative factor will facilitate failure in soft - tissue grafting to the degree that smoking does. Smoking causes constriction of capillaries, diminished blood flow to the area, poor oxygenation of tissue causing sloughing of the graft. Thus, patient is instructed to quit smoking immediately preoperatively and abstain for the first week (preferably for 2 weeks).

- *Sutures removal:* Sutures are removed after 7-10 days.

Drawbacks of epithelialized palatal graft for the root coverage procedure are:
- Blood supply to the graft is available on only one surface, rather than two, as with the connective tissue graft.
- Color match of the tissues is a problem between the grafted area and the adjacent tissues.
- Palatal wound is more invasive, more prone to hemorrhage and slower to heal.
- It is sensitive and time consuming technique.

Healing after Grafting Procedure **(Fig. 50.1)**

Phase I. *Plasmatic circulation (0-3 days):* A thin layer of exudate is present between the graft and the recipient bed. The grafted tissue survives with an avascular "plasmatic circulation" from the recipient bed. The epithelium of the free graft degenerates early in the initial healing phase and subsequently, it becomes desquamated. The area of the graft over the avascular root surface receive nutrients from the connective tissue bed that surrounds the recession.

Phase II. *Vascularization (2-11 days):* Anastomoses establish between the blood vessels of the recipient bed and those in the grafted tissue which is characterized by capillary proliferation. Thus, the circulation of blood is re-established in the pre-existing blood vessels of the graft. Epithelium from the adjacent tissues proliferates causing the re-epithelialization of the graft.

Phase III. *Organic union (11- 42 days):* Tissue maturation phase- The vascular system of the graft appears normal. The epithelium gradually matures with the formation of a keratin layer during this stage of healing.

The two ways of root coverage are primary root coverage and secondary root coverage. Primary root coverage is found initially after grafting whereas; secondary root coverage is through creeping attachment. In 1964, Goldman et al noted a second mechanism of gaining root coverage by phenomenon of creeping attachment. This occurs between 1 month to 1 year which is the result of coronal migration of newly grafted attached gingiva over the portions of a previously denuded root. Factors associated with incomplete coverage are:
  i. Improper classification of marginal tissue recession
 ii. Improper preparation of recipient site: Inadequate root planing or failure to treat planed root with citric acid.
iii. Graft factors: Inadequate graft size or graft thickness, dehydration of graft, inadequate adaptation of graft to root and remaining periosteal bed, failure to stabilize the graft, excess or prolonged pressure in coadaptation of the graft.

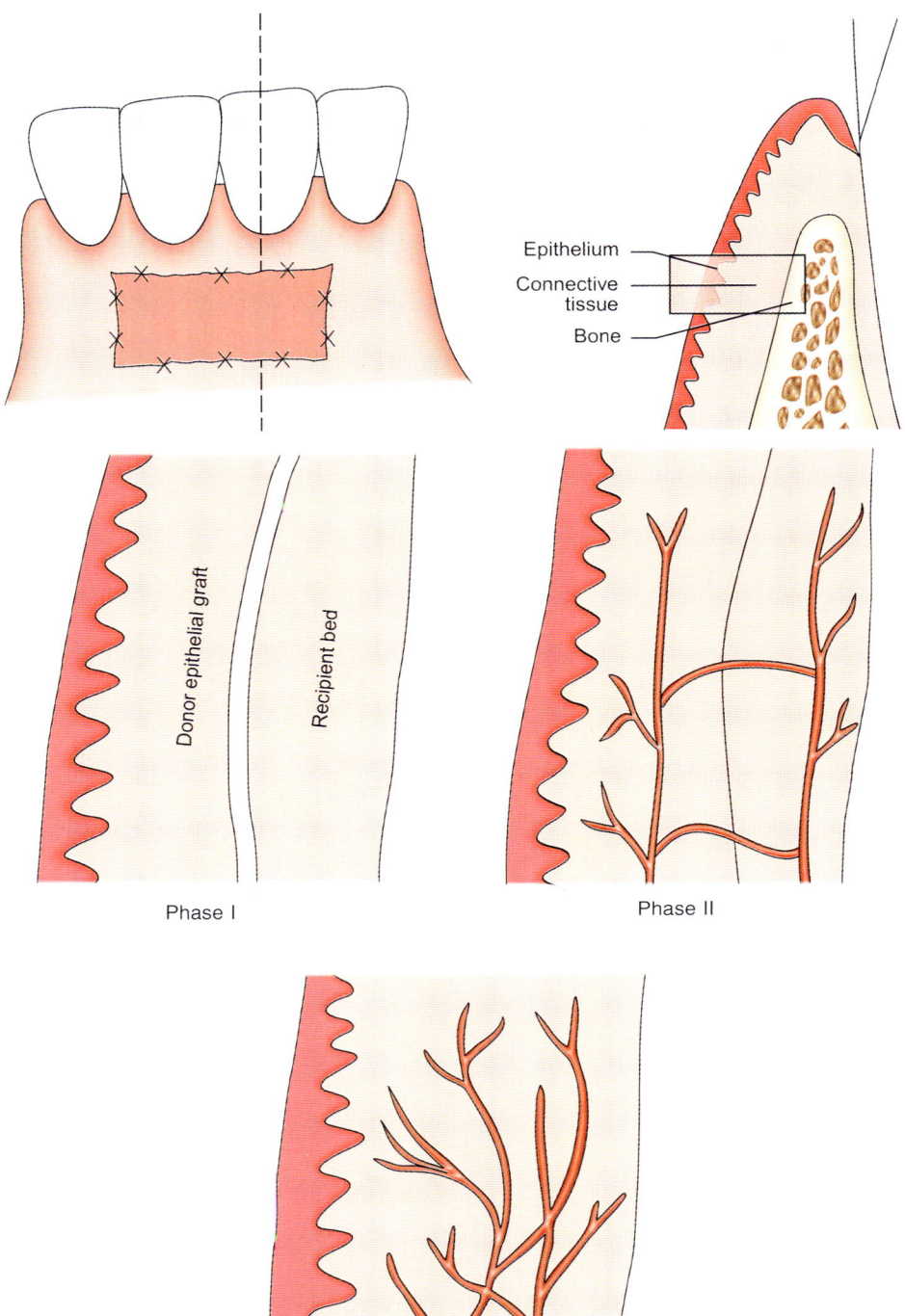

Epithelium

Connective tissue

Bone

Donor epithelial graft

Recipient bed

Phase I

Phase II

Phase III

Fig. 50.1: Healing of free epithelial graft

iv. Patient factors: Excessive smoking, alcohol or non compliance.

TECHNIQUES FOR ROOT COVERAGE

Indications for root coverage procedure are to reduce root sensitivity, to improve esthetics and to manage defects resulting from root caries removal or cervical abrasions.

Etiological Factors of Marginal Tissue Recession

I. Anatomical/Developmental factors:
   A. Dehiscence: Abnormal direction of tooth eruption, malposition of teeth, buccolingual thickness of root more than crestal bone thickness, morphotypes having narrow long teeth and orthodontic tooth movement.
   B. Fenestration
   C. Lack of attached gingiva
   D. Abnormal path of tooth eruption
   E. Individual tooth shape
   F. Tooth eruption compensation
   G. Abnormal tooth position in the arch
II. Physiological factors:
   A. Senile atrophy/aging process
   B. Genetic predisposition
   C. Orthodontic movement of teeth – Controlled and Erratic
III. Pathological factors:
   A. Gingivitis/Periodontitis
   B. Chronic trauma: Impaction of foreign bodies against gingiva and factitious injuries, fingernail scratching of the gums, over rigorous and incorrect tooth brushing and occlusal injury.
   C. Frenal pull
   D. Tobacco chewing
   E. Acute traumatic injuries
   F. Psychological factors – stress and emotions

Etiopathogenesis of Gingival Recession

It is based on inflammation and subsequent destruction of connective tissue of free gingiva. The oral epithelium migrates to the borders of destroyed connective tissue. The thickening of gingival and sulcular basal lamina reduces the quantity of connective tissue between them. Thus, blood supply is reduced, negatively influencing the repair of initial lesion. As the lesion progresses, connective tissue disappears and oral epithelium fuse with junctional or sulcular epithelium. In recession caused by plaque and calculus, initial ulcer appears in the junctional epithelium of sulcus and destruction of connective tissue occurs from inside out. In toothbrush trauma lesions, destruction occurs from outside in.

Classification of Marginal Tissue Recession

I. According to Miller (1985): The marginal tissue recession was classified as (Figs 50.2A to H):
   Class I: Marginal tissue recession not extending to the mucogingival junction. No loss of interdental bone/soft tissue.
   Class II: Marginal tissue recession extends to or beyond the mucogingival junction. No loss of interdental bone/soft tissue.
   Class III: Marginal tissue recession extends to or beyond the mucogingival junction. Loss of interdental bone/soft tissue or there is malpositioning of the tooth.
   Class IV: Marginal tissue recession extends beyond the mucogingival junction. Loss of interdental bone and soft tissue loss interdentally and/or severe tooth malposition.
II. According to Sullivan and Atkins (1968): Gingival recession was classified as follows;
   • Shallow – narrow
   • Shallow – wide
   • Deep – narrow
   • Deep – wide

Classification of Soft Tissue Procedures used for Root Coverage

Cohen classified soft tissue grafting procedures as:
1. Free soft tissue autografts:
   a. Epithelial graft
   b. Subepithelial connective tissue graft
2. Contiguous/Pedicle soft tissue flap:
   a. Rotational flap:
      • Laterally positioned flap
      • Oblique rotated flap
      • Double papillae flap
   b. Advanced flap:
      • Coronally positioned flap

Subepithelial Connective Tissue Graft

It was described by Langer and Langer in 1985. This procedure is indicated for larger and multiple defects with good vestibular depth and gingival thickness to allow a split thickness flap to be elevated. Adjacent to the denuded root surface, the donor connective tissue is sandwiched between the split flap.

Procedure

• *Incisions and Flap Reflection:* Raise a partial-thickness flap with a horizontal incision 2 mm away from the tip of the papilla and two vertical incisions 1 to 2 mm

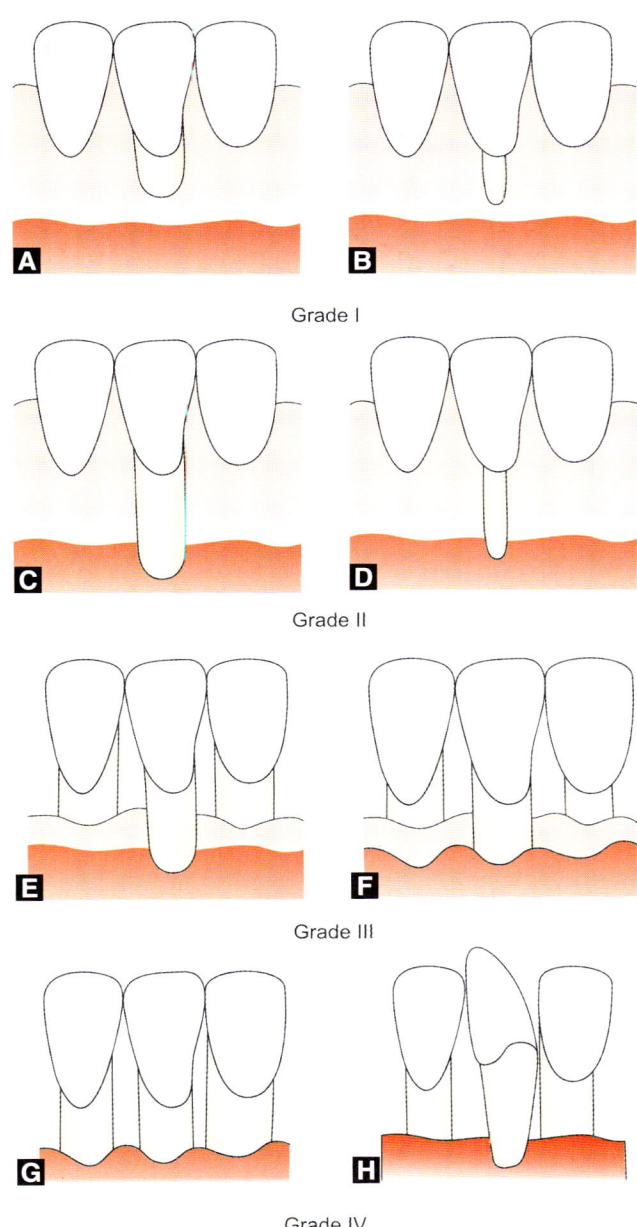

Grade I

Grade II

Grade III

Grade IV

Figs 50.2A to H: P.D Miller's classification of marginal tissue recession

away from the gingival margin of the adjoining teeth. These incisions should extend at least one half to one tooth wider mesiodistally than the area of gingival recession. Extend the flap to the mucobuccal fold without perforations that could affect the blood supply.

- *Scaling and Planing:* Thoroughly scale and plane the root surface, reducing any prominence of the root surface.

- *Obtaining the Graft:* From the palate, obtain connective tissue graft by means of a horizontal incision 5 to 6 mm from the gingival margin of molars and premolars. The connective tissue is carefully obtained and all adipose and glandular tissue are removed. The donor site is sutured after the graft is removed.
- *Transferring the Graft:* Place the connective tissue on the denuded root. Suture it with resorbable sutures to the periosteum. Good stability of the graft must be attained with adequate sutures.
- *Suturing:* Cover the graft with the outer portion of the partial-thickness flap and suture it interdentally. At least one half to two thirds of the connective tissue graft must be covered by the flap for the exposed portion to survive over the denuded root.
- *Covering the Graft:* Cover the grafted site with dry aluminium foil and periodontal dressing. After 7 days, the dressing and sutures are removed.

Laterally Positioned Pedicle Flap

It was originally developed by Grupe and Warren in 1956.

Procedure (Figs 50.3A to D)

- *Incisions:* Make an incision, resecting the gingival margin around the exposed root . Remove the resected soft tissue and scale and plane the root surface. With the blade held at right angles to the surface of the gingiva, a horizontal incision to the depth of the bevel of the blade is made 1-2 mm below the free margin of the gingiva of the donor tooth and extending nearly to the proximal line angle of the next tooth. From that proximal line angle, a vertical incision is made into connective tissue parallel to the exposed root.
- *Prepare the Flap:* A split thickness flap is then prepared by sharp dissection within the area delineated by these incisions so that a layer of connective tissue is left covering the bone in the donor area when the flap is laterally displaced over the denuded root surface.
- *Cut back incision* is given at the distal corner of the flap into the alveolar mucosa, pointing in the direction of the recipient site.
- *Transfer the Flap:* Slide the flap laterally onto the adjacent denuded root, making sure that it lies flat and firm without excess tension on the base. Suture the flap to the adjacent gingiva and alveolar mucosa with interrupted sutures. Sling suture is made around

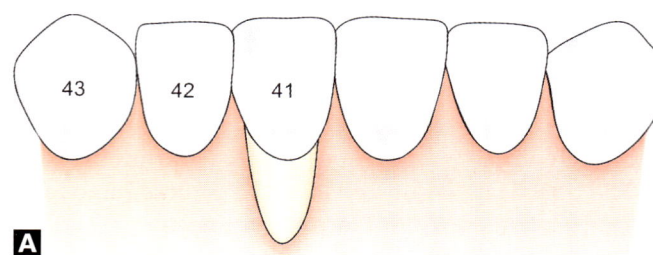

Grade I recession on 41; 42, 43 are donor sites with sufficient amount of attached gingiva

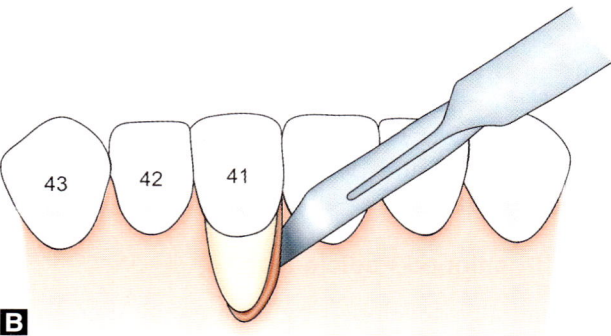

Resecting gingival margin around the exposed root of 41

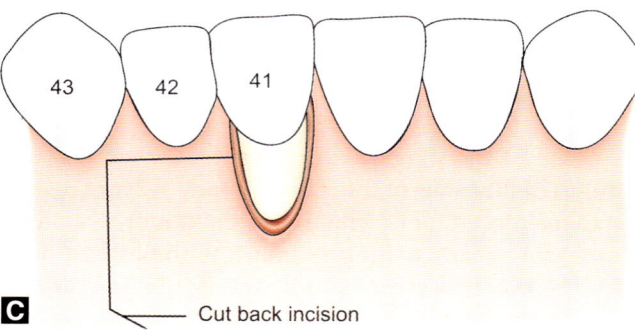

Vertical and horizontal incisions around the donor sites 42 and 43

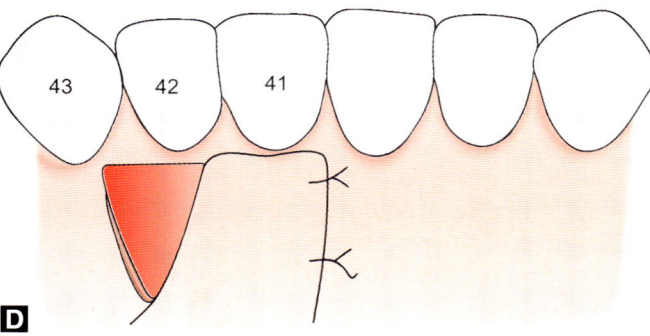

Flap laterally displaced from 42, 43 to 41 and sutured

Figs 50.3A to D: Laterally displaced flap procedure

the involved tooth to prevent the flap from slipping apically.

- *Protect the flap and donor site:* Cover the operative field with aluminium foil and periodontal dressing, extending it interdentally and onto the lingual surface to secure it.
- Postoperative instructions are given thereafter.

Advantages

- Single surgical site
- Aesthetic, close colour blend
- Good vascularity

Disadvantages

- Dehiscence or fenestration at the donor site
- Possibility of recession at donor site
- Limited to one or two teeth with recession

Contraindications

- Shallow vestibule
- Lack of keratinized attached gingiva
- Excessive root prominence
- Presence of deep interproximal pockets
- Deep or extensive root abrasion/erosion
- Significant loss of interproximal bone height

Double Papilla Flap Procedures

It is a variant of lateral pedicle flap in which the basic technique is similar except that the donor tissue is mobilized from the two adjacent papillae rather than from a single adjacent tooth papilla.

Indications

- When the interproximal papillae adjacent to the mucogingival problem are sufficiently wide.
- When the attached gingiva on an approximating tooth is insufficient to allow for a laterally positioned flap.
- When periodontal pocket is not present.

Procedure: (Figs 50.4A and B)

- *Incision:* V – shaped incision is made around the margin of the recessed gingiva to expose connective tissue at its edge. The incision is extended to the depth of, but not including the periosteum. V – section (wedge of gingiva) is then removed and the root surface is scaled thoroughly.

- The lateral releasing/vertical incisions are made at the mesiofacial and distofacial line angles of the adjacent teeth. Horizontal incisions are made across the top of papillae.
- *Flap reflection:* The two papillary tissues is grasped with rat – tail tissue pliers and gently lifted as it is separated from its underlying tissue by means of surgical blade no. 15. Care must be taken not to lift the periosteum, puncture or severe the flap. The two papillary flaps are raised and repositioned to cover the exposed root.
- *Suturing:* The flaps are sutured together. Suture needle is passed through the outer surface of the first papilla and on through the undersurface of the second papilla. Resorbable 5 – 0 medium gut sutures are used for suturing.
- Postoperative instructions are given thereafter.

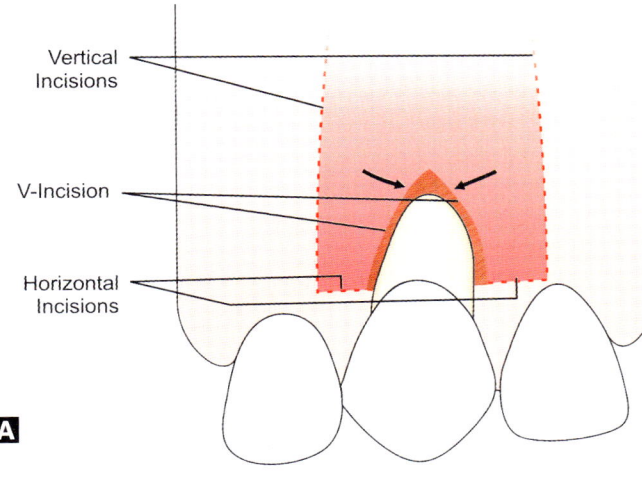

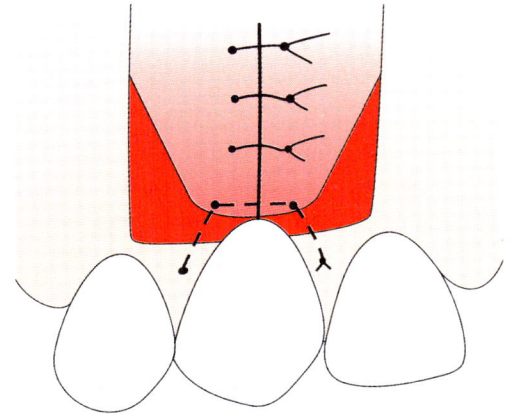

Figs 50.4A and B: Double papilla flap procedure

Advantages

- Risk of resorption of alveolar bone is minimized because interdental bone is more resistant to loss than is radicular bone.
- Clinical predictability of the procedure is good.
- Papilla usually supplies a greater width of attached gingiva than radicular surface of tooth.
- Less tension is placed on the donor tissue.

Disadvantages

- Two flaps are sutured over root surface.
- Manipulation of freed papilla during suture is difficult.

Coronally Displaced Flap

The purpose of the coronally displaced flap is to create a split thickness flap in the area apical to the denuded root and position it coronally to cover the root.

Indication

- Cover denude root surface with adequate width of keratinized gingiva.

Procedure

- *Incisions:* Internal bevel incision is given from the gingival margin to the bottom of the pocket on the selected site. At each end of internal bevel incision, vertical incisions are given beyond the mucogingival junction, to delinate the flap.
- *Flap reflection*: Partial thickness flap is raised with surgical blade no.11 or 15.
- *Scaling and planing:* Scaling and planing is done on the root surface with the help of curettes.
- *Suturing:* The flap is then sutured to the level coronal to pretreatment position to cover the recession. Cover the area with periodontal pack.

Semilunar Coronally Repositioned Flap

This technique was given by Tarnow. The technique is very simple and predictably provides 2 to 3 mm of root coverage which is successful for the maxilla. It is not recommended for mandibular teeth.

Procedure (Figs 50.5A to C)

- *Incision:* A semilunar incision is made following the curvature of the receded gingival margin and ending about 2 to 3 mm short of the tip of the papillae, so that the flap derives all of its blood supply from the papillary areas.

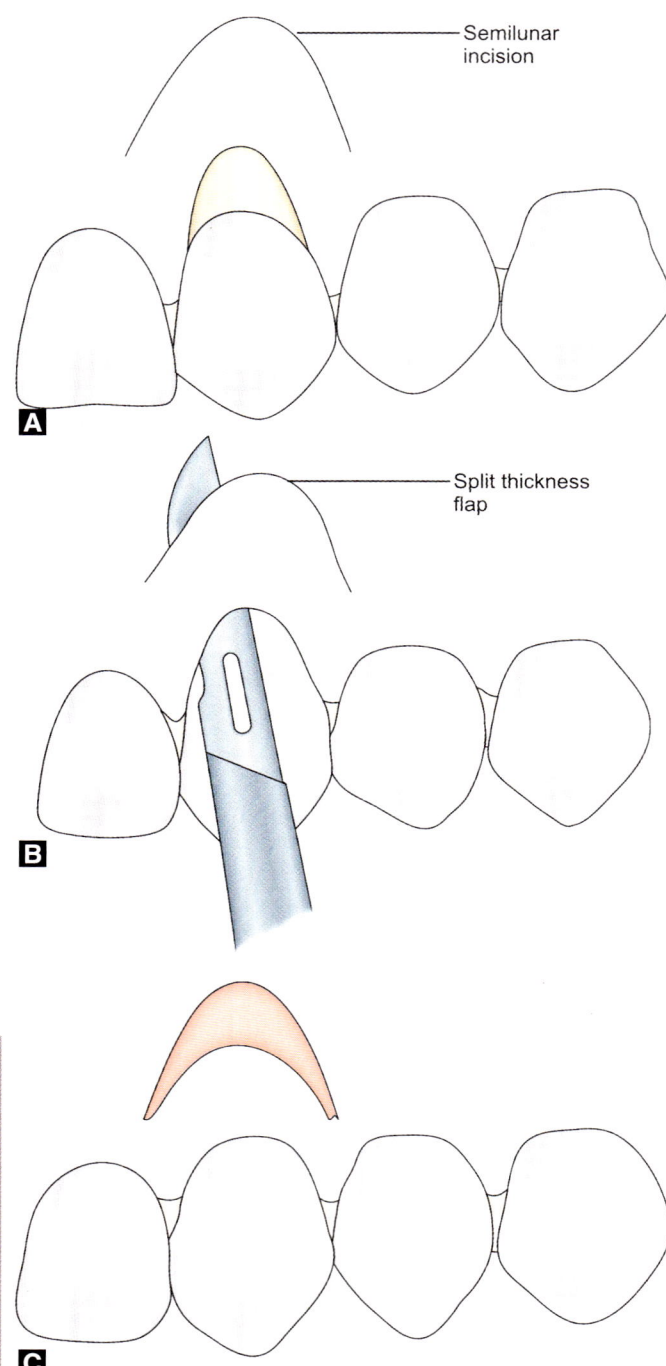

Figs 50.5A to C: Semilunar coronally displaced flap procedure

- *Perform a split thickness* dissection of the facially located tissue by an intracrevicular incision extending apically to the level of the semilunar incision.
- The tissue collapse coronally, covering the denuded root. It is then held in its new position and stabilized by light pressure for 5 minutes; there is no need to suture or to pack.

Advantages

- No shortening of vestibule.
- Can treat multiple areas of recession.
- Flaps are not under tension and require no sutures.

Disadvantages

- Fails if adjacent papillae are not wide enough because flap derives its blood supply from adjacent papillae.
- Cannot be used in mandibular teeth with narrow interdental papillae.

TECHNIQUES FOR THE REMOVAL OF ABERRANT FRENUM (FRENECTOMY)

Frenectomy

Frenectomy is the complete removal of the frenum, including its attachment to the underlying bone whereas frenotomy is the incision of the frenum.

Indications

1. *Gingival or papillary frenal attachment:* Where frenal fibres radiate into marginal gingiva producing gingival retraction and localized gingival recession.
2. *High frenum attachment:* Where oral hygiene is hindered by shallow vestibule caused by high frenum attachment.
3. When lingual frenum interferes with speech.

Instruments: Mosquito forceps/hemostat, Surgical handle Bard Parker no.3 with detachable and replacable surgical blades no. 15/11.

Procedure

- *Anesthesia:* Local infiltration is given to anesthesize the selected site.
- The lip is extended and the frenum is gripped with mosquito forceps/hemostat to the depth of the vestibule.
- *Incisions:* Incisions are made above and below the instrument, the triangular frenum tissue is removed **(Figs 50.6A to C)**. Underlying fibrous attachment to the bone is exposed **(Fig. 50.6D)**. Horizontal incision is given onto these fibers separating and dissecting from the bone.
- *Suturing:* The edges of the wound are undermined slightly and approximated without creating tension and suture only the mucosal extent of incision. The gingival extent is not closed and allowed to heal by secondary intention. Cover the area with dry aluminium foil and then periodontal pack is placed.

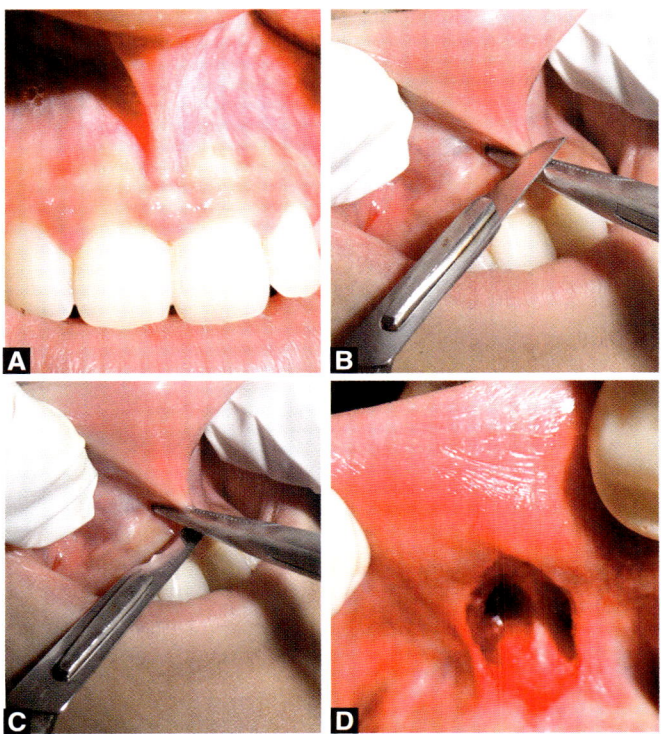

Figs 50.6A to D: Frenectomy (*Courtesy:* Dr Deepak)

- *Postoperative instructions:* The most important postoperative instruction is to ask the patient not to stretch the lip again and again thus, avoiding vigorous lip movements after the frenectomy procedure. Rest postoperative instructions are given in chapter no. 43 General Principles of Periodontal Surgery.

TECHNIQUES TO DEEPEN THE VESTIBULE

The shallow vestibule was one of three original mucogingival problems cited by Friedman in the late 1950's that required the increased apicocoronal dimension of gingiva. The termination of the orofacial muscles into the soft tissues covering the alveolar process forms the vestibular fornix. Shallow vestibular depth usually interferes with oral hygiene procedures causing ineffective plaque control. There are three basic procedures for extending the gingiva into the vestibule.

i. Gingival extension using periosteal fenestration
ii. Vestibuloplasty using modified Edlan – Mejchar procedure
iii. Gingival extension with a free epithelial graft.

Vestibuloplasty is a procedure designed to extend the vestibular fornix.

Objectives:
- To enhance plaque control by allowing space for effective use of plaque control aids.
- To gain more retention for removable prosthetic appliances by expanding the prosthesis bed.

Gingival extension using Periosteal Fenestration

Indications for vestibular extension with periosteal fenestration include areas where a shallow vestibule puts tension on a broad region of the gingival margin, leading to progressive gingival recession. It is also indicated prior to construction of partial prosthesis where expansion of the prosthesis bed is needed.

Procedure: After adequate LA, an incision is made at or near the mucogingival junction, retaining all of the attached gingiva from the mucogingival junction to the margin of gingiva. A split thickness flap is then reflected using a broad surgical blade, with reflection beginning at the mucogingival junction. The muscle fibers and tissue are sharply dissected from the periosteum, freeing the mucosal flap; which is then sutured in the depth of the vestibule. Once the sutures are completed, a strip of the exposed periosteum is removed across the entire surgical area at the level of the original mucogingival junction; leaving a periosteal fenestration exposing bone. A dressing is placed over the surgical site to minimize patient discomfort. Following healing, the vestibular depth is maintained by scar tissue formed in the area of the fenestration.

Vestibuloplasty Using the Edlan-Mejchar Procedure

The Edlan-Mejchar procedure for vestibular deepening results in an increased width of attached mucosa extending into the fornix. No new attached gingiva develops from this procedure; however, it can provide a widened band of alveolar mucosa extending into the deepened vestibule and fixed to the underlying tissue.

Indications for this procedure include the need for expansion of the prosthesis bed and cases of generalized recession over a large arch segment. This procedure is also indicated for treatment of localized recession or for elimination of a broad, high frenum.

The Edlan-Mejchar procedure is contraindicated if a wide band of attached gingiva is needed to cover a recession area.

Procedure (**Figs 50.7A to E**)*:* Two vertical incisions are made from the gingival margin to outline the area of the

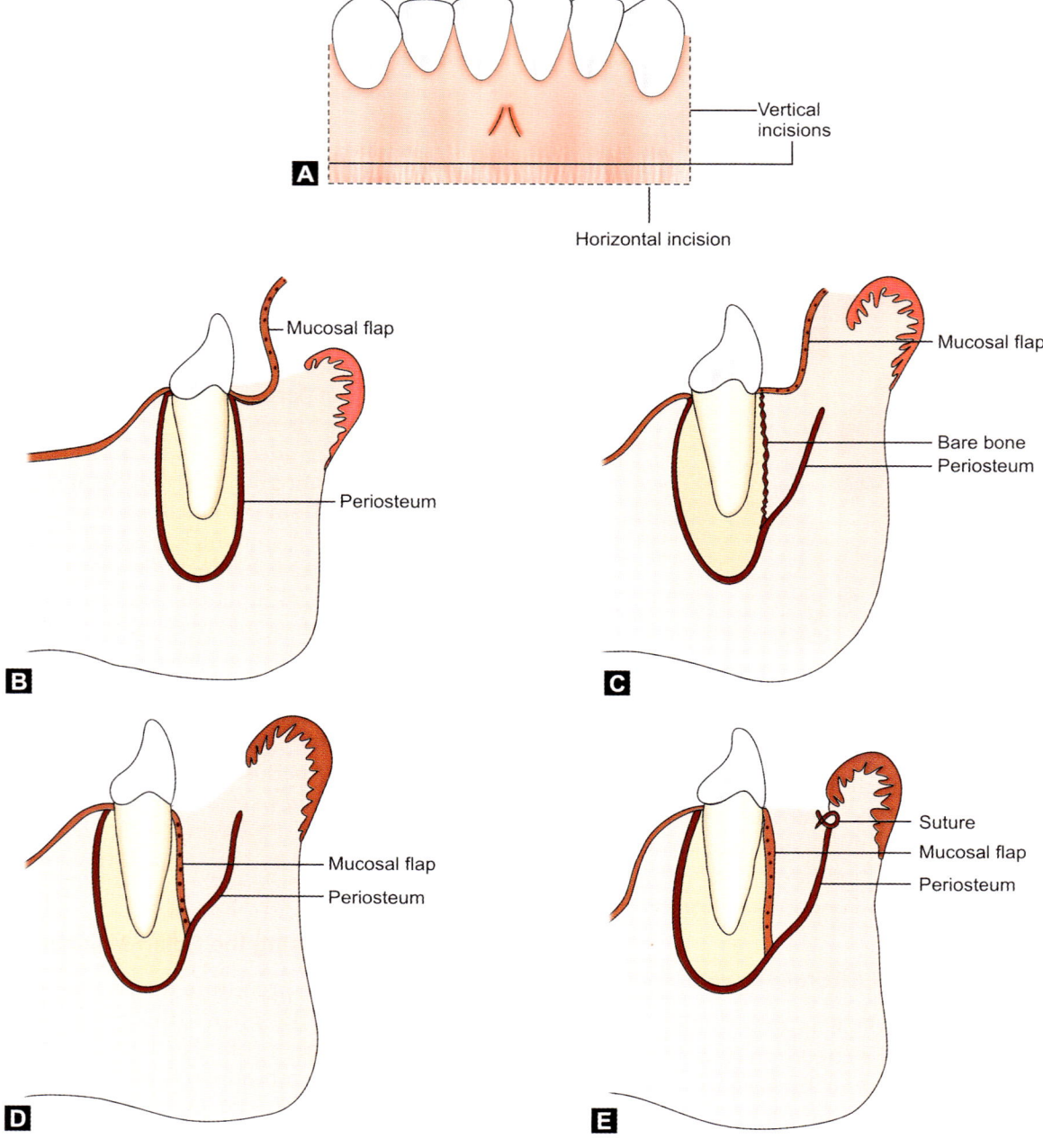

Figs 50.7A to E: Vestibuloplasty (*Courtesy:* Dr SK Salaria)

Edlan-Mejchar operation
A. Two vertical incisions are joined by horizontal incision
B. Mucosal flap elevated, exposing periosteum
C. Periosteum separated from bone
D. Mucosal flap folded down over the bone
E. Periosteum is transposed to lip and sutured

operative field. This is followed by a horizontal incision 10 to 12 mm from the alveolar margin into the depth of the vestibule. A mucosal flap is elevated, exposing the periosteum. The periosteum is then separated from the bone beginning at the margin of the alveolar crest; including the muscle fibers. The periosteal flap is then transposed to the lip and the margins of the flap are sutured to the margin of the incision on the lip. Next the mucosal flap is sutured at the depth of vestibule. Caution should be exercised during incisions and flap reflection in the area of the area of the mental foramen to prevent trauma to the mental nerve or severing the blood vessels in this region. To help adaptation of the mucosal flap to the denuded bone, a moist gauze square is applied to the flap and held for 3 to 5 minutes with gentle pressure. This will help to control hemorrhage, reducing the chance of the flap being dislodged by a blood clot. A periodontal dressing is placed and carefully adapted to the vestibular contours.

TECHNIQUES FOR PAPILLA RECONSTRUCTION

The loss of a key papilla in an aesthetic zone and the presence of a black triangle is an indication for evaluation for papillary reconstruction. The complete regeneration of lost papillae is unpredictable; therefore, retention of papilla is of great importance when an esthetic result is desired from surgical procedures.

Classification of Papillary Height

According to Nordland and Tarnow (1998) **(Fig. 50.8)**:
- *Normal:* The interdental papilla occupies the entire embrassure space apical to the interdental contact point/area.
- *Class I:* The tip of the interdental papilla is located between the interdental contact point and the level of the CEJ on the proximal surface of the tooth.
- *Class II:* The tip of the interdental papilla is located at or apical to the level of the CEJ on the proximal surface of the tooth but coronal to the level of the CEJ mid – buccally.
- *Class III:* The tip of the interdental papilla is located at or apical to the level of CEJ mid – buccally.

The causes of loss of interdental papilla are tooth extraction, excessive surgical periodontal treatment and localized progressive gingival and periodontal lesion.

The effects of loss of interdental papilla are cosmetic deformities, phonetic problems and lateral food impaction.

The various methods to create interdental papilla are:
A. *Non - surgical papilla creation*:
- If interdental papilla is absent because of diastema – Orthodontic closure is the treatment of choice
- Orthodontic forced eruption
- Repeated scaling, root planing and curettage procedure.
B. *Surgical papilla creation*:
- Pedicle graft technique ultilizing the soft palatal tissues of the interdental area
- Semilunar coronally repositioned papilla
- Envelope type flap with connective tissue graft.

TECHNIQUES FOR ALVEOLAR RIDGE AUGMENTATION

Classification of Ridge Defects

I. According to Seibert (1983) **(Fig. 50.9)**:
   Class I: Loss of buccolingual width but normal apicocoronal height.
   Class II: Loss of apicocoronal height but normal buccolingual width.
   Class III: A combination of loss of both height and width of the ridge.
II. According to Allen et al, a modification of Seibert classification:
   Type A: Apicocoronal loss of ridge contour.
   Type B: Buccolingual loss of ridge contour.
   Type C: Combined loss of ridge contour in both apicocoronal and buccolingual dimensions.
III. According to depth of defect:
   Mild: less than 3 mm
   Moderate: 3 to 6 mm
   Severe: greater than 6 mm

The various approaches for utilization of soft tissues for ridge augmentation are:
I. Pedicle graft procedure
- Roll flap procedure
II. Free graft procedures
- Pouch graft procedure
- Interpositional graft procedure **(Figs 50.10A to D)**
- Onlay graft procedure

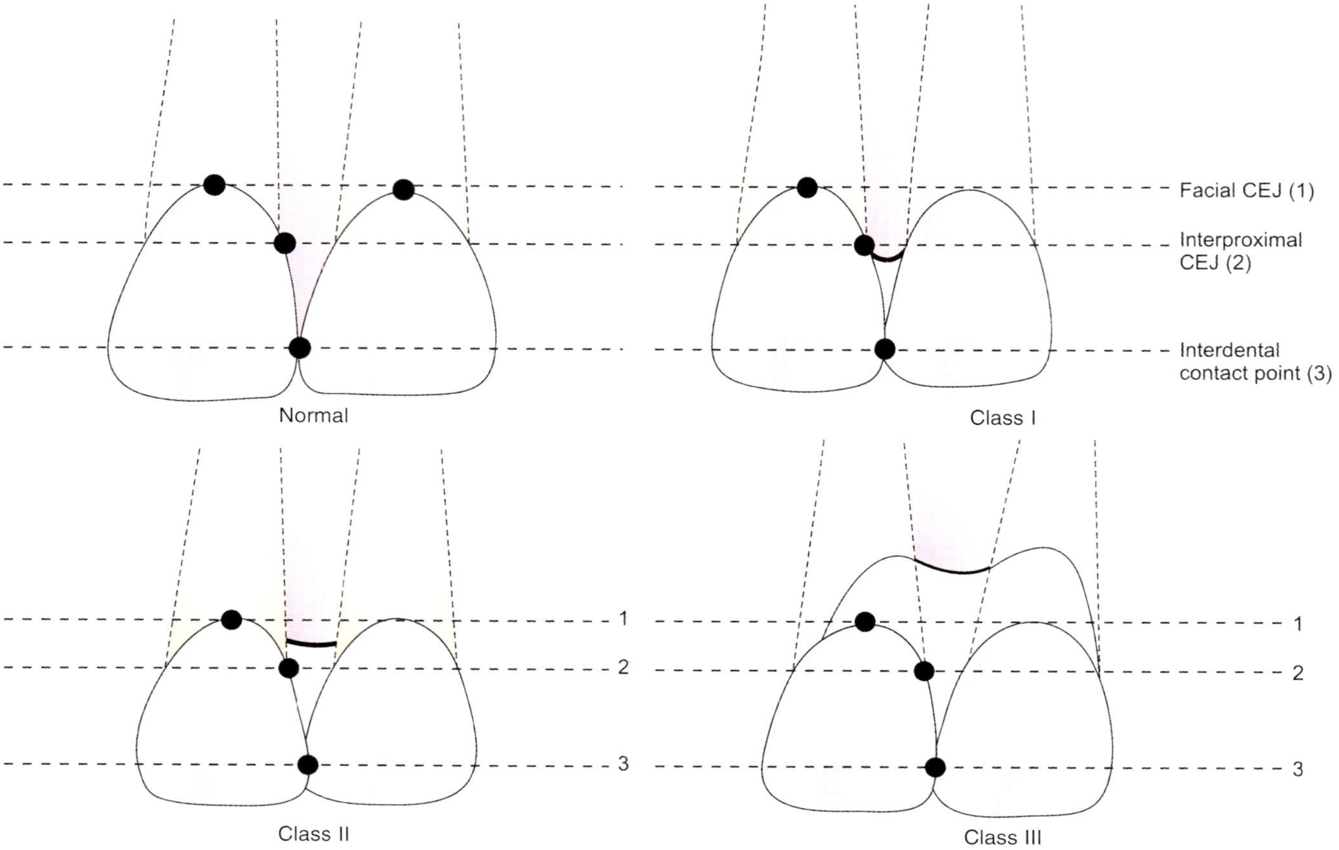

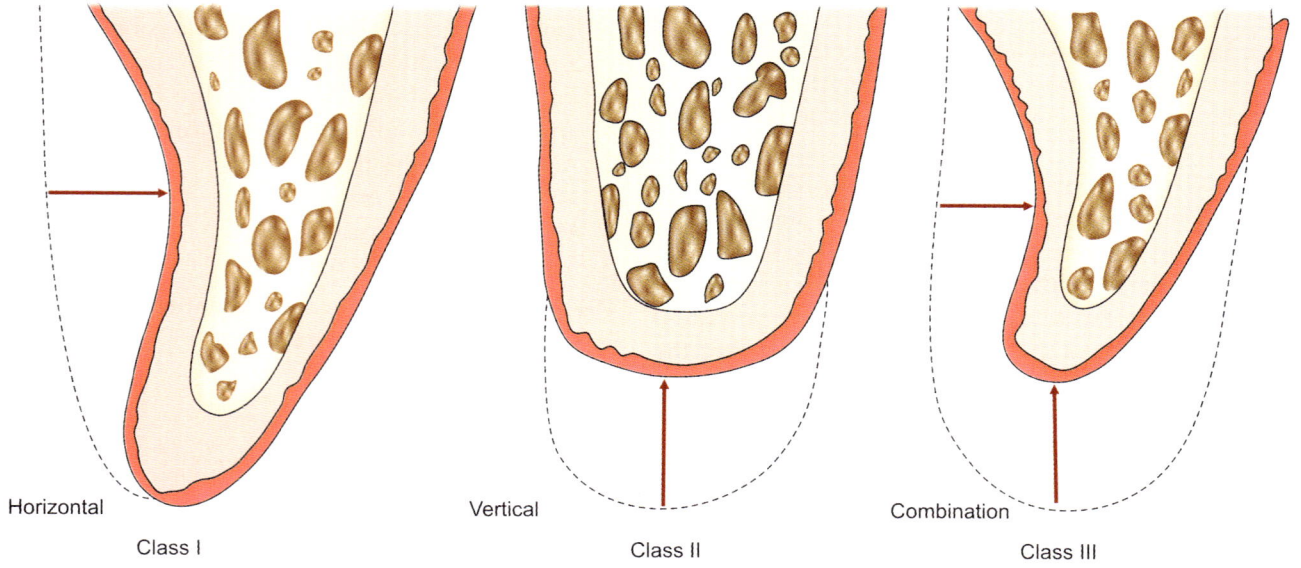

Facial CEJ (1)
Interproximal CEJ (2)
Interdental contact point (3)
Normal
Class I
1
2
3
Class II
1
2
3
Class III

Fig. 50.8: Classification of papillary height

Horizontal
Class I
Vertical
Class II
Combination
Class III

Fig. 50.9: Classification of ridge defects

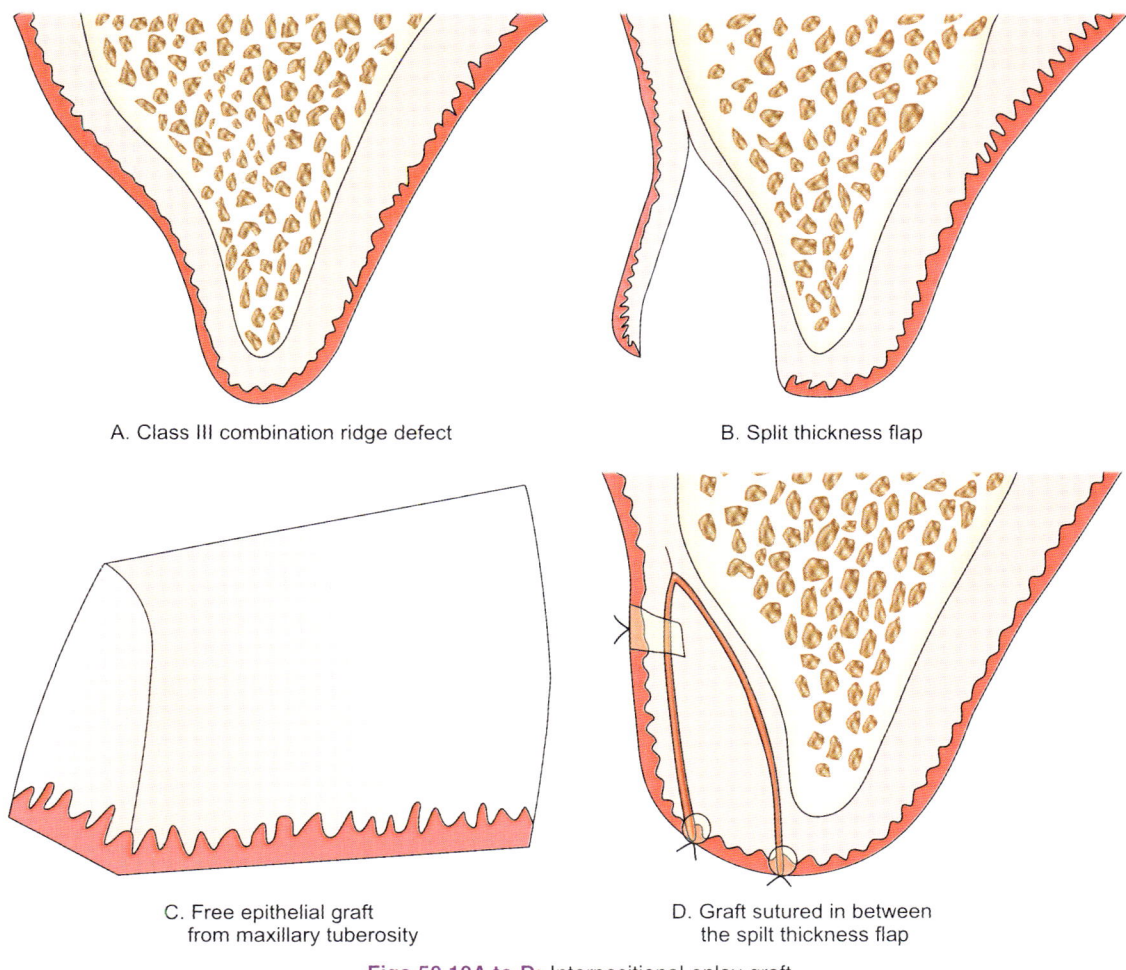

A. Class III combination ridge defect

B. Split thickness flap

C. Free epithelial graft from maxillary tuberosity

D. Graft sutured in between the spilt thickness flap

Figs 50.10A to D: Interpositional onlay graft

POINTS TO PONDER

✓ Cut back incision is given at the distal corner of the lateral displaced flap into the alveolar mucosa, pointing in the direction of the recipient site.

✓ The free epithelial graft is usually covered by whitish mass, termed as ghost graft, which consists of sluffing epithelial cells after 7-10 days postoperatively. This matter can be rinsed away with gentle stream of water.

BIBLIOGRAPHY

1. Abrams L. Augmentation of the residual edentulous ridge for fixed prosthesis. Comp Cont Educ Gen Dent 1980;1:205-14.
2. Azzi R, Etienne D, Carranza F. Surgical reconstruction of the interdental papilla. Int J Periodontics Restorative Dent 1998;18:467-73.
3. Beagle JR. Surgical reconstruction of the interdental papilla: Case report. Int J Periodontics Restorative Dent 1992;12:144-51.
4. Genco RJ, Rosenberg ES, Evian C. Periodontal surgery. In, Genco RJ, Goldman HM, Cohen DW. Contemporary Periodontics. CV Mosby Company 1990;554-84.
5. Glover ME. Periodontal plastic and Reconstructive surgery. In, Rose LF, Mealey BL, Genco RJ, Cohen DW. Periodontics, Medicine, Surgery and Implants. Elsevier Mosby 2004; 405-87.
6. Grant DA, Stern IB, Listgarten MA. Mucogingival surgery. In, Periodontics 6th ed CV Mosby Company 1988;883-910.
7. Hall WB. The Free Gingival graft. In, Pure mucogmgival problems - Etiology, Treatment and prevention. Quintessence publishing Co. Chicago 1984;127-52.
8. Han TJ, Takei HH. Progress in gingival papilla reconstruction. Periodontol 2000 1996;11:65-8.
9. Hiatt WH, Genco RJ. Regenerative therapy in Periodontics. In, Genco RJ, Goldman HM, Cohen DW. Contemporary Periodontics. C.V Mosby 1990,585-604.
10. Miller PD Jr, Allen EP. The development of the periodontal plastic surgery. Periodontol 2000 1996;11:7-17.

11. Miller PD Jr. Periodontal plastic surgery. Curr Opin Periodontol 1993;136-43.
12. Miller PD Jr. Root coverage using a free soft tissue autografts following citric acid application. A successful and predictable procedure in areas of deep wide recession. Int J Periodontics Restorative Dent 1985;5:15-37.
13. Miller PD. Periodontal Plastic Surgical Techniques for Regeneration. In, Polson AM. Periodontal Regeneration Current status and Directions.Quintessence Publishing Co, Inc 1994; 53-70.
14. Miller PD. Regenerative and Reconstructive Periodontal plastic surgery. Dent Clin North Am 1988;32:287-306.
15. Mormann W, Schaer F, Firestone AC. The relationship between success of free gingival grafts and transplant thickness. J Periodontol 1981; 52:74.
16. Nordland WP, Tarnow DP. A classification system for loss of papillary height. J Periodontol 1998;69:1124-26.
17. Oliver RG, Loe H, Karring T. Microscopic evaluation of the healing and re-vascularization of free gingival grafts. J Periodontal Res 1968;3:84-95.
18. Ramfjord SP and Ash MM. Mucogingival surgery. In, Periodontology and Periodontics. Modern Theory and Practice.1st ed AITBS Publisher and Distributor India 1996;305-26.
19. Seibert JS. Soft tissue grafts in periodontics. In, Robinson PJ and Guernsey LH. Clinical transplantation in dental specialties. St.Louis C V Mosby Co, 1980.
20. Takei HH, Azzi RR. Periodontal plastic and esthetic surgery. In, Newman, Takei, Carranza. Clinical Periodontology 9th ed WB Saunders 2003;851-75.
21. Wennstrom JL, Pini Prato GP. Mucogingival Therapy - Periodontal Plastic Surgery. In, Lindhe J, Karring T, Lang NP. Clinical Periodontology and Implant dentistry. 4th ed Blackwell Munksgaard 2003;576-649.

MCQS

1. Ideal thickness of graft should be:
   A. 1.0 to 1.5 mm
   B. 0.25 to 0.5 mm
   C. 0.5 to 1 mm
   D. 2 to 3 mm
2. Mucogingival defect with recession beyond mucogingival line with no loss of bone or soft tissue is:
   A. Class I defect   B. Class II defect
   C. Class III defect   D. Class IV defect
3. Langers technique is used in:
   A. Subepithelial connective tissue grafts
   B. Free soft tissue autografts
   C. Fenestration operation
   D. Vestibular extension operation
4. Vestibular extension procedure results in:
   A. Increase in width of keratinized attached gingiva
   B. Decrease in width of keratinized attached gingiva
   C. Increase in width of nonkeratinized attached gingiva
   D. Decrease in width of nonkeratinized attached gingiva
5. The flap technique for pocket elimination and to increase in width of attached gingiva:
   A. Modified widman flap
   B. Lateral pedicle flap
   C. Apically displaced flap
   D. Coronally repositioned flap
6. In a free gingival graft, what happens to epithelium of the graft?
   A. Degenerates
   B. Proliferates
   C. Remain as such
   D. Has to be removed by surgeon
7. The flap technique procedure which does not increase the width of attached gingiva:
   A. Free gingival graft
   B. Apically displaced flap
   C. Fenestration operation
   D. Undisplaced flap

Answers

1. A	2. B	3. A	4. C	5. C
6. A	7. D			

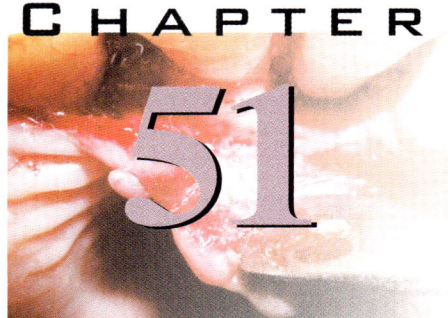

CHAPTER 51

Periodontal Microsurgery

Vikram Jeet Singh Dhingra, Shalu Bathla

INTRODUCTION

It is defined as refinements in existing basic surgical techniques that are made possible by the use of the surgical microscope and subsequent improved visual acuity.

Microsurgery can also be defined as a refinement in operative technique by which visual acuity is enhanced through the use of the surgical operating microscope.

In microsurgery, there is great reduction in surgical damage to the tissues due to the excellent visualization of the operative field through microscope, this least traumatic surgical approach being possible because of magnified surgical field and enhanced dexterity of the surgeon leading to less injury and more meticulous tissue handling.

MAGNIFICATION SYSTEMS

Basically, there are two types of optical magnification available:
I. Magnifying loupes
   - Simple loupes
   - Compound loupes
   - Prism telescopic loupes
II. Surgical microscope

Magnifying Loupes

Three types of loupes are commonly used. Each type may differ widely in lens construction and design.

Simple Loupes: Simple loupes consist of a pair of single, positive, side-by-side meniscus lenses. Each lens has two refracting surfaces. Cost is the sole advantage of simple loupe. Disadvantages are – a) They are highly affected by spherical and chromatic aberration,which distorts the image of the object that is being viewed; b) They have no practical dental application beyond a magnification range of 1.5 diameter, where working distances and depths of field are compromised.

Compound Loupes: Compound loupes use converging multiple lenses with intervening air spaces to gain additional refracting power, magnification, working distance and depth of field. Achromatic lenses consist of two glass lenses, joined together with clear resin. Compound loupes are commonly mounted in or on eyeglasses **(Fig. 51.1)**. Multi-element compound loupes become optically inefficient at magnifications above 3.0 diameters.

Prism Telescopic Loupes: These are the most optically advanced type of loupes **(Fig. 51.2)**. These loupes employ Schmidt or rooftop prisms to lengthen the light path through a series of switchback mirror reflections within

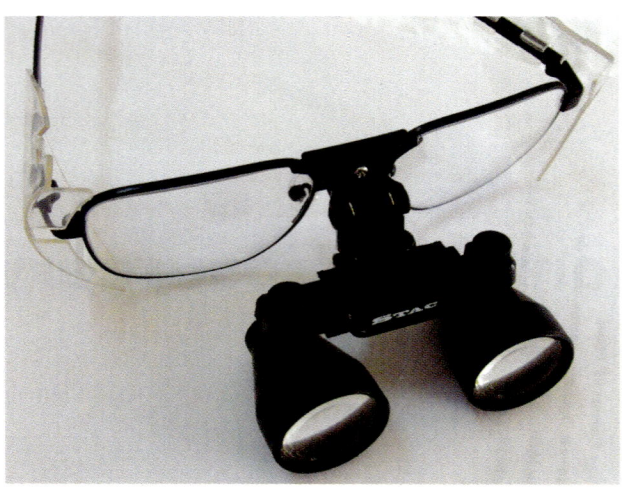

Fig. 51.1: Galilean compound loupe (3.5 × 420 mm)

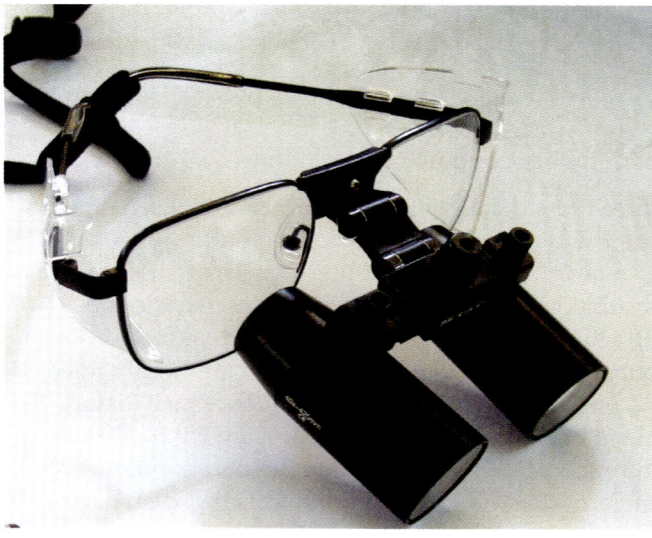

Fig. 51.2: Prismatic loupe (4.0 × 420 mm)

the lens elements, vitually folding the light so that the barrel of the loupe can be shortened. Advantages are – a) better magnification; b) wider depths of field; c) longer working distances; and d) larger fields of view than other types of loupes. The barrels of prism loupes are short enough to be mounted on either eyeglass frames or headbands. However, the increased weight of prism telescopic loupes with magnification above 3x makes headband mounting more comfortable and stable than eyeglass frame mounting.

Surgical Microscope

The surgical microscope (OPM) is a complicated system of lenses that allow binocular viewing at a magnification of approximately x4 to ×40. In contrast to loupes, both light beams fall parallel onto the retinas of the observer so that no eye convergence is necessary and the demand of the eye muscle is minimal. The OPM consists of the magnification changer, objective lenses, lighting unit, binocular tubes and eyepieces **(Fig 51.3)**. It can be fixed to the floor or mounted on the wall or ceiling.

Benefits of microscopes: Operating microscopes offer three distinct advantages to the clinician: illiumination, magnification, and increased precision in the delivery of surgical skills. Collectively these advantages are referred to as the "microsurgical triad". The advantages of microscopes over loupes is that of greater operator comfort and same view can be shared with the students or reflected on to a monitor for teaching and achieve better team work, or even record the surgery.

MICROSURGICAL INSTRUMENTS

Design of the microinstruments: They should be approximately 18 cm long but are much smaller, often by ten-fold. Using these smaller instruments under magnification allows surgeons to refine their movements with the end result of enhanced surgical skills. Their handles have a round cross – sectional diameter to enhance rotary movements using the precision grip. The weight of each instrument should be a maximum of 15 to 20 g to avoid hand and arm muscle fatigue. They are made of titanium

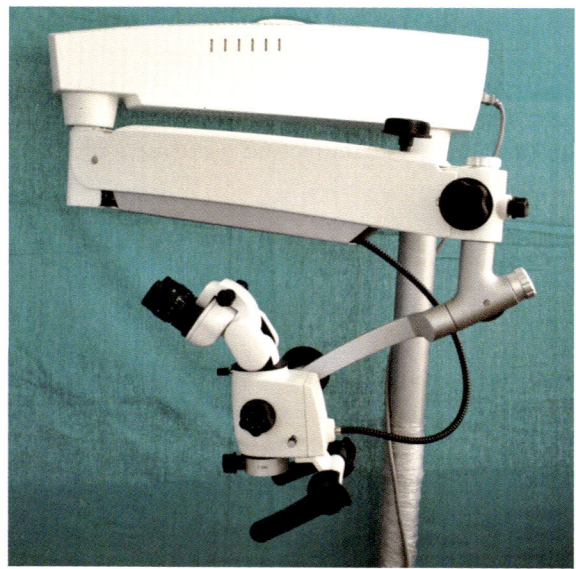

Fig. 51.3: Surgical operating microscope *(Courtesy:* Dr Suresh DK)

to reduce weight and prevent magnetization. In order to avoid an unfavorable metallic glare under the OPM, these instruments have a colored coating surface.

Scalpel and blades: Ophthalmic scalpel, blades and castroviejo microsurgical scalpel are used. Ophthalmic knives offer the dual advantages of extreme sharpness and minimal size. Because ophthalmic knives are chemically etched rather than ground, their sharper blades produce a more precise wound edge **(Fig. 51.4)**.

Suture material requisites: Atraumatic suture consists of a strand that is firmly connected to the needle through a press - fit swage. The needle consists of a swage, body, and tip. Reverse cutting needles with precision tips or spatula needles with micro tips are preferred. Reverse cutting needles have a greater degree of firmness than do round-body needles, which is advantageous for the penetration of coarse gingiva. The diameter of the needle body should be flattened in order to stabilize the needle in its holder for periodontal microsurgery, the 3/8" circular needle generally ensures optimum results. The lengths, as measured along the needle curvature from the tip to the proximal end of the needle lock, extend from 5 to 13 mm depending on their area of application. Needle length should range from 11 to 13 mm for a papilla suture. A spatula needle is 6.6 mm in length and has a curvature of 140°. The needle track is shallow and the needle purchase point is precise. These characteristics allow extremely accurate apposition, closure and immobilization of the connective tissue graft.

7-0 to 9-0 microsutures are used. Needle angle of entry and exit is slightly less than 90°. Sutures pass across the incision line at oblique/acute angles rather than perpendicularly. Bite size is 1.5 times the tissue thickness. Polypropylene, a water proof isotactile thread that is hydrolytically unchanged in the tissues of the body, is the optimum suture material for microsurgery.

Needle holder: The needle holder should be equipped with a precise working lock that should not exceed a locking force of 50 g. High locking forces generate tremor and reduce the feeling for the movement **(Fig. 51.5)**.

Surgical and anatomical forceps: As an innovation, the surgical forceps is designed as a combination

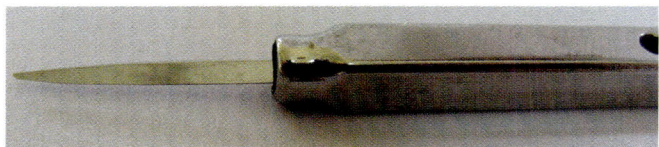

Fig. 51.4: Scalpel

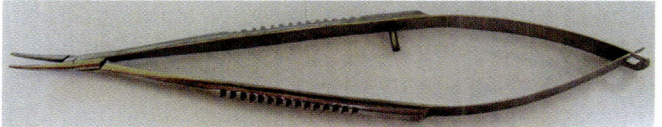

Fig. 51.5: Microneedle holder

instrument. It is an anatomical forceps that converts into a surgical forceps at its end **(Fig. 51.6)**. This combination enables mucosal flaps to be seized and the ensuing thread to be knotted without a change of instruments. In order to avoid sliding of the thread when knotting, the tips of the forceps have flat surfaces or can be finely cross - hatched. The latter should be designed to grip fine and rough needles. When closed, no light must pass through the tips. Locks aid in the execution of controlled rotation movements on the instrument handles without pressure. The tips of the forceps should be approximately 1 to 2 mm apart when the instrument lies in the hand without any pressure.

Scissors: Laschal microscissor with small beak scissor are used **(Fig. 51.7)**.

Storage of instruments: In order to prevent damage, microinstruments are stored in a sterile container or tray. The tips of the instruments must not touch each other during sterilization procedures or transportation.

REQUIREMENTS OF THE SURGEON

Microsurgical training attempts to improve the fine tuning of the motor muscles of the hand and arm and

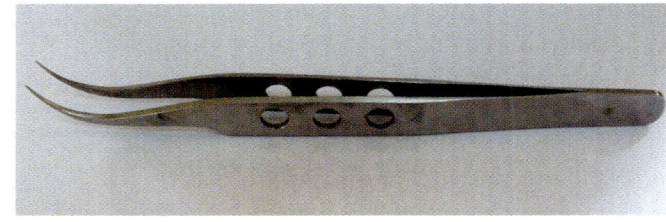

Fig. 51.6: Curved Jeweler microforcep

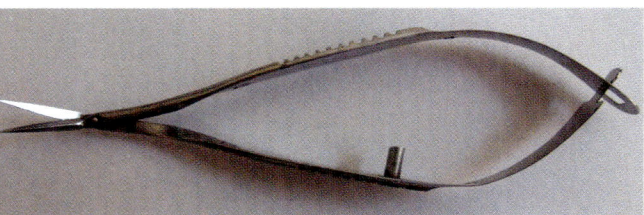

Fig. 51.7: Microscissor
(*Courtesy:* Dr Sudhir Kumar Mehta)

PERIODONTICS REVISITED

the training of the clinician's cognitive abilities. One to two hours of training per week for approximately 3 months is recommended for the beginners. Using the time knotting technique, instrument handling and dexterity can be standardized so that the surgeon can totally concentrate on the surgical procedure.

The clinicians seated position should be adjusted so that the upper part of the body balances symmetrically and the lower arms and hands are well supported. Treatment chairs designed specifically for microsurgeons are useful as they allow fine tuning of the arm supports. In the learning phase, folded cloth rolls may be placed on the patient's shoulders to enable sufficient hand support.

ROLE OF MICROSURGERY IN PERIODONTAL PROCEDURES

The reason microsurgery has gained acceptance among some periodontists is not due to the reduced morbidity but rather, the end-point appearance of microsurgery is simply superior to that of conventional surgery. The difference is shown in cleaner incisions, closer wound apposition, reduced hemorrhage and reduced trauma at the surgical site.

Periodontal Plastic Surgery: In periodontal plastic surgery, the aesthetic and functional results are equally important. Due to microsurgical technique, optimal aesthetics can be obtained in micro gingival surgery when numerous parameters are maintained: the theoretical and practical training of the surgeon, the necessary viewing aids, the instruments and the suture technique.

Various microgingival surgical procedures are:
  i. Tissue grafting procedure to correct gingival recession
     a. Free epithelial grafting
     b. Subepithelial connective tissue grafting
 ii. Papilla reconstruction procedure
iii. Establishing an esthetic smile line: The creation of an ideal esthetic smile with harmonious gingival contours involves many factors including lip position, symmetry and relative gingival levels of adjacent teeth. Complex periodontal plastic microsurgery involving removal of tissue on some teeth and replacement on others may be required.

 iv. Restoring the edentulous ridge: Ridge augmentation can involve a variety of techniques, including guided bone regeneration, block and particulate grafts, soft tissue grafts and a combination of these.

Advantages of periodontal microsurgery
* Improved cosmetics
* Rapid healing
* Minimal discomfort
* Less invasive - As there is reduced incision size, lessened need for vertical releasing incisions and smaller surgical sites thus, periodontal microsurgery is considered less invasive procedure
* Reduces surgical fatigue and development of spinal and occupational pathology of the operator
* Enhanced patient acceptance.

POINTS TO PONDER

✓ Carl Nylen is considered the father of microsurgery.
✓ Advantages of loupes over microscopes: i. Less expensive to purchase; ii. Easier to use; iii. Loupes tend to be less cumbersome in operating field and less likely to breech a clean operative field; and iv. They are handy in free – lancing practice.
✓ Disadvantage of loupes over microscopes is that the individual light source is required for loupes.
✓ In periodontal surgery a magnification of × 4.5 to ×5 for loupe spectacles and ×10 to ×20 for surgical microscope appears to be ideal.

BIBLIOGRAPHY

1. Belcher JM. A Perspective on Periodontal Microsurgery. Int J Periodontics Restorative Dent 2001;21:191-6.
2. Burkhardt R, Hurzeler MB. Utilization of the surgical microscope for advanced plastic periodontal surgery. Pract Periodont Aesthet Dent 2002; 12(2):171-80.
3. GH Shanelec DA. Periodontal Microsurgery. J Esthet Restor Dent 2003;15:18-23.
4. Shanelec DA. Principles of Periodontal Plastic Microsurgery. In, Rose LF, Genco RJ, Mealey BL, Cohen DW. Periodontics, Medicine, Surgery and Implant. Elsevier Mosby 2004;488-501.
5. Shanelec DA, Tibbetts LS. Recent advances in surgical technology. In, Newman, Takei, Carranza. Clinical Periodontology 9th ed WB Saunders 2003;876-81.
6. Tibbetts LS, Shanelec D. Periodontal microsurgery. Dent Clin North Am 1998; 42:339-59.

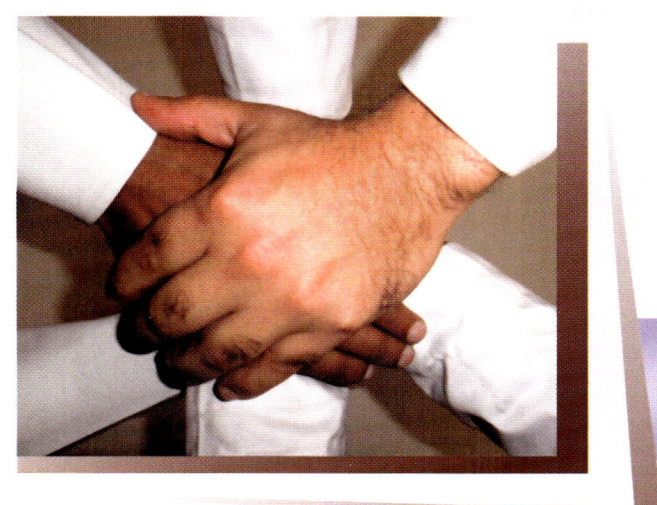

SECTION

SEVEN

INTERDISCIPLINARY
APPROACH

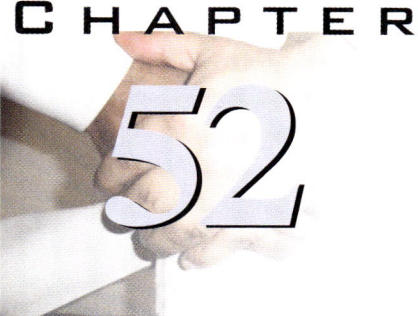

CHAPTER 52

Periodontics-Prosthodontics

Sushant Garg, Shalu Bathla

INTRODUCTION

The relationship between periodontal health and the restoration of teeth is intimate and inseparable. For restorations to survive long term, the periodontium must remain healthy so that the teeth are maintained. For the periodontium to remain healthy, restorations must be critically managed in several areas so that they are in harmony with their surrounding periodontal tissues.

SEQUENCE OF TREATMENT

In patients with mutilated dentitions and extensive periodontal disease, the sequence of treatment can be modified as follows:

First of all hopeless teeth are extracted which is followed by construction of a temporary partial denture and then, periodontal therapy is performed. Approximately 2 months after periodontal treatment, when gingival health is restored and the location of the gingival sulcus is established, the preparations are modified to relocate the margins in proper relation to the healthy gingival sulcus, and final restorations are constructed.

APPLICATION OF PERIODONTICS IN PROSTHETIC DENTISTRY

Preprosthetic Periodontal Care

Periodontal tissues should be in a state of health prior to preparation of a tooth for any restoration. Inflammation alters the contour, shape, volume and consistency of the marginal gingiva and the interdental papilla, so that when inflammation is present, it is impossible to accurately prepare the tooth because of lack of reference points for the correct placement of the cervical margin of the preparation, and ease of bleeding of the pocket wall. The gingiva should therefore be treated first and after healing has been completed, the preparation should be done. It is the periodontal health that determines when the tooth preparation can be started. Once gingival inflammation and periodontal pockets have been eliminated, the gingival margin will change position and shape. The possibilities of gingival recession after placement of restoration are minimized if the procedure is started with healthy periodontal tissues.

Periodontal disease must be eliminated prior to prosthetic treatment because of the following reasons:

1. Margins of restorations covered by inflamed gingiva shrinks after periodontal treatment. Thus, to locate and determine the gingival margin of restoration properly, the position of the healthy and stable gingival margin must be established prior to tooth preparation.

2. The position of teeth is frequently altered in periodontal disease. Resolution of inflammation and regeneration of periodontal ligament fibers after treatment cause the teeth to move again, often back to their original position.

3. Inflammation of the periodontium impairs the capacity of abutment teeth to meet the functional demands made on them.

4. Partial prosthesis constructed on casts made from impressions of diseased gingiva and edentulous mucosa do not fit properly when periodontal health is restored. When the inflammation is eliminated, the contour of gingiva and adjacent mucosa is altered. Shrinkage creates spaces beneath the pontics of fixed bridges and the saddle areas of removable prosthesis again resulting in plaque accumulation.

5. Tooth mobility and pain interfere with mastication and function of restored teeth.

Gingival massage is adviced to the patient for better healing after extraction. Thus, preprosthetic periodontal treatment and care should create healthy gingivomucosal environment and osseous topography necessary for the proper function of single-tooth restorations, fixed prosthesis and removable partial prosthesis.

Preprosthetic Periodontal Surgery

The procedure which aims to treat the periodontal condition and preparing the mouth for the ensuing esthetic, restorative and prosthetic therapy is called as preprosthetic periodontal surgery.
This includes:
• Crown lengthening
• Ridge augmentation

Crown – lengthening Surgery

The surgical procedure to expose adequate clinical crown to prevent the placement of the crown margin into the area of the biologic width is called as crown–lengthening surgery.

Biologic width is defined as the dimension of healthy gingival tissue, which is attached to the tooth coronal to the crest of the alveolar tissue. Average length of connective tissue attachment is 1.07 mm and of junctional epithelium is 0.97 mm which makes total biologic width of 2.04 mm **(Fig. 52.1)**. Significance of biologic width: If the restorative margin is placed into biologic width area there will be gingival inflammation, pocket formation and loss of crestal bone to reestablish the biologic width.

Indications for Crown – lengthening surgery:
• Subgingival caries or fracture
• Inadequate clinical crown length for retention
• Unequal/unesthetic gingival height

Apically positioned flap with ostectomy removes the tooth-supporting bone to lengthen the clinical crown. There should be atleast 3 mm distance between the apical extension of restoration and crest of the alveolar bone **(Figs 52.2A and B)**. This space allows sufficient room for the supracrestal collagen fibers that are part of the periodontal support mechanism, as well as providing a gingival crevice of 2 to 3 mm. The margin of the crown is finally positioned at its correct level, approximately halfway down the gingival crevice. Failure to allow sufficient space between the crown margin and the alveolar crest height means that the finished restoration is positioned deep in the periodontal tissues and results in increased inflammation and pocket formation **(Fig 52.3)**.

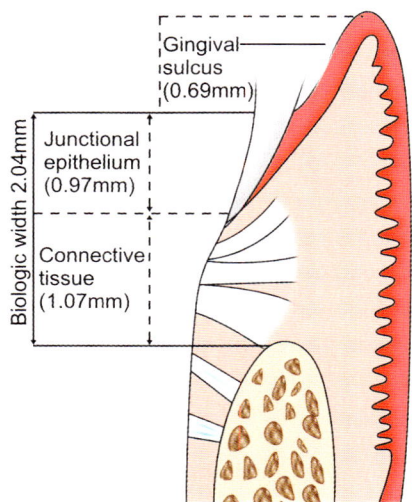

Fig. 52.1: Biologic width

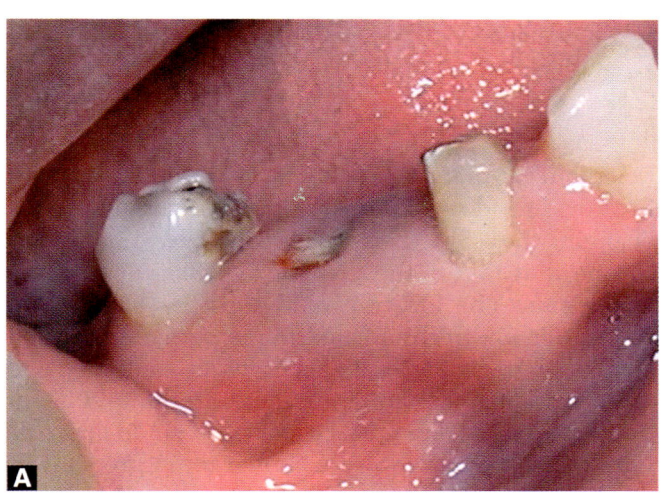 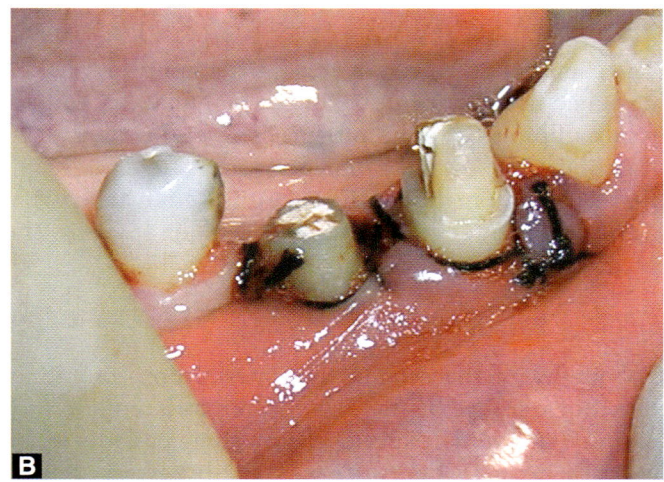

Figs 52.2A and B: Crown – lengthening procedure

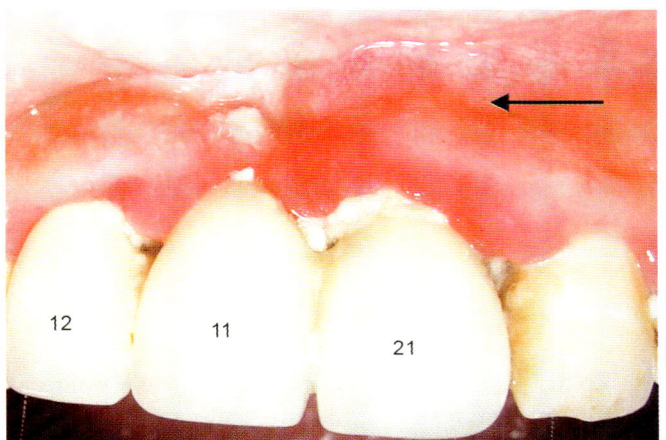

Fig. 52.3: Violation of biologic width—Inflammatory changes on gingiva of crown 21

Ridge Augmentation

These procedures correct the excessive loss of alveolar bone that sometimes occurs in the anterior region. This excessive bone loss complicate the prosthetic reconstruction as large space may result in either a long pontic or a space between the apical end of the pontic and the resorbed ridge. These osseous defects may occur in a coronoapical or buccolingual direction or in both directions.

The roll technique by Abrams manage moderate tissue loss in the buccolingual direction. The epithelium on the palatal side of the defect is removed. After a split thickness incision, the flap denuded of the epithelial covering is rolled beneath the buccal split flap. The rolled portion of the palatal split flap augments the ridge in a buccal direction. If the ridge defect is more extensive subepithelial connective donor tissue from the palate can be placed in tunnel created at the recipient site. Vertical incisions at the two ends of the defect and a tunnel made in both the horizontal and vertical directions create a recipient site that provides excellent blood supply to the donor tissue. This tissue is positioned with gut sutures from the palatal side. The vertical augmentation achieved by this surgery provides an excellent soft tissue environment for an esthetic fixed restoration. In larger defects bone grafts in the form of a monocortical block using fixation screws can be placed.

PERIODONTAL CONSIDERATIONS IN COMPLETE DENTURE AND REMOVABLE PARTIAL DENTURE PROSTHODONTICS

Impression Materials

In general, completely set hydrocolloid (both reversible and irreverible), polysulfide, and silicone impression materials have not been shown to cause any detrimental tissue reactions. The main concern with reversible hydrocolloid is the possibility of burning soft tissue if the material has not been conditioned at the proper temperature. The catalyst of the silicone materials has been known to be chemically irritating. Care should be exerted not to inadvertently leave any impression material, especially the rubber base type, in the gingival crevice. Such residual impression material may lead to a foreign body reaction with severe periodontal implications.

PERIODONTICS REVISITED

Design of the Prosthesis

The components of removable partial denture must be designed and fabricated in such a way that the gingiva is not impinged by the prosthesis. Major connector in maxillary and mandibular are kept at 6 and 3 mm respectively from the gingival margin. Removable partial dentures covering gingival tissue favour the accumulation of plaque.

Denture Plastics

Polymethyl methacrylate is the material most commonly used for denture bases. The chronic inflammation, or denture stomatitis, experienced by some patients in the mucosa beneath dentures was attributed to allergic reaction to the components of denture base plastic. Some of the constituents (polymer, benzoyl peroxide, hydroquinone, or the dye pigment) could indeed individually cause chemical irritation. Therefore, incompletely cured polymers could cause some inflammation to oral tissue. Partial dentures that are worn night and day induce more plaque formation than those worn only during day time. The presence of removable partial dentures induces not only quantitative changes in dental plaque but also qualitative changes promoting the development of spirilla and spirochetes.

Partial Denture Framework Alloys

Some patients have been observed to develop mucosal contact stomatitis, general dermatitis or combinations of the two. Reactions have varied from severe to minor. The predominant culprits in these alloys have been nickel, although cobalt and chromium have also been responsible on occasions.

PERIODONTAL CONSIDERATIONS IN FIXED PARTIAL DENTURE PROSTHODONTICS

The ideal goal for prosthodontic work should be to make conditions adjacent to fixed single crowns and bridges as favorable as around natural teeth and not to initiate pathologic processes that may endanger the longevity of abutment teeth.

Certain factors to be consider are:
1. Tooth preparation in relation to the gingival margin
2. Gingival management for making impressions
3. Contour of restoration
4. Occlusal surface
5. Pontic design
6. Cementation
7. Impression materials

Tooth Preparation in Relation to the Gingival Margin

Overhanging margins contribute to periodontal disease by providing ideal locations for plaque accumulation and changing the ecologic balance of the gingival sulcus area to one that favors the growth of disease-associated organisms. The location of the gingival margin of restoration is directly related to the periodontal health status. Subgingivally located margins are associated with large amounts of plaque, more severe gingivitis and deeper pockets. Care must be exercised not to injure the gingival tissues during subgingival tooth preparation, especially where gingiva is thin and delicate. When there is minimal attached gingiva, injuries are more likely to cause recession. The epithelial attachment is the most vulnerable to all the supporting structures and procedural trauma can initiate its apical migration and result in periodontitis or recession. In crown preparation, a basic general principle should be followed:

- Sufficient tooth structure should be removed so that there is a definite cervical area to accommodate a restoration that will reconstruct the anatomy of the tooth in harmony with dental and periodontal environment
- Subgingival finish lines should be terminated at least 0.5 mm short of epithelial attachment
- Rotary instruments can severely injure or obliterate the gingiva, resulting in esthetically poor soft tissue contours, which can produce problems in maintaining periodontal health
- The type of subgingival finish line being formed is related to the potential for gingival trauma. A shoulder finish line can be established subgingivally while keeping the entire rotary instrument diameter within the peripheral tooth contours
- The formation of chamfers and beveled shoulders requires that part of rotary instrument diameter be located outside peripheral tooth contours, with greater potential for gingival trauma.

Gingival Management for Making Impressions

For subgingival preparation margin extending to the appropriate depth in the sulcus, gingival tissue must be protected from abrasion. Tissue management is achieved with gingival retraction cords of the appropriate size to achieve the required displacement. Electrosurgery can also be used to remove any overlying tissue in the retraction process. A fine wire-tip electrode is held parallel to the tooth and against the margin in the sulcus and moved through the overhanging tissue, opening up the margin and the retraction cord to visual access.

Contours

Overcontoured crowns and restorations tend to accumulate plaque and prevent self - cleansing mechanisms of adjacent cheek, lips and tongue. Inadequate or improperly located proximal contacts and failure to reproduce the normal protective anatomy of the occlusal marginal ridges and developmental grooves lead to food impaction. The facial and lingual contours of restorations are also important in the preservation of gingival health. In patients in whom periodontal disease causes the gingival margin to be in a much more apical position than it was during health, the facial and lingual contours become even more significant. In this particular case the bulge on the facial contour of the crown, which normally would be subgingival, appear supragingivally. In class III and IV furcation defect, it is important that the restoration be contoured in such a way as to facilitate access for oral hygiene. In these cases, it is important to emphasize the mid - facial groove of the crown so that this groove is confluent with the furcation.

Occlusal Surface

Occlusal surfaces should be designed to direct masticatory forces along the long axis of the teeth. The anatomy of the occlusal surface should provide well - formed marginal ridges and occlusal sluiceways to prevent interproximal food impaction. Thus, restorations that do not conform to the occlusal patterns of the mouth cause occlusal disharmonies that may be injurious to the supporting periodontal tissues.

Pontic Design

From a periodontal point of view, pontics in fixed bridges represents a hygienic problem. Therefore, in designing pontic the following requirement should be met—(a) All surfaces should be smooth, polished and convex. Soldered points must be polished. (b) Pontics should be constructed to permit adequate oral hygiene measures. Principally there should be no contact between the undersurface and the soft tissue, the embrasure should be wide, and the shape of the pontic should be convex in buccolingual as well as mesiodistal direction. There are four pontic design: sanitary, ridge-lap, modified ridge-lap, and ovate pontic designs. The key differences between the four pontic designs relate to the esthetics and access for hygiene procedures. The shape of the undersurface of pontic determines the ease with which plaque and food debris can be removed. The sanitary and ovate pontics have convex undersurfaces that facilitate cleaning whereas ridge-lap and modified ridge-lap designs have concave surfaces which are more difficult to access with dental floss. The ovate pontic serves important periodontal function by maintaining the interdental papilla next to abutment teeth after extraction. Becker et al. stated that the modified ridge-lap in the posterior region and ridge lap facing design in the anterior region offer minimal tissue contact, acceptable cosmetic value, proper check support, and accessibility for adequate oral hygiene. This design will allow for a mechanical cleansing of the undersurface and interproximal surfaces of the pontic with an interdental brush. (c) Embrasure spaces should be large enough to provide some self cleansing and allow woodstick to clean through. (d) The occlusal table should be the same width as that of the abutment teeth, and food shedding surfaces of the pontic in harmony with those of the abutments.

Cementation

Restoration must be seated as close to the tooth preparation as possible during cementation. A minimal cement line at the margin reduces plaque formation. All excess cement should be removed from the sulcus after cementation. Retained cement particles causes gingival inflammation.

Impression Materials

Inflammatory gingival responses related to the use of alloys containing nickel in dental restorations have been reported. Glass ceramics and porcelain veneers offer a clear advantage over any other type of restorative material in the maintenance of gingival health. Their fine marginal fit results in a thin cement line, which lessens gingival irritation. More importantly, tissues respond more to the differences in surface roughness of the material rather than the composition of the material. Moreover, nonporous surface of porcelain does not allow bacteria to adhere significantly.

PERIODONTAL MAINTENANCE IN THE PROSTHETIC PATIENT

A patient should be instructed to evaluate the effectiveness of his home care periodically. Plaque –

PERIODONTICS REVISITED

disclosing agents are commonly used for this purpose. However, prolonged staining of the oral mucosa, restoration margins, fingernails or the wash basin are often undesirable side effects of this procedure and are motivational deterrents. The patient should be given written instructions for the care, cleansing, and maintenance of the prosthesis.

Fixed Partial Prosthesis (FPD)

- *Tooth brushing*: Microbial debridement of the apical third or neck of the crown has been emphasized in the natural or intracoronally restored dentition because that area represents the major site of microbial activity that is detrimental to the tooth and its periodontium. Charters tooth brushing technique is helpful in cleaning the gingival surface of the pontic from the facial aspect. The filaments can be directed under the pontic to clean the gingival surface. For removal of plaque from proximal crown margins, the use of an interdental cleanser is necessary to reach the middle third of mesial and distal tooth surface. The specific aids indicated for proximal tooth cleaning depend on the size of the gingival embrasures between crowns and on the manual dexterity of the patient. Dental floss is used to remove plaque and loose debris between the abutment and pontic. With dentifrice, dental floss is used with moderate pressure on the undersurface/gingival surface of pontic to remove bacterial plaque. Floss threader are used to position yarn or gauze bandage strip around an abutment and under fixed prosthesis. Super floss are used for cleaning the under surface of fixed prosthesis **(Fig. 52.4)**. Knitting yarn may also be used for the same. Interdental brushes, single end tuft brushes are also used for cleaning interproximal areas. For cleaning crown margins adjacent to extremely large embrasures or sanitary pontics, unitufted brushes are preferred over bottle – brush cleansers.

- A nonabrasive dentifrice is indicated to prevent the possibility of abrasion when pontic or crown facings are made of acrylic. Fluoride containing dentifrice is important for the protection of remaining tooth surfaces, particularly exposed cementum. Acidulated Fluoride preparations are contraindicated for porcelain and composite restorations.

- *Oral irrigators*: In dentition with excessive fixed restorations that often provide less than ideal interproximal access for oral hygiene aids, daily oral irrigation with a pulsating stream of water is useful for removing food lodged between crowns and underneath pontics. However, water irrigators are not capable of removing any appreciable amounts of stainable plaque from tooth surfaces and, therefore, should not be recommended for prevention of caries, gingivitis, or periodontitis.

Removable Partial Prosthesis (RPD) and Complete Dentures

- Separate denture brush should be used for cleaning removable prosthesis **(Fig. 52.5)**. These are specially designed brush having one group of tufts in a large round arrangement that permits access to the thinner, curved impression surface of the denture. The second group of tufts is arranged to form a rectangular brush for convenient adaptation to the polished and occlusal denture surfaces. These brushes have round end filaments. Edentulous gingiva under removable denture is cleaned by soft manual/power assisted toothbrush and digital massage.

- Power assisted brush can also be used but not in about the intricate clasps of removable prosthesis.

- Short brushing strokes further minimize the risk of catching a clasp with the brush. An abrasive dentifrice

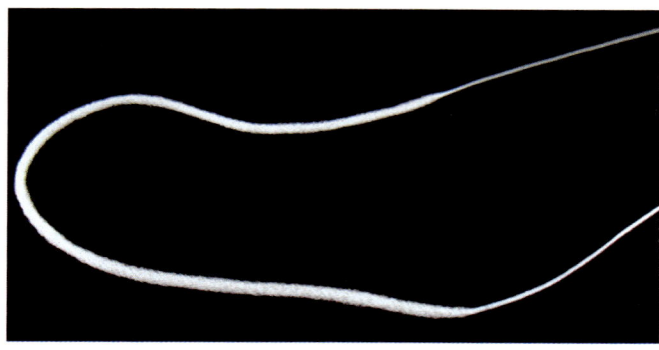

Fig. 52.4: Superfloss

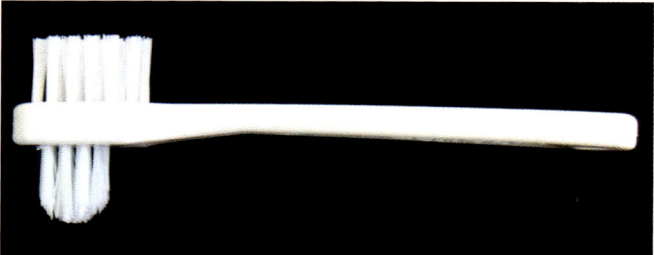

Fig. 52.5: Denture brush

should be used to maximize the cleaning effect. All debris and dentifrice residues on the prosthesis must be brushed off thoroughly under running water before replacing the appliance. This prevents irritation of the oral mucosa. A commercial denture cleaning solution can be used to supplement, but not substitute for, mechanical debridement. Cetyl dimethiocone copolymer inhibit the formation of plaque and stain on the surface of acrylic dentures.

- Specially designed narrow, tapered cylindrical brush about 2 inches long that can be adapted to the inner surface of clasps are recommended. Grasp of a partial prosthesis should not be too tight otherwise it may bend or fracture the clasp or bar. Partial filling of the sink with water or lining of the sink with a face towel is necessary to prevent accidents that cause breakage of prosthesis.

Recall schedule: The individual schedule for each patient is determined on the basis of relevant information gathered during the active treatment phase, such as complexity of prosthetic reconstructions, caries activity, formation rate of plaque and calculus, level of manual skills and motivation, and periodontal and general state of health.

BIBLIOGRAPHY

1. Ahmad I. Anterior dental aesthetics: Gingival perspective. Br Dent J 2005;199:195-202.
2. Becker CM. Current theories of crown contour, margin placement, and pontic design. J Prosthet Dent 2005;93:107-15.
3. Caputo AA. Biological Implications of dental materials. Dent Clin North Am 1980;24:331-42.
4. Ehlrich J. Alteration on crown contour- Effect on gingival health in man. J Prosthet Dent 1980;41:523-5.
5. Goodacre CJ. Gingival esthetics. J Prosthet Dent 1990;64:1-12.
6. Hall WB. Periodontal preparation of the mouth for restoration. Dent Clin North Am 1980;24:195-214
7. Manson JD. Restorative and Prosthetic Procedures. In, Periodontics 4th ed Wright 1980 Henry Kimpton Publishers; 262-74.
8. McGuire MK. Periodontal-Restorative interrelationship. In, Carranza and Newman. Clinical Periodontology 8th ed WB Saunders1996;723-42.
9. Orkin DA. et al. The relationship of the position of crown margins to gingival health. J Prosthet Dent 1987;57:421-4.
10. Padbury JA, et al. Interaction between the gingival and the margin of restorations. J Clin Periodontol 2003;30:379-85.
11. Schmid MO. The maintenance phase of dental therapy. Dent Clin North Am 1980;24:379-93.
12. Seibert JS. Surgical preparation for fixed and removable prostheses. In, Genco RJ, Goldman HM and Cohen DW. Contemporary Periodontics. CV Mosby Company 1990;637-52.
13. Spear FM, Cooney JP. Periodontal restorative interrelationship. In, Newman, Takei, Carranza. Clinical Periodontology 9th ed WB Saunders 2003;949-65.
14. Takei HH, Azzi RR, Han TJ. Preparation of the periodontium for restorative dentistry. In, Newman, Takei, Carranza. Clinical Periodontology 9th ed WB Saunders 2003;943-8.
15. Thayer HH, Kratochavil FJ. Periodontal Considerations with removable partial dentures. Dent Clin North Am 1980;24:357-68.

MCQs

1. Average biologic width is approx:
   A. 2.04 mm
   B. 3 mm
   C. 0.15 mm
   D. 3.5 mm
2. Superfloss are used for cleaning:
   A. Under surface of fixed prosthesis
   B. Removable prosthesis
   C. Implant
   D. None of the above
3. The least distance between the apical extension of restoration and crest of the alveolar bone:
   A. 3 mm
   B. 4 mm
   C. 6 mm
   D. 1 mm
4. How much time after periodontal plastic surgery, the restoration can be placed:
   A. 3 months   B. 2 months
   C. 6 months   D. 9 months
5. The tooth preparations are needed to be extended into gingival sulcus due to:
   A. Esthetics in maxillary anterior region
   B. Extensive carious lesions
   C. Replacement of defective and extensive restoration
   D. All of the above

Answers

1. A   2. A   3. A   4. B   5. D

Periodontic-Endodontics

Seema Nayyar, Shalu Bathla

INTRODUCTION

Since 1964, when Simring and Goldberg first described the relationship between periodontal and endodontic disease, the term 'endo-perio' has become an integral part of the dental vocabulary. The relationship between pulpal and periodontal disease can be traced to embryological development since the pulp and the periodontium are derived from a common mesodermal source of the developing tooth bud. Ectomesenchymal cells proliferate to form the dental papilla and follicle, which are the precursors of the pulp and the periodontium respectively. This embryonic development gives rise to anatomical connections, some of which remain patent throughout life.

PATHWAYS OF COMMUNICATION

There is a very close relationship between the pulpal and periodontal tissues and the disease transmission between these two is strongly supported by many studies, which showed significant microbiological similarities between infected root canals and advanced periodontitis. Other than these microbial findings, similarities in the composition of cellular infiltrates also suggest the existence of communication between the pulp and the periodontal tissues. The possible pathways for ingress of bacteria and their products into these tissues can broadly be divided into: anatomical and nonphysiological pathways.

Anatomical pathways: These include vascular pathways such as the apical foramen, lateral canals and tubular pathways **(Fig. 53.1).**

Apical foramen: The apical foramen is the principal and most direct route of communication between the periodontium and the pulp. Although periodontal disease has been shown to have a cumulative damaging effect on the pulp tissue, total disintegration of the pulp can occur only, if bacterial plaque involves the main apical foramen, compromising the vascular supply. Irritants from a diseased pulp may permeate readily through the apical foramen resulting in periapical pathosis. This results in destruction of periodontal tissue fibers and resorption of the adjacent alveolar bone and root.

Accessory canals: In addition to the apical foramen, which is the main route of communication, there are a

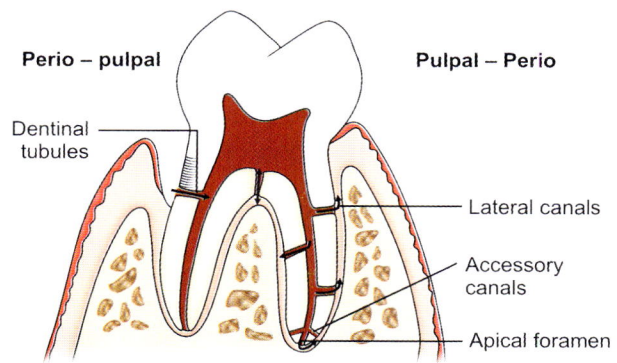

Fig. 53.1: Pathways between pulp and periodontium

multitude of branches connecting the main root canal system with the periodontal ligament. These ramifications are now currently termed as 'accessory canals'. As the root develops, ectomesenchymal channels get incorporated, either during the dentin formation around existing blood vessels or when there is break in the continuity of the Hertwig's epithelial root sheath, to become lateral or accessory canals. The majority of the accessory canals are found in the apical part of the root and the molar furcation areas. Bender et al. stated that periodontal endodontic problems were much more frequent in the molars than in the anterior teeth because of the greater number of accessory canals present in the molars. The percentage of lateral canals in the furcation is 46% in first molars and 50 to 60% in any multirooted teeth. Gutmann (1978) found 25.5% accessory canals in the furcation areas. Patent accessory canals are the potential pathways for the spread of microorganisms and their toxic byproducts, as well as other irritants, from the pulp to the periodontal ligament and vice versa, resulting in an inflammatory process in the involved tissues.

Tubular pathways: Passage of microorganisms between the pulp and periodontal tissues is possible through the patent dentinal tubules, when the cementum layer is denuded. This is usually attributed to various developmental defects such as incomplete union of cementum and enamel at cementoenamel junction (CEJ), disease processes or surgical procedures involving root surfaces like scaling and root planing. Exposed dentinal tubules, in areas of denuded cementum may serve as communication pathways between pulp and the periodontal ligament.

Nonphysiological pathways: These include iatrogenic root canal perforations, vertical root fractures caused by trauma, pathway created due to resorption etc. The incidence of root fractures is more in the roots that are filled with lateral condensation technique and the teeth restored with intracanal posts.

ETIOPATHOGENESIS OF PERIO-ENDO LESIONS

Effect of Periodontal Lesions on the Pulp

Microbial agents: These are the main cause in the evolution of perio-endo lesions along with the other etiologic factors. The formation of bacterial plaque on denuded root surfaces, following periodontal disease has the potential to induce pathologic changes in the pulp through lateral or accessory canals. The effect of periodontal lesions on the pulp can result in atrophic and other degenerative changes like reduction in the number of pulp cells, dystrophic mineralization, fibrosis, reparative dentin formation, inflammation and resorption.

Atrophic changes: The pulp tissue of a periodontally involved tooth has cells which are small and have more collagen depositions than normal. Due to impaired nutrition, the pulp cells slowly degenerate. The death of the cells is so gradual that morphologic evidence sometimes appears to be lacking. The cause of these atrophic changes is the disruption of blood flow through the lateral canals, which leads to localized areas of coagulation necrosis in the pulp. These areas are eventually walled off from the rest of the healthy pulp tissue by collagen and dystrophic mineralization. With slowly advancing periodontal disease, cementum deposition may act to obliterate lateral canals before pulpal irritation occurs. This may explain why, not all periodontally involved teeth demonstrate pulpal atrophy and canal narrowing. Pressure atrophy may also occur because of the mobility of these periodontally involved teeth.

Inflammatory changes: The causative agents of periodontal disease are found in the sulcus and are continually challenged by host defenses. An immunologic or inflammatory response is elicited in response to this microbiologic challenge. This results in the formation of granulomatous tissue in the periodontium. When periodontal disease extends from the gingival sulcus towards the apex, the inflammatory products attack the elements of the periodontal ligament and the surrounding alveolar bone.

PERIODONTICS REVISITED

A clear cut relationship between progressive periodontal disease and pulpal involvement, however, does not invariably exist. The most common periodontal lesion produced by the pulp disease is the localized apical granuloma. It is produced by the diffusion of bacterial products through the root apex, with the formation of vascular granulation tissue. Subsequently, resorption of the alveolar bone and occasionally of the root itself may occur.

Resorption: Resorption of the sides of the roots is frequently found adjacent to the granulation tissue overlying the roots. When the periodontal lesions are deep, resorption may also be found within the root canals, often opposite lateral canals, and at the apical foramen. Since this resorptive process extends into the dentin peripherally towards the pulp, and the activating factors are produced from the periodontal lesion, a name which reflects the etiology of this phenomenon, peripheral inflammatory root resorption (PIRR) was proposed.

Effects of Periodontal Treatment Procedures on the Dental Pulp

Scaling and root planing: This procedure removes the bacterial plaque and calculus. However, improper root planing procedures can also remove cementum and the superficial parts of dentin, thereby exposing the dentinal tubules to the oral environment. Subsequent microbial colonization of the root dentin may result in bacterial invasion of the dentinal tubules. As a consequence, inflammatory lesions may develop in the pulp. The initial symptom is sharp pain of rapid onset that disappears once the stimulus is removed.

Acid etching: During periodontal regenerative therapy, root conditioning using citric acid helps to remove bacterial endotoxin and anerobic bacteria and to expose collagen bundles to serve as a matrix for new connective tissue attachment to cementum. Though beneficial in the treatment of periodontal disease, citric acid removes the smear layer, an important pulp protector. Application of citric acid may have a detrimental effect on the dental pulp.

Effects of Endodontic Infection on the Periodontium

It has been demonstrated that intrapulpal infection tends to promote epithelial downgrowth along a denuded dentin surface. Also, experimentally induced periodontal defects around infected teeth were associated with 20% more epithelial downgrowth than noninfected teeth. Noninfected teeth showed 10% more connective tissue

coverage than infected teeth. Therefore, it is essential that pulpal infections should be treated first, before undertaking periodontal regenerative procedures.

CLASSIFICATION OF PERIO-ENDO LESIONS

A. Classification according to Weine, based on etiology of the disease:

Class 1 - Tooth in which symptoms clinically and radiographically simulate periodontal disease but are in fact due to pulpal inflammation and/or necrosis.

Class 2 - Tooth that has both pulpal or periapical disease and periodontal disease concomitantly.

Class 3 - Tooth that has no pulpal problem but requires endodontic therapy plus root amputation to gain periodontal healing.

Class 4 - Tooth that clinically and radiographically simulates pulpal or periapical diseases but in fact has periodontal disease.

B. The most accepted classification was given by Simon, Glick and Frank in 1972. According to this classification, perio-endo lesions can be classified into:

1. Primary endodontic lesion
2. Primary periodontal lesion
3. Primary endodontic lesion with secondary periodontal involvement
4. Primary periodontal lesion with secondary endodontic involvement
5. True combined lesion

Primary Endodontic Lesion

An acute exacerbation of a chronic apical lesion on a tooth with a necrotic pulp may drain coronally through the periodontal ligament into the gingival sulcus **(Figs 53.2 and 53.3)**. This condition may clinically mimic the presence of a periodontal abscess. In reality, however, it would be a sinus tract originating from the pulp that opens into the periodontal ligament. Primary endodontic lesions usually heal following root canal therapy. The sinus tract extending into the gingival sulcus or furcation area disappears at an early stage, if the necrotic pulp has been removed, the root canals are well sealed.

Primary Periodontal Lesion

These lesions are caused primarily by periodontal pathogens **(Fig. 53.4)**. In this process, chronic periodontitis

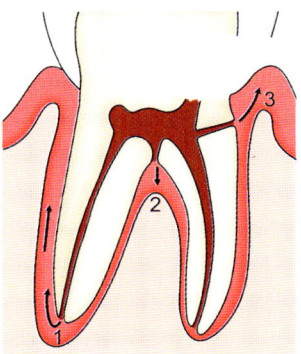

Endodontic origin-Pulpal infection spread through:
1. Apical foramen to periodontal ligament;
2. Accessory canals to furcation;
3. Accessory canals to gingiva

Fig. 53.2: Primary endodontic lesion

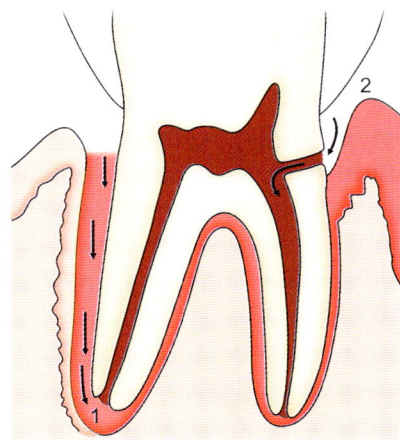

Perio-origin-Periodontal infection spread through: 1. apical formen and 2. lateral canal to pulp

Fig. 53.4: Primary periodontal lesion

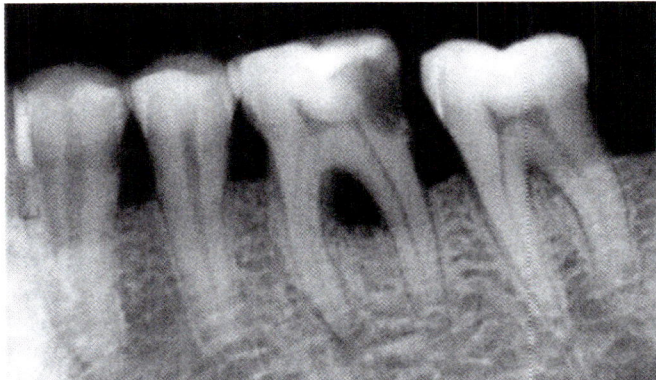

Fig. 53.3: Radiograph showing primary endodontic lesion

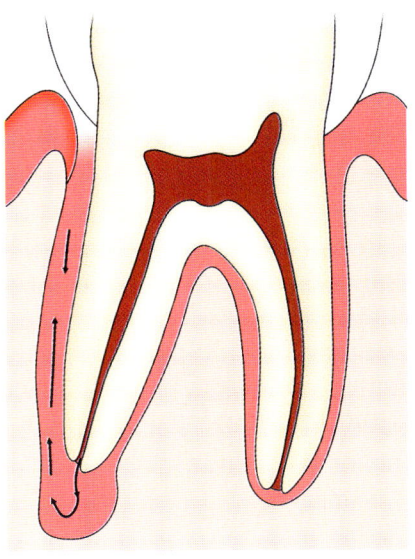

Fig. 53.5: Retrograde periodontitis

progresses apically along the root surface. In most cases, pulpal tests indicate a clinically normal pulpal reaction. There is frequently an accumulation of plaque and calculus and the presence of deep pockets may be detected.

Combined Diseases

Primary Endodontic Lesion with Secondary Periodontal Involvement

If a primary endodontic lesion remains untreated, it may become secondarily involved with periodontal breakdown. Long – standing periapical lesion draining through the periodontal ligament can become secondarily complicated leading to retrograde periodontitis **(Fig. 53.5)**

Plaque accumulation at the gingival margin of the sinus tract leads to plaque induced periodontitis in this area. When plaque and calculus are detected, the treatment and prognosis of the teeth are different from those teeth involved with only endodontic disease. The tooth now requires both endodontic and periodontal treatment.

Primary endodontic lesion with secondary periodontal involvement may also occur as a result of root perforation during root canal treatment, or where pins and posts may have been misplaced during restoration of the crown. Symptoms may be acute, with periodontal abscess formation associated with pain, swelling, pus or exudates, pocket formation, and tooth mobility. A more chronic response may occur without pain, and involves the sudden appearance of a pocket with bleeding on probing or exudation of pus. Root fractures may also present as primary endodontic lesions with secondary periodontal involvement. These typically occur in root canal treated teeth, often with posts and crowns. The signs may range from a local deepening of periodontal pocket to a more acute periodontal abscess formation.

Primary Periodontal Disease with Secondary Endodontic Involvement

Bacterial and inflammatory products of periodontitis could gain access to the pulp via accessory canals, apical foramen and dentinal tubules and this reverse effect is called as retrograde pulpitis. The apical progression of a periodontal pocket may continue until the apical tissues are involved. In this case, the pulp may become necrotic as a result of infection entering through lateral canals or the apical foramen. In single-rooted teeth, the prognosis is usually poor. In molar teeth, the prognosis may be better. Since not all the roots may suffer the same loss of supporting tissue, root resection can be considered as a alternative treatment.

If the blood supply circulating through the apex is intact, the pulp has good prospects for survival. It has been reported that pulpal changes resulting from periodontal disease are more likely to occur when the apical foramen is involved. In these cases, bacteria originating from the periodontal pocket are the most likely source of root canal infection.

The treatment of periodontal disease can also lead to secondary endodontic involvement. Lateral canals and dentinal tubules may be opened to the oral environment by scaling and root planing or surgical flap procedures. It is possible for a blood vessel within a lateral canal to be severed by a curette and for the micro-organisms to be pushed into the area during treatment, resulting in pulp inflammation and necrosis.

True Combined Lesion

True combined endodontic-periodontal disease occurs less frequently than other endodontic-periodontal problems. It is formed when an endodontic lesion progress coronally and joins an infected periodontal

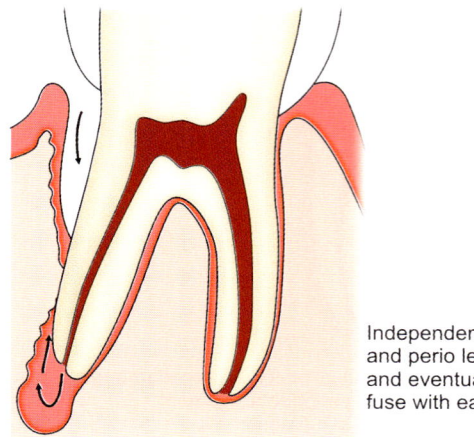

Independent endo and perio lesions coexist and eventually fuse with each other

Fig. 53.6: True combined lesion

pocket progressing apically **(Fig. 53.6)**. The degree of attachment loss in this type of lesion is invariably large and the prognosis is guarded. This is particularly true in single-rooted teeth. In molar teeth, root resection can be an alternative treatment. The radiographic appearance of combined endodontic periodontal disease may be similar to that of a vertically fractured tooth. If a sinus tract is present, it may be necessary to raise a flap to determine the etiology of the lesion.

DIAGNOSIS

It is important to determine whether the primary lesion is pulpal or periodontal, otherwise wrong treatment may be chosen or there may be unnecessary overtreatment. Following diagnostic measures are undertaken to establish the correct diagnosis:

1. *Vitality tests*: The first step would be to examine for vitality by pulp testing and with heat and cold. A nonvital tooth may indicate primary pulpal involvement, although at times, it can indicate secondary pulpal disease. Endodontic treatment (root canal therapy) is required in this situation. A vital tooth indicates primary periodontal involvement, and does not require endodontic therapy. Clinician should be cautious about the possibility of false positive results also.

2. *Radiographic evaluation*: Radiograph may exhibit loss of bone at the alveolar crest, an apical radiolucency, or a continuous bone loss involving both sites. Apical radiolucency indicates primary pulpal disease. Bone loss confined to coronal one third of the tooth is associated with primary periodontal disease. Finding

the cause is more difficult when bone loss is present at both sites. If the tooth has a radiographic furcation involvement that cannot be detected clinically, there is likelihood of pulpal involvement. Gutta-percha points used as probes in sinus tracts can be a valuable aid in tracing the origin of a draining lesion.

3. *Pain and abscess formation*: Clinical signs and symptoms will help to differentiate between endodontic and periodontal lesions.
   a. Pulpal pain is usually sharp. Periodontal abscess may produce a dull, more even pain which is accompanied by a feeling of fullness in the area.
   b. Pulpal lesion may be difficult to localize when the symptoms start. The periodontal lesion is usually easy to localize.
   c. Pulpal lesion usually drain by a fistula through the alveolar mucosa or gingiva, it rarely fistulates through the sulcus. The periodontal abscess usually drains through the lumen of the pocket.

4. *Probing*: The presence of a deep solitary pocket in the absence of periodontal disease may indicate the presence of a lesion of endodontic origin or a vertical root fracture. Periodontal probing helps in differentiating between endodontic and periodontal disease. It can also be used to track a sinus resulting from an inflammatory periapical lesion that extends cervically through the periodontal ligament space. In periodontal lesions, numerous osseous defects are present throughout the mouth and subgingival calculus can be detected. A pocket that does not extend to the apical one third of the root in a periodontally involved mouth also indicates primary periodontal disease.

5. *Mobility*: When mobility is present around one isolated tooth, the source of the problem can be endodontic, periodontal, or occlusal. In the acute stage of an endodontic infection, mobility involves a single tooth. Generalized mobility, however, involving many teeth suggests periodontal or occlusal origin.

6. *Percussion and palpation*: Results of percussion and palpation tests are usually negative in an individual tooth with a periodontal problem. When a periodontal abscess is present, these clinical entities may be positive; however, other tests indicate a vital pulp. A tooth with an endodontic problem usually produces definite tenderness and pain on percussion and palpation.

TREATMENT AND PROGNOSIS OF PERIODONTAL-ENDODONTIC LESIONS

Treatment and prognosis of primarily endodontic and primarily periodontal disease is very straight forward. However, prognosis of combined forms of the lesions is more difficult to predict. Endodontic therapy is more predictable and completion of this therapy before periodontal procedures has a positive effect on periodontal healing. It is essential to understand that in perio-endo lesions, the endodontic treatment is the more predictable of the two. However the success of endodontic therapy is dependent on the completion of periodontal therapy. The complete treatment of both aspects of perio-endo lesions is essential for successful long-term results.

Primary endodontic lesion:

Treatment	Root canal treatment
Prognosis	Good

Primary periodontal lesion:

Treatment	Periodontal treatment
Prognosis	Depends upon periodontal treatment and patient's response

Primary endodontic-secondary periodontal lesion:

Treatment	Root canal treatment first followed by periodontal treatment after 2-3 months
Prognosis	Depends upon endodontic and periodontal treatment and patient's response

Primary periodontal-secondary endodontic lesion:

Treatment	Endodontic and periodontal treatment (GTR)
Prognosis	Depends upon severity of the periodontal disease and periodontal tissue response to treatment

True Combined lesion:

Treatment	Endodontic and periodontal treatment procedures including surgical procedures like amputation, hemisection or bicuspidization
Prognosis	More guarded prognosis

BIBLIOGRAPHY

1. Ammons WF Jr, Harrington GW. The periodontic-endodontic continuum. In, Newman, Takei, Carranza. Clinical Periodontology 9th ed WB Saunders 2003;840-50.
2. Bergenholtz G, Hasselgren G. Endodontic and Periodontic. In, Lindhe J, Karring T, Lang NP. Clinical Periodontology and Implant dentistry. 4th ed Blackwell Munksgaard 2003;318-51.
3. Bergenholtz G, Lindhe J. Effect of experimentally induced marginal periodontitis and periodontal scaling on the dental pulp. J Clin Periodontol 1978;5:59-73.
4. DeDeus QD. Frequency, location and direction of the lateral, secondary and accessory canals. J Endod 1975;1:361-6.

PERIODONTICS REVISITED

5. Gold S, Hasselgren G. Peripheral inflammatory root resorption: A review of literature with case reports. J Clin Periodontol 1992;19:523-34.
6. Kipioti A, Nakou M, Legakis N, Mitis F. Microbiological findings of infected root canals and adjacent periodontal pockets in teeth with advanced periodontitis. Oral Surg Oral Med Oral Pathol 1984;58:213-20.
7. Kobayashi T, Hayashi A, Yoshikawa R, Okuda K, Hara K. The microbial flora from root canals and periodontal pockets of non vital teeth associated with advanced periodontitis. Int Endod J 1990;23:100-6.
8. Rahmat A, Barkhordar, Stewart GG. The potential of periodontal pocket formation associated with untreated accessory root canals. Oral Surg Oral Med Oral Pathol 1990;70:769-72.
9. Rossman LE. Endodontic – Periodontic Consideration. In, Rose LF, Mealey BL, Genco RJ, Cohen DW. Periodontics, Medicine, Surgery and Implants. Elsevier Mosby 2004;772-89
10. Simon JH, Glick DH, Frank AL. The relationship of endodontic-periodontic lesions. J Clin Periodontol 1972;43:202.
11. Simring M, Goldberg M. The pulpal pocket approach: Retrograde periodontitis. J Periodontol 1964;35:22-48.
12. Vertucci FJ, Williams RJ. Furcation canals in the human mandibular first molars. Oral Surg 1990;69:743.
13. Zehnder M, Gold SI, Hasselgren G. Pathologic interaction in pulpal and periodontal tissues. J Clin Periodontol 2002;29:663-71.

MCQs

1. Following are the various developmental pulpal-periodontal communications *except*:
   A. Dentinal tubules
   B. Lateral canals
   C. Apical foramina
   D. Developmental grooves
   E. CEJ
2. Iatrogenic causes of Perio-Endo lesions are:
   A. Root perforation   B. Vertical root fractures
   C. None of the above   D. Both A and B
3. Retrograde periodontitis is:
   A. Long – standing periapical lesion draining through the periodontal ligament
   B. The apical progression of a periodontal pocket to reach apical tissues and pulp via accessory canals, apical foramen
   C. Both A and B
   D. None of the above

Answers

1. E   2. D   3. A

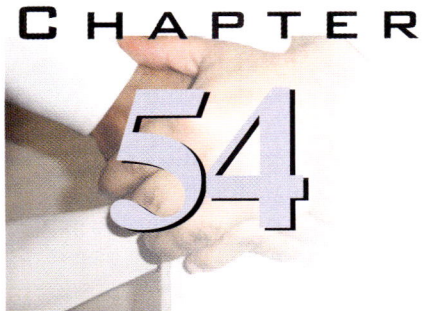

CHAPTER 54

Periodontics-Restorative Dentistry

Seema Nayyar, Shalu Bathla

INTRODUCTION

Properly constructed restorations are of therapeutic value. Restorations, when improperly constructed, can become etiologic factor for the periodontal disease. The outer surface of a restoration is of significance from periodontal viewpoint. Proper contact, contour, occlusion, marginal adaptation and surface finish are as important to periodontics as they are to restorative dentistry. Also, periodontal health is critical for both the preservation of the natural dentition and the success of any restorative procedure. Thus, periodontium and the restoration of teeth are intimate and inseparable.

APPLICATION OF PERIODONTICS IN RESTORATIVE DENTISTRY

- Pre-restorative periodontal care
- Periodontal surgery for the placement of restoration

Pre-restorative Periodontal Care

Active periodontal disease must be treated and controlled prior to any restorative procedure because margins of restorations covered by inflamed gingiva shrinks after periodontal treatment. Thus, to locate and determine the gingival margins of restorations properly, the position of the healthy and stable gingival margin must be established prior to tooth preparation.

Periodontal Surgery for the Placement of Restoration

Free gingival graft and full crown restoration- When the attached gingiva is totally absent and the soft tissue-crown interface has been compromised by recession or inflammation, surgical augmentation to provide a collar of attached gingiva is beneficial. Periodontal plastic surgery (free gingival graft) should be carried out atleast 2 months before placement of dental restorations. This allows time for mature tissue to form in the gingival margin so that restorative procedures do not cause the return of clinical inflammation.

Crown lengthening procedures- This procedure is usually done in cases of subgingival caries, fracture and when there as inadequate clinical crown length for retention. When severe caries approaches or extends below the alveolar crest, a full thickness flap extending to adjacent teeth and osseous reduction to gain sound tooth structure are required. The apically positioned flap with ostectomy is an excellent means of preserving and often gaining attached gingiva. Atleast 3 mm should be the least distance between the apical extension of restoration and crest of the alveolar bone otherwise law of biologic width is compromised.

APPLICATION OF RESTORATIVE DENTISTRY IN PERIODONTICS

- Excavation of dental caries and restoration
- Restorative correction of open gingival embrasures
- Management of gingival embrasure form with periodontal recession
- Restoration of root-resected teeth
- Splinting

Excavation of Dental Caries and Restoration

Caries destroy tooth structure, creating open contacts, poor embrasure form and plunger cusps all of which encourage food impaction, plaque retention and periodontal disease. Thus, the removal of dental caries and the restoration of sound tooth structure are necessary components of early treatment (Phase I) of a patient with periodontal disease. Restoration of dental caries should be conservative with normal interproximal contacts and proper embrasure space preventing plaque accumulation and creating environment conducive to periodontal health **(Fig. 54.1)**.

Restorative Correction of Open Gingival Embrasures

There are two causes of open gingival embrasures: Either the papilla is inadequate in height due to bone loss, or

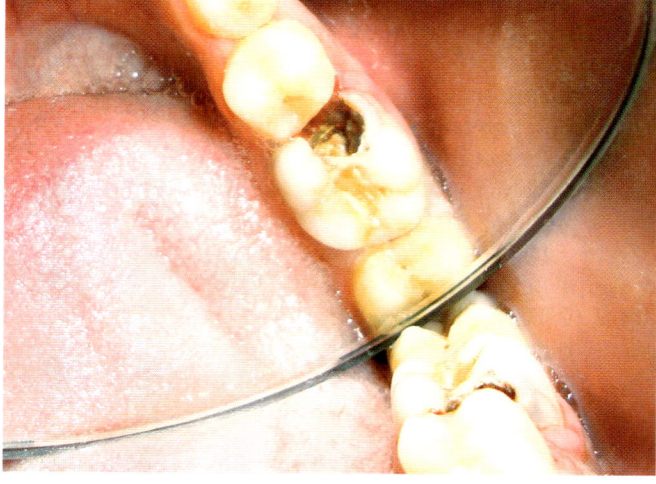

Fig. 54.1: Carious lesion acting as plaque retentive area

the interproximal contact is located too high coronally. If the open gingival embrasures is due to high contact and the roots are parallel with the normal papilla, then the problem is probably related to tooth shape, specifically, an excessively tapered form. Restorative dentistry can correct this problem by moving the contact point to the tip of the papilla. Thus, the margins of direct bonded restoration is carried subgingivally 1 to 1.5 mm, and the emergence profile of the restoration is designed to move the contact point towards the papilla while blending the contour into the tooth below the tissue.

Management of Gingival Embrasure form with Periodontal Recession

In esthetic areas, it is necessary to carry the interproximal contacts apically toward the papilla to eliminate the presence of large open embrasures. With multiple unit restorations, it is possible to bake porcelain papillae directly on the restoration using tissue-colored ceramics.

Restoration of Root-resected Teeth

The removal of a root alters the direction of occlusal forces on the remaining resected teeth. Occlusion of that tooth is evaluated and adjusted and then the crown is placed. But before giving permanent restoration the quality of the endodontic filling, residual ledges should be examined radiographically and clinically. A cast post and core may be indicated to create an adequate foundation for the final restoration. Because the remaining roots are often very thin mesiodistally, it is difficult to cement prefabricated posts and have adequate bulk to place a foundation core on the mesial and distal of the post. That is why the one-piece cast post and core restoration is placed. Heavy convexities should be avoided for restoring these teeth for hygiene access. Facially and lingually, the contours should be essentially a straight line from the margin coronally, whereas interproximally, the contour emerges from the margin as a straight line or is slightly convex as it slopes up to the contact point. The gingival embrasure form created in the restoration must be fluted into these areas so that the surfaces can be accessed with an interdental brush.

Splinting

Splinting stabilize mobile teeth during periodontal surgery and also during the healing period following surgery. Various restorative materials can be used for intracoronal and extracoronal splinting such as amalgam, acryclic or composite. Explained in Chapter no. 42—Splinting.

PERIODONTAL CONSIDERATIONS IN RESTORATIVE DENTISTRY

1. Margins of restorations
2. Gingival management for making impressions
3. Contour of restoration
4. Occlusal surface
5. Surface finish of restorative materials
6. Restoration of hemisected and resected tooth
7. Restorative procedures
8. Materials
9. Restorative design features for periodontally treated teeth

1. *Margins of restorations*: In restoring a tooth with any plastic filling material, accurately contoured and placed matrix bands stabilized by triangular wood or plastic wedge are essential to avoid overhanging margins. In cross-section, the base of the triangle will be in contact with the interdental papillae, apical to gingival margin of the proximal cavity. The two sides of triangle coincide with the corresponding two sides (mesial and distal) of the gingival embrasure. The apex of wedge should coincide with the gingival start of the contact area. Thus, wedge defines the gingival extent of the contact area thereby, assuring the health of proximal periodontal tissues. Overhanging margins contribute to periodontal disease by providing ideal locations for plaque accumulation and changing the ecological balance of the gingival sulcus area to one that favors the growth of disease-associated organisms **(Fig. 54.2)**. Overhanging can be removed with the help of files, enamel shavers or EVA prophylaxis system. When overhang cannot be

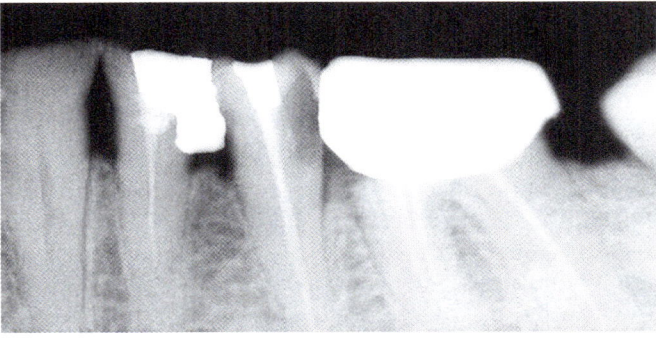

Fig. 54.2: Overhanging restoration leading to interproximal bone loss

removed, restoration should be replaced. The location of the gingival margin of restoration is directly related to the periodontal health status. Subgingivally located margins are associated with large amounts of plaque, more severe gingivitis and deeper pockets.

2. *Gingival management for making impressions*: For subgingival preparation margin extending to the appropriate depth in the sulcus, gingival tissue must be protected from abrasion. Tissue management is achieved with gingival retraction cords of the appropriate size to achieve the required displacement. Electrosurgery can also be used to remove any overlying tissue in the retraction process. A fine wire-tip electrode is held parallel to the tooth and against the margin in the sulcus and moved through the overhanging tissue, opening up the margin and the retraction cord to visual access.

3. *Contours*: Overcontoured crowns and restorations tend to accumulate plaque and prevent self - cleansing mechanism of adjacent cheek, lips and tongue. The facial and lingual contours of restorations are also important in the preservation of gingival health. In patients in whom periodontal disease causes the gingival margin to be in a much more apical position than it was during health, the facial and lingual contours become even more significant **(Figs 54.3A to C)**. In this particular case, the bulge on the facial contour of the crown, which normally would be subgingival, appear supragingival. In class III and IV furcation defects, it is important that the restoration be contoured in such a way so as to facilitate access for oral hygiene. In these cases, it is important to emphasize the mid facial groove of the crown so that this groove is confluent with the furcation.

4. *Occlusal surface*: Failure to reproduce the normal protective anatomy of the occlusal marginal ridges and developmental grooves lead to food impaction. Occlusal surfaces should be designed to direct masticatory forces along the long axis of the teeth. The anatomy of the occlusal surface should provide well formed marginal ridges and occlusal sluiceways to prevent interproximal food impaction. Thus, restorations that do not conform to the occlusal patterns of the mouth cause occlusal disharmonies that may be injurious to the supporting periodontal tissues.

5. *Surface finish*: The surface of restoration should be smooth so as to limit plaque accumulation. Rough

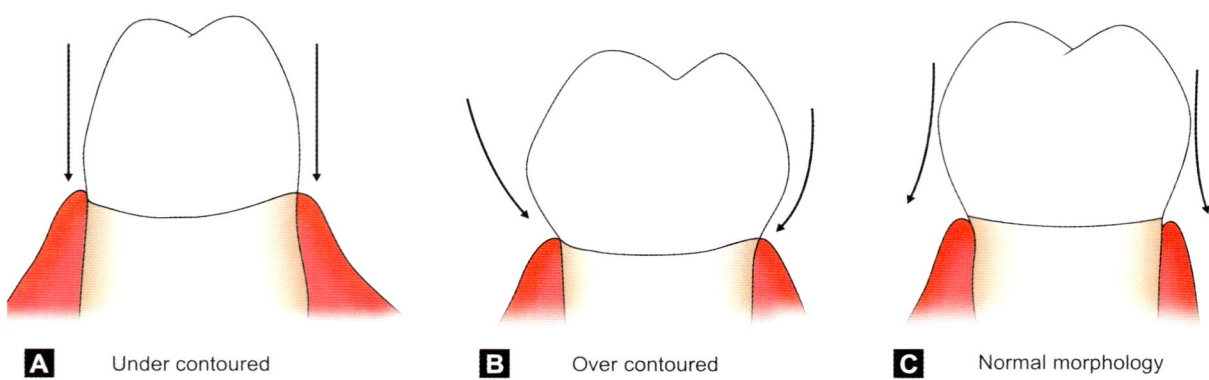

| A | Under contoured | B | Over contoured | C | Normal morphology |

Figs 54.3A to C: Crown morphology

restorative surface in subgingival region result in plaque accumulation and thus, results in gingival inflammation. Therefore, all restorative materials placed in gingival environment must have the highest possible polish.

6. *Restoration of hemisected and resected tooth:*

Mandibular molar- If both parts of hemisected tooth are to be retained, it is essential that an adequate embrasure space must be created between the two halves of the tooth, as it is too narrow. Hemisected teeth are prepared for restorative procedures, adequate tooth material is removed in the areas between the roots, so that a wide embrasure space is constructed, which will allow passage of an oral hygiene device. When a mandibular molar is hemisected and one portion is extracted, the remaining portion serves as an abutments for a three-unit bridge.

Maxillary molars- When a mesiobuccal or distobuccal root has been resected, it is necessary to hollow out the crown contours in the area coronal to the area where root was resected so that adequate access is available for oral hygiene procedures. When palatal root has been resected, the crown is made thinner buccopalatally, with a groove running in the midpalatal surface resembling a mandibular molar.

7. *Restorative procedures*: Injudicious tooth separation injure the supporting tissues of the periodontium. The use of rubber dam clamps, copper bands, matrix bands and discs may lacerate the gingiva resulting in gingival inflammation. Excessive vigorous condensing of gold foil restorations may also be the source of injury to the periodontium.

8. *Materials*: Inflammatory gingival responses related to the use of alloys containing nickel in dental restorations have been reported. Glass ceramics and porcelain veneers offer a clear advantage over any other type of restorative material in the maintenance of gingival health. Their fine marginal fit results in a thin cement line, which lessens gingival irritation. More importantly, tissues respond more to the differences in surface roughness of the material rather than the composition of the material. Moreover, nonporous surface of porcelain does not allow bacteria to adhere significantly.

9. *Restorative design features for periodontally treated teeth*: Restoration of badly broken down, periodontally involved teeth or periodontally treated teeth pose a challenge to clinician. Gingival margins of tooth preparation should be placed supragingivally. If the restoration is to replace all occluding surface, the width of occlusal table should be reduced to minimize the amount of forces to be received by the periodontally involved tooth.

PERIODONTAL MAINTENANCE IN THE RESTORATIVE PATIENT

- *Restored teeth:* A nonabrasive dentifrice is indicated to prevent the possibility of abrasion of acrylic. Fluoride containing dentifrice is important for the protection of remaining tooth surfaces, particularly exposed cementum. Acidulated fluoride preparations are contraindicated for porcelain and composite restorations.

- *Root-resected restored teeth*: The interproximal areas of root-amputated and hemisected teeth often present with surface concavities on the root trunk, and these areas cannot be adequately cleaned with floss, thus the gingival embrasure form created in the restoration must be fluted into these areas so that the surfaces can be accessed with an interdental brush.

BIBLIOGRAPHY

1. Casullo DP. Periodontal considerations in restorative dentistry. In, Genco RJ, Goldman HM and Cohen DW. Contemporary Periodontics. CV Mosby Company 1990;619-35.
2. Grant DA, Stern IB, Listgarten MA. Restorative and prosthetic dentistry. In, Periodontic 6th ed CV Mosby Company 1988;1045-55.
3. McGuire MK. Periodontal restorative interrelationship. In, Newman, Takei, Carranza. Clinical Periodontology 8th ed WB Saunders 1996;723-42.
4. Ramfjord SP, Ash MM. Periodontal considerations in restorative and other aspects of dentistry. In, Periodontology and Periodontics. Modern Theory and Practice 1st ed AITBS Publisher and distributor India1996;339-51.
5. Restorative and Prosthetic Procedures. In, Manson JD. Periodontics 4th ed Wright 1980 Henry Kimpton Publishers; 262- 74.
6. Spear FM, Cooney JP. Periodontal restorative interrelationship. In, Newman, Takei, Carranza. Clinical Periodontology 9th ed WB Saunders 2003;949-65.
7. Takei HH, Azzi RR, Han TJ. Preparation of the periodontium for restorative dentistry. In, Newman, Takei, Carranza. Clinical Periodontology 9th ed WB Saunders 2003;943-48.

PERIODONTICS REVISITED

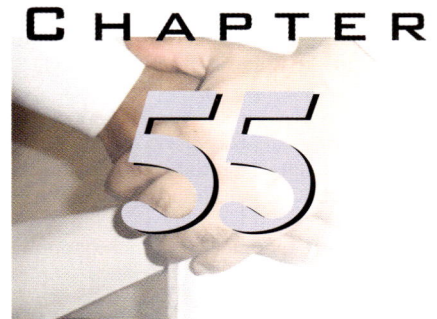

CHAPTER 55

Periodontics-Orthodontics

Shalu Bathla

INTRODUCTION

Periodontal therapy has entered a new era because of the innovations in adult tooth movement. Severe crowding that strangles the embrasure spaces, and tilted and tipped molars, can be resolved by orthodontic treatment. In addition, very difficult surgical situations can be minimized or even eliminated by this multidisciplinary approach of combining periodontal and orthodontic therapy. Thus, orthodontic treatment may be adjunctive to periodontal therapy.

Every orthodontic intervention has a periodontal dimension. Orthodontic biomechanics and treatment planning are basically determined by periodontal factors, such as length and shape of the root, the width and height of alveolar bone and structure of the gingiva. Orthodontics is a non surgical approach to enhance hard and soft tissue volume and height before the placement of an implant. Forced eruption can be used not only as a means of atraumatically extracting hopeless teeth, but of "carrying" the surrounding bone and soft tissue into

a more coronal position. Periodontal maintenance visits are scheduled in orthodontic visits and mechanical aids such as powered toothbrushes, interdental brushes are advised at the time.

INDICATIONS

Orthodontic treatment for individuals with periodontal disease may be indicated in the following situations

1. *Basic malocclusion*: Crowded, malposed teeth may result in poor gingival form. Deep overbites are accompanied by trauma to maxillary palatal gingiva, and mandibular labial gingiva.
2. *Migration*: Tooth migration can contribute to further periodontal breakdown by producing alteration in occlusion. Tooth migration can be caused by habits such as tongue thrusting, trauma, aggressive periodontitis and gingival hyperplasia.
3. *Bony defects*: Bony defects sometimes are treated better by combined periodontal - orthodontic measures than by periodontal treatment alone.

4. *Preparation for reconstruction*: Fixed splinting requires parallel abutments, pontic require sufficient width and open embrasure. Thus, tilted and protruded teeth are uprighted. If adjacent teeth have drifted into edentulous spaces, orthodontics is often helpful to provide the ideal amount of space for implants and subsequent restorations.

5. *Esthetic improvement*: Migration which is evident in periodontal disease may be the cause of embarrassment and may compel the patient to seek orthodontic treatment.

CONTRAINDICATIONS

1. Lack of inflammatory control prior to, or lack of maintenance of periodontal health during tooth movement. A far worse situation may be created if inadequate anchorage due to extensive bone loss is lost. Thus, the presence of active periodontal disease or existing extensive periodontal destruction is contraindicated to adult tooth movement.

2. Lack of occlusal control (occlusal traumatism, parafunctional habits) for periodontally susceptible individuals.

3. Short root or idiopathic root resorption.

BENEFITS OF ORTHODONTICS FOR A PERIODONTAL PATIENT

Orthodontic therapy can provide several benefits to the adult periodontal patient in the following manner:

1. *Reducing plaque retention*: Aligning crowded or malposed maxillary or mandibular anterior teeth permits the adult patient better access to adequately clean all surfaces of their teeth.

2. *Improving osseous form*: Vertical orthodontic tooth repositioning can improve certain type of osseous defects in periodontal patients. Often, the tooth movement eliminates the need for resective osseous surgery.

3. *Improving gingival form*: Orthodontic treatment can improve the esthetic relationship of the maxillary gingival margin levels before restorative dentistry. Aligning the gingival margin orthodontically, avoids gingival recontouring, which potentially could require bone removal and exposure of the roots of the teeth.

4. *Facilitating prosthetic replacements*: The other benefit of orthodontics is for the patient who has suffered a severe fracture of a maxillary anterior tooth, which requires forced eruption to permit adequate restoration of the root. In this situation, erupting the root allows the crown preparation to have sufficient resistance form and retention for the final restoration.

5. *Improving esthetics*: Orthodontic treatment allows open gingival embrasures to be corrected to regain lost papilla. If these open gingival embrasures are located in the maxillary anterior region, they can be unesthetic. In most patients, these areas can be corrected with a combination of orthodontic root movement, tooth reshaping, and/or restoration.

6. Orthodontic treatment could improve adjacent tooth position before implant placement or tooth replacement. This is especially true for the patient who has missing teeth for several years and has drifting and tipping of the adjacent dentition.

PERIODONTAL RESPONSE TO VARIOUS KINDS OF TOOTH MOVEMENT IN PERIODONTALLY COMPROMISED PATIENTS

1. Extrusion
2. Intrusion
3. Tipping
4. Bodily movement

1. *Extrusion*: Extrusion is the bodily movement of the tooth out of the socket. Least hazardous kind of tooth movement as far as periodontium is considered. Extrusion followed by equilibration of the clinical crown has been shown to reduce infrabony defects and pockets **(Fig. 55.1)**. Extrusive tooth movement in areas of one- and two-wall bony pockets leads to a coronal (favorable) positioning of intact connective tissue attachment and a shallowing of the bony defect. These changes in attachment and bone levels are a key factor in uprighting tipped molars **(Fig. 55.2)**. The use of light, well-controlled forces enables fractured teeth and hemiseptal defects to be treated more easily.

2. *Intrusion*: Intrusion is the bodily movement of a tooth into the socket and into the bone. Some consider that intrusion may results in deepening of infrabony pockets, root resorption and bone defects. Thus, benefits of intrusion for improvement of the periodontal condition around teeth are controversial.

3. *Tipping*: Heavy forces at the alveolar crest results in severe destruction of the epithelial attachment and crestal bone loss. Controlled tipping also produces high forces in the periodontal ligament as the fulcrum shifts more and more apically with increasing

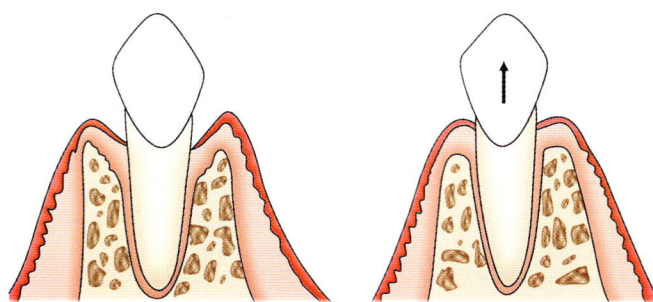

Fig. 55.1: Extrusion reducing infrabony defect and pocket

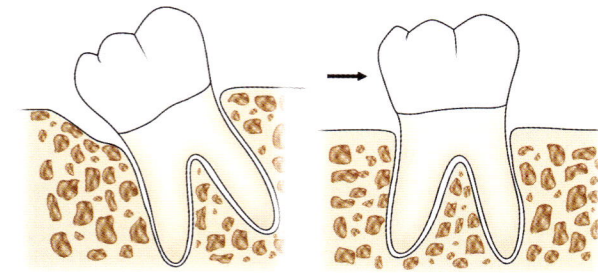

Fig. 55.2: Uprighting

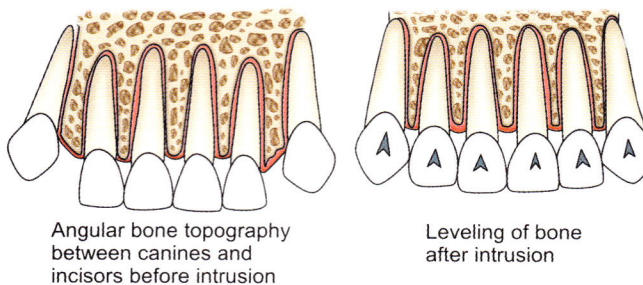

Angular bone topography between canines and incisors before intrusion

Leveling of bone after intrusion

Fig. 55.3: Intrusion

amounts of bone loss. Infact cases have been documented where a gingival lesion has been converted into a periodontal lesion by the injudicious use of tipping movement. Mild gingival changes associated with orthodontic appliances are transitory. These cause no periodontal damage and resolve on their own.

4. *Bodily movement:* Moving a tooth bodily into a periodontal defect has been believed to carry the bone along with the tooth resulting in improvement of the defect. However, recent studies have shown that this is only an illusion because it causes only an improved connective tissue attachment and infact worsens the bony defect. Hence, until new evidence surfaces this is contraindicated.

APPLICATION OF ORTHODONTICS IN PERIODONTICS

Orthodontic Treatment of Osseous Defects

1. *Hemiseptal defects*: Hemiseptal defects are one- or two-wall osseous defects that often are found around mesially tipped teeth or teeth that have supraerupted. Usually, these defects can be eliminated with the appropriate orthodontic treatment. In the case of the tipped tooth, uprighting and eruption of the tooth levels the bony defect. If the tooth is supraerupted, intrusion and leveling of the adjacent cementoenamel junctions can help to level the osseous defect **(Fig. 55.3)**.

2. *Furcation defects*: Class III furcation defect can be eliminated by hemisecting the crown and root of the tooth. However, this procedure requires endodontic, periodontal and restorative treatment. Hemisected roots when separated orthodontically permit favorable restoration and splinting. Hemisection, endodontic therapy and periodontal surgery must be completed before the start of orthodontic treatment. Bands or brackets and coil springs are placed on the root fragments to be separated. About 7 or 8 mm of space created between the roots of the hemisected molar. This process eliminates the furcation defects and allows the patient to clean the area with greater efficiency.

3. *Root proximity*: When roots of posterior teeth are in close proximity, the ability to maintain periodontal health and accessibility for restoration of adjacent teeth may be compromised. By orthodontic therapy, the roots can be moved apart and bone will be formed between the adjacent roots. Thus, open embrasure beneath the tooth contact provides additional bone support and enhances the patient's access to the interproximal region for hygiene. Brackets must be placed obliquely to facilitate orthodontic movement to separate the roots. Generally, 2 to 3 mm of root separation provides adequate bone and embrasure space to improve periodontal health.

4. *Fractured teeth/ forced eruption*: If the fracture extends beneath the level of the gingival margin and terminates at the level of the alveolar bone, then erupt the fractured root out of the bone and move the fracture margin coronally so that it can be properly restored. If a tooth fracture extends to the level of the bone, it must be erupted at 4 mm. The first 2.5 mm

moves the fracture margin far enough away from the bone to prevent a biologic width problem. The other 1.5 mm provides the proper amount of ferrule for adequate resistance form of the crown preparation. The orthodontic mechanics necessary to erupt the tooth can vary from elastic traction to orthodontic banding and bracketing. If a large portion of the tooth is still present, then orthodontic bracketing is necessary. If the entire crown has fractured, leaving only the root, then elastic traction from a bonded bar may be possible.

5. *Hopeless teeth maintained for orthodontic anchorage*: Hopeless teeth can be useful for orthodontic anchorage if the periodontal inflammation is controlled. Flaps are reflected for debridement of the roots to control inflammation around the hopeless tooth during the orthodontic process. The hopeless tooth may be so improved after orthodontic treatment that it is retained.

Orthodontic Treatment of Gingival Discrepancies

1. *Uneven gingival margins*: The relationship of the gingival margin of the six maxillary anterior teeth plays an important role in the esthetic appearance of the crowns. Four factors contribute to ideal gingival form:
   - The gingival margin of the two central incisors should be at the same level.
   - The gingival margin of the central incisors should be positioned more apically than the lateral incisors and at the same level as the canines.
   - The contour of the labial gingival margin should mimic the CEJs of the teeth.
   - A papilla should exist between each tooth, and the height of the tip of the papilla is usually halfway between the incisal edge and the labial gingival height of contour over the center of each anterior tooth. Therefore, the gingival papilla occupies half of the interproximal contact, and the adjacent teeth form the other half of the contact. Evaluate the relationship between the shortest central incisor and the adjacent lateral incisors. If the shortest central is still longer than the lateral incisors, the longer central incisor is extruded and then incisal edge is equilibrated. This moves the gingival margin coronally and eliminates the gingival margin discrepancy.

2. *Significant attrition and overeruption*: If the patient had a protrusive bruxing habit that had caused severe attrition and overeruption of the maxillary anterior teeth, resulting in the loss of over half of the crown length of the incisors, intrusion movement is applied on the four incisors which level the gingival margin apically. Then the incisal edges are restored and final crowns are placed.

3. *Open gingival embrasures*: Advanced periodontal disease with loss or cratering of interdental alveolar crest may result in the loss of the papilla. In these cases, there is no means of "resurrecting" the gingival papillae, but the esthetics of the situation may be greatly improved by a tooth movement. As these teeth are moved together orthodontically, the gingival tissue between the teeth squeezes into the shape of an interdental papilla. Missing papilla may result from overdivergence of adjacent roots. This is seen frequently in orthodontic cases where mistakes were made in initial bracket placement. In these cases, as soon as this discrepancy is noted, it is prudent for the operator to immediately verify the mesiodistal root tip with periapical radiographs. The "missing papilla" can then be prevented by simple repositioning of the orthodontic brackets or by judicious wire bending countering the exaggerated root divergence.

Correction of Pathologic Migration

Three basic appliances that are used for intra arch tipping movements are Hawley appliance, Crozat appliance and Spring retainer, thus correcting pathologic tooth migration.

Implant Placement

Orthodontic extrusion of a single tooth that needs to be extracted is an excellent method for improvement of the marginal bone level before the surgical placement of single implant **(Figs 55.4A to D)**. Not only the bone, but also the soft supporting tissues will move vertically with the teeth during orthodontic extrusion. Orthodontic extrusion of a " hopeless" incisor is therefore a useful method also for esthetic improvement of the marginal gingival level associated with the placement of implants. Through controlled movement of hopeless teeth, the orthodontist can establish an environment that will ultimately house a functional and esthetic restoration. This facilitates immediate implant placement after tooth

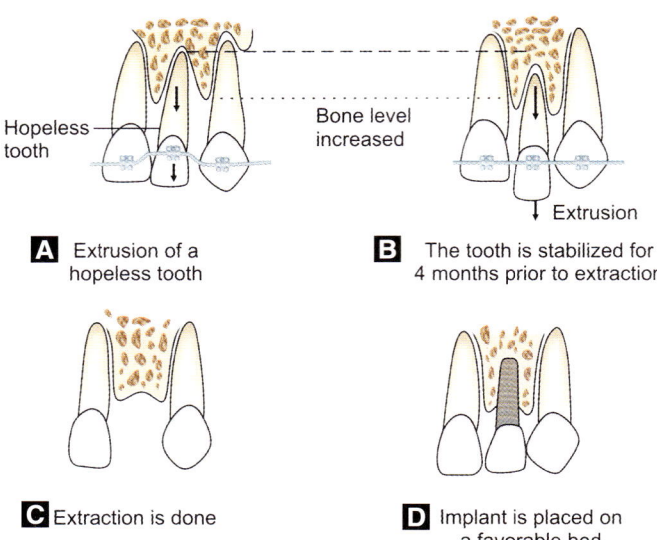

Hopeless tooth

Bone level increased

A Extrusion of a hopeless tooth

B The tooth is stabilized for 4 months prior to extraction

Extrusion

C Extraction is done

D Implant is placed on a favorable bed

Figs 55.4A to D: Implant placement

extaction because an increased volume of peri-implant bone and soft tissue are available.

APPLICATION OF PERIODONTICS IN ORTHODONTICS

I. **Preorthodontic osseous surgery:** The extent of the periodontal osseous surgery depends on the type of defect (i.e. crater, hemiseptal defect, three-wall defect and furcation lesion).

  Osseous craters: An osseous crater is an interproximal, two-wall defect that usually does not improve with orthodontic treatment. Some shallow craters (i.e. 4 to 5-mm pocket) may be maintainable nonsurgically during orthodontic treatment. But deep craters are first corrected surgically by reshaping the defect and reducing the pocket depth. This in turn enhances the ability to maintain these interproximal areas during orthodontic treatment. Thus, by eliminating the crater before orthodontics, the patient could maintain the area during and after orthodontic treatment.

  Three-Wall intrabony defects: Regenerative periodontal therapy including bone grafts and barrier membranes has been successful in regenerating the lost periodontium and filling three-wall defects. If the result of periodontal therapy is stable 3 to 6 months after periodontal surgery, orthodontic treatment may be initiated.

II. **Fiberotomy:** It reduces the occurrence of rotational relapse. Two soft-tissue periodontal entities which may influence the stability are the principal fibers of the periodontal ligament and the supra-alveolar fibers. Whereas the fibers of the periodontal ligament and transseptal groups remodel efficiently and histologically completely in only 2 to 3 months after orthodontic rotation of teeth whereas the supra-alveolar fibers are apparently more stable, with a slow turnover. Since the gingival soft tissues are composed primarily of non-elastic collagenous fibers, the exact mechanism by which the gingival soft tissues may apply a force capable of moving the teeth is as yet unknown. From a practical and clinical point of view, however, the supracrestal gingival tissues seemingly do contribute to rotational relapse, as evidenced by the effect of the circumferential supracrestal fiberotomy (CSF) technique. Basically, this technique consists of inserting a scalpel into the gingival sulcus and severing the epithelial attachment surrounding the involved teeth. The blade also transects the transseptal fibers by interdentally entering the periodontal ligament space.

III. **Frenectomy:** The contribution of the maxillary labial frenum to the etiology of a persisting midline diastema, and to re-opening of diastemas after orthodontic closure, is controversial. (Procedure is explained in Chapter no. 50 Periodontal Plastic Surgery.)

IV. **Preorthodontic grafting:** During tooth movement, the periodontal tissues should maintain a stable relationship around the cervical area of the tooth. An adequate amount of attached gingiva is necessary to be compatible with the gingival health and to allow orthodontic forces without creating bone loss and gingival recession. The thin, delicate tissue is far more prone to exhibit recession during orthodontics than is normal to thick tissue. In such cases, free gingival grafting is done before beginning orthodontic movement.

EFFECT OF ORTHODONTIC TOOTH MOVEMENT ON PERIODONTAL HEALTH

1. *Loss of periodontal attachment and bone relative to orthodontic therapy*: In the absence of periodontal disease and in the presence of excellent oral hygiene (including adults with reduced, but healthy, periodontium), proper orthodontic treatment causes no significant long-term effects on periodontal attachment and bone levels. Conversely, in patients (mostly adults)

with active periodontitis (that is, plaque-infected deep pockets evidenced by bleeding on probing), orthodontic tooth movement may accelerate the disease process, even when good oral hygiene is practiced. Because of the reduced volume of the periodontal ligament space in advanced periodontitis, orthodontic forces should be lighter than those used with periodontally healthy teeth. Orthodontic band placement causes an overall increase in salivary bacterial counts especially *Lactobacillus*, *Prevotella intermedia* and *Porphyromonous gingivalis*.

2. *Gingival recession relative to orthodontic therapy*: An adequate amount of attached gingiva is necessary to be compatible with gingival health to allow appliances (functional and orthopedic) to deliver orthodontic forces without gingival recession. Orthodontic tooth movement per se does not cause gingival recession. In areas of thin labial tissue, however, labial orthodontic tooth movement can result in bone dehiscence, creating an environment in which plaque and/or toothbrush trauma may cause sudden recession.

3. *Gingival hyperplasia relative to orthodontic therapy*: In the presence of excellent oral hygiene (provided that the appliances are properly placed, without excessive adhesive flash), no significant hyperplasia should develop as a result of orthodontic tooth movement in adolescents or adults. However, fixed orthodontic appliances in the presence of consistently poor oral hygiene can lead to moderate to severe hyperplasia, especially in the lower incisor region **(Figs 55.5 and 55.6)**. Severe cases of gingival hyperplasia may lead to attachment loss. Proper band fit or bonding of etching material is necessary so that the patient is able to continue adequate oral hygiene procedures.

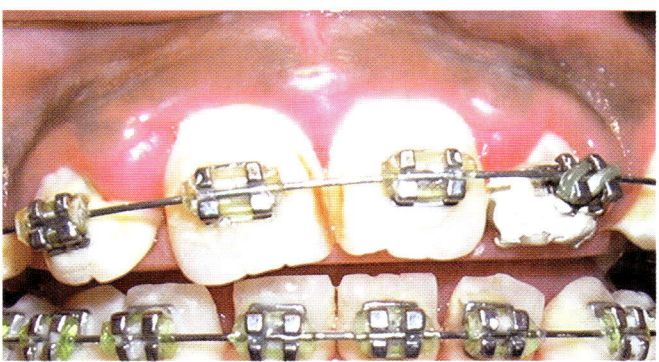

Fig. 55.6: Gingival hyperplasia in upper incisors during fixed orthodontic treatment

4. Kokich delineates three unesthetic situations that may develop during orthodontic treatment: gingival margin discrepancies, the missing papilla and the gummy smile.

PERIODONTAL MAINTENANCE IN THE ORTHODONTIC PATIENT

Plaque control: The presence of fixed orthodontic appliances make plaque control measures difficult. The orthodontic patient should be reinforced at each visit with the oral hygiene techniques. Soft special bi-level orthodontic brush with rounded end filaments is generally recommended **(Fig. 55.7)**. These brushes are designed with spaced rows of soft nylon filaments with

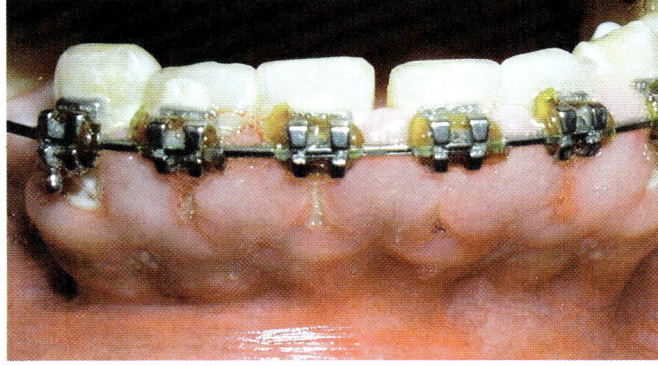

Fig. 55.5: Gingival hyperplasia in lower anteriors during fixed orthodontic treatment

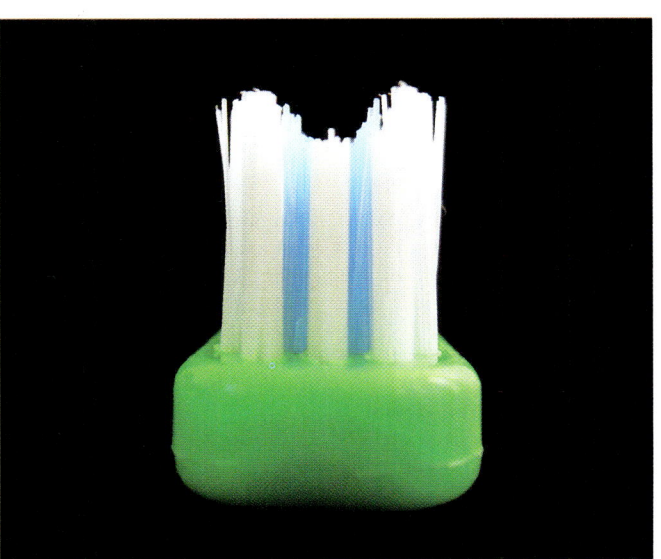

Fig. 55.7: Orthodontic bi-level toothbrush

PERIODONTICS REVISITED

a middle row that is shorter and can be applied directly over the fixed appliance. It is used with a short horizontal stroke. Sometimes, power assisted toothbrushes are recommended. Tufted dental floss or yarn used in the floss threader remove plaque more efficiently from the proximal tooth surfaces than regular dental floss. Most orthodontic patients can benefit from the regular use of an irrigator for removal of loose bacterial plaque and food debris and prevention of gingival inflammation. Removable appliances are cleaned after each meal and before retiring. Brush and rinse teeth and gingival tissue under the appliance each time the appliance is removed. The orthodontic appliance has to be properly designed. It must provide stable anchorage without causing tissue irritation, and must be esthetically acceptable. To counteract the tendency of orthodontic appliances to increase the accumulation of plaque on the teeth, attempts should be made to keep the appliances and mechanics simple, and avoid hooks, elastomeric rings and excess bonding resin outside the bracket bases.

The use of steel ligatures is recommended on all brackets, since elastomeric rings have been shown to be significantly more plaque attractive than steel ties.

Bonds are preferred over bands, as bonded molars show less plaque accumulation, gingivitis and loss of attachment interproximally. Thus, every attempt must be made to have the oral tissues in health and the patient motivated to perform thorough daily plaque removal.

The effects of orthodontic treatment on periodontium:
Favour plaque accumulation
Modify the gingival ecosystem
Gingival recession and hyperplasia
Excessive force causes necrosis of periodontal ligament and alveolar bone

BIBLIOGRAPHY

1. Carranza FM, Murphy NC. Orthodontics considerations in periodontal therapy. In, Carranza and Newman. Clinical Periodontology. 8th ed WB Saunders1996;559-64.
2. Grant DA, Stern IB, Listgarten MA. Orthodontic measures in periodontal therapy. In, Periodontics 6th ed CV Mosby Company 1988;1017-44.
3. Keim RG. Aesthetics in clinical orthodontic-periodontic interactions. Periodontol 2000 2001; 27: 59-71.
4. Kokich VG, Kokich VO. Orthodontic therapy for the periodontal-restorative patient. In, Rose LF, Mealey BL, Genco RJ, Cohen DW. Periodontics, Medicine, Surgery and Implants. Elsevier Mosby 2004; 718-44.
5. Kokich VG. Esthetics: the orthodontic-periodontic restorative connection. Semin Orthod 1996; 2: 21-30.
6. Kokich VG. The Role of Orthodontics as an Adjunct to Periodontal Therapy. In, Newman, Takei, Carranza. Clinical Periodontology 9th ed WB Saunders 2003;704-18.
7. Sanders NI. Evidence-based care in orthodontics and periodontics: A review of the literature JADA 1999;130:521-27.
8. Vanarsdall RL. Tooth movement as an adjunct to periodontal therapy. In, Genco RJ, Goldman HM and Cohen DW. Contemporary Periodontics. CV Mosby Company 1990;505-19.
9. Wilkins EM. Care of Dental Prostheses. In, Clinical practice of the Dental hygienist. Lippincott Williams and Wilkins. 8th ed 395-409
10. Zachrisson BU. Orthodontics and Periodontics. In, Lindhe J, Karring T, Lang NP. Clinical Periodontology and Implant dentistry 4th ed Blackwell Munksgaard 2003;744-80.

MCQs

1. Brush recommended to orthodontic patient:
   A. Soft special bi-level brush
   B. Novel design brush
   C. Small toothbrush
   D. Powdered toothbrush
2. Fibers transected in the circumferential supracrestal fiberotomy (CSF) technique are:
   A. Transseptal fibers   B. Apical fibers
   C. Interradicular fibers   D. None of the above
3. The orthodontic treatment may effects the periodontium by:
   A. Favouring plaque accumulation
   B. Modifying the gingival ecosystem
   C. Gingival recession
   D. All of the above
4. Gingival discrepancy in anterior teeth can be corrected by:
   A. Gingivectomy
   B. Intrusion and incisal restoration/porcelain laminate veneer
   C. Extrusion and fiberotomy and porcelain crown
   D. Surgical crown lengthening by flap procedure and osteotomy/osteoplasty of bone
   E. All of the above

Answers

1. A   2. A   3. D   4. E

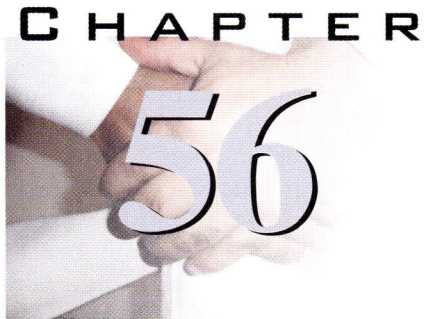
Periodontics-Oral Surgery

Atul Sharma, Shalu Bathla

INTRODUCTION

Oral surgery deals with diagnosis and treatment of oral conditions of the jaw and mouth structures that require surgical intervention. This specialty is related to the surgical removal of teeth and treatment of diseases, deformities and defects of the jaws and associated structures. Because of the close proximity, maxillofacial surgeons have to work in area which also is under the domain of other surgical specialties like neurosurgery, otorhinolaryngology, ophthalmology and orthopedics. Apart from this oral surgeons have to work in an area where other specialties of dentistry have to work afterwards for the complete rehabilitation of the patient such as prosthodontics, orthodontics, endodontics and periodontics. Though relationship of oral surgery with medical specialties, prosthodontics and orthodontics is much talked about in literature, we don't find much literature on relationship of periodontics and oral surgery.

PERIO-ORAL SURGERY RELATIONSHIP

While doing surgical procedures in the maxillofacial region surgeon is likely to injure the tooth supporting structures like the gingiva, periodontium and alveolar bone leading to plaque retention, gingivitis, pocket formation and alveolar bone loss. Thus, perio-oral surgery relationship becomes very important for a successful clinical practice. We can divide perio-oral surgery relationship into two main headings:

I. Inadvertent injury to periodontium during oral surgical procedures
II. Spread of infection during oral surgical procedures

Inadvertent Injury to Periodontium During Oral Surgical Procedures

The most common oral surgical procedures which can cause inadvertent injury to periodontium include:
1. Removal of an impacted tooth
2. Fixation of maxillo-mandibular fixation apparatus on the teeth

   1. Removal of an impacted tooth: Removal of an impacted tooth is considered as bread and butter procedure for maxillofacial surgeons. Though much has been discussed in literature about prevention of major postoperative complications such as fracture of the jaw, pain, swelling, infection, trismus, etc. The greatest periodontal hazard in oral surgery is development of distal pocket on second molars following extraction of impacted third molars.

Iatrogenic damage to the gingiva of the mandibular second molar is an often overlooked complication. During impaction surgery, the peripheral gingival soft tissues may be damaged on flap elevation, during bone removal or tooth sectioning with rotary instruments. Loss of the often thin band of keratinized gingiva of the second molar predisposes patient to pain. The surgically induced bone defect associated with impaction removal exacerbates the aforementioned problems. When the tooth is unerupted, the distal part of the second molar is often adjacent to the anterior border of the ascending ramus with almost no distobuccal collar of keratinized gingiva clinically evident. Only a thin band of keratinized gingiva (often less than 1 mm in width) may be noticeable on the buccal aspect of the tooth. In such cases, flap reflection and removal of the impacted mandibular third molar occasionally lead to destruction of what little attached gingiva was present before surgery. Disruption of the gingival attachment of the second molar and destruction of the fragile attached gingival collar will cause an immediate loss in vestibular depth because of the pull of the buccinator muscle insertions on the flap. This often prevents cervical reattachment of the gingiva to the second molar, hindering healing of the remaining nonkeratinized gingiva, which leads to plaque retention, inflammation, and pocket formation, requiring periodontal therapy secondarily.

2. Fixation of maxillomandibular fixation apparatus on the teeth: The goal of maxillomandibular fixation (MMF) is to provide indirect stabilization of fractures of the maxilla, mandible or both. With the technique of using arch bars, generally 16-22 interdental wires are passed. The patient has to keep his mouth closed from 4 to 6 weeks. Passing of wires and presence of arch bar in the neck of the tooth causes injury to the periodontium. Prolonged maxillomandibular fixation also leads to poor oral hygiene status which further aggravates the condition. Though ivy eyelet wiring is a good alternative but still some wires have to be passed through the neck of the teeth leading to injury of periodontium and also there is difficulty in maintaining oral hygiene. It has some limitations like we cannot use this method in severely displaced and impacted fractures as elastic traction cannot be given.

Another alternative can be the use of transalveolar screws. The technique of intraoral transalveolar bone screw fixation begins with local anesthetic administration, followed by the use of a curved mosquito hemostat to perforate the mucosa to the level of the periosteum, then elevation with a periosteal elevator. A 2·1 mm drill bit is used to perforate the bone before the insertion of 2·7 mm self-tapping screws. 18-20 mm long screws are used in the maxilla while 20 mm long screws are chosen for the mandible. It has many advantages including increased patient compliance, improved oral hygiene, decreased rate of infection and no penetration of wires through gingiva.

Spread of Infection During Oral Surgical Procedures

As incidence of periodontal diseases are very high in a developing country like India, a patient requiring maxillofacial surgical procedure may also be suffering from some periodontal disease. Thus, chances of spread of infection from infected periodontium to surgical site are high. As a rule thorough oral prophylaxis should be done prior to any oral surgical procedure. When multiple extractions are to be done first maxillary teeth should be extracted so that specks of calculus don't fall into fresh mandibular extraction sockets. Whenever cyst or tumor removal warrants extraction of the involved tooth prior oral prophylaxis should be done so that debris from extracted tooth should not contaminate to surgical area.

Pericoronitis is one of the most common condition where patient is either referred to oral surgeon or periodontist. Operculectomy should only be done in soft tissue impactions where there is no hindrance in eruption of tooth either from adjacent bone or tooth, otherwise removal of impacted tooth should be sought.

PERIODONTAL CONSIDERATIONS IN PERFORMING ORAL SURGICAL PROCEDURES

Atraumatic extraction of infected teeth: Teeth should be extracted in an atraumatic manner to conserve alveolar bone. If bone is to be removed to avoid fracturing a tooth or the alveolus, it is best to remove the tooth through a lingual or palatal approach to conserve the remaining buccal plate of bone. The extreme challenge to conserve the soft and hard tissues of the ridge arises when tooth to be extracted have fractured or decayed to the level of gingival margins or crestal bone. The design of soft tissue flaps and plans for osseous resection must be thought carefully to prevent the formation of a deformity in the healed residual ridge. Surgical elevators and forceps must be used with extreme caution in such conditions.

Postextraction management of socket area: Extraction sockets should be inspected carefully for any sign of infection after the teeth or remaining roots have been removed. Granulomatous tissue should be curetted to remove it from its attachment to the walls or the base of the sockets, and the area should be irrigated thoroughly to ensure removal of all debris and loose bony spicules. Earlier, clinician used to apply pressure at the crest of the socket to compress the rim of the alveolar bone. But this practice should be avoided as it results in the collapse of the remaining buccal plate of bone and also hastens the formation of a deformity within the ridge.

PERIODONTAL MAINTENANCE OF ORAL SURGERY PATIENT

Preparation of the mouth prior to general inhalational anesthesia: Plaque control and professional instrumentation aid in reducing the oral bacteria count. Because the mouth is an entrance to the respiratory chamber, the possibility always exists that debris and fluids may be inhaled from the mouth during the administration of an anesthetic or when the patient coughs.

Patient with intermaxillary fixation: Every attempt should be made to keep patient's mouth as clean as possible for comfort and sanitation and as plaque-free as possible for disease prevention. When the temporomandibular joint is injured, the patient wearing fixation appliances that involve only the mandible has difficulty in applying a toothbrush to the lingual surfaces of teeth. The extent of possible care depend on the appliances; the condition of the lips, tongue and other oral tissue; and the cooperation of the patient. Encouragement must be given to the patient to begin toothbrushing as soon as possible after the surgical procedure, but until the patient is able, a plan for care is outlined for a caregiver. The limited access for personal oral care procedures and the effect of the liquid diet required for most cases define the need for special dental hygiene care for the patient with intermaxillary fixation. After removal of appliances, all patients have a degree of muscular trismus that hinders toothbrushing and mastication. When the patient can open mouth normally then plaque control procedures are initiated, complete scaling and planing can be performed.

BIBLIOGRAPHY

1. Motamedi MHK. A technique to manage gingival complications of third molar surgery. Oral Surg Oral Med Oral Pathol Oral Radiol Endod 2000;90:140-3.
2. Ramfjord SP and Ash MM. Periodontal considerations in restorative and other aspects of dentistry. In, Periodontology and Periodontics. Modern Theory and Practice 1st ed AITBS Publisher and distributor India1996;339-51.
3. Richardson DT, Dodson TB. Risk of periodontal defects after third molar surgery: An exercise in evidence-based clinical decision-making. Oral Surg Oral Med Oral Pathol Oral Radiol Endod 2005;100:133-7.
4. Seibert JS. Treatment of Moderate Localized Alveolar Ridge Defects: Preventive and Reconstructive Concepts in Therapy. In, Interdisciplinary Periodontal Surgery. Dent Clin North Am 1993; 37(2):265-80.
5. Wilkins EM. The Oral and Maxillofacial Surgery Patient. In, Clinical practice of the Dental Hygienist. Lippincott Williams and Wilkins. 8th Ed 1999;707-20.

PERIODONTICS REVISITED

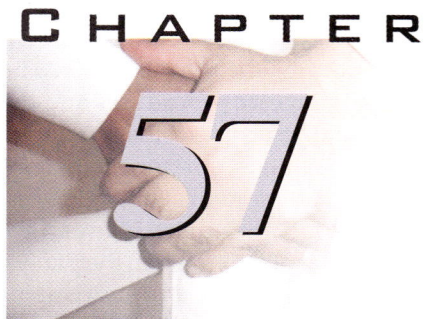

CHAPTER 57

Periodontics-Psychiatry

JC Bathla, Manish Bathla, Shalu Bathla

INTRODUCTION

Periodontists have demonstrated the etiological significance in chronic periodontitis of biological and behavioral risk factors, including a range of systemic conditions, smoking, oral cleanliness and age. However, a significant proportion of the variation in disease severity cannot be explained taking only these factors into consideration. The remaining variance, at least in part, may be explained by important psychosocial factors. Freud's oral stage of psychoanalytic theory places great importance on the relationship of the oral cavity to the psyche. It is also hypothesized that the psychologic and social factors are involved in diseases of the oral cavity.

PARAFUNCTIONAL HABITS

Parafunctional means altered/abnormal function. These habits represent perversion of occlusion that is potentially injurious to the periodontal tissues, masticatory muscles and temporomandibular joint. They are referred to as "parafunction" which designates tooth contacts in other than chewing and swallowing.

Classification of Parafunctional Habits

I. According to the cause, these are classified in three ways:
   • Tooth to tooth function, e.g. bruxism.
   • Tooth to soft tissue, e.g. digit – sucking.
   • Tooth to foreign object, e.g. chewing of pens and pencils.
II. According to Sorrin and Cheek, the habits are classified into:
   A. Neurosis:
      • Lip biting
      • Fingernail biting
      • Tongue thrusting
      • Pencil/pen biting
   B. Occupational habits:
      • Holding of nails in the mouth by cobblers, upholsterers and carpenter.
      • Pressure of a reed during the playing of musical instruments.
   C. Miscellaneous habits:
      • Mouth breathing
      • Thumb sucking
      • Pipe/cigarette smoking
      • Incorrect methods of toothbrushing

Bruxism, Clenching and Tapping

Bruxism consists of aggressive, repetitive or continuous grinding or gritting of the teeth during the day or night or both, i.e. constant or intermittent occlusal contact of the teeth, aside from mastication, swallowing or speech. Bruxism often occurs without any neurolgical disorders or defects and can be viewed as a phenomenon present in healthy individuals. The patient may be completely unaware of these repeated and sustained forced contacts of the teeth that seem to have no functional significance in humans. Certain types of individuals seem to be predisposed to bruxism.

Clenching is a continuous or intermittent closure of the jaws under pressure.

Tapping/doodling is repetitive tooth contact made on isolated prominent tooth surfaces or dental restorations when mandible is in eccentric occlusion.
Etiology:
- Occlusal disharmonies or prematurities represent struggling movements of the mandible in an attempt to wear away or push aside the offensive tooth surfaces. This is accompanied by abnormal muscle activity and both disappear when occlusal disharmonies are corrected.
- Emotional tension, anxiety and deep-seated aggression could cause or aggravate bruxism, clenching and tapping. Thaller and associates (1976) define the profile of the bruxistic patient as a person who tends to be anxious, with intrinsic hostility, and unable to vent frustration outwardly. Psychiatrists explain these neurosis as the oral outlet for subconscious aggression.
- The psychological explanation for bruxism- All persons have drives that are associated with life goals. When these drives are blocked the resultant frustration produces rage. Rage must have an outlet; for instance, an enraged child does not hesitates to bite. When the child learns that such biting behavior is socially unacceptable, the biting is repressed. Since the rage cannot be suppressed, new outlets for its dissipation must be found. Substitute satisfaction (sublimation) may be employed. When the substitution is inadequate, one may still resort to biting to gain satisfaction. This satisfaction may be gained surreptitiously and symbolically on an unconscious level by bruxing or clenching or tapping.

Symptoms: Patients are usually unaware of the habit, but may complain of pain or tired feeling in the jaws or muscles, particularly upon arising in the morning, which may radiate to the head and neck and a burning sensation in the muscles or head.
Consequences of bruxism on periodontium:
- Excessive tooth wear characterized by polished facets on tooth surfaces with exaggerated facets in normal functional areas.
- Flat inclined planes.
- Widening of occlusal surfaces.
- Reduction in vertical dimension.
- Eccentric occlusion and mandibular deviation.
- The periodontium often responds favorably to the increased function by thickening of the periodontal ligament and increased density of the alveolar bone.
- Aggravates existing periodontal diseases.
- Causes tooth mobility.
- Muscle fatigue.
- Causes temporomandibular joint disorders secondary to hypertonicity of masticatory muscles.

Treatment for these habits includes bite appliances (anterior and posterior bite plane), selective grinding, orthodontic therapy, restorative therapy and use of psychotherapy or psychotherapeutic drugs.

Lips, Cheek and Tongue Biting

The inadvertent habit of biting or chewing of lips, cheek, or tongue can affect periodontal health. Chewing the mucosa on the interior lip or cheek usually results in a keratinized bite line in the affected area. In a Class II Division I occlusion, the degree of overjet frequently carries the incisal edges of maxillary incisor past the vermilion border of the lower lip. This establishes a wedging force from the labial and circumoral musculature against the lingual aspects of maxillary anteriors. Migration, mobility, and degeneration of the labial attachment apparatus can occur.

Thumb Sucking

Thumb or hand sucking can be a problem in periodontics only if it continues into the post childhood years as seen in some congenital diseases or mental retardation. Thumb or hand sucking has profound effect in childhood and contributed to arch displacement and malocclusion. The periodontal result will be the same as those seen in lip, tongue or cheek biting.

Tongue Thrusting

It entails persistent forceful wedging of tongue, against the teeth particularly in the anterior region. Instead of placing the tongue against the palate with the tip behind the maxillary teeth during swallowing, the tongue is thrust forward against the mandibular anterior teeth, which tilt and also spread laterally. It is usually associated with an abnormal swallowing habit (reverse swallow). Tongue thrusting may develop in infancy as a result of bottle feeding or nasopharyngeal diseases.

Consequences: Causes excessive lateral pressure, which may be traumatic to the periodontium.

- Spreading and tilting of anterior teeth with open bite anteriorly, posteriorly or in premolar area **(Fig. 57.1)**.
- Altered inclination of maxillary anterior teeth results in the change in direction of functional forces, which aggravates the labial drift and undesirable labiolingual rotational forces.
- The antagonism between the forces that direct the tooth labially, and inward pressure from the lip, may lead to tooth mobility.
- Altered inclination of the teeth also interferes with food excursion and favors the accumulation of food debris at gingival margin.
- Loss of proximal contact leads to food impaction.
- Pathological tooth migration.

Treatment of tongue thrust can be performed with appliance therapy, myofunctional and speech therapy, or a combination. Restorative therapy alone will not resolve the damage caused by tongue thrusting. The treatment of the overt anterior thrust must include comprehensive attention to the circumoral as well as the glossal musculature.

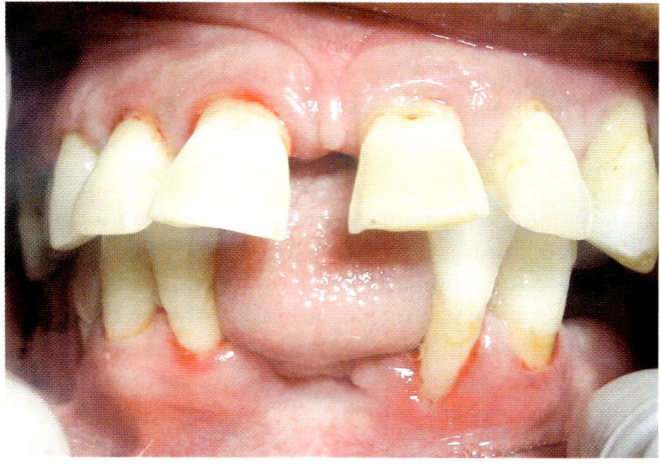

Fig. 57.1: Tongue thrusting leading to pathologic tooth migration

Mouth Breathing

Gingivitis is often seen associated with mouth breathing. The gingival changes include erythema, edema, enlargement and a diffuse surface shineness in the exposed areas. Maxillary anterior region is the commonest site of involvement. Its harmful effect is generally attributed to irritation from surface dehydration.

Factitial Habits

A self-inflicted injury of the periodontal tissues can occur with repeated voluntary trauma to a localized area. This injury can be caused by pacifiers, fingernails, pens, pencils, eyeglass stems, and many other provocative objects. Factitial habits, as they are called, can cause a local mechanical injury that invites bacterial contamination and results in inflammatory disease. These habits could proceed from localized recession to bone loss if left unattended. The psychological profile of an individual with a factitial habit should be considered in the treatment plan.

Cigarette Smoking

Smoking potentially acts by affecting tissue moisture or temperature that has been related to the etiology for NUG and other oral diseases as well. Smoking is also inversely related to many psychosocial variables associated with mental health. Understanding the cytotoxic effects of tobacco use as well as the nature of nicotine dependence is essential for adequate patient management. Nicotine is a highly psychoactive tertiary amine. Chronic exposure to nicotine stimulates release of dopamine into the central nervous system (CNS), neuronal cleft, and other sites and proliferation of nicotinic acetylcholine receptors on postsynaptic neurons. Brain metabolism initially increases and then stabilizes in the presence of nicotine. With repeated exposure, CNS stimulation by nicotine gradually decreases and the presence of nicotine becomes necessary to ward off withdrawal symptoms. Nicotine dependence is not only a "risk factor" for other diseases, but is a disease requiring treatment in its own way.

Dental Problems Associated with Musical Wind Instruments

Wind instruments create forces on the teeth that may injure the periodontium and cause loosening and pathological migration of teeth.

PSYCHOSOMATIC DISORDERS AND FACTORS

Harmful effects that result from psychic influence on the organic control of tissues are known as psychosomatic disorders.

There are two ways, in which psychosomatic disorder may be induced in the oral cavity:

a. Through the development of habits that are injurious to the periodontium and

b. By the direct effect of the autonomic nervous system on the physiologic tissue balance **(Fig. 57.2)**

Psychosomatic Factors

- Stress
- Oral hygiene negligence
- Changes in dietary intake
- Smoking and other harmful habits
- Oral habits
- Bruxism
- Gingival circulation
- Alteration in salivary flow and components
- Lowered host resistance

1. **Stress:** Selye coined the term "Stress". Stress is defined as a total transaction from demand to resolution in response to an environmental encounter that requires appraisal, coping and adaptation by the individual. Coping is the response of the individual to stress (emotionally and physically). Selye proposed that the initial Hypothalamic- pituitary -adrenal axis (HPA) axis response to stress was beneficial but that prolonged mental or physical stress can be detrimental to the human body by exhausting or diminishing the ability to respond to a perceived threat or challenge. Selye defined this as the General Adaptation Syndrome (GAS), a set of non-specific physiologic reactions to stress. Response to prolonged stress is a part of the individual's adaptive mechanism which may lead to clinical signs and symptoms called the GAS. The pioneers who suggested that psychological stress might play a role as an etiological agent of periodontal disease were Dean and Dean (1945) and Schluger (1949). Stress, distress and coping behaviors are regarded as important indicators for periodontal disease. Psychosocial factors can modify the periodontal status through behavioral changes regarding oral hygiene, smoking, dietary intake, bruxism and drug use.

Stress and psychosomatic influences are considered to be separate but parallel factors in the causation of disease. The pituitary and adrenal hormones play a role in regulating the response to

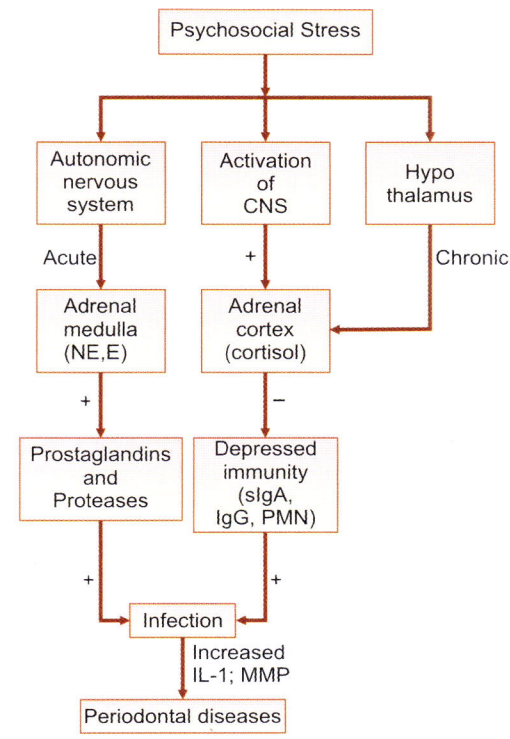

Fig. 57.2: The effects of stress on periodontal diseases. CNS- Central Nervous System; NE- Norepinephrine; E- Epinephrine; MMP- Matrix metalloproteinase; IL-1- Interleukin-1

stress, involving a feed back mechanism. Psychosocial stress has been found to influence host defenses exerting an immunosuppressive effect and affecting one's vulnerability to periodontal disease. **Figure** 57.2 demonstrates the potential role of psychosocial stressors in initiating a cascade of events in hypothalamic – pituitary – adrenal axis, the autonomic nervous system and the central nervous system. The physiologic consequences of which are to depress immunity enhancing likelihood of periodontal disease.

The consequences of behavioral change, extending from neglect of oral hygiene to dietary inadequacies, poor sleep patterns, use of tobacco products and other substance abuse constitute an important class of psychosocial stressors that contribute to the 'vicious cycle' of increasingly severe forms of advanced periodontal inflammation and disease. The less common form of periodontal disease – aggressive periodontitis, periodontal disease associated with diabetes are similarly associated with a myriad of intra- and interpersonal stressors that are significant risk

PERIODONTICS REVISITED

factors for exacerbating the underlying periodontal disease condition **(Fig. 57.3).**

2. **Oral hygiene:** Proper oral hygiene is partially dependent on the mental health status of the patient. Some patients may be so disturbed or distracted psychologically that personal hygiene is neglected. It has been reported that psychological disturbances can lead patients to neglect oral hygiene and the resultant accumulation of plaque is detrimental to the periodontal tissues. Other patients may intentionally ignore oral hygiene to fulfill deep neurotic needs. Oral hygiene may be neglected during depression, deep anxiety and rebellion against authority or may be a result of passive aggression. Dependent individuals may exhibit chronic neglect as if they were expecting such care to be the responsibility of others. The dentist's instructions concerning oral hygiene may be ignored as a form of "parental defiance".

3. **Diet and appetite:** Psychologic factors affect the choice of foods, the physical consistency of diet, and the consumption of excessive quantities of refined carbohydrates and softer diets, requiring less vigorous mastication and therefore predisposing to plaque accumulation at the proximal risk sites.

These factors may have a direct or indirect influence on the periodontium.

4. **Smoking and other harmful habits:** Explained in Chapter no.16 Smoking and Periodontium.

5. **Oral habits:** Neurotic needs find oral expression. The mouth may be used to obtain satisfaction, to express dependency or hostility, and to inflict or receive pain.

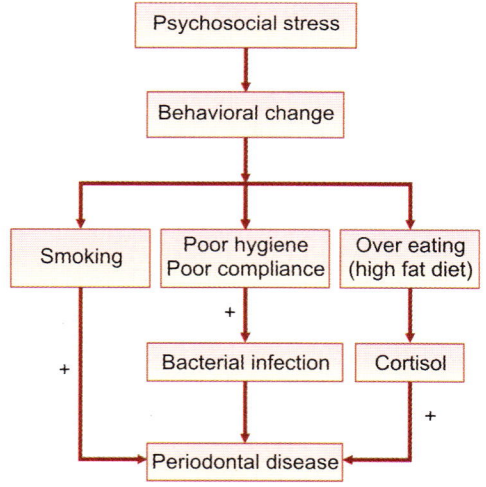

Fig. 57.3: Psychosocial stress and its effect on behavior as manifested by alterations in periodontal disease

Sucking, biting, sensing, and feeling may become habitual, as in thumb sucking, tongue thrusting, infantile swallowing, and biting of tongue, lip, cheek, or finger nail. These actions also figure in bruxing, clenching, tooth doodling, and smoking. Such habits may lead to tooth migration, occlusal traumatism and occlusal wear.

Coffee drinking is another habit that may act extrinsically (through thermal or chemical properties) and intrinsically (through caffeine content). Coffee drinking is more frequent among smokers and has also been shown to be greater among patients with NUG than among those with healthy gingiva.

It has been reported that depression had little direct effect on plaque accumulation between groups of individuals with aggressive or chronic periodontitis.

6. **Bruxism:** Explained earlier in this chapter.

7. **Gingival circulation:** The tonus of smooth muscle of blood vessels may be altered by the emotions by way of the autonomic nervous system, e.g. prolonged contraction could alter the supply of oxygen and nutrients to the tissues. Smoking and stress have been implicated in reducing gingival blood flow which in turn could increase the possibility of necrosis of tissues, with subsequent reduced resistance to plaque.

8. **Saliva:** Phrases like 'spitting mad,' "frothing at the mouth," and "drooling in anticipation" shows that salivation has psychiatric implications. Psychological factors are known to influence the rate of secretion and composition of saliva. Saliva, in turn, relates to plaque formation, calculus deposition, anti-bacterial and proteolytic activities, all of which may have a bearing on periodontal disease. Mental activity, stress, muscular efforts or emotional disturbances produce a transient reduction of salivary flow and changes in the salivary enzyme count, making the individual more susceptible to oral diseases and disorders. Level of pH has also been observed to go up as salivation increases. These relationships between salivary physiology and psychologic status do not necessarily demonstrate causation of periodontal disease, but they show a pathway in which periodontal health is influenced by salivary changes.

9. **Lowered host resistance:** Stress and its biochemical mediators may modify the immune response to microbial challenge, which is an important defense against periodontal disease. Under stress, the release of adrenaline and nor-adrenaline may not only induce

a decrease in blood flow, but possibly also those blood elements necessary for maintaining resistance to disease related microbes.

10. **Other factors:** Patients may have unrealistic attitudes or protective mechanisms that lead them to deny their dental illness. Some patients seeking cosmetic surgery or dental surgery because of somatic delusions may displace their dissatisfaction on the therapist. The acceptance of treatment and its course and success for some patients depends on the therapist's interaction with the patient and management of their psychological status.

RELATIONSHIP BETWEEN NECROTIZING ULCERATIVE GINGIVITIS AND STRESS

Necrotizing ulcerative gingivitis (NUG) is a disease that may have an emotional basis. The disease often occurs in association with stressful situations **(Fig. 57.4)**. Psychological disturbances, as well as increased adrenocortical secretion are common in patients with the disease. Significant correlation between disease incidence and two personality traits, i.e dominance and abasement, suggests the presence of a NUG-prone personality. The mechanisms whereby psychologic factors create or predispose to gingival damage have not been established, but alterations in digital and gingival capillary responses suggestive of increased autonomic nervous activity have been demonstrated in patients with NUG. It can be concluded that opportunistic bacteria are the primary etiologic agents of NUG in patients that demonstrate immunosuppression. Stress, smoking and pre-existing

gingivitis are common predisposing factors. The incidence of NUG increases during periods of physiologic and emotional stress and, as a result, stress has long been recognized as one of the contributing factors for NUG. The negative effect of stress on the periodontium can be due to either altered behaviors, such as poor oral hygiene and smoking or impaired immune function, leading to increased susceptibility to infection. Smoking is very common in this patient population. Increased smoking may be stress related and may induce vasoconstriction and localized ischemia.

Study on gingivitis volunteers by Deinzer et al. also suggested that proinflammatory cytokine levels are increased in stressed subjects. These data strongly suggest that stress may be a contributing factor not only for NUG, but also for other periodontal diseases, such as gingivitis and chronic periodontitis, and may also modify the response to periodontal treatment. The intervening physiologic mechanisms between stress and increased susceptibility to periodontal disease are not well documented but are probably related to impaired immune function and altered oral health behaviors.

PERIODONTAL ASPECTS OF PSYCHIATRIC PATIENTS

1. *Effect of depression on periodontal health*:
   Direct effect of stress affects host resistance factors. Indirect effects of stress:
   * negligence in performing oral hygiene procedures
   * failure to seek dental care
   * increased smoking and use of alcohol
   * altered food intake
   * clenching, grinding of the teeth (Bruxism)
2. *Effect of anxiety on periodontal health*: Oral health problems associated with anxiety disorders include canker sores, dry mouth, lichen planus (lacy white lines, mouth ulcers, burning mouth syndrome, and temporomandibular joint disorders). People with anxiety disorders may disregard their oral health altogether and are at an increased risk for periodontal disease and bruxism. Being anxious of a needle can also complicate periodontal procedure.
3. *Effect of mental retardation and Down's syndrome on periodontal health*: People with Down's syndrome are prone to the same degree of dental disease as the general population but develop more severe forms of periodontal disease than the general population.

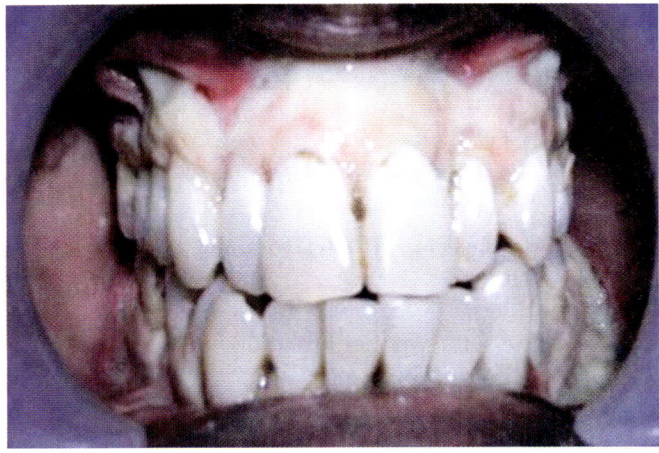
Fig. 57.4: Necrotizing ulcerative gingivitis (NUG)

PERIODONTICS REVISITED

Down's syndrome associated with mental retardation is characterized by aggressive and generalized periodontitis, with the subsequent destruction of the supporting tissues and loss of teeth at an early age. Bruxism occurs in people with Down's syndrome and may be triggered by a state of chronic anxiety, dental malocclusion, temporomandibular joint dysfunction due to laxity of the supporting ligaments, and/or underdeveloped nervous control. Dental trauma is frequently experienced due to lack of motor development. Fracture or luxation of the anterior teeth is frequent and often involves loss of tooth vitality.

PERIODONTAL ASPECTS OF PSYCHIATRIC MEDICATIONS

Following are the oral adverse effects of psychiatric medications:

1. *Gingival enlargement*: One of the most serious side effects encountered with the use of phenytoin is phenytoin - induced gingival enlargement (PIGO), which may occur in approximately 50% of the patients on long-term use of phenytoin. Phenytoin - induced gingival enlargement has been reported to be most marked on the labial surfaces of anterior teeth **(Fig. 57.5)**. Edentulous areas are usually not affected. The first 6 months appear to be critical for the initiation of gingival enlargement. With regular dental prophylaxis and frequent recalls for reinforcement of plaque control, clinically significant gingival enlargement is preventable for patients who are cooperative. This means that the patients must be aware of this possible side effect of phenytoin therapy and be referred to a dentist for appropriate treatment. Several studies have suggested that initiation of meticulous oral care prior to the beginning of phenytoin therapy will prevent gingival enlargement. Elimination of plaque after the lesion is present, appears only to modify the size of PIGO. Other anticonvulsant drugs causing gingival enlargement are: Phenobarbital, Carbamazepine, Sodium Valproate, Primidone and Felbamate.

2. *Xerostomia*: Reduced saliva secretions as a consequence of anti-depressant medication has been widely reported, dry mouth being a common adverse effect of tricyclic antidepressants (TCAs) as well as selective serotonin reuptake inhibitors (SSRIs).

3. *Altered taste sensation*: Following are the psychiatric medications causing altered taste sensation:
   - *Anticonvulsants*: Carbamazepine, Phenytoin
   - *Antidepressants*: Amitriptyline, Clomipramine, Desipramine, Doxepin, Imipramine, Nortriptyline
   - *Mood stabilizer*: Lithium
   - *Antipsychotics*: Clozapine, Trifluoperazine

4. *Halitosis*: Following are the psychiatric medications causing halitosis:
   - *Antianxiety*: Lorazepam, Hydroxyzine, Chlordiazepoxide, Diazepam, Alprazolam
   - *Anticonvulsants*: Carbamazapine, Lamotrigine
   - *Antidepressants*: Amitriptyline, Desipramine, Doxepin, Imipramine, Amoxapine, Fluoxetine, Bupropion, Clomipramine, Fluvoxamine
   - *Antipsychotics*: Clozapine, Haloperidol, Pimozide, Trifluoperazine, Chlorpromazine
   - *Sedatives*: Flurazepam

5. *Dental caries*: Increased caries activity has been found in depressed patients receiving antidepressants.

6. *Bruxism*: Buspirone, Citalopram, Fluoxetine, Paroxetine, Sertraline and Venlafaxine are the psychiatric drugs causing bruxism.

DOCTOR PATIENT RELATIONSHIP

Interview

Rapport: The doctor—patient relationship begins to form when the patient first meets the dentist. The interview gives the dentist an opportunity to establish rapport, to introduce patient education, and to make the patient familiar with the way in which the practice is conducted.

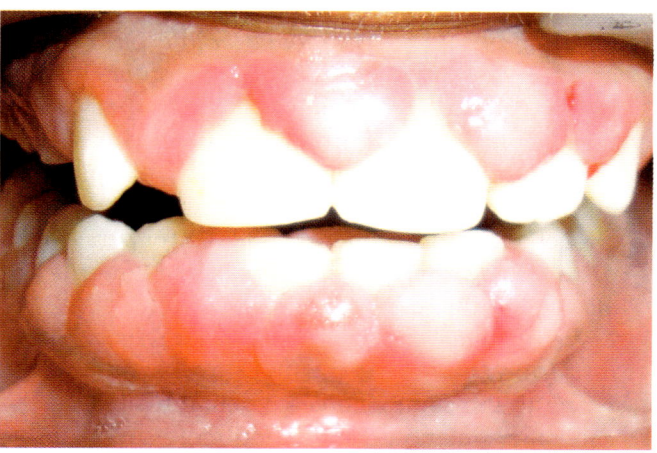

Fig. 57.5: Phenytoin induced gingival enlargement

During the interview the chief complaint, the medical history and the dental history are obtained. Simultaneously the patient is observed for the purpose of making a preliminary evaluation of the individual.

Observation: A good share of observation consist of being attentive to the patient's manner of response. Patient's choice of words; voice tone, pitch, tempo; facial expression and movements during the time of interview. These reactions tend to be heightened in the dental office, since a visit to a dental clinic represents a stressful situation to many patients. Do not lecture the patient on the subject of dentistry.

Questioning: When the patient asks questions concerning dentistry, he/she may be expressing anxiety rather than an interest in dentistry. The more experienced practitioner will sense this anxiety and reassure the patient. Do not deliver long details on dentistry that does not satisfy the patient's need, leaving the patient with a feeling of frustration.

Psychological Factors

Qualities of sensitivity, perception, and insight can be nurtured by devoting adequate time to the interview. Some knowledge of these qualities is as important to the dentist as it is to the physician.

Responses are clues to the unconscious mind. The unconscious is generally well hidden, and the patient is unaware of its influence on his/her behavior, but the observer can detect the behavior and through it interpret the unconscious mind.

The dentist must deal with the patient's psychological structure and the mouth as a center for emotional manifestations.

Psychiatric Manifestations During Therapy

Value judgments: The dentist should treat the patient with friendliness and respect, not with criticism or condemnation. The patient should be treated with tact and courtesy. The dentist must be sincerely concerned with the welfare of the patient and this should take precedence over dentistry as a business. He/she should try to understand the patient as well as the patient's dental illness. The dentist is often not sufficiently well prepared to meet the psychological demands of the patient or guide the development of new attitudes in patients concerning treatment and health. Although the dentist should conduct a practice in a psychologically sensitive manner, he/she should not attempt psychotherapy per se.

Referral: If the dentist perceives a rising level of nervousness or anger, he/she would be best advised to try to determine what he/she or the patient may be doing to precipitate this state of events and if possible deal with its basic cause. When the situation appears to be unmanageable, the patient should be referred to another dentist or physician. The dentist feels less angry when there is no compulsion to comply with impossible demands. This can be done by setting limits for the patient's behavior. The dentist should not view the patient as a threat to himself/herself or his/her competence. The patient should be reassured, not threatened.

Patient Compliance in Health Care

No other area in health care has more psychological overtones than patient compliance with prescription for medication, smoking, drinking and plaque control. Measures to increase patient compliance with home care instructions are needed. Self-care motivation is a necessary basis for successful preventive dentistry.

LANDMARK STUDIES RELATED

Deinzer R, Forster P, Fuck L, Herforth A, Stiller-Winkler R, Idel H. Increase of crevicular interleukin 1β under academic stress at experimental gingivitis sites and at sites of perfect oral hygiene. Journal of Clinical Periodontology 1999;26:1-8.

This randomized controlled split-mouth trial involved inducing experimental gingivitis and measuring levels of interleukin-1β in a group of students undergoing academic stress as compared to a non-stressed control group. The experimental group was found to have significantly higher levels of the immunological mediator at the sites of experimental gingivitis than the control group and also higher levels at sites of experimental gingivitis as compared to sites of perfect oral hygiene. This not only showed a relationship between psychosocial stress and periodontal conditions, but also suggested a synergistic relationship for the increase of interleukin-1β via stress and presence of plaque.

Renate D, Stefan R, Ole M, Armin H. Increase in gingival inflammation under academic stress. Journal of Clinical Periodontology 1998; 25(5): 431-33.

PERIODONTICS REVISITED

In this study 26 medical students participating in a major exam and the same number of medical students not participating in any exam throughout the study period were taken up for the study. Bleeding on probing was assessed 4 weeks prior to the exam period (baseline) and at the last day of the exam. Severe deterioration in gingival health from baseline to the last exam day were observed more frequently in exam students than in controls (p=0.014). Six exam students but only one control person developed a severe gingivitis at atleast one formerly healthy tooth throughout the study period. These results further support the hypothesis that psychological stress is a significant risk factor for periodontal inflammation.

Maupin CC, Bell WB. The relationship of 17-hydroxycorticosteroid to acute necrotizing ulcerative gingivitis. Journal of Periodontology 1975;46(12):721-22.

This study was conducted on 11 patients presenting with ANUG, collected 24 hours urine sample before and after the course of ANUG. They measured 17 – Hydroxy corticosteroid content in urine which is a physiological measure of stress. They concluded that patients had a significant high level of 17 – Hydroxycorticosteroid during the course of ANUG.

Genco RJ, Ho AW, Grossi SG, Dunford RG, Tedesco LA. Relationship of stress, distress and inadequate coping behaviors to periodontal disease. Journal of Periodontology 1999; 70: 711–723.

A cross-sectional epidemiological study was conducted on 1426 adults, aged 25–74 years. Results indicated a significant role for financial strain in relation to greater alveolar bone and periodontal attachment loss, after adjusting not only for age and gender, but also for smoking. Interestingly, those individuals with a problem solving coping style for managing the stressors of daily living fared better than those who exhibited a more emotionally focused and less adequate coping response to psychosocial strain. The pattern of results from this study suggests that effects of psychosocial stress on periodontal disease can be modulated by adequate coping behaviors. Ability to cope with psychological stressors has been thought to influence onset and progression of periodontal disease because ineffectiveness of coping with the stress may lead to neglect in oral hygiene, yielding increased levels of the most common forms of adult periodontitis as well as exacerbating the less frequently occurring rapidly progressive periodontitis.

BIBLIOGRAPHY

1. Axtelius B, Soderfeldt B, Nilsson A, Edwardsson S, Attstrom R. Therapy-resistant periodontitis. Psychosocial characteristics. J Clin Periodontol 1998;25:482-91.
2. Breivik T, Thrane PS, Murison R, Gjermo P. Emotional stress effects on immunity, gingivitis and periodontitis. Eur J Oral Sci 1996;104: 327-34.
3. Chandna S, Bathla M. Stress and Periodontium: A review of concepts. J Oral Health Comm Dent 2010;4(Spl):17-22.
4. Croucher R, Marcenes WS, Torres MC, Hughes F, Sheiham A. The relationship between life-events and periodontitis. A case-control study. J Clin Periodontol 1997; 24:39-43.
5. Deinzer R, Forster P, Fuck L, Herforth A, Stiller-Winkler R, Idel H. Increase of crevicular interleukin 1β under academic stress at experimental gingivitis sites and at sites of perfect oral hygiene. J Clin Periodontol 1999;26:1-8.
6. Genco RJ, Ho AW, Kopman J, Grossi SG, Dunford RG, Tedesco LA. Models to evaluate the role of stress in periodontal disease. Ann Periodontol 1998;3:288-302.
7. Genco RJ, Ho AW, Grossi SG, Dunford RG, Tedesco LA. Relationship of stress, distress and inadequate coping behaviors to periodontal disease. J Periodontol 1999; 70: 711-23.
8. Karlsson E, Lymer U-B, Hakeberg M. Periodontitis from the patient's perspective, a qualitative study. Int J Dent Hygiene 2009;7:23-30.
9. Koyama K, Yasui T. Epidemiological analysis of periodontal disease. Analysis of junior high school and high school students. Meikai Daigaku Shigaku Zasshi 1990; 19(3): 323-39.
10. LeResche L, Dworkin SF. The role of stress in inflammatory disease, including periodontal disease: Review of concepts and current findings. J Clin Periodontol 2001; 30:91-103.
11. Maupin CC, Bell WB. The relationship of 17-hydroxycorticosteroid to acute necrotizing ulcerative gingivitis. J Periodontol 1975 ;46(12):721-2.
12. Mengel R, Bacher M, Flores-de-Jacoby L. Interactions between stress, interleukin-1β, interleukin-6 and cortisol in periodontally diseased patients. J Clin Periodontol 2002; 29:1012-22.
13. Monteiro da Silva AM, Newman HN, Oakley DA. Psychosocial factors in inflammatory periodontal diseases: A review. J Clin Periodontol 1995;22: 516-26.
14. Monteiro da silva AM, Oakley DA, Newman HN, Nohl FS, Lloyd HM. Psychosocial factors and adult onset rapidly progressive periodontitis. J Clin Periodontol 1996;23:789-94.
15. Renate D, Stefan R, Ole M, Armin H. Increase in gingival inflammation under academic stress. J Clin Periodontol 1998;25:431-33.

MCQs

1. Which of the following is a parafunctional habit?
   A. Bruxism
   B. Chewing of pencil
   C. Holding of nails in the mouth by cobblers/carpenters
   D. All of the above

PERIODONTICS REVISITED

2. Who coined the term "Stress"?
   A. Hippocrates
   B. Selye
   C. Carranza
   D. Genco
3. Psychosocial factors can modify the periodontal status through behavioral changes regarding:
   A. Oral hygiene
   B. Smoking
   C. Dietary intake
   D. All of the above
4. Which of the following is not a oral adverse effect of psychiatric medications?
   A. Xerostomia
   B. Altered taste sensation
   C. Pain in teeth and MPDS
   D. All of the above
5. Depression affects oral health by:
   A. Neglect of oral hygiene
   B. Altered immune mechanism
   C. Increase smoking
   D. All of the above
6. Which of the following drug cause gingival enlargement?
   A. Alprazolam   B. Phenytoin
   C. Lithium   D. Amitriptyline
7. Which of the following is a consequence of bruxism?
   A. Excessive tooth wear
   B. Widening of occlusal surfaces
   C. Injury to periodontium
   D. All of the above
8. Which of the following is not a consequence of tongue thrusting?
   A. Loss of proximal contact
   B. Pathological tooth migration
   C. Tooth mobility
   D. Deep bite

Answers

1. D	2. B	3. D	4. C	5. D
6. B	7. D	8. D		

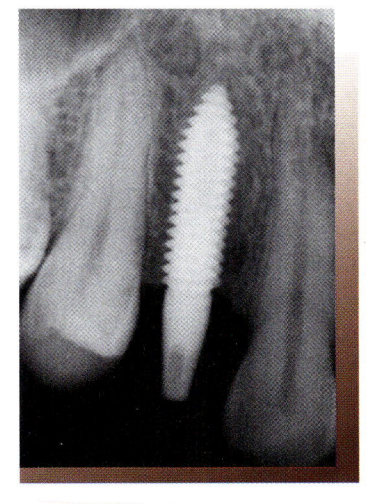

SECTION

EIGHT

IMPLANTOLOGY

Basic Aspects of Implants

Shalu Bathla

INTRODUCTION

Implants are now routinely considered as an option in the treatment of partial or complete edentulism. Implant procedures are very technique sensitive and therefore should be undertaken by adequately trained periodontists/surgeons/prosthodontists. A primary reason to consider dental implants to replace missing tooth is the maintenance of alveolar bone. The dental implant placed into the bone serves both as an anchor for the prosthetic device and as one of the better preventive maintenance procedure. One basic principle in implant dentistry is that implants are used as replacement for the natural roots. It is therefore, important to understand the similarities and differences between implants and teeth to create strategies that will achieve predictably superior results. Implants and tooth roots have some important similarities and dissimilarities.

TERMINOLOGY (FIG. 58.1)

Body: The body is that portion of the implant designed to be surgically placed into the bone.

Cover screw: In two-stage implant, the first-stage cover screw is placed on the top of the implant to prevent bone and soft tissue from invading the abutment connection area during healing.

Healing abutment/ permucosal extension: In two-stage implant, a second surgical procedure is performed to expose implant and to attach a transepithelial portion. This transepithelial portion is called permucosal extension. These are designed to heal or shape tissues after the uncovery procedures. It's purpose is to create an emergence profile in the gingival tissue for the future implant crown.

Abutment: The abutment is the portion of the implant that serves to support and/or retain the prosthesis or implant superstructure.

There are 3 main categories of implant abutment, according to the method by which the prosthesis or superstructure is retained to the abutment:
1. An abutment for screw, uses a screw to retain the prosthesis or superstructure.
2. An abutment for cement, uses dental cement to retain the prosthesis or superstructure.
3. An abutment for attachment, uses an attachment device to retain a removable prosthesis.

Each of the three types of abutments may be further classified into straight or angled abutment, describing the axial relationship between the implant body and the abutment.

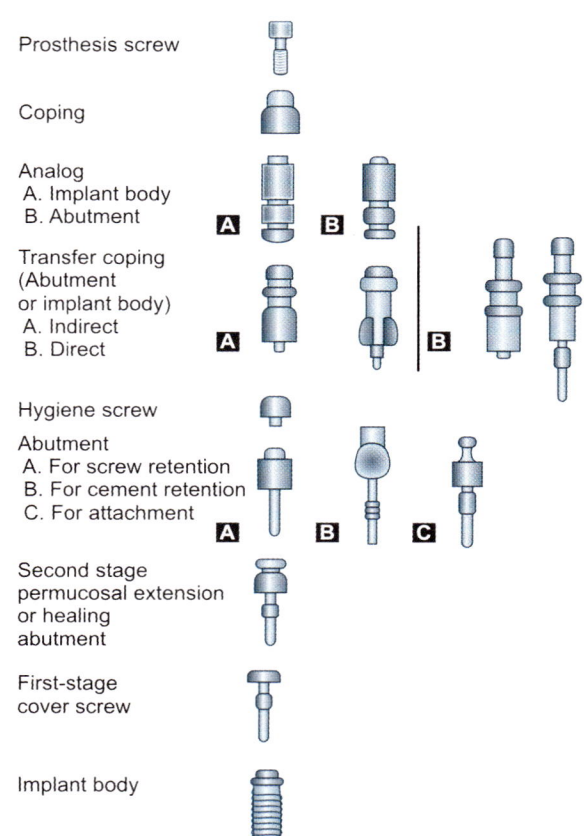

Prosthesis screw

Coping

Analog
A. Implant body
B. Abutment

Transfer coping
(Abutment
or implant body)
A. Indirect
B. Direct

Hygiene screw

Abutment
A. For screw retention
B. For cement retention
C. For attachment

Second stage
permucosal extension
or healing
abutment

First-stage
cover screw

Implant body

Fig. 58.1: Terminology related to implant

An abutment for screw uses a hygiene cover screw placed over the abutment between prosthetic appointments to prevent debris and calculus from entering the internally threaded portion of the abutment.

Superstructure: A superstructure is defined as a metal framework that fits the implant abutment (or abutments) and provides retention for the prosthesis.

Transfer coping: It is used to position an analog in an impression.

Analog: An implant analog is used in the fabrication of the master cast to replicate the retentive portion of the implant body or abutment.

Coping: A coping is a thin covering, usually designed to fit the implant abutment and serve as the connection between the abutment and the prosthesis or superstructure. A screw retained prosthesis or super-structure is secured to the implant body or abutment with a coping screw.

INDICATIONS

1. Edentulous patient: One of the first indication for dental implant treatment is to treat complete edentulism.

2. Partially Edentulous patient.
3. Single tooth loss: Implant maintains bone volume after tooth extraction.
4. Anchorage for the maxillofacial prosthesis: Patients with maxillofacial deformities uses implant for the maxillofacial prosthesis.
5. For rehabilitation of congenital and developmental defects like cleft palate, ectodermal dysplasia, etc.
6. For orthodontic anchorage.

CONTRAINDICATIONS

Following are the extraoral and intraoral contraindications for implant therapy:
1. Immunologically compromised patients: Systemic diseases such as developing cancer and AIDS.
2. Cardiac diseases: Implant surgery should be carefully considered in patients with heart valve replacements and should not be performed on patients having suffered from recent infarcts, i.e. within the latest 6 months period.
3. Deficient hemostasis and blood dyscrasias.
4. Anticoagulant medications.
5. Certain psychiatric disorders: Patients with psychological disorders have difficulties in cooperating and maintaining sufficient oral hygiene.
6. Uncontrolled acute infections, as in the respiratory tract, may negatively influence the surgical procedure or may affect the treatment result and are thus, a contraindication for surgical treatment.
7. Recent history of orofacial irradiation: Irradiation of the jaw may be another potential risk factor for implant treatment, specifically if the jaw has been exposed to irradiation over the level of 50 Gy.
8. Heavy smoking and alcohol abuse.
9. Various intraoral contraindications are xerostomia, macroglossia and unfavorable intermaxillary occlusal relationship.

CLASSIFICATION

Implants can be classified as follows:
I. According to the shape and position in the jaws:
   1. Subperiosteal implant
   2. Transosteal implant
   3. Endosseous implant
   Subperiosteal implant: Custom fabricated framework of metal that is supraalveolar (on top of the bone) but beneath the oral tissues.

Transosteal implant: These are nonosseointegrated staple implant which are used in mandibular anterior sextant.

Endosseous implant: Implant is placed directly into the socket which is prepared by using a series of specially prepared drills.

II. According to their body shapes (macrodesign) **(Fig. 58.2)**
1. *Threaded implant*: These implants are threaded into bone recipient site like a screw with a handpiece or wrench after drilling a hole slightly smaller in diameter than the implant **(Fig. 58.3)**. The threaded implants are more widely used because they usually provide superior initial stability in bone and vertical positioning of the implant during placement can be more precisely controlled. Conical threaded implants are useful in placing implants into anterior extraction sockets immediately.
2. *Threadless/ Smooth implant*: The cylinder shaped, threadless implants are tapped into a recipient hole that is similar to the diameter of the implant body.

III. According to surface characteristics (microdesign)
1. *Additive surface treatment*:
   i. Titanium plasma spraying (TPS)
   ii. Hydroxyapatite (HA) coated surface
2. *Substractive surface treatment*:
   i. Blasting with titanium oxide/aluminium oxide
   ii. Acid etched surface
3. *Modified surface treatment*:
   i. Laser induced roughened surfaces
   ii. Ion implantation
   iii. Oxidized surface treatment

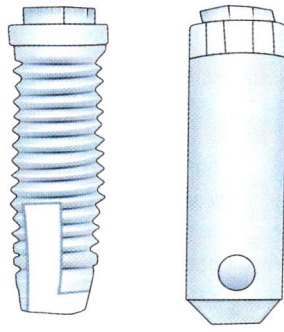

A. Threaded implant   B. Smooth implant

Fig. 58.2: Macrodesign of implants

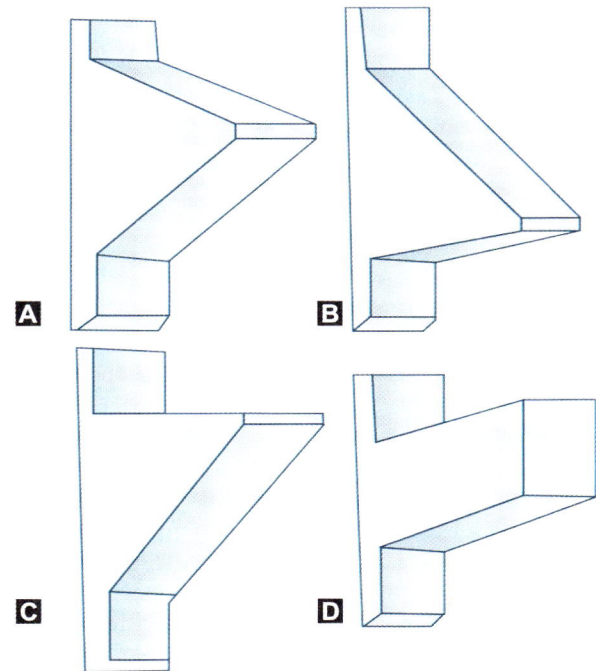

Fig. 58.3A to D: The four basic thread shapes for implant design include: (A) V-thread, (B) Buttress thread, (C) Reverse buttress thread, and (D) Square thread

- *Titanium plasma spray:* The Titanium plasma spray (TPS) surface has been reported to increase the surface area of the bone – implant interface and acts similarly to a three – dimensional surface, which may stimulate adhesion osteogenesis. TPS - porous or rough titanium surfaces have been fabricated by plasma spraying a powder form of molten droplets at high temperatures. Molten particles of titanuim powder of 0.05 to 0.1 mm diameter is projected at high velocity of 600 m/sec at 15,0000°C onto metal or alloy substrate **(Fig. 58.4)**. The plasma-sprayed layer after solidification provide a thickness of 0.04 to 0.05 mm.
- *Hydroxyapatite coatings*: Hydroxyapatite coatings have a similar roughness and increased functional surface area as TPS. A direct bone bond shown with HA coatings and the strength of the HA to bone interface is greater than titanium to bone and even greater than TPS to bone. Hydroxyapatite coated implants have been recommended for compromised bone sites, because the HA coating accelerates bone apposition to the implant surface in the early healing period and significantly improves the anchorage in bone.

PERIODONTICS REVISITED

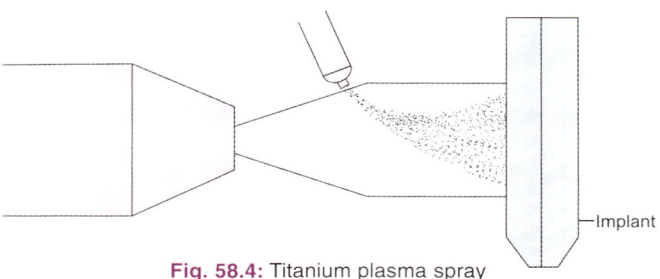

Fig. 58.4: Titanium plasma spray

- *Blasted surface*: The surface is blasted with TiO_2 particles or Al_2O_3 particles. Blasting technique is used to enhance implant surface topography with micro to macroscopic hills, valley, and indentations.
- *Acid–etched surfaces*: Acid etching is performed by bathing titanium base in hydrochloric acid (HCl), sulfuric acid (H_2SO_4), HF and nitric acid (HNO_3) in different combinations. The roughness before etching, the acid mixture, the bath temperature and the etching time all effect the acid – etching process.
- *Sandblasted and Acid–etched surfaces*: Implants are blasted with 250 to 500 µm corundum grit followed by acid etching in a hot solution of hydrochloride acid and sulfuric acid. Sandblasting produces macroroughness onto which acid etching superimposes microooroughness.
- *Laser*: Laser ablation is a technique that can be used to produce a surface with predetermined reproducible characteristics. Implants are modified to produce a controlled, micron – sized surface, with topographical features on the flanks of the threads. Excimer laser is used to create roughness over the implant surface.

BIOMATERIALS

Many biologically compatible materials can be used for the manufacturing of implants. There are three basic types of biomaterials for dental implants:

I. *Metals and alloys*:
   a. Commercially pure titanium (cpTi): Titanium is a reactive metal. In air, water or any other electrolyte, an oxide is spontaneously formed on the surface of the metal. This mechanism is unique for titanium and other elements of valency IV, such as silicon and zirconium.
   b. Ti-6Al-4V-(90% Ti, 6% Al, 4% V): This reactive group of metals and alloys form tenacious oxides in air or oxygenated solutions. Titanium oxidizes (passivates) on contact with room air and normal tissue fluids, which is favourable for dental implant devices.
   c. Co-Cr-Mo-based alloys: These are used to make custom designs such as subperiosteal frames. Chromium provides corrosion resistance through the oxide surface. Molybdenum provides strength and bulk corrosion resistance.
   d. Fe-Cr-Ni: The surgical stainless steel alloy is high strength and high ductility alloy. This alloy should be avoided in patients allergic or hypersensitive to nickel.
   e. Other metals and alloys are:
      - Gold
      - Niobium
      - Tantalum

II. *Polymers*: These include cross-linked polymers such as polymethyl-methacrylate, silicone rubber, and polyethylene. These polymers lack adhesion property to living tissues and they sometime show adverse immunological reactions.

III. *Ceramics and Carbon*: These are inorganic, non-metallic materials manufactured by compacting and sintering at elevated temperatures. This group includes aluminium oxide (alumina and sapphire) ceramics, carbon and carbon-silicon compounds. Hydroxyapatite has been proposed as a solid material and as a surface coating, which is also widely used. Zirconia (ZrO_2) is a ceramic material used in implantology because of its biocompatibility, esthetics (because its colour is similar to the teeth) and mechanical properties, which are better than alumina. Implants produced with ZrO_2 are biocompatible, bioinert, radiopaque and they present a high resistance to corrosion, flexion and fracture.

SOFT TISSUE—IMPLANT INTERFACE/ PERI-IMPLANT MUCOSA

Clinical features of peri-implant mucosa: The clinically healthy gingiva and peri-implant mucosa has a pink color and a firm consistency.

Radiographic features of peri-implant mucosa: The alveolar bone crest is usually located about 1 mm apical to a line connecting the cementoenamel junction of neighboring teeth. The marginal termination of the bone crest is usually close to the junction between the abutment and fixture part of the implant system.

Histological features of peri-implant mucosa: The mucosal tissues around intraosseous implants form a tightly adherent band consisting of a dense collagenous lamina propria covered by stratified squamous keratinizing epithelium. The junctional and barrier epithelia are about 2 mm long and the zones of supra-alveolar connective tissues are between 1 and 1.5 mm high. Both epithelia are via hemidesmosomes attached to the implant surface. The main attachment fibers (the principal fibers) invest in the root cementum of the tooth, but at the implant site the corresponding collagen fibers are nonattached and run parallel to the implant surface, owing to the lack of cementum. The sulcus around an implant is lined with sulcular epithelium that is continuous apically with the junctional epithelium.

IMPLANT—BONE INTERFACE

The relationship between endosseous implants and bone consists of one of the two mechanisms namely: fibrosseous and osseointegration.

1. *Fibrosseous integration*: It is the integration in which soft tissues such as fibers and/or cells, are interposed between the two surfaces of implant and bone **(Fig. 58.5)**.
2. *Osseointegration*: Originally, it was defined as direct bone deposition on the implant surfaces, a fact also called "functional ankylosis". In a more comprehensive way osseointegration is characterized as a direct structural and functional connection between ordered living bone and the surface of a load - bearing implants. Branemark defined osseointegration phenomenon as the "direct contact between the living bone and a functionally loaded implant surface without interposed soft tissue at the light microscope level." **(Fig. 58.6)**.

Stages of osseointegration: Osseointegration follows a common, biologically determined program that is subdivided into 3 stages:
1. Incorporation by woven bone formation.
2. Adaptation of bone mass to load (lamellar and parallel - fibered bone deposition); and
3. Adaptation of bone structure to load (bone remodeling).

Key factors responsible for successful osseointegration are **(Fig. 58.7)**:

METHODS TO EVALUATE OSSEOINTEGRATED IMPLANT OR IMPLANT STABILITY

Perio Test

The Perio test method was developed by Schulte and coworkers at the University of Tubingen. The Perio test is an electronic device designed to perform quantitative

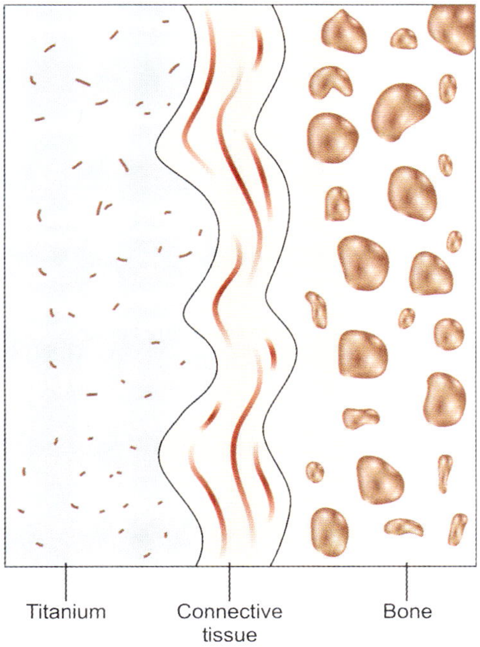

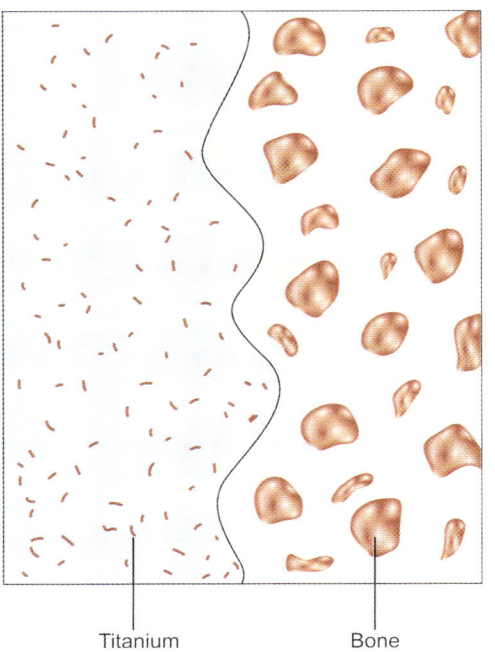

Fig. 58.5: Fibrosseous integration

Titanium   Connective   Bone
                   tissue

Titanium   Bone

Fig. 58.6: Osseointegration

Various Implant Systems

	System	Design	Surface	Number of surgery stages
1.	Nobel Biocare (Branemark)	Screw and tapered screw	Pure Ti machined and Ti-unite	Two
2.	Nobel Biocare (Steri – Oss)	Screw, cylinder and tapered screw	Acid – etched, Ti and HA plasma – sprayed	Two and one
3.	ITI Straumann	Screw, cylinder and basket	Ti plasma-sprayed and SLA	One
4.	Paragon/ Core-Vent	Screw, cylinder, hollow basket	Acid – etched Ti + HA plasma – sprayed	Two
5	Friadent	Tapered cylinder and screw	Acid – etched Ti	Two
6.	Astra	Screw	Pure Ti blasted	Two
7.	3i	Screw, cylinder	Osseotite and Ti + HA plasma sprayed	Two and One

Ti- Titanium; HA-Hydroxyapatite; SLA-Sandblasted acid etched;   ITI-International Team for Oral Implantology

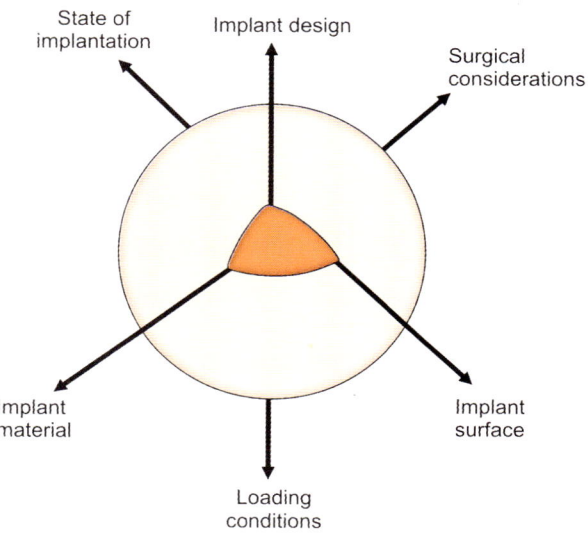

Fig. 58.7: Key factors for osseointegration

Comparison of Tooth and Implant Support Structures

	TOOTH (Fig. 58.8)	IMPLANT (Fig. 58.9)
Connection	Cementum, bone, periodontal ligament	Osseointegration, bone functional ankylosis
Connective tissue	Thirteen groups: perpendicular to tooth surfaces	Only two groups: parallel and circular fibers. No attachment to the implant surface and bone
	↓ Collagen, ↑ fibroblasts	↓Collagen, ↑ fibroblasts
Biologic width	JE: 0.97-1.14 mm (approx.)	JE: 1.88 mm (approx.)
	CT: 0.77-1.07 mm	CT: 1.05 mm
	BW: 2.04 -2.91 mm	BW: 3.08 mm
Vascularity	Greater; supraperiosteal and periodontal ligament	Less; supraperiosteal
Probing depth	3 mm in health (Fig. 58.10A)	2.5 to 5.0 mm (depending on soft tissue depth) (Fig. 58.10B)
Bleeding on probing	More reliable	Less reliable

↓-decrease; ↑-increase; JE-junctional epithelium; CT-connective tissue; BW-biologic width

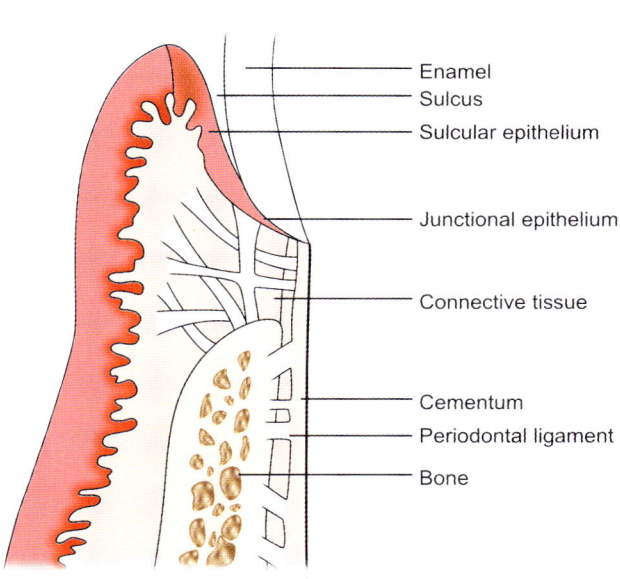

Fig. 58.8: Attachment apparatus of tooth

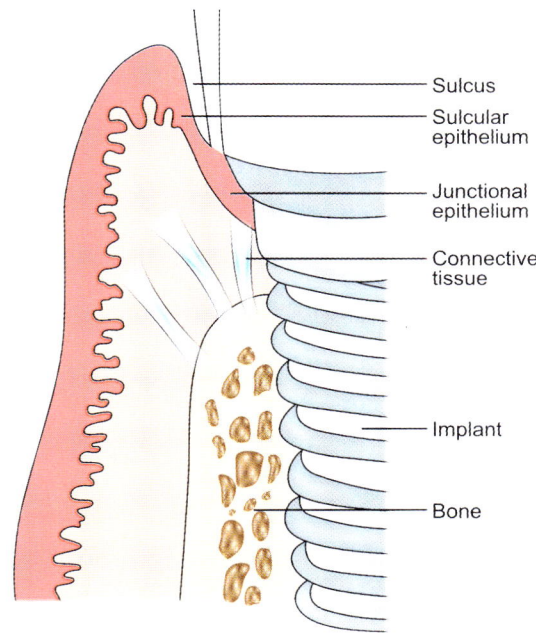

Fig. 58.9: Attachment apparatus for implant peri-implant mucosa. (No periodontal ligament fibers and cementum)

measurements of the damping characteristics of the periodontium, thereby establishing a value for implant mobility. This device measures the braking time following a reproducible impact applied to a tooth crown or implant abutment. The handpiece of the Periotest contains a rod inside, held in a low friction bearing that is accelerated until it reaches a nominal speed. The rod flies at a constant speed of 2 m/s which is maintained

by compensation for friction and gravitation until contact with the surface of the implant is made. The rod is then automatically drawn back to its starting point and again re-accelerated, achieving 16 defined and reproducible impacts, 4 times/sec. The tapping head of the rod contains a miniature accelerometer, which records the impacts deacceleration during the contact time (braking effect). The greater the stability, the higher the damping effect and faster the de-acceleration. The braking time between the implant and the tapping head of the rod is the signal used for analysis by the system. The braking time ranges between 0.3 to 2.3 ms which corresponds to Periotest values - 8 to 50 **(Fig. 58.11)**.

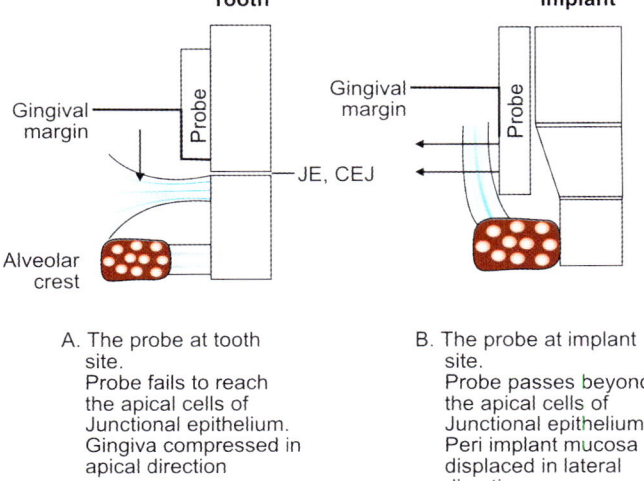

A. The probe at tooth site.
   Probe fails to reach the apical cells of Junctional epithelium. Gingiva compressed in apical direction

B. The probe at implant site.
   Probe passes beyond the apical cells of Junctional epithelium. Peri implant mucosa displaced in lateral direction

Fig. 58.10A and B: Probe in position at A). Tooth site B). Implant site (No periodontal ligament fibers and cementum)

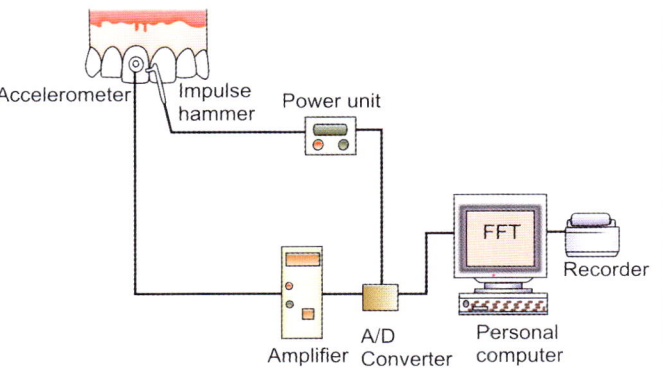

Fig. 58.11: Perio test

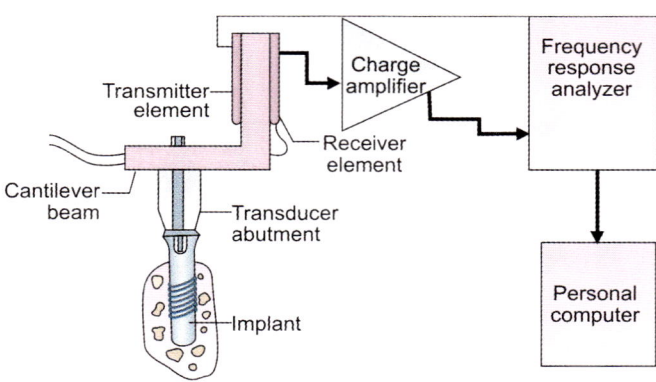

Fig. 58.12: Resonance frequency analysis

Resonance Frequency Analysis

A method based on a steady - state, swept frequency technique termed Resonance Frequency Analysis (RFA) has been developed by Meredith and co-workers. The method utilizes a small transducer, which is screwed onto an implant or abutment. The transducer is excited by steady - state signal and its response is measured **(Fig. 58.12)**. The resonance frequency value of an implant is a function of its stiffness in the surrounding bone and the level of the marginal bone. The overall stiffness of an implant placed in the recipient bone is influenced by the stiffness of the implant itself, the implant - tissue interface and the surrounding bone.

DIAGNOSIS AND TREATMENT PLANNING

Information acquired by medical history, dental history, clinical examination, laboratory tests, diagnostic casts, diagnostic wax-up and diagnostic imaging plays an important role in developing patients treatment plan.

Medical History: A thorough medical history is fundamental in preparation for dental implant treatment. Medical history identifies the factors that potentially poses a risk to the patient during the course of periodontal reconstructive and implant surgery. Such factors are history of myocardial infarction, compromised immune system and prolonged use of steroids, uncontrolled endocrine disorders, alcohol and excessive smoking.

Dental history: The timing of and reason for the previous dental extractions will predict the adequacy of bone which is necessary for implant placement. Dental history is necessary to determine the patient's compliance as maintenance is crucial for long term implant success. It is also important to know how the extraction socket was treated at the time of extraction.

Oral examination: The examination should include a detailed dental and soft tissue evaluation to rule out infection, pathology and deformities. In oral examination following information should be considered:

- Periodontal status and prognosis
- Tooth mobility
- Amount of interocclusal space
- Position of teeth
- Root configuration and crown - to - root ratio
- Space availability
- Ridge morphology width
- Esthetics.

Diagnostic cast: The study of articulated casts help in diagnosing arch form and arch relationship and implant sites in relation to the remaining teeth. A diagnostic wax-up of the final restoration help in finalizing the treatment plan and in determining the position and number of implants necessary to achieve the desired restoration. The ideal surgical guide is fabricated from a full diagnostic wax – up that is completed on properly mounted diagnostic cast. The cast assists in implant site selection and angulation requirement during surgical phase. Surgical templates are also designed from the diagnostic casts.

Surgical template: When adapting the template for surgical use, holes are created in the template to accommodate the various drills used in preparing the implant osteotomy. Thus, surgical template ensures proper implant angulations and positioning relative to adjacent teeth or implants. It should fit passively after surgical flap reflection. Thus, it dictates the implant body placement.

Diagnostic imaging (Presurgical imaging): The potential sites for implant placement and the number, length and width of implants to be placed to accomodate the prosthetic design are made with the aid of radiographs. Thus, radiographs are used:

i. To determine bone quality and quantity
ii. To determine implant position and orientation
iii. To identify the disease
iv. To verify the absence of pathology
v. To identify vital structures such as the floor of the nasal cavity, maxillary sinus, mandibular canal and mental foramen.

Based on its radiographic appearance and the resistance at drilling, bone quality has been classified in to four categories by Lekholm and Zarb **(Fig. 58.13)**:

Type 1 bone in which almost the entire bone is composed of homogenous compact bone. This type of

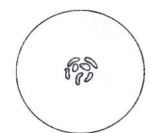
Type I
Most of the bone
consist of homogenous
cortical bone

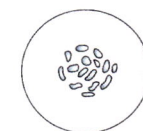
Type II
Thick compact bone
surrounds highly
trabecular core

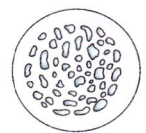
Type III
Thin cortical bone
surrounds highly
trabecular core

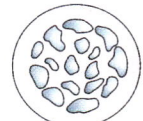
Type IV
Thin cortical bone
surrounds loose
spongy core

Fig. 58.13: Bone quality (Lekholm and Zarb classification 1985)

bone has less blood supply than all of the rest of the types of bone. The blood supply is required for the bone to harden or calcify the bone next to the implant. Therefore, it takes approximately 5 months for this type to integrate with an implant;

Type 2 bone in which a thick layer of compact bone surrounds a core of dense trabecular bone. This type of bone usually takes 4 months to integrate with an implant;

Type 3 bone in which a thin layer of cortical bone surrounds a core of dense trabecular bone. Six months time is suggested before loading an implant placed in this type of bone;

Type 4 bone characterized as a thin layer of cortical bone surrounding a core of low density trabecular bone of poor strength. This type takes the longest length of time to integrate with the implant after placement, which is usually 8 months.

These differences in bone quaility can be associated with different areas of anatomy in the upper and lower jaw. Mandibles generally are more densely corticated than maxillas and both jaws tend to decrease in their cortical thickness and increase in their trabecular porosity as they move posteriorly.

Following are the types of imaging modalities
Two-dimensional imaging modalities are:
1. Periapical radiography
2. Panoramic radiography
3. Occlusal radiography
4. Cephalometric radiography
Threedimensional imaging modalities are:
1. Computed tomography (CT)
2. Magnetic resonance imaging (MRI)
3. Interactive computed tomography (ICT)

Computed tomography (CT) produces images made up of individual units known as voxels. The density of the image is measured in Hounsfield units, named for the inventor of CT Sir Godfrey Hounsfield. Water has a Hounsfield value of 0 and is the standard for comparison. It is possible to relate the density of the CT image in Hounsfield units to the density of the bone. The Housefield units used in CT scan improve the diagnosis of bone quality by providing radiologic densitometric readings of bone.

A computerized tomography scan such as Dentascan, can provide an accurate 3-dimensional representation of maxilla and mandible . In Dentascans axial scans are obtained parallel to the occlusal plane at 1 mm intervals

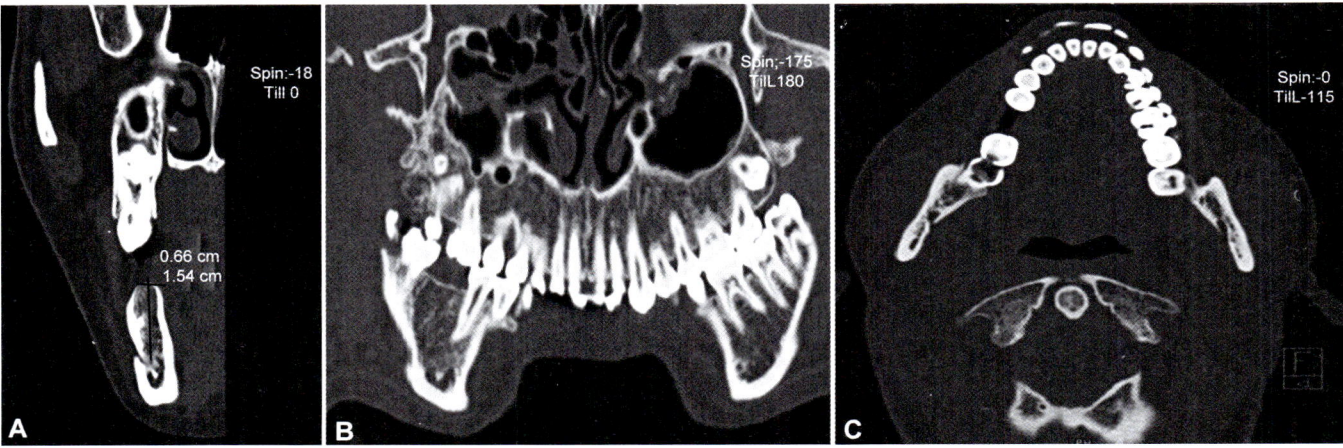
A. Axial View   B. Panoramic View   C. Cross-sectional View
Fig. 58.14A to C: Dentascan (*Courtesy:* Dr Rachna Garg)

PERIODONTICS REVISITED

through maxilla or mandible. Then, the software program produces a segmental oblique cross-sections every 2 or 3 mm around the entire curvature of alveolar lidge. Each of the cross - sections is sequentially numbered and matched to tick marks on the axial views. Thus, Dentascans helps in planning the position, angulations and size of implant **(Fig. 58.14).**

POINTS TO PONDER

✓ *Osseocalescence*: It is defined as the chemical integration of implants in bone tissue.

✓ *Angled abutment*: Due to constrain in bone availability and clinical error, implants may be placed in unfavourable angulation/inclination. To correct this inclination in desired position of screw access holes in superstructure, angulated abutments may be used. For this purpose these days various abutments with various angles (up to 30°) are available which places the superstructure in line with rest of the dentition.

BIBLIOGRAPHY

1. Bernard GW, Carranza FA, Jovanovic SA. Biologic Aspects of Dental Implants. In, Newman, Takei, Carranza. Clinical Periodontology 9th ed WB Saunders 2003;882-88.
2. Iacono VJ. Dental Implants. In, Genco RJ, Goldman HM, Cohen DW. Contemporary Periodontics CV Mosby Company 1990; 653-70.
3. Lemons JE. Dental implants and biomaterials. JADA 1990;12:716-19.
4. Misch CE. Generic Root Form Component Terminology. In, Misch CE Contemporary Implant Dentistry. 3rd ed Mosby 2008; 26-37.
5. Piattelli A, Misch CE, Pontes AEF, Iezzi G, Scarano A, Degidi M. Dental implant surfaces: A review. In, Misch CE. Contemporary Implant Dentistry 3rd ed Mosby 2008; 599-620.
6. Resnik RR, Kircos LT, Misch CE. Diagnostic Imaging and Techniques. In, Misch CE. Contemporary Implant Dentistry. 3rd ed Mosby 2008;38-67.
7. Rose LF, Minsk L. Dental implants in the periodontally compromised dentition. In, Rose LF, Mealey BL, Genco RJ Cohen DW. Periodontics, Medicine, Surgery and Implants. Elsevier Mosby 2004;610-75.
8. Sarment DP, Misch CE. Diagnostic Casts and Surgical templates. In, Misch CE. Contemporary Implant Dentistry 3rd ed Mosby 2008;276-92.
9. Schenk RK, Buser D. Osseointegration: a reality. Periodontol 2000 1998;17:22-35.

MCQs

1. Following are the contraindications for dental implants *except*:
   A. Uncontrolled diabetes
   B. Controlled diabetes
   C. Heavy smoking
   D. Anticoagulant therapy
2. Following implant system is one - staged system:
   A. Mobel Biocare – Branemark
   B. Astra
   C. Paragon
   D. ITI Strausmann
3. Factors responsible for successful osseointegration:
   A. Implant design characteristic
   B. Implant surface characteristic
   C. Implant material biocompatibility
   D. All of the above
4. Vascular supply of Periimplant mucosa is:
   A. Supraperiosteal
   B. Vessels of periodontal ligament
   C. Vessels of cementum
   D. None of the above
5. Implant stability can be evaluated by:
   A. Resonance frequency analysis (RFA)
   B. Periotron
   C. Diamond probe
   D. DNA probe

Answers

1. B   2. D   3. D   4. A   5. A

CHAPTER 59

Surgical Aspects of Implants

Shalu Bathla

INTRODUCTION

A well-performed surgical protocol, based on preoperative examinations and treatment planning, constitutes the prerequisite for a successful future implant treatment result. The placement of the implant within tooth position, both in mesiodistal and buccolingual dimensions, is of prime importance.

SURGICAL PROTOCOL

Endosseous implant systems can be categorized as either the traditional two - stage (submerged) or one stage (non-submerged) **(Figs 59.1A to B)**.

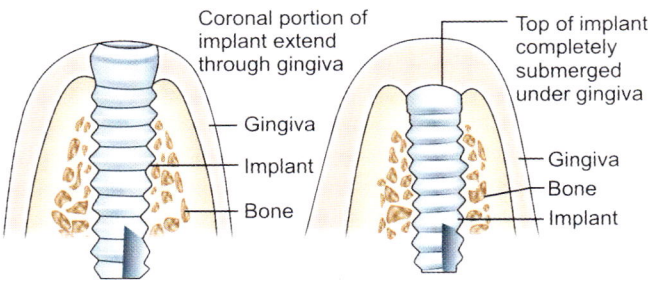

A. One stage implant surgery   B. Two stage implant surgery

Figs 59.1A and B: One-stage implant versus two-stage implant surgery

Two-stage implant system: The implant is placed and then covered with soft tissue and allowed to be osseointegrated for the defined period. The top of the implant is completely submerged under gingiva and thus also called as submerged implant system. In the second - stage surgical procedure, the implant is exposed to oral environment by using a temporary healing abutment. The two-stage surgical approach is recommended when there is extensive bone loss at the implant site or when vertical bone augmentation is necessary, or when bone quality is poor.

One-stage implant system: In this system, the coronal portion stays exposed through gingiva during the healing period. The advantages of the one-stage surgical approach are that: i) the mucogingival management around the implant is easier, ii) patient comfort increases because fewer surgeries are involved and iii) the esthetic management is easier in many cases.

TWO-STAGE IMPLANT SYSTEM (FIGs 59.2A TO D)

1. *Flap design*
   - *Incisions*: Crestal incision is used in the wider alveolar crest while in high and narrow crest, buccal approach is used. For the crestal design flap, the incision is made along the crest of the ridge bisecting the existing zone of keratinized mucosa.

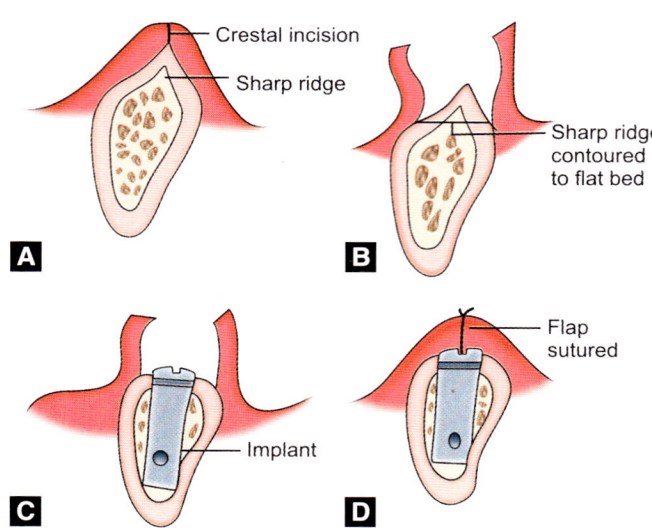

A. Crestal incision
B. Full-thickness flap is raised and sharp ridge is surgically contoured
C. Implant placed on flat bed
D. Crestal flap sutured

Figs 59.2A to D: Two stage implant surgery

- *Flap reflection*: A full-thickness flap is raised buccally and lingually to the level of the mucogingival junction, exposing the alveolar ridge of the implant sites. Elevated flaps may be sutured to the buccal mucosa or the opposing teeth to keep the surgical site open during the surgery.

2. *Preparation of osteotomy site*: Once the flap is reflected, a surgical guide or stent is placed intraorally, and a small round bur or spiral drill is used to mark the implant site. The stent is then removed, and the site is checked for their appropriate faciolingual location. Osteotomy site is prepared with intermittent drilling and under profuse saline irrigation because osteocyte damage occurs above 47°C. A small spiral drill of 2mm diameter is used to establish depth and align the axis of the implant recipient site. Internal or external irrigation continually wash away bone chips and keeps the drill bits clear of debris. A wider-diameter pilot drill is used to increase the size of the recipient site. A final size drill is used to finish the preparation of the recipient site. A countersink drill is then used to widen the entrance of the recipient site. A tap is used to create screw threads. Various drills to be used for preparing osteotomy sites are shown in **figure 59.3.**

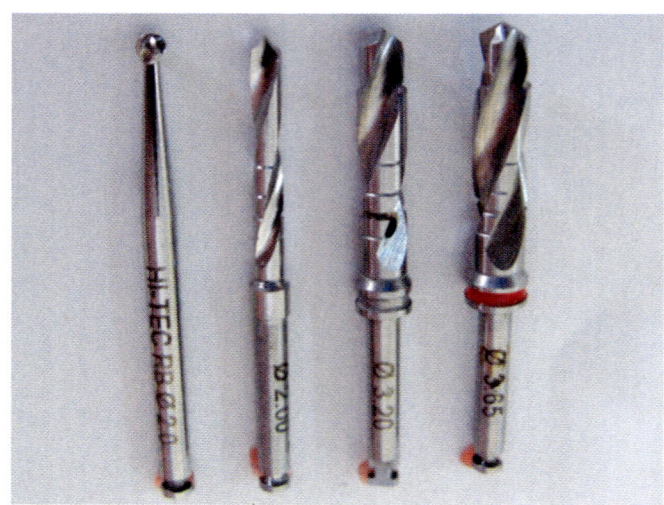

Fig. 59.3: Various drills used during osteotomy of implant recipient site

3. *Implant placement*: Following are the parameters that are correctly addressed to achieve optimal aesthetic results and biologic health –

Vertical positioning: As a general recommendation, inserted implant should whenever possible be placed so that they engage two cortical layers, i.e. one at the marginal and another at the apical level of the implant.

Buccolingual positioning: It is usually not a critical issue for implant supported overdentures, but is extremely important for the placement of implants for crown and bridge restorations in areas demanding high aesthetic results. The maxillary anterior implant must be positioned far buccally to provide proper esthetics, but not compromising over the thin buccal plate. This bone is responsible for supporting the overlying gingiva, which in turn affects the esthetics of the restoration by providing soft tissue framing. The general principle is still to place the implants within tooth position, which means that normally the long axis of the implant should be directed through the crown. The long axis of mandibular implants will mainly be directed towards the limbus part of the incisors or the palatal cusps of the teeth in the maxilla. For implants placed in the maxilla, the corresponding inclination should be towards the incisive edges of incisors or the buccal cusps of the premolars or molars of the mandible **(Figs 59.4A and B).**

Mesiodistal positioning: For the mesiodistal dimension, the rule is that the implant site closest to the last tooth is placed parallel to the long axis of the root of that

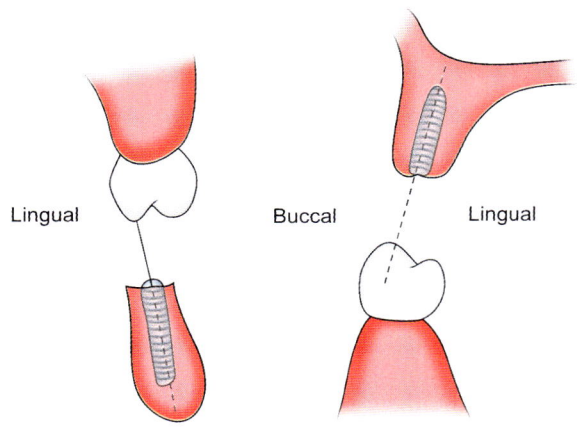

A. For placement of mandibular implant

B. For placement of maxillary implant

Figs 59.4A and B: Implant positioning

tooth. In the mandible, it is recommended that the most distal implants be placed in a slightly mesial direction to facilitate the connection of the abutments and the fabricated fixed bridge construction. Correspondingly, when working in the premolar regions of the maxilla, the last implant could be directed slightly distally in order to follow the mesial wall of the maxillary sinus, thereby allowing a longer implant to be placed.

Depending on the specific condition of each site, the surgeon selects the most suitable type of implant. Whenever possible, the longest implant should as a rule be inserted, as shorter implants have a tendency to show less favorable survival rates than longer ones. Consequently, it is the bone quality and not the implant length that is of importance for the outcome of the implant treatment.

The implant is screwed into the recipient site, and the cover screw is placed.

Principles of implant positioning:
- Vertical positioning of the implant in bone
- Buccolingual positioning of the implant in bone
- Mesiodistal placement of the implant in bone
- Trajectory or angle of the implant

4. *Closure of the flap*: Once the implant is screwed in and the cover screw is placed, the flap is closed with inverted mattress and interrupted sutures over the implant. The inverted mattress sutures keep the bleeding edges of the flap close together, while the interrupted sutures seal the edges.

5. *Postoperative care*: Written postoperative instructions should be clearly explained and given to the patient. To prevent infection postoperative antibiotics (Amoxicillin 500 mg tid) starting immediately before the surgery and continuing it for 7 to 10 days. Patient should apply ice packs extraorally intermittently for the first 24 hours. The surgical site should be kept as clean as possible. Chlorhexidine gluconate mouthrinses should be used twice daily. Analgesics are dispensed before surgery and continued after surgery. Patients should have a liquid or semisolid diet for the first few days and then gradually return to normal diet. Patients should also refrain from tobacco and alcohol use for 1 to 2 weeks postoperatively.

6. *Healing period*: The general and original principle has been that the softer the bone the longer the healing time. For mandibular implant, the standard length of healing is 3-4 months for bone of good quality and for the maxilla the corresponding time is 5-6 months, as the bone is normally more cancellous in that jaw.

7. *Second stage surgery:* It is done to expose the submerged implant ensuring proper abutment seating. Gingiva covering the head of the implant can be punched out or a full thickness flap can be raised to expose the implant. The cover screw is then removed, the head of the implant is thoroughly cleaned of any soft or hard tissue overgrowth and the healing abutment or standard abutment is placed on the fixture.

Surgical preparation
- Elevation of a full mucoperiosteal flap
- Placement of surgical stent
- Preparation of implant site
- Placement of implant
- Placement of over-screw or healing abutment
- Wound closure
- Adjustment and replacement of temporary prosthesis

ONE-STAGE IMPLANT SYSTEM

Surgical protocol for one-stage implant system is similar to two-stage implant system with the following exception:

i. The flap design is always a crestal incision bisecting the existing keratinized tissue. Vertical incisions may be needed in one or both ends.

ii. The only difference in the placement of the implant is that the implant or the healing abutment extension of the implant is placed in such way that the head of

PERIODONTICS REVISITED

the implant protrudes about 2 to 3 mm from the bone crest in one stage implant system.

IMMEDIATE IMPLANT PLACEMENT

Following tooth removal, a variable amount of ridge collapse takes place because of bone resorption. This bone resorption either buccolingual or apicocoronal, reduces bone available for implant placement. To correct these defects, complex regenerative procedures requiring additional treatment time are required. To avoid these problems, a technique involving simultaneous tooth extraction and immediate implant placement has been introduced.

The decision regarding immediate implant placement is determined by 3 factors:

1. Absence of acute noncontained infection
2. Achievement of initial stability of the implant
3. Sufficient quantity and quality of bone present.

Following are advantages for immediate placement of implant:

- Reduction of surgical procedure
- Reduction in treatment time
- Maintenance of ideal soft tissue contour
- Preservation of alveolar bone
- Better implant placement
- Improvement in the patient's psychological outlook for implant therapy.

Disadvantages:

i. Possibility of infection
ii. Thin tissue biotype may compromise optimal outcome
iii. Procedure is technique sensitive.
iv. Potential lack of keratinized mucosa for flap adaptation.

Procedure:

- LA is administered at the selected surgical site.
- *Incision and flap reflection:* Blade no. 15 or 12 is used to create a sulcular incision along the buccal aspect of the planned implant site and a vertical releasing incision to share the adjacent papillae. Full thickness flap is elevated and extended beyond the anticipated apical extension of the preplanned implant length. This permits careful evaluation of any pathology present at the periapical region of the tooth to be extracted.
- *Tooth Extraction:* Questioned tooth is extracted involving minimal trauma to the bone and surrounding soft tissues. The extraction is accomplished using a periotome directing along the proximal and buccal surfaces of the tooth root. Care is taken not to fracture the thin buccal plate in case of type I thin gingival phenotype.
- *Site preparation:* Socket is then thoroughly degranulated with curettes and diamond rotatory instrumentation to remove all remnants of periodontal ligament and granulation tissue. Depth gauges of various diameters is inserted to ascertain the socket architecture before the initiation of the osteotomy. Initiation of the osteotomy should be performed in a standard fashion with the initial penetration point for the anterior maxillary teeth approximately 2 mm coronal to the extraction apex and along the palatal wall. The initial bur penetration point for maxillary premolars and all mandibular single rooted teeth is directed towards the exact apex of the extraction socket.
- *Implant placement:* Following implant insertion, an appropriate healing cap is selected depending on the desire for a submerged, nonsubmerged healing approach.
- *Graft placement:* If gap between the wall of extraction socket and surface of implant is more than 2 mm, then osseous grafting membrane is done. To increase soft - tissue volume, a connective tissue graft is placed before flap closure, if required
- *Suturing:* Suture material of 5 - 0 is used to tie interrupted suture.

DENTAL IMPLANT FAILURE AND COMPLICATIONS

From a therapeutic point of view, the distinction between ailing implants, failing implants, failed implants and biologic complications are critical. Ailing implant has been defined as a clinically stable implant showing soft tissue inflammatory signs, pocketing or mild bone loss. Peri-implant mucositis involves inflammatory changes confined to the soft tissue surrounding an implant. Therefore, an implant exhibiting peri-implant mucositis is an ailing implant. In some instances, the ailing implant may have exhibited early bone loss along with soft tissue pocketing. An implant that is progressively losing its bone anchorage, but is still clinically stable can be defined as failing. If properly recognized and treated, a "failing" implant might be saved. The major difference between an ailing and a failing implant is the outcome of the therapy.

In other words, the term ailing implies a somewhat more favorable prognosis than failing.

Clinically, lack of osseointegration is generally characterized by implant mobility. Therefore, a mobile implant is a failed implant.

The classification of dental implant failure is divided into seven categories :

A. According to the etiology
B. According to timing of the failure
C. According to condition of failure
D. According to responsible personnel
E. According to failure mode
F. According to the tissues involved
G. According to the origin

Category A: According to the etiology

It is concerned with the etiologic reasons of implant failures, which include failure because of host factors, surgical placement, implant selection and restorative problems.

I. Host factors
- Medical status: Osteoporosis and other bone disease, uncontrolled diabetes
- Habits: smoking, parafunctional habits
- Oral status: Poor home care, irradiation therapy

II. Surgical placement
- Off – axis placement (severe angulation)
- Lack of initial stabilization
- Impaired healing and infection because of improper flap design or others
- Overheating the bone and exerting too much pressure
- Minimal space between implants
- Placing the implant in immature bone grafted sites
- Placement of implant in an infected socket or a pathologic lesion
- Contamination of the implant body before insertion

III. Implant selection
- Improper implant in improper bone type
- Length of the implant (too short, crown – root ratio unfavorable)
- Improper width of the implant
- Incorrect number of implants
- Improper implant design

IV. Restorative problems
- Excessive cantilever
- Improper fit of the abutment
- Improper occlusal scheme

Category B: According to timing of failure

I. Before Stage II: It usually occurs as a result of implant malplacement (e.g. placement of the implant in an infected socket, pathological lesion, or immature bone previously augmented or placement of a contaminated implant in the osteotomy), infection or soft tissue complications, lack of biocompatibility, excessive surgical trauma and/or lack of primary stabilization of the implant.

II. At Stage II: It can fail at the second stage of surgery, during healing or head placement, at abutment connection and before prosthetic placement.

III. After restoration: This particular timing of failure is the most common. It starts after an integrated implant is loaded. The most common cause is occlusal trauma.

Category C: According to origin of infection

I. Peri-implantitis (Infective process, bacterial origin) Peri-implantitis was defined by Meffert as the progressive loss of peri-implant bone as well as soft tissue inflammatory changes. Tonetti and Schmid divided the host's reaction to bacterial invasion into two groups: peri-implant mucositis, which implies that the inflammatory changes are localized only to the surrounding soft tissue and peri - implantitis, in which the reaction affects the deeper soft tissue and surrounding bone.

II. Retrograde peri-implantitis

Category D: According to condition of failure (clinical & radiographic status).

Meffert proposed a classification of failure including ailing, failing and failed implants.

Category E: According to responsible personnel

The success and integrity of the dental implant rely on cooperation among dental team that consists of the general dentist, surgeon, prosthodontist, periodontist, laboratory technician and the patient.

Category F: According to failure mode

I. Lack of osseointegration
II. Unacceptable esthetics
III. Functional problems
IV. Psychological problems

Category G: According to supporting tissue type

I. Soft tissue problems (lack of keratinized tissues, inflammation)
II. Bone loss (radiographic changes, etc.)
III. Both soft tissue and bone loss

POINTS TO PONDER

✓ The drilling of the osteotomy site should be performed with a pumping action, in which the drill is moved up and down along the same axis, allowing for bone chips to be expelled and bone tissue and drill to be cooled.

✓ At immediate implant placement site, if peri-implant osseous defects resulting in a gap measurable from the wall of extraction socket to the surface of the implant is more than 2 mm, augmentation with bone grafts and membrane are required.

✓ Tapered implant is the implant of choice in fresh extraction sites as these implants mimic the shape of natural tooth root.

BIBLIOGRAPHY

1. Al- Sabbagh M. Implants in the esthetic zone. Implantology. WB Saunders Dent Clin North Am 2006;50:391-407.
2. Arvidson K. A subsequent two - stage dental implant system and its clinical application. Periodontol 2000 1998;17:96-105.
3. Askary ASE, Meffert RM, Griggin T. Why do dental implants fail? Part I. Implant dentistry 1999;8:173-83.
4. Askary ASE, Meffert RM, Griggin T. Why do dental implants fail? Part II. Implant dentistry 1999;8:265-75.
5. Beagle JR. The immediate placement of Endosseous Dental implants in fresh extraction sites. Dent Clin North Am 2006;50(3):375-89.
6. Buser D, Belser UC, Lang NP. The original one stage dental implant system and its clinical application. Periodontol 2000 1998;17:1106-08.
7. Esposito M, Hirsch JM, Lekholm U, Thomsen P. Differential Diagnosis and Treatment Strategies for Biologic Complications and Failing Oral Implants: A Review of the Literature. Int J Oral Maxillofac Implants 1999;14:473-90.
8. Han TJ, Park KB. Surgical Aspects of Dental Implants. In, Newman, Takei, Carranza. Clinical Periodontology 9th ed WB Saunders 2003;897-904.
9. Lekholm U. The surgical site. In, Lindhe J, Karring T, Lang NP. Clinical Periodontology and Implant dentistry. 4th ed Blackwell Munksgaard 2003;852-65.
10. Steenberghe DV, Navert I. The first two stage dental implant system and it's clinical application. Periodontol 2000 1998;17:89-95.
11. Wilson TG Jr, Schenk R, Buser D, et al. Implants placed in immediate extraction sites: a report of histologic and histometric analysis of human biopsies. Int J Oral Maxillofac implants 1998;13(3):333-41.

MCQs

1. Following is true about surgical template *except*:
   A. Ensures proper implant angulations
   B. Ensures implant positioning
   C. Should fit actively after surgical flap reflection
   D. Dictates the implant body placement.

2. Two-stage implant surgeries are recommended for patients who have:
   A. Abundant bone at implant site
   B. Good quality bone at implant site
   C. The need for bone grafting
   D. All of the above

3. The first drill used at osteotomy site for implant placement should be of a diameter of:
   A. 2 mm   B. 3 mm
   C. 4 mm   D. 1 mm

4. The minimum distance to be maintained between implants is:
   A. 5 mm   B. 2 mm
   C. 4 mm   D. 3 mm

5. Tapping of the bone before placing the implants is not recommended in:
   A. Anterior mandible   B. Anterior maxilla
   C. Posterior maxilla   D. Posterior mandible

Answers

1. C   2. C   3. A   4. D   5. C

Advanced Implant Surgery

Shalu Bathla

INTRODUCTION

Periodontal bone loss, tooth extraction and long term use of removable appliances typically result in advanced alveolar bone loss that prevents the placement of implants in an optimal prosthetic position. Fortunately, continuous innovations in surgical techniques have resulted in advanced implant procedures and bone augmentation procedures to overcome anatomic deficiencies for the optimal placement of dental implants.

GUIDED BONE REGENERATION (GBR)

Guided Bone Regeneration (GBR) was originally developed by Hurley et al. in 1959 and Boyne in 1964. They introduced the use of a microporous cellulose acetate filter for covering bone defects, and were thus able to achieve bone regeneration. Because the objective of GBR is to regenerate a single tissue, namely bone, it is theoretically easier to accomplish than GTR, which strives to regenerate multiple tissues in a complex relationship.

Barrier Membranes

Barrier membranes are bio-inert materials that serve to protect the blood clot and prevent soft tissue cells (epithelium and connective tissue) from migrating into the bone defect, allowing osteogenic cells to be established. The ideal properties of a barrier membrane are: (i) biocompatibility, (ii) space maintenance, (iii) cell-occlusiveness, (iv) good handling properties, and (v) resorbability.

A. *Nonresorbable Barrier Membranes*: Space can be maintained under a barrier membrane with bone graft material or tenting screws, thereby facilitating the regeneration of bone. Stiffer membranes are able to promote significant amount of new bone and maintain sufficient space without the use of supportive devices. Ridge augmentation can be enhanced with a titanium reinforced membrane in conjunction with implant placement in localized bone defects. The disadvantage of a nonresorbable barrier membrane is that subsequent surgical procedure is required to remove it.

B. *Resorbable Barrier Membranes*: The primary advantage of a resorbable membrane is the elimination of a surgical reentry for a membrane removal. In case of subsequent implant placement procedure (or exposure surgery), this may not be a significant advantage.

The disadvantage associated with resorbable membrane is that it sometimes degrades before bone formation is completed and the degradation process is associated with varying degrees of inflammation. Another disadvantage is that resorbable membranes lack in stiffness which results in the collapse of membrane into the large defect area.

Bone Graft Materials

Bone graft materials have been used to facilitate bone formation within a given space by occupying that space and allowing the subsequent bone growth (and graft replacement) to take place.

- *Osteogenesis* occurs when living osteoblasts are part of the bone graft. Given an adequate blood supply and cellular viability, these transplanted osteoblasts form new centers of ossification within the graft like autogenous bone grafts.
- *Osteoinduction* involves new bone formation via stimulation of osteoprogenitors from the defect (or from the vasculature) to differentiate into osteoblasts and begin forming new bone.
- *Osteoconduction* is the formation of bone by osteoblasts from the margins of the defect on the bone graft material. Materials that are osteoconductive serve as a scaffold for bone growth. They do not inhibit bone formation, nor do they induce bone formation.

Autogenous Bone Harvesting

Intraoral sources of autogenous bone include edentulous spaces, maxillary tuberosity, mandibular ramus, mandibular symphysis and extraction sites.

Basic principles that should be followed to harvest autogenous bone graft are:

- Critical radiographic evaluation prior to surgery identifies individuals with the branches of inferior alveolar nerve extending anteriorly beyond the mental foramen.
- Use extreme care in making incisions laterally towards the mental nerve, and dissect the area with blunt instruments to locate the foramen.
- Do not elevate and reflect muscle attachments beyond the inferior border of the mandible.

- Avoid overheating of bone and do not exceed temperature beyond 47° C which cause bone necrosis.
- Limit bone cuts to an area at least 5 mm away from the tooth apices, the inferior border of the mandible, and the mental foramen. Do not extend cuts or harvest bone deeper than 6 mm, and do not include both labial and lingual cortical plates.
- Suturing should be done in layers (muscle and overlying mucosa separately) to prevent postoperative wound separation.

RIDGE AUGMENTATION

Flap Management for Ridge Augmentation

Soft tissue management is a critical aspect of bone augmentation procedures. Incisions, reflection and manipulation should be designed to optimize blood supply and wound closure.

Following are the principles associated with flap management for ridge augmentation:

- Incisions should be remote relative to the placement of barrier membranes (e.g. vertical releasing incisions should be given atleast one tooth away from the site to be grafted.)
- The use of vertical incisions should be minimized wherever possible.
- Full mucoperiosteal flap elevation atleast 5 mm beyond the edge of the bone defect is desirable.
- Wound closure should incorporate a combination of mattress sutures to approximate connective tissues and interrupted sutures to adapt wound edges.

Bone Expansion

Ridge bone expansion is the procedure which is used to increase the horizontal dimension of the alveolar bone. In 1992, Simion and colleagues reported the use of a split crest technique in patients receiving immediate implant placement in alveolar ridges that had significantly reduced width.

Procedure:

- After giving local anaesthesia, elevate full-thickness buccal and lingual mucoperiosteal flap to expose the alveolar ridge.
- Curette the cortical bone to remove all connective tissue and periosteum.
- Before implant placement, split alveolar ridge longitudinally into two parts, with the help of a small chisel creating a greenstick fracture.

- To spread the two cortical plates, tap the bone with the chisel and mallet, which is then used as a lever. Extend the surgical fracture to a depth of 5 to 7 mm leaving atleast 3 to 4 mm of intact bone apical to the fracture to allow proper implant site preparation and to achieve primary stabilization of the implants.
- Care should be taken to avoid sharp and complete vertical or horizontal fractures of the buccal, palatal, or lingual bone plates.
- Cover the implants with a contoured nonresorbable barrier membrane extending 3 to 4 mm over the bone margin of the defects.
- Remove the membranes at the abutment – connection, in Stage 2 surgery after 6 months of healing.

Distraction Osteogenesis

The process of generating new bone by stretching is referred to as distraction osteogenesis. It was introduced by Ilizarov. In distraction osteogenesis, no second surgical site is needed to harvest bone and the newly created bone has native bone at the crest, which can withstand forces better than fully regenerated bone. This surgical technique has been developed to increase vertical bone height in the deficient jaw site and is in contrast to the more conventional method of bone grafting with or without membranes.

Growth Factors for Bone Augmentation

Bone morphogenetic proteins (BMPs): Another adjunct to regenerative therapy is osteogenic stimulating substrates to enhance bone formation. One group is the bone morphogenetic proteins (BMPs), belonging to the transforming growth factor β (TGF-β) superfamily. Of this family, recombinant human bone morphogenetic protein (rhBMP-2) has shown significant signs of bone enhancing potential.

Platelet-rich plasma (PRP): It is an autologous source of platelet derived growth factors and transforming growth factors that is obtained by sequestering and concentrating platelets by centrifugation. The PRP contains a high mixture of platelets and a concentration of growth factors. This PRP mixture is added to the autologous bone graft and has shown to increase the quality of and reduce the time needed for bone regeneration.

SINUS ELEVATION AND SINUS BONE GRAFTING

Maxillary antroplasty: The maxillary sinus lift grafting procedure that was originally designed and described by Hilt Tatum, Bob James and Phil Boyne is not the same procedure that is performed today. The maxillary sinus is a 15-ml volume airspace that resembles a slopped paperweight, with its largest and only flat side composing the medial wall (which is also the lateral wall of the nasal cavity). The bony walls of the sinus are thin, except for its anterior wall and the alveolar ridge in the dentate individual. In the edentulous person, the alveolar bone is atrophied and may be only 1 to 2 mm thick, making it unsuitable as an implant site. Thus, the purpose of sinus lift surgery is to restore a sufficient amount of alveolar bone so that implants can be successfully placed. The maxillary sinus is lined with pseudo stratified columnar epithelium, which is also called the Schneiderian membrane. The thickness of the maxillary sinus correlates with the degree of pneumatization. Sinus pneumatization will often minimize or completely eliminate the amount of vertical bone available for endosteal implant placement.

Grafting materials that are currently being used for antral floor augmentation include autogenous bone graft, bone allograft, and alloplasts such as tricalcium phosphate and resorbable and non-resorbable hydroxyapatite (HA). Autogenous bone has long been considered the gold standard and remains the best grafting material because of its high osteogenic, osteoinductive and osteoconductive properties.

Indication: Sinus lift procedure is indicated in maxilla, where insufficient bone height is present.

Contraindications:
1. An absolute contraindication is previous sinus surgery like the Caldwell - Luc operation, which often leaves a scar tissue.
2. Maxillary sinus diseases such as chronic polypous sinusitis comprise a contraindication for sinus lifting.
3. A relative contraindication for sinus lifting is the presence of Underwood's septa/severe sinus floor convolutions.

Preoperative evaluation: Panoramic and sinus radiographic and computed tomography scans are taken to determine the available maxillary alveolar bone height, the location of sinus floor convolutions (septi) and the surgical entry site.

PERIODONTICS REVISITED

Surgical technique of the sinus lift procedure:

- The surgery can be performed with local anesthesia i.e posterosuperior alveolar and greater palatine nerve blocks combined with infiltration.

- A horizontal incision is made on the crest or palatal aspect of the edentulous ridge and incision is carried forward beyond the anterior border of the sinus. A vertical releasing incision in the canine fossa will help to reflect the flap and expose the bone and will also ensure soft tissue closure over the bone. The lateral wall of the maxilla is exposed by reflecting the mucoperiosteal flap superiorly to the level of the molar buttress.

- After the lateral maxillary wall has been completely exposed, a No. 8 round diamond bur should be used at a low speed (100 rpm) to make an oval or semicircular osteotomy in the lateral wall of the maxillary sinus **(Fig. 60.1)**.

- An oval osteotomy is recommended instead of a rectangular or trapezoidal osteotomy to minimize sharp edges on the bony window, which can cause tears in the underlying Schneiderian membrane.

- To ensure that the bone has been penetrated all the way around the oval osteotomy, it should be tapped gently and any movement is noted.

- Thus bone can be either pushed in to serve as the root of the graft or removed to create a window for better visualization and access.

- At this point, the underlying Schneiderian membrane is exposed. Meticulous care should be taken to reflect the Schneiderian membrane superiorly without perforating it **(Fig. 60.2)**. The Schneiderian membrane is then carefully elevated from the floor interiorly, anteriorly, and posteriorly through the osteotomy sites thus, creating an empty chamber superior to the residual alveolar bone **(Fig. 60.3)**. The newly created space i.e. inferior maxillary antrum is then augmented with various types of bone graft materials. These materials may be autografts, allografts, alloplasts or a combination.

- Postoperative instructions: The postoperative instructions are similar to those for most periodontal implant surgery. A chlorhexidine mouthrinse should be used twice a day for 2 weeks to reduce the chances of infection. Blowing the nose, sucking liquid through a straw (which creates negative pressure) and smoking cigarettes should be avoided for at least 2 weeks after surgery. Smoking can also compromise healing. Coughing or sneezing should be done with

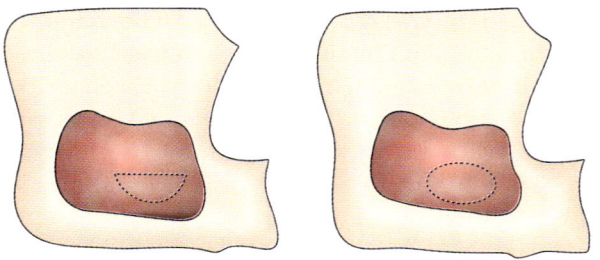

Semicircular window   Oval or round configuration of antral window

Fig. 60.1: Osteotomy in the lateral wall of maxillary sinus

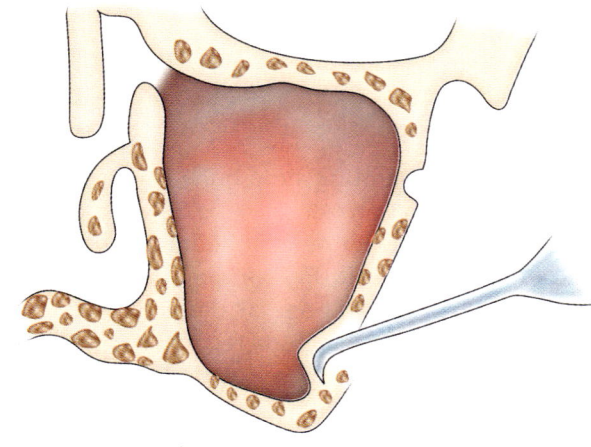

Fig. 60.2: Sinus membrane is scrapped off the bone

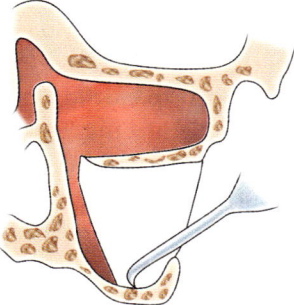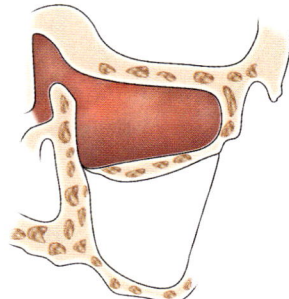

Sinus curette scratches the floor of the antrum to the medial wall

The distance from the crest of the ridge to the elevated sinus is increased

Fig. 60.3: Sinus lift procedure

an open mouth to relieve pressure. Antibiotic therapy, such as Augmentin 500 mg bid for 7 to 10 days, is continued postoperatively. Before the prosthetic phase begins, 4 to 6 months should be allowed for the bone graft and implants to integrate. During this period, the patient can wear a conventional prosthesis that has been modified with a soft relining material.

Complications: The first and most common complication is the perforation of the Schneidarian membrane. Another complication may be loss of graft or loss of implants into the sinus, which occurs when there is sinus mucosa perforation. Sinus graft is a technique sensitive procedure, which requires surgical and prosthodontic skills.

NERVE REPOSITIONING

To avoid injury to the Inferior alveolar nerve (IAN), some authors have advocated the use of local anesthesia as infiltration agents only, rather than as nerve blocks, to leave the patient with some sensation. The damage to the IAN can be lessened by using computer based navigational systems for drilling in the posterior mandible. Nerve avoidance tactics, such as slanting the implants in the posterior mandible so that they incline downward and laterally from the crestal cortical bone to engage the buccal cortical plate at a lower level. These have been termed transverse alveolar implants. In the partially edentulous mandibular arch with severely resorbed ridges, a mandibular nerve repositioning is an option. This procedure requires extensive manipulation of the mandibular nerve and often results in extended periods of paresthesia and dysesthesia of the lower lip. In most cases, the patient returns to normal sensation in about 6 months. Patients should be carefully selected for these procedures and clearly informed in writing of all possible side effects.

Two related procedures are:
i.   Inferior alveolar nerve lateralization
ii. Distalization of mental neurovascular bundle.

Alveolar Nerve Lateralization

Procedure:
- Anesthesia: Intravenous sedation or general anesthesia is required for alveolar nerve lateralization. Infiltration and block local anesthesia are also used for the purpose of both vasoconstriction and postoperative pain management.
- Incision: Soft tissue incision is initiated slightly buccal to the crest of the residual alveolar ridge. Incision is carried forward to the mesial portion of the cuspid tooth, where a vertical releasing incision is made. Anterior vertical releasing incision is carried to the mesial portion of the cuspid tooth to reduce the trauma to the anterior component of the mental neurovascular bundle.
- Full thickness flap is reflected to the inferior border of the mandible. The inferior alveolar canal is usually 2 mm below the level of mental foramen in its distal path through the body of the mandible.
- Anterior border of the osteotomy is created 3 to 4 mm distal to the mental foramen and extending positively 4 to 6 mm distal to the most distal implant position.
- With the help of bur in straight hand piece, trabecular bone is removed with the help of bone chisel to gain access to the cortical bony layer of inferior alveolar canal. The nerve hook retractor is used to free the inferior alveolar nerve from its position in canal **(Fig. 60.4)**. Then, elastic type retractor is passed around the nerve bundle and is used to lateralize and retract the neurovascular bundle.
- Osseous receptor site is prepared using appropriate burs for the placement of implant. The apical end of the preparation must be positioned inferior to osteotomy site to ensure stabilization and immobilization of implant in bone.
- After the implant is placed, nerve is repositioned over the lateral aspect of implant.

Distalization of the Mental Neurovascular Bundle

- Incision, flap design and reflection is similar to the procedure for lateralization of nerve.
- For distalization of mental neurovascular bundle, the osteotomy is made at the distal wall of the mental foramen. Once the inferior alveolar nerve is located, remaining osseous structure between the mental foramen and the osteotomy site is removed by creating a thin groove. As these bony cuts are created, the mental neurovascular bundle is retracted distally,

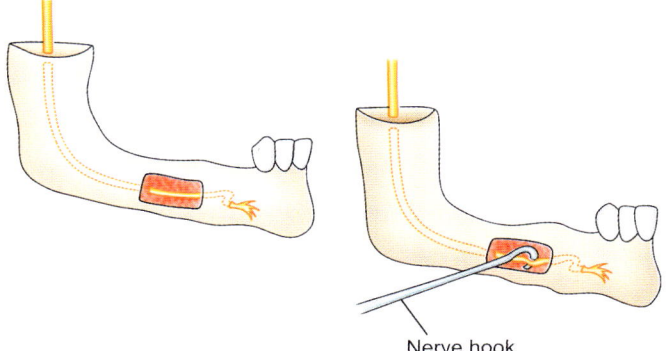

Nerve hook

Fig. 60.4: Inferior alveolar lateralization

away from the area of the cut using the Nerve hook instrument.

POINTS TO PONDER

✓ A condition referred to as "Witch's chin" occur when the facial muscles and overlying skin of the chin fall, causing a disfiguring sag of facial tissues after autogenous bone harvesting surgery from the mandibular symphysis.

✓ In maxillary sinus lift grafting, the configuration of maxillary antrum is changed by rotating the osteotomized window medially and superiorly. The sinus membrane is elevated, creating an empty chamber superior to the residual alveolar bone. The newly created space, i.e. inferior maxillary antrum is then augmented with various types of bone graft materials.

BIBLIOGRAPHY

1. Babbush CA. Inferior alveolar nerve lateralization and mental neurovascular distalization. Dental implants - The art and science. WB Saunders.
2. Bruggenkate CM, Vanden Bergh JPA. Maxillary sinus floor elevation: a valuable pre - prosthetic procedure. Periodontol 2000 1998;17:176-82.
3. Garg AK. Augmentation Grafting of the Maxillary sinus for placement of dental implants: Anatomy, Physiology and procedures. Implant Dent 1999;8:36-46.
4. Goldberg PV, Higginbottom FL, Wilson TG. Periodontal considerations in restorative and implant therapy. Periodontol 2000 2001;25:100-109.
5. Hammerle CHF, Karring T. Guided bone regeneration at oral implant sites. Periodontol 2000 1998;17:151-75.
6. Klokkevold PR, Jovanovic SA. Advanced Implant Surgery and Bone Grafting Techniques. In, Newman, Takei, Carranza. Clinical Periodontology 9th ed WB Saunders 2003; 905-21.
7. Misch CE, Resnik RR, Dietsch FM. Maxillary sinus anatomy, pathology and Graft surgery. In, Misch CE. Contemporary Implant Dentistry 3rd ed Mosby 2008;905-74.
8. Misch CE, Suzuki JB. Tooth extraction, socket grafting and barrier membrane bone regeneration. In, Misch CE. Contemporary Implant Dentistry 3rd ed Mosby 2008;870-904.
9. Tiwana PS, Kushner GM, Haug RH. Maxillary Sinus augmentation. Dent Clin North Am 2006;50:409-24.
10. Worthington P. Injury to the Inferior Alveolar nerve during implant placement: A Formula for protection of the patient and clinician. Int J Oral Maxillofac Implants 2004;19:731-34.

MCQs

1. The implants that are placed into anterior sockets immediately after extraction are preferably:
A. Cylindrical
B. Basket-like
C. Conical
D. Blade shaped
2. When osseous grafts are used along with implant placement, a relatively low success rate occurs with:
A. Medium textured implants
B. Smooth surface implants
C. Hydroxyapatite implants
D. Plasma sprayed titanium surfaces
3. Procedure used to regain bone in vertical direction:
A. Distraction osteogenesis
B. Sinus elevation
C. Inferior alveolar nerve lateralization
D. None of the above
4. The main objective of Guided Bone Regeneration (GBR) is to:
A. Regenerate cementum, alveolar bone and periodontal ligament
B. Periodontal ligament
C. Cementum
D. Alveolar bone

Answers

1. C   2. B   3. A   4. D

CHAPTER

61

Peri-implantitis

Mayank Hans, Veenu Madaan Hans

INTRODUCTION

Implants are being used extensively these days for the replacement of the missing teeth. Despite the observed long-term success of osseointegrated implants, there are complications that are associated with them. Pathological changes around implants may develop during or after healing period. If these pathological changes are present in the soft tissue, these are termed peri-implant mucositis and if bone is also involved then it is termed peri-implantitis.

DEFINITIONS

Pathologic changes of the peri-implant tissues can be placed in the general category of peri-implant disease.
- Inflammatory changes, which are confined to the soft tissue surrounding an implant, are diagnosed as peri-implant mucositis.
- Progressive peri-implant bone loss in conjunction with a soft tissue inflammatory lesion is termed peri-implantitis.

The term peri-implantitis was introduced in 1987 by Andrea Mombelli to describe a destructive inflammatory process affecting the soft and hard tissues around the osseo-integrated implants leading to formation of peri-implant pocket and loss of supporting bone.

PERI-IMPLANT MUCOSITIS

Etiology

The etiology for peri-implant mucositis is similar to gingivitis, which is bacterial plaque. The bacterial plaque induces an inflammatory response in peri-implant mucosa similar to that in gingiva around tooth.

Clinical Features

The clinical features of peri-implant mucositis are similar to gingivitis. The symptoms of inflammation like swelling and redness are also present in peri-implant mucosa. The differences in morphology of peri-implant mucosa and gingiva around tooth and lack of light transmission through metal may mask visible signs of inflammation. Assessment of peri-implant mucositis includes assessment of bleeding following probing and suppuration. Presence of bleeding on probing indicates presence of inflammation in peri-implant sulcus. Suppuration and slight increase in probing pocket depth may also be present in peri-implant mucositis.

PERI-IMPLANTITIS

Etiology

The cause of peri-implant tissue breakdown is multifactorial, but bacterial infection and biomechanical overload are considered to be the major factors.

1. *Bacterial infection:* The plaque is formed similarly around the implants as it forms around the teeth. If the plaque accumulates around an implant, the subepithelial connective tissue becomes infiltrated with inflammatory cells. If the plaque migrates further apically, clinical and radiographic appearance of tissue destruction is seen around implants. The subgingival flora around diseased implants is different from that around healthy implants. It is suggested, that the microbiology associated with implants are related to the bacteria already residing in the oral cavity, that is, the remaining teeth act as reservoirs for seeding of bacteria in the peri-implant tissues. An early study, which compared the microbiota surrounding successful and failing titanium implants found that failing sites had a significantly higher proportion of microorganisms traditionally associated with periodontal diseases. Specifically, gram negative anaerobic rods, spirochetes and fusiform bacteria were found in higher proportions at peri-implantitis sites as compared with healthy sites, which were predominantly composed of coccoid forms.

2. *Biomechanical factors:* Biomechanical forces also play an important role in success, survival or failure of dental implants. Excess of these forces may lead to high stress and microfractures in coronal bone to implant contact. On persistence of excess biomechanical forces, loss of osseointegration around neck of implant occurs. This cause is particularly important in case of insufficient bone, poor bone quality, parafunctional activities and misfit of prosthesis. In contrast to bacteria related peri-implantitis, bone loss caused by mechanical overload is not associated with a primary inflammatory response of the surrounding mucosal tissues. As the bone loss progresses, a combination of bacteria-related and loading-related bone loss is seen when the bone loss creates deep pocket that collect plaque, resulting in a secondary microbial-related inflammatory reaction leading to bone loss.

3. *Other co-factors are:*
   a. The relationship between the influence of surface roughness of implants and bacterial colonization has been clinically assessed. There seems to be a clear proportional relationship between surface roughness and the rate of bacterial colonization in regards to both supragingival and subgingival plaque.
   b. Smoking is an established risk factor for chronic periodontitis and undoubtedly contributes to an increased risk of implant loss.
   c. Compromised host response.
   d. Traumatic surgical technique.

Classification

Spiekermann has given the following classification of the peri-implant bone loss:

Class 1: Slight horizontal bone loss with minimal peri-implant defect.

Class 2: Moderate horizontal bone loss with isolated vertical defect.

Class 3: Moderate to advanced horizontal bone loss with broad circular bony defect.

Class 4: Advanced horizontal bone loss with broad circumferential vertical defects as well as loss of oral and/or vestibular bony wall.

Diagnosis

The well advanced peri-implantitis lesion may be clearly identifiable but, it is the early lesion that poses the greatest challenge to the clinician and is undoubtedly of greatest value in order to avoid further bone resorption and subsequent loss of the implant. Diagnosis of peri-implantitis relies on same parameters as for diagnosing periodontal diseases. The parameters include clinical signs, peri-implant probing, bleeding on probing (BOP), suppuration, mobility and peri-implant radiography.

1. *Clinical assessment:* Swelling and redness of the peri-implant mucosa have been reported from peri-implant infections. The amount of plaque around an implant should always be evaluated. Suppuration has been linked with inflammation of the peri-implant tissues, suggesting that suppuration may be a sign of peri-implantitis. Implant mobility is an indication of lack of osseointegration, but it is of no use in diagnosing early implant disease, rather it shows the final stages of de-integration.

2. *Peri-implant probing:* Probing the peri-implant sulcus with a blunt, straight plastic periodontal probe **(Fig. 61.1)** allows for assessment of peri-implant probing depth, distance between the soft tissue margin and a reference point on the implant for measuring hyperplasia or recession along with bleeding and suppuration. Probing around oral

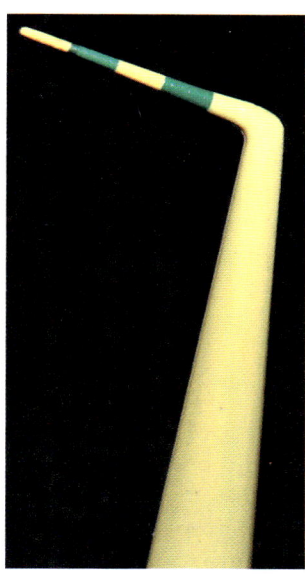

Fig. 61.1: Plastic probe

implants should be considered a reliable and sensitive parameter for the long term monitoring of peri-implant mucosal tissues. A probing depth of more than 4 mm may be suggestive of peri-implant disease. Bleeding on probing indicates inflammation in the pocket or sulcus and is an indicator of ongoing inflammatory process.

3. *Peri-implant radiography:* The distance from implant shoulder or apical termination of the cylindrical part to the alveolar bone crest is a reliable parameter, provided the radiographs are properly standardized. However, in conventional radiography minor changes in bone morphology may not be noticed until they reach a significant size. Radiographic evidence of bone to implant contact does not indicate osseointegration. Digital subtraction radiography can increase the sensitivity significantly and has been successfully applied.

TREATMENT OF PERI-IMPLANT PATHOLOGY

The early diagnosis and management of peri-implant pathology is important to prevent further bone loss and subsequent loss of implant. Mombelli has suggested five considerations in the therapy of peri-implantitis:

1. The disturbance and/or removal of the bacterial biofilm in the peri-implant pocket.
2. Decontamination and conditioning of the surface of the implant.
3. Correction via reduction or elimination of sites that cannot be adequately maintained by oral hygiene measures.
4. Establishment of an effective plaque control regime.
5. Re-osseointegration.

The treatment of peri-implantitis is divided in to an initial therapeutic phase and surgical phase.

Initial Therapeutic Phase

1. *Occlusal therapy:* Analysis of prosthesis and occlusal evaluation is an important aspect of peri-implant diagnosis as excessive forces could also contribute to peri implant bone loss. Therefore, prosthesis design change, improvement in implant number and position can contribute to the arrest of peri-implant tissue breakdown progression.
2. *Anti-infective therapy:* The removal of plaque deposits with plastic instruments and polishing of all accessible surface with pumice initiates the non surgical anti-infective therapy for peri-implantitis and peri-implant mucositis. Additionally peri-implant pockets can be irrigated with the help of 0.12% chlorhexidine or local antimicrobials. As for periodontal diseases this initial phase of therapy may be sufficient for re-establishing peri-implant health or may have to be followed by surgical phase.
3. *Systemic antibiotics:* Systemic antibiotics can be administered as a supportive therapy for treatment of peri-implant disease. Frequently used antibiotics for this purpose are doxycycline, metronidazole or a combination of amoxicillin and metronidazole.
4. *Implant surface preparation:* In peri-implantitis, the implant surface gets contaminated with bacteria and bacterial by products. Due to this contamination the wound healing is compromised which inhibit the regeneration of bone and re-osseointegration in the area. Therefore, for desirable outcome of bone regeneration implant surface preparation has to be done. This can be achieved by use of air powder abrasive which is a mixture of sodium bicarbonate and sterile water. This does not change surface topography of implant and has no adverse effect on cell adhesion. Implant surface preparation can also be done with the application of tetracycline HCl for 30 to 60 seconds and more recently, use of CO_2 lasers has been advocated for implant surface decontamination and preparation.

PERIODONTICS REVISITED

Surgical Phase

1. *Peri-implant resective therapy:* Peri-implant lesion with horizontal bone loss or moderate vertical bone defects (<3 mm) are suitable choice for resective therapy. Full thickness flap is raised to access the surgical area, degranulation of the defect is done and if required bone around implant is re-contoured. Later, implant surface is prepared and flap is apically repositioned and sutured.

2. *Peri-implant regenerative therapy:* Use of guided bone regeneration is recommended in cases where moderate to deep vertical defects are seen in peri-implant bone. The surgical therapy includes removal of granulation tissue after elevation of flap, implant surface preparation and use of bone graft and barrier membrane on the defect. The membrane is extended 3-4 mm beyond the defect and flap is closed over it.

3. *Re-osseointegration:* The treatment goal of peri-implant regenerative therapy is *de novo* bone formation at the portion of implant that has lost its osseointegration in the inflammatory process. This increase in height of the bone leads to marginal shift of mucosa thereby, enhancing the soft tissue esthetics.

CUMULATIVE INTERCEPTIVE SUPPORTIVE THERAPY (CIST)

The "cumulative interceptive supportive therapy" (CIST), suggests a protocol for the monitoring of healthy implants and the interception of peri-implant diseases. This protocol relies on probing depth, bleeding on probing and radiographic evidence of bone loss. As each parameter becomes more severe, more complex treatment is introduced, with each subsequent treatment incorporating that of the previous protocol.

I. *CIST protocol A (Mechanical debridement):* If the probing depth is <4 mm, oral hygiene can be improved by using soft scalers, rubber cup and paste.

II. *CIST protocol A+B (Antiseptic therapy):* If the probing depth is 4-5 mm, antiseptic therapy (chlorhexidine rinse or topical chlorhexidine gel daily) is used along with step A.

III. *CIST protocol A+B+C (Antibiotic therapy):* If the probing depth is ≥ 6 mm, tetracycline fibers for 10 days and systemic antibiotics for 10 days (amoxicillin + metronidazole) are used along with step A+B.

IV. *CIST protocol A+B+C+D (Regeneration and Resective therapy):* If the CIST protocol A+B+C is used and still considerable amount on bone loss and probing pocket depth are present, surgical therapy is used along with step A+B+C. Regenerative approach (barrier membrane, nonsubmerged) or resective approach (osteoplasty + apically positioned flap) is opted depending on esthetic considerations and morphological characteristics of the lesion.

The goal of this cumulative treatment approach is to intercept peri-implant tissue destruction as early as possible.

MAINTENANCE

Maintenance procedures performed by the patient:

Plaque control should be started immediately after the implant is exposed to the intraoral environment and monitored over time. Implant superstructures are often bulky and overcontoured, which makes traditional home care procedures more difficult. Patients may find smaller diameter toothbrush heads to be beneficial in areas of difficult access. When single tooth implant is present, it can generally be cleaned just like tooth with a toothbrush and dental floss but when restorations are attached to multiple implants in a splinted fashion, or when hybrid—type prosthesis are present, oral hygiene can become much more difficult for the patient.

- Toothbrush should be round ended with soft filaments to prevent damage to peri-implant tissue.
- Dentifrice or other cleaning agents should not be used as it causes abrasion of the titanium or other implant material. Titanium implants are corroded by acidic fluoride preparations.
- Yarn or gauge strips with floss threader are used to clean crossbar of subperiosteal implant and proximal surface of endosseous implants abutment.
- Irrigators can also be used as adjunctive aids.
- Gauze strips can be easily used to clean under posterior cantilever areas using a shoeshine technique.

Maintenance procedures performed by the therapist:

Patient recall should be at 3-month intervals for the first year and then on a semi-annual basis. Some patients may require more frequent follow-up care. Recall visits should include an (i) evaluation of oral hygiene compliance, (ii) occlusal harmony, (iii) implant and prosthesis stability, (iv) overall soft and hard peri-implant tissue health and (v) radiographic follow up. The recommended instrumentation for implant debridement includes plastic, nylon, or special alloy instruments that will not alter the implant surface **(Fig. 61.2)**. Sonic or ultrasonic scalers that

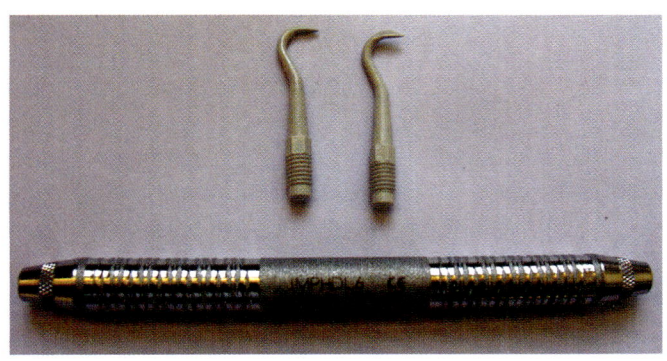

Fig. 61.2: Implacare implant instrument

use a plastic cap over the metal tip have been shown to be safe and effective. Titanium tipped curettes has been developed for removal of calculus on implant surface.

Instruments used for assessment and calculus removal from implant should be made of a material that is softer than the implant material; plastic instrument is most commonly used; some plastic instrument can be sterilized by autoclave for several cycles; follow manufacturer's instructions for sterilization and reuse.

BIBLIOGRAPHY

1. Askary ASE, Meffert RM, Griggin T. Why do dental implants fail? Part I. Implant dent 1999;8:173-83.
2. Askary ASE, Meffert RM, Griggin T. Why do dental implants fail? Part II. Implant dent 1999;8:265-75.
3. Berglundh T, Lindhe J, Lang NP, Mayfield L. Mucositis and Peri-implantitis. In, Lindhe J, Karring T, Lang NP. Clinical Periodontology and Implant dentistry. 4th ed Blackwell Munksgaard 2003;1014-23.
4. Esposito M, Jan Hirsch J, Lekholm, Thomsen P. Differential Diagnosis and Treatment Strategies for Biologic Complications and Failing Oral Implants: A Review of the Literature. Int J Oral Maxillofac Implants 1999;14:473-90.
5. Han TJ, Park KB. Surgical Aspects of Dental Implants. In, Newman, Takei, Carranza. Clinical Periodontology 9th ed WB Saunders 2003;897-904.
6. Humphrey S. Implant Maintenance. Implantology. Dent Clin North Am WB Saunders 2006;50:391-407.
7. Jovanovic SA. Diagnosis and Treatment of Periimplant Complications. In, Newman, Takei, Carranza. Clinical Periodontology 9th ed WB Saunders 2003;931-42.
8. Klinge B, Hultin M, Berglundh T. Peri-implantitis. Periodontology; Present status and Future Concepts. Dent Clin North Am WB Saunders 2005;50:661-76.
9. Lang NP, Lindhe J. Maintenance of the Implant Patient. In, Lindhe J, Karring T, Lang NP. Clinical Periodontology and Implant dentistry. 4th ed Blackwell Munksgaard 2003;1024-30.
10. Lekholm U. The surgical site. In, Lindhe J, Karring T, Lang NP. Clinical Periodontology and Implant dentistry. 4th ed Blackwell Munksgaard 2003;852-65.
11. Muller E, Odont D, Gonzalez YM, Andreana S. Treatment of Peri-implantitis: Longitudinal Clinical and Microbiological findings - A Case Report. Implant Dent 1999;8:247-54.
12. Roos-Jansaker AM, Renvert S, Egelberg J. Treatment of peri-implant infections: A literature review. J Clin Periodontol 2003;30:467-85.

MCQs

1. Peri-implant mucositis is:
   A. Reversible
   B. Irreversible
   C. Peri-implantitis
   D. None of the above
2. Cumulative interceptive supportive therapy (CIST) is:
   A. Divided into 4 protocol
   B. This protocol relies on probing depth, bleeding on probing and radiographic evidence of bone loss
   C. All of the above
   D. None of the above
3. While treating peri-implantitis, the plaque deposits on the implant surface are removed with:
   A. Ultrasonic scaler
   B. Stainless steel curettes
   C. Plastic curettes/instruments
   D. Micromotor
4. Which one of the following is recommended for preventive maintenance with dental implants?
   A. Ultrasonic scaler
   B. Acidic fluoride preparations
   C. Coarse polishing paste
   D. Chlorhexidine
5. Following should not be used in implant patient:
   A. Rounded end, soft filaments toothbrush
   B. Acidic fluoride preparations
   C. Yarn or gauge strips with floss threader
   D. Irrigators
   E. Gauze strips

Answers

1. A   2. C   3. C   4. D   5. B

PERIODONTICS REVISITED

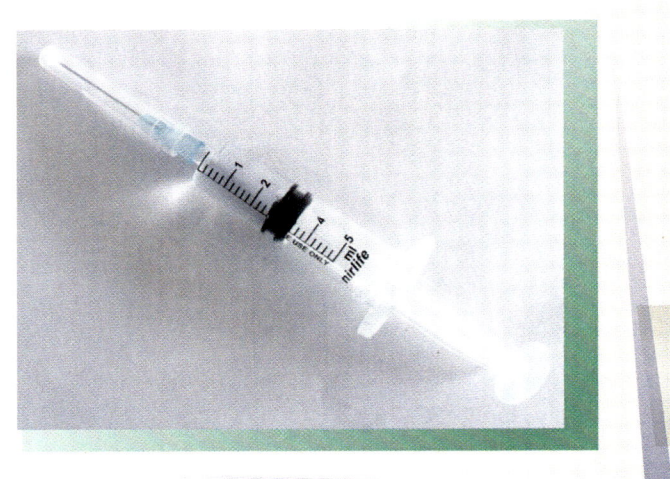

SECTION

NINE

ADVANCES

Recent Advancements

Veenu Madaan Hans, Shaveta Sood, Shalu Bathla

- Lasers
- Photodynamic Therapy
- Tissue Engineering
- Gene Therapy

- Nanotechnology
- Periodontal Vaccine
- Minimally Invasive Surgery

LASERS

1. Introduction
2. Historical Perspective
3. Basic Structure of a Laser Device
4. Laser Delivery Systems
5. Classification
6. Laser Energy and Tissue Temperature

7. Laser-tissue Interactions
8. Laser Wavelengths Used in Periodontics
9. Laser uses in Periodontics
10. Dental Laser Safety
    - Types of Hazards
    - Safety Precautions

INTRODUCTION

The word LASER is an acronym for Light Amplification by Stimulated Emission of Radiation.

Light: Laser light is monochromatic that is, it is of one specific color and that color may be visible or invisible. In addition, it has other characteristics of collimation and coherency. Collimation means that beam has specific spatial boundaries, which ensures that there is a constant size and shape of the beam emitted from the laser cavity. Coherency means that the light waves produced are all in phase with one another and have identical wave shapes; that is, all the peaks and valleys are equivalent.

Amplification: The mirrors at each end of the active medium of a laser device reflect photons back and forth to allow further stimulated emission and increase the power of the photon beam.

Stimulated emission: The term "stimulated emission" has its basis in the quantum theory of physics. A quantum, the smallest unit of energy, is absorbed by the electrons of an atom or molecule, causing a brief excitation; then a quantum is released and process is called spontaneous emission. Albert Einstein theorized that an additional quantum of energy travelling in the field of the excited atom that has the same excitation energy level would result in a release of two quanta, a phenomenon he termed stimulated emission. These photons are able to energize more atoms, which further emit additional identical photons, stimulating more surrounding atoms **(Fig. 62.1)**.

Radiation: Radiation refers to the light waves produced by the laser as a specific form of electromagnetic energy. All available dental laser devices have emission wavelengths of approximately 0.5 μm (or

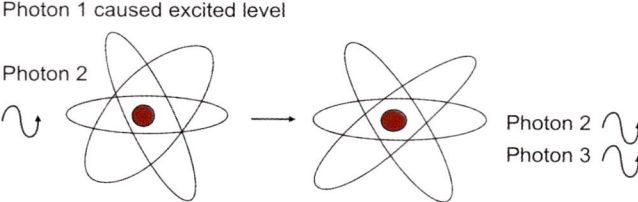

Fig. 62. 1: Stimulated emission

500 nm) to 10.6 μm (or 10,600 nm). They are therefore, within the visible or the invisible infrared nonionizing portion of the electromagnetic spectrum and emit thermal radiation.

HISTORICAL PERSPECTIVE

Maiman developed the first laser prototype in 1960. Maiman's device used a crystal medium of ruby that emitted a coherent radiant light from the crystal when stimulated by energy. Thus, the ruby laser was created. Shortly thereafter, in 1961, Snitzer published the prototype for the Nd:YAG laser. The first application of a laser to dental tissue was reported by Goldman, et al. However, the current relationship of dentistry with the laser takes its origins from an article published in 1985 by Myers and Myers describing the *in vivo* removal of dental caries using a modified ophthalmic Nd:YAG laser. Four years later, it was suggested that the Nd:YAG laser could be used for oral soft tissue surgery, which ultimately lead to the present relationship between lasers and clinical periodontics.

BASIC STRUCTURE OF A LASER DEVICE

An optical cavity is at the center of the device. The core of the cavity is comprised of chemical elements, molecules or compounds and is called the active medium. Lasers are generically named for the material of the active medium, which can be a container of gas, a crystal, or a solid-state semiconductor. There are two gaseous active medium lasers used in dentistry: argon and CO_2. The remainder that are available are solid-state semiconductor made with multiple layers of metals such as gallium, aluminium, indium and arsenic or solid rods of garnet crystal grown with various combinations of yttrium, aluminium, scandium and gallium and then doped with the elements of chromium, neodymium, or erbium. There are two mirrors, one at each end of the optical cavity, placed parallel to each other. Surrounding this core is an excitation source, either a flash lamp device or an electrical coil, which provides the energy into the active medium. There is some heat generated in the process and the optical cavity must be cooled. A cooling system, focusing lenses and other controls complete the mechanical components. The parallelism of the mirrors ensures that the light is collimated. One of the mirrors is selectively transmissive, allowing light of sufficient energy to exit the optical cavity **(Fig. 62.2)**.

LASER DELIVERY SYSTEMS (Fig. 62.3)

1. *Articulated arm:* Articulated arm delivery systems consist of a series of rigid hollow tubes with mirrors at each joint (called a knuckle) that reflect the energy down the length of the tube. The disadvantages are that they are bulky, have noncontact systems and there is difficulty in removing discrete lesions within the oral cavity.
2. Flexible hollow waveguide or tube has an interior mirror finish. The laser energy is reflected along this tube and exits through a handpiece at the surgical end with the beam striking the tissue in a noncontact fashion. An accessory tip of sapphire or hollow metal can be connected to the end of the waveguide for contact with the surgical site.
3. *Glass fiberoptic cable:* This cable is more pliant than the waveguide and has a corresponding decrease in weight and resistance to movement and is usually smaller in diameter. Although the glass component is encased in a resilient sheath, it can be fragile and cannot be bent into a sharp angle. The fiber fits snugly into a handpiece and can be used in contact or noncontact mode.

Laser Emission Modes

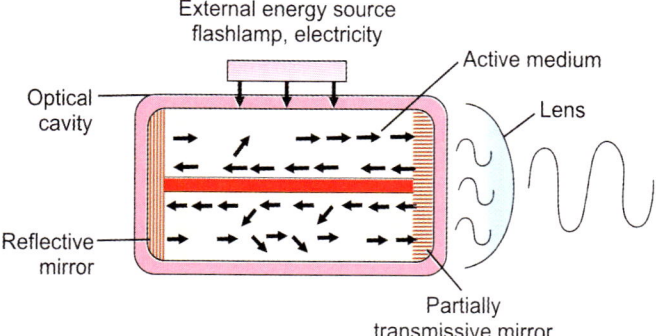

Fig. 62. 2: Basic component of laser

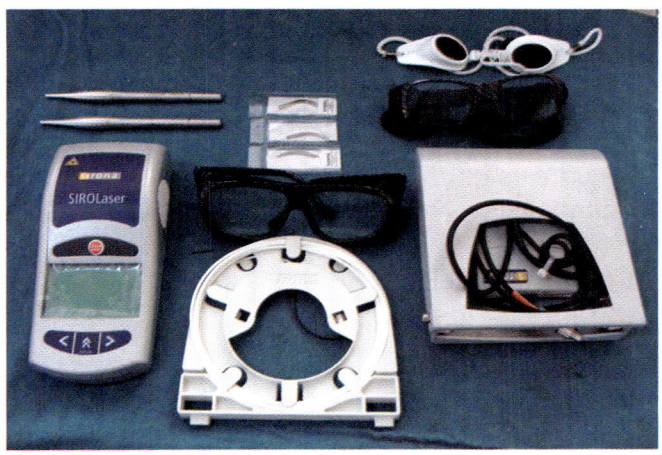

Fig. 62. 3: Laser parts

The dental laser device can emit the light energy in two modalities as a function of time:

a. Continuous wave meaning that the beam is emitted at only one power level for as long as the operator presses the foot switch.

b. Pulsed on and off.

  i. Gated-pulse mode, meaning that there are periodic alternations of the laser energy, much like a blinking light.

  ii. Free-running pulsed mode, sometimes referred to as "true pulsed." This emission is unique in that large peak energies of laser light are emitted for a short time span, usually in microseconds, followed by a relatively long-time in which the laser is off.

The important principle of any laser emission mode is that the light energy strikes the tissue for a certain length of time, producing a thermal interaction. If the laser is in a pulsed mode, the targeted tissue has time to cool before the next pulse of laser energy is emitted. In continuous wave mode, the operator must cease the laser emission manually so that thermal relaxation of the tissue may occur. Similarly, when using hard-tissue lasers, a water spray helps to prevent microfracturing of the crystalline structures and reduces the possibility of carbonization.

CLASSIFICATION

I. Based on state of the medium:
  • Solid
  • Gas
  • Excimer
  • Diode

II. Based on Output energy:
  • Low output, soft or therapeutic – A thermic low energy laser emitted at wavelength which is supposed to stimulate cellular activity. For example He – Ne, Ga – As, Ga – Al – As.
  • High output, hard or surgical – A thermic laser emitted at wave length in visible, infrared and U.V range utilized to cut, coagulate, vaporize and carbonize. For example CO_2 - Ar, Nd: YAG

III. Based on Oscillation mode:
  • Continuous wave
  • Pulsed wave

LASER ENERGY AND TISSUE TEMPERATURE

The principle effect of laser energy is photothermal. This thermal effect of laser energy on tissue depends on the degree of temperature rise and the corresponding reaction of the interstitial and intracellular water. As the laser energy is absorbed, heating occurs.

Tissue temperature (°C)	Observed Effect
37º – 50º	Hyperthermia
60º – 70º	Coagulation, Protein denaturation
70º – 80º	Welding
100º – 150º	Vaporization, Ablation
> 200º	Carbonization

The first event, hyperthermia occurs when the tissue temperature is elevated above normal temperature but is not destroyed. At temperatures of approximately 60°C, proteins begin to denature without any vaporization of the underlying tissue. This phenomenon is useful in surgically removing diseased granulomatous tissue because if the tissue temperature can be controlled, the biologically healthy portion can remain intact. Soft tissue edges can be "welded" together with a uniform heating at 70°C to 80°C where there is adherence of the layers because of the stickiness of collagen molecules. When the target tissue containing water is elevated to a temperature of 100°C, vaporization of the water within tissues occurs, this process is called ablation. If the tissue temperature continues to be raised to about 200°C, it is dehydrated and then burned in the presence of air. Carbon, as the end product, absorbs all wavelengths. Thus, if laser energy continues to be applied, the surface carbonized layer absorbs the incident beam, becoming a heat sink and preventing normal tissue ablation.

PERIODONTICS REVISITED

LASER-TISSUE INTERACTIONS

Laser light can have four different interactions with the target tissue, depending on the optical properties of that tissue **(Fig. 62.4)**.

1. **Absorption** of the laser energy by the intended tissue. The amount of energy that is absorbed by the tissue depends on the tissue characteristics, such as pigmentation and water content, and also on the laser wavelength and emission mode.
2. **Transmission:** Laser energy directly passes through the tissue with no effect on the target tissue, the inverse of absorption. This effect is highly dependent on the wavelength of laser light.
3. **Reflection:** It is the beam redirecting itself off of the surface, having no effect on the target tissue. This reflection can be dangerous because the energy is directed to an unintentional target, such as the eyes; this is a major safety concern for laser operation.
4. **Scattering** of the laser light, weakening the intended energy and possibly producing no useful biologic effect. Scattering of the laser beam could cause heat transfer to the tissue adjacent to the surgical site and unwanted damage could occur.

LASER WAVELENGTHS USED IN PERIODONTICS

Laser devices that have applications in periodontics are described in **Table 62.1**

LASER USES IN PERIODONTICS

1. Lasers in Diagnosis
   - *Caries detection*: Caries detection with laser works on the principle of differential florescence between healthy and diseased tooth. Such a system has become commercially available (Diagnodent). It operates at a wavelength of 655 nm. At this specific wavelength, clean healthy tooth structure exhibits little or no fluorescence, resulting in very low scale readings on the display. However, carious tooth structure will exhibit fluorescence, proportionate to the degree of caries, resulting in elevated scale readings on the display.
   - *Calculus detection*: Same laser wavelength of 655 nm can also be used for calculus detection. The commercially available device for caries detection provides a separate tip for the detection of calculus in the subgingival area. Calculus fluoresce (glow)

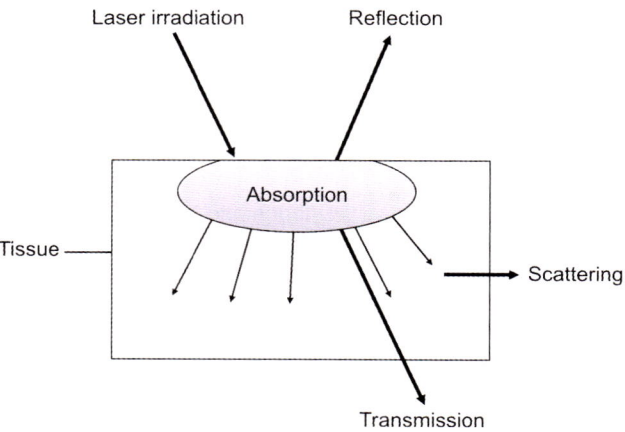

Fig. 62. 4: Laser tissue interactions

TABLE 62.1: Laser wavelengths used in periodontics

Laser	Wavelength	Wave form	Delivery Tip	Application
Argon	488-514 nm	Gated or continous	Flexible fibre optic system	Soft tissue incision and ablation
Diode	635-950 nm	Gated or continous	Flexible fibre optic system in contact mode for most of the procedures	Soft tissue incision and ablation, soft tissue curettage and bacterial elimination
Neodymium: yttrium-alumnium-garnet	1,064 µm	Pulsed	Flexible fiber optic system: contact mode for most procedures	Soft tissue incision and ablation; subgingival curettage and bacterial elimination
Erbium: yttrium-aluminum-garnet	2.94 µm	Free running pulsed	Flexible fiber optic system or hollow waveguide; contact mode for most procedures	Soft tissue incision and ablation; subgingival curettage; scaling of root surfaces: osteoplasty and ostectomy
Holnium: yttrium-aluminum-garnet	2.1 µm	Pulsed	Flexible fiber optic system: contact mode for most procedures	Soft tissue incision and ablation; subgingival curettage and bacterial elimination
Carbon dioxide	10.6 µm	Gated or continous	Hollow waveguide; beam focused when I to 2 mm from target surface	Soft tissue incision and ablation; subgingival curettage

differently than healthy tissue. The device senses the difference and sends the signal to the numerical display and also presents an audible signal, indicating that calculus has been identified.

- *Mobility assessment*: Laser has also been applied for the assessment of the mobility of teeth. Laser Doppler vibrometry can be used to assess even small movement in the tooth. This technique is being developed for commercial purposes.

2. Lasers in prevention

   Laser toothbrush: Laser toothbrush is designed to provide an antibacterial effect in oral cavity using an irradiating laser beam of 630 nm low output semiconductor laser. It works with a programmed tooth management system that turns on the laser for a recommended treatment period with one-touch mode switch. The laser toothbrush does not need toothpaste but directly radiates laser on teeth. This semiconductor medical laser helps to decrease plaque, relieves dentinal sensitivity, toothache and inflammation. It also treat halitosis and can be used in dental bleaching.

3. Lasers in nonsurgical Pocket therapy

   - *Laser Bacterial Reduction (LBR)*: It is a simple non-surgical procedure to eliminate or at least reduce the number of viable bacteria in the gingival sulcus. In this procedure a diode laser is used with a thin fiber optic fiber. Photonic laser energy is then emitted in to the sulcus through this optic fiber reducing the microbes and periodontal pathogens present within.

   - *Calculus removal*: The most difficult step that ultimately determines the success or failure of the periodontal therapy is the removal of the diseased tissue from the surgical site. If the calcified accretions on the root surface are not removed, the therapy is doomed to fail. Lasers now are being used for this procedure. Not only does the laser remove the calculus on the root surface, it also alters the cementum surface in such a way that it makes it favorable for fibroblast attachment. Diode and Nd:YAG lasers may be used for initial periodontal therapy but both of these wavelengths have a significant interaction with the root surface and may produce craters on it. Er:YAG treatment leaves no craters on the root surface. Also, the Er:YAG laser provides selective subgingival calculus removal on a level equivalent to that provided by scaling and root planing. Studies

have shown the ability of the Er:YAG laser to remove lipopolysaccharides, smear layer and calculus from root surfaces. The American Academy of Periodontology has stated that the Er:YAG laser demonstrated the best application of laser use directly on hard tissue, leaving the least thermal damage and creating a surface biocompatible for soft tissue attachment.

- *Photodynamic therapy*: The use of photoactivatable compounds or photosensitizers to cause photodestruction of oral bacteria has been demonstrated, indicating that photodynamic therapy (PDT) could be a useful alternative to mechanical means in eliminating periopathogenic bacteria. Photodynamics involves the application of a dye to the treatment area. The dye is termed photosensitizer because the dye after absorbing the light sensitizes the organisms to visible light inducing damage. Application of light results in the production of free oxygen radicals. These oxygen radicals are cytotoxic and destroy cellular constituents. Periowave™ is a photodynamic disinfection system that utilizes low intensity lasers (Diode) and wavelength-specific, light-activated compounds to specifically target and destroy microbial pathogens and reduce the symptoms of disease.

- *Lasers in treatment of hypersensitivity*: Low level laser therapy (LLLT) has been shown to have anti-inflammatory, analgesic and cellular effects in both hyperemia and inflammation of the dental pulp. For the treatment of hypersensitivity, a 780nm diode Laser can be used at power of 30mW, or Nd: YAG laser at low power can be used. The effect of laser therapy on hypersensitive teeth are: (1) Primary or immediate effect - remission of painful symptoms; and (2) secondary or late effect - intense cellular metabolic activity, proliferation of odontoblasts, and production of dentin. LLLT interferes with transmission of peripheral nerve signals to the central nervous system, where the signals are interpreted. The maintenance of this analgesic state of the dentin comes from sealing of dentinal tubuli, which impedes the internal communication of the pulp with external oral fluids. This sealing results from the coagulation of the hydroxyapatite crystals as well as formation of reparative dentin following laser stimulation.

4. Lasers in Surgical therapies

Most soft tissue laser procedures can be categorized into one of three simple processes: incision, excision, or ablation. Whether the dentist is using any of these, the basic process is the same regardless of the wavelength. The difference depends on the ability of the target tissue to absorb the laser energy which depends on its pigmentation, vascularity and water content.

Advantages of Laser Therapy

Wigdor et al described the advantages of lasers over conventional surgical procedures as:
- Dry and bloodless surgery
- Instant sterilization of the surgical site
- Reduced bacteremia
- Reduced mechanical trauma
- Minimal postoperative swelling and scarring
- Minimal postoperative pain.

Other advantages being high patient acceptance, less need for suturing and faster healing.

The type and wavelength of laser for a particular procedure depends on the personal preference of the clinician. Some may prefer diode laser for its compact size and portability while other may prefer Nd:YAG for its deeper depth of penetration. Many dentists are now prefering the erbium family of lasers for soft tissue due to their high absorption in water and lack of thermal penetration. Following procedures can be carried out with the use of above mentioned lasers.

- LNAP (laser new attachment procedure): In this procedure, laser is used to remove the epithelial lining of the sulcus as well as junctional epithelium. With the use of laser, it has been observed that there is retardation of epithelial downgrowth providing more time for connective tissue attachment on the root surface.
- Subgingival curettage: In this procedure, granulation tissue is removed from within the sulcus and pocket area without raising a flap with the help of a soft tissue laser.
- Minor surgeries: Nonosseous gingival surgeries, like frenectomy, frenotomy, gingivectomy, gingivoplasty and operculectomy can be performed.
- Biopsy and excision of soft tissue pathologies
- De-epithelialization: The use of lasers to retard epithelial downgrowth has been investigated. CO_2 laser has been used for this purpose. The epithelialization of the CO_2 irradiated side is delayed by at least 7 days, allowing for new connective tissue to grow. CO_2 laser de-epithelialization technique has the ability to obtain new clinical attachment with bone fill in previously diseased sites. The results are even better than that obtained through conventional osseous grafting alone. Also, this technique is less technically demanding and more time efficient than other currently known methods of epithelial retardation.

- Osseous recontouring: The only wavelengths cleared by the FDA for osseous surgery are the erbium family of lasers. Er:YAG and Er:Cr:YSGG are the only wavelengths that have the ability to ablate osseous tissue safely.

- Removal of granulation tissue: Soft tissue lasers are a good choice for removal of granulation tissue. The soft tissue lasers -argon (488 nm, 514 nm), diode (800-830 nm, 980 nm) and Nd:YAG (1064 nm) are well absorbed by melanin and hemoglobin and other chormophores present in periodontally diseased tissues. The laser energy is transmitted through water and poorly absorbed in hydroxyapatite. These properties of the soft tissue lasers make them an excellent choice to use in a periodontally involved sulcus that has dark inflamed tissue and pigmented bacteria.

- Periodontal regeneration surgery: Lasers are also being used for periodontal regenerative procedures. The most effective method of regenerative periodontal surgical techniques is a double-wavelength technique. This technique uses the Er:YAG to debride the open surgical site, clean and sterilize the root surface and prepare the root surface for the adhesion of fibroblasts. The CO_2 laser would remove the epithelium, which would allow the fibroblasts to adhere and proliferate, creating new attachment. Such a procedure will result in new attachment on previously diseased site.

5. Lasers in esthetic surgeries
- *Depigmentation*: Laser peel can be used for depigmentation of gingiva. A CO_2 laser can be used at continuous wave in a defocused mode. By using the laser in this manner, it is possible to separate the epithelium from the underlying connective tissue by creating a blister. Because the melanocytes are found in the basement membrane of the epithelium, they will be permanently eliminated with the tissue that is removed providing a long term result.

- Crown lengthening/soft tissue management around abutments
- Formation of ovate pontic sites and modification of soft tissue around laminates
- Bleaching
- Graft retrieval from palate
6. Lasers in Implants
   - *Second-stage recovery*: The tissue over the implant can be ablated using a CO_2 laser. Because the surgical site is so small, the area tends to form a char layer quickly. This char must be removed during surgery. If the char is not removed during surgery, then absorption of the laser energy will cease and scattering of the laser beam will occur, possibly heating up the tissue surrounding the implant and possibly damaging the implant. After the implant is exposed, the cover screw can be removed and a healing abutment placed. The advantage of using a laser to uncover the implant is that it avoids an incision that would extend through the interproximal papillae located next to the adjacent teeth. By avoiding this incision, a better cosmetic result can be assured.
   - *Peri-implantitis*: Er-YAG laser can be used for managing periimplantitis, because Er-YAG laser is very well suited for both hard and soft tissue treatment. Also, it disinfects implant along with implant surface treatment. The objective is to have a "surgically clean" interface; one that is indistinguishable from the sterile implant when it was originally placed. The ablative laser is the only instrument that can accomplish this. Lasers kill the microbes during the cleaning of infected area leaving the area free from infection. Even CO_2 laser is being researched for this purpose. Pulsed or continuous CO_2 laser is effective in removing the granulation and infected tissue. It does not cause overheating of the implant even if the laser beam hits on the implant within reasonable time and power settings.
7. Lasers in residual ridge modification
   - Tuberosity reduction
   - Torus reduction

DENTAL LASER SAFETY

Laser Hazard Classification according to ANSI and OSHA Standards:
Class I—Low powered lasers that are safe to view

Class IIa—Low powered visible lasers that are hazardous only when viewed directly for longer than 1000 sec.
Class IIb—Low powered visible lasers that are hazardous when viewed for longer than 0.25 sec.
Class IIIa—Medium powered lasers or systems that are normally not hazardous if viewed for less than 0.25 sec without magnifying optics
Class IIIb—Medium powered lasers (0.5W max) that can be hazardous if viewed directly.
Class IV—High powered lasers (>0.5W) that produce ocular, skin and fire hazards.

The types of hazards can be grouped as follows:

1. *Ocular injury*: Potential injury to the eye can occur either by direct emission from the laser or by reflection from a mirror like surface or high polished, convex curved instruments. Damage can be manifested as injury to sclera, cornea, retina and aqueous humor and also as cataract formation.
2. *Tissue damage*: Laser induces damage to skin and other non target tissues which results from the thermal interaction of radiant energy with tissue proteins. Temperature elevation of above normal body temp (37°C) can produce cell destruction by denaturation of cellular enzymes and structural proteins.
3. *Environmental hazards*: This involves potential inhalation of airborne biohazardous materials which results from surgical application of lasers. Chemicals like formaldehyde, methane and benzene are present in the laser plume which can be injurious if inhaled.
4. *Combustion hazards*: Flammable solids, liquids and gases used within the clinical setting can be easily ignited if exposed to the laser beam.
5. *Electrical hazards*: This is due to the very high currents and high voltage required to use the present dental lasers. These can be electrical shock hazards or electrical fire or explosion hazards.

Safety Precautions

- *Beam alignment*: Beam should be aligned properly at the treatment area before switching Laser on, to prevent undue injuries to patient as well as practitioner.
- *Laser control*: Foot pedal control of Laser should have a protective hood to prevent an accidental depression by assisting staff.
- *Reflected energy*: Anodized instrument should be used to prevent reflection of laser light. Also, mirror should be avoided in path of laser beam.
- *Fire protection*: All the flammable substances should be kept away from the operating area to prevent accidental fire hazard.

PERIODONTICS REVISITED

- *Eye protection*: Safety goggles should be worn by the operating person as well as the assistant. If safety goggles are not available for patient wet gauge pieces should be kept on closed eyes of the patient for prevention.

- *Plume control*: Laser filtration masks should be worn by the clinician as well as the assistant. The pore size of 0.1 µm has been shown to be effective. A high volume evacuator or a special laser plume evacuator should be used for the purpose.

PHOTODYNAMIC THERAPY

1. Introduction
2. Historical Perspective
3. Materials Used for Photodynamic Therapy (PDT)
4. Applications of Photodynamic Therapy
5. Photodynamic Antimicrobial Chemotherapy (PACT)

INTRODUCTION

The susceptibility of microorganisms to the damaging action of visible light in the presence of a dye has been known since 20th century when microbiologist started using acridine. More recently, photodynamic therapy (PDT) has been introduced for its antimicrobial action and also for selective killing of tumor cells. Photodynamic therapy (PDT), also known as photoradiation therapy, photo-therapy, or photochemotherapy, uses a photoactive dye (photosensitizer) that is activated by exposure to light of a specific wavelength in the presence of oxygen, forming free radical species that kill targeted microbes.

PDT is now being considered as a possible treatment for periodontal diseases, which are caused by the overgrowth of pathogenic microflora around teeth. PDT can be a valuable alternative to traditional scaling and root planing as well as antibiotic therapy. PDT offers a new treatment modality that is required since periodontal infection tends to recur after scaling and root planing and also because of wide spread drug resistance to antibiotics.

HISTORICAL PERSPECTIVE

Photodynamic therapy was discovered accidently at the beginning of the 20th century and was then applied in the medical field for the light induced inactivation of cells, microorganisms or molecules. The term 'photodynamic action' ('Photodynamische Wirkung') was introduced in 1904 by one of the pioneers of photobiology: Professor Hermann von Tappeiner. It is not clear why he called the process 'dynamic'; it might have been to distinguish this biological phenomenon from the reactions taking place in the photographic process that had been discovered a few years earlier. The very first attempt to apply PDT in treatment of tumors and other skin diseases, such as lupus of the skin and chondyloma of the female genitalia, were performed by the group of Von Tappeiner in 1903-1905.

PDT was first approved by the Food and Drug Administration in 1999 to treat pre-cancerous skin lesions of the face or scalp. Applications of PDT in dentistry are growing rapidly in the treatment of oral cancer, as well as bacterial and fungal infections and in the photodynamic diagnosis (PDD) of the malignant transformation of oral lesions.

MATERIALS USED FOR PHOTODYNAMIC THERAPY (PDT)

1. *Light source:* A diode laser system is commonly used for photodynamic therapy since it is easy to handle, portable and cost effective. For treatment of larger areas, noncoherent light sources such as tungsten filament, quartz halogen, xenon arc, metal halide and phosphor-coated sodium lamps are used. These days, LEDs are being used because they are small, lightweight, highly flexible and less expensive than typical light sources.

2. *Delivery unit:* The light from the source is delivered according to the location and morphology of the lesion. Usually, fiber optic catheters are used. These fiber tips can be made into various shapes, allowing for diffusion in all directions.

3. *Photosensitizers:* Photosensitizers are usually dyes which get activated in presence of light of specific

wavelength to form free radicals which kill the unwanted microbes or tumor cells.

Classification of photosensitizers:

First generation photosensitizers: Phenothiazine dyes, porphyrin-chlorin-phthalocyanine platforms, hemato-porphyrin derivatives.

Second generation photosensitizers: 5-aminolevulinic acid (ALA), benzoporphyrin derivative, lutetium texaphyrin, temoporfin (mTHPC), tinethyletiopurpurin and talaporfin sodium.

An ideal photosensitizer should display local toxicity only after illumination. The majority of the sensitizers used clinically are phenothiazine dyes or porphyrin-chlorin-phthalocyanine platforms. Photofrin (dihemato-porphyrin ether) is the most extensively studied and clinically used photosensitizer. Foscan (temoporfin), the most potent second-generation photosensitizer, has been found to be 100 times more active than Photofrin in animal studies.

APPLICATIONS OF PHOTODYNAMIC THERAPY

Applications of this technique in dentistry may include:
a. *Photodynamic diagnosis (PDD) of malignant transformation of oral lesions:* A relatively new approach in the diagnosis of oral lesions is topical application of ALA.
b. *Treatment of premalignant and malignant oral lesions:* Topical ALA-based photodynamic therapy has been used to treat premalignant and malignant lesions in the oral cavity. Photodynamic therapy already has shown potential in the treatment of oral leukoplakia, oral lichen planus and squamous cell carcinoma of the tongue and lip. Photodynamic therapy of the oral mucosa causes superficial necrosis, leaving little scarring and no cumulative toxicity. ALA-based photodynamic therapy appears to be an effective treatment for oral leukoplakia. This may be attributed to its low invasiveness, good tolerance, excellent cosmetic effects, ability to treat multifocal lesions and low risk of toxicity after repeated use.
c. *Chemotherapy (PACT) for biofilms:* Dental plaque is a complex aggregation of microorganisms found on the tooth surface in the form of a biofilm; that is, the organisms are embedded in an extracellular polymeric matrix. Biofilm-associated bacteria have increased resistance to antibiotics, to environmental stresses and to the immune defense mechanisms of their host. The limited access of topical agents into the plaque and the development of antibiotic resistance have stimulated the search for new strategies to control plaque and to treat caries, gingivitis and periodontal disease. PACT is equally effective against antibiotic-resistant and susceptible bacteria. Repeated photosensitization does not induce the selection of resistant strains.
d. *Oropharyngeal candidiasis:* It is a widespread opportunistic infection in immunocompromised patients, such as HIV infected individuals. In addition, *Candida* associated denture stomatitis is a common disease in denture wearers. The ability of *C. albicans* to form biofilms on mucosal surfaces and on prosthetic devices contributes to recurrent infections and to the failure of antifungal therapy. The increasing resistance of *C. albicans* to antifungal agents has stimulated an interest in photodynamic treatments. Similarly to other yeasts, *C. albicans* is more difficult to kill by PACT than gram-positive bacteria. Recently, Ryan F. Donnelly and his colleagues at Queen's University Belfast in the UK reported that mucoadhesive patches containing toluidine blue O as a potential delivery system in oral candidiasis.

PHOTODYNAMIC ANTIMICROBIAL CHEMOTHERAPY (PACT)

It represents an alternative antibacterial, antifungal, and antiviral treatment for drug-resistant organisms. It is unlikely that bacteria would develop resistance to the cytotoxic action of singlet oxygen or free radicals. Bacteria that grow in biofilms, are also susceptible to PACT.

Mechanism of Action

In photodynamic therapy, a photosensitizer or its metabolic precursor is administered to the patient. Most photosensitizers are activated by light between 630 and 700 nm. Upon irradiation with light of a specific wavelength, the photosensitizer undergoes a transition from a low-energy ground state to an excited singlet state. Subsequently, the photosensitizer may decay back to its ground state, with emission of fluorescence, or may undergo a transition to a higher-energy triplet state. The triplet state can react with endogenous oxygen to produce singlet oxygen and other radical species, causing a rapid and selective destruction of the target micro organisms.

PERIODONTICS REVISITED

PACT in Periodontitis

PACT can be applied in periodontics by using low intensity lasers and wavelength-specific, light-activated compounds to specifically target and destroy microbial pathogens and reduce the symptoms of disease. The photosensitive compounds are topically applied in the gingival sulcus and the laser is used to activate the compounds and complete the disinfection.

The photosensitivity of bacteria appears to be related to the charge of the sensitizer. In general, neutral or anionic photosensitizers bind efficiently to and inactivate gram-positive bacteria, while they bind to some extent to the outer membrane of gram negative bacteria, but do not inactivate them after illumination. A relatively porous layer of peptidoglycan and lipoteichoic acid outside the cytoplasmic membrane of gram-positive species allows the photosensitizer to diffuse into sensitive sites. The outer membrane of gram negative bacteria acts as a physical and functional barrier between the cell and its environment. The affinity of negatively charged photosensitizers for gram negative bacteria may be enhanced by linking the sensitizer to a cationic molecule (e.g. poly-L-lysine-chlorin e6), by the use of membrane-active agents (e.g. treatment with Tris-EDTA), or by conjugating the sensitizer with a monoclonal antibody that binds to cell-surface-specific antigens.

Advantages of PACT

- Because the antimicrobial activity of photosensitizers is mediated by singlet oxygen, PACT has a direct effect on extracellular molecules. Thus, these polysaccharides of an extracellular polymeric matrix are susceptible to photodamage. This activity, not displayed by antibiotics, represents a significant advantage of PACT.
- The development of resistance to PACT appears to be unlikely, since, in microbial cells, singlet oxygen and free radicals interact with several cell structures and have different metabolic pathways.
- PACT is equally effective against antibiotic-resistant and antibiotic-susceptible bacteria and repeated photosensitization has not induced the selection of resistant strains.
- The potencies of some key virulence factors (lipopolysaccharide and proteases) have also been shown to be reduced by photosensitization.
- Antioxidant enzymes, such as superoxide dismutase and catalase, protect against some oxygen radicals, but not against singlet oxygen.
- It is non-invasive and convenient for the patient.
- PACT can be performed in outpatient or day-care (inpatient) settings.
- PACT can be targeted accurately and selectively in localized diseases.
- Repeated doses can be given without the need for total-dose limitations.

Photosensitizers Used for PACT

Platform	Example
Phenothiazine dyes	Methylene blue, Toluidine blue O
Phthalocyanines	Aluminium disulphonated phthalocyanine cationic, Zn (II)-phthalocyanine
Chlorines	Chlorine 6, Sn (IV) chlorine 6, Chlorine 6-2.5, Nmethyl-d-glucamine, polylysine and Polyethyleneimine conjugates of chlorine 6
Porphyrins	Hematoporphyrin HCl, Photofrin(di hematoporphyrin ether), Aminolevulinic acid (ALA)
Xanthenes	Erythrosine
Monoterpene	Azulene

TISSUE ENGINEERING

1. Introduction
2. Principles of Tissue Engineering
3. Scaffolds for Tissue Engineering
4. Cells for Tissue Engineering
5. Biological Mediators and Signaling Molecules for Tissue Engineering
6. Requirement for Successful Periodontal Tissue Engineering

INTRODUCTION

Tissue engineering is an emerging field of science aimed at developing techniques for the fabrication of new tissue to replace damaged tissues and is based on principles of cell biology, development biology and biomaterial science. The term tissue engineering was initially coined to denote the construction in the laboratory of a device containing viable cells and biological mediators in a synthetic or biological matrix that could be implanted in patients to facilitate regeneration of a particular tissue. More recently the definition has been broadened to refer to any attempt to regenerate tissues whether in laboratory or patients by adding appropriate biologic mediators and matrices.

PRINCIPLES OF TISSUE ENGINEERING

Strategies to tissue engineering: Currently, strategies employed to engineer tissue can be categorized into three major classes: conductive, inductive and cell transplantation approaches. Conductive approaches utilize biomaterials in a passive manner to facilitate the growth or regenerative capacity of existing tissue. An example of this is the use of barrier membranes in guided tissue regeneration. The inductive approach uses a biodegradable polymer scaffold as a vehicle to deliver growth factors and genes to the host site. The growth factors or genes can be released at a controlled rate based on the breakdown of the polymer which induces regeneration at the site. The cell transplantation strategy uses a similar vehicle for delivery in order to transplant cells and partial tissues to the host site.

The main requirements for producing an engineered tissue are the appropriate levels and sequencing of regulatory signals, the presence and numbers of responsive progenitor cells and an appropriate extracellular matrix or cellular carrier construct. The regeneration of peridontium requires recruitment of progenitor cells which have the potential to differentiate into specialized regenerative cells, followed by proliferation of these cells and synthesis of specialized components which are to be repaired. The tissue engineering strategy for periodontal regeneration will thus, require growing these cells within a three dimensional construct and subsequent implantation in to the defect.

Reconstruction of lost periodontal tissue requires the combination of cells, scaffolds, signaling molecules, and blood supply. Each of these elements plays a fundamental role on the healing process and is interconnected into the generation of new tissues **(Fig. 62.5).** A limiting factor in the achievement of periodontal regeneration is the presence of microbial pathogens that contaminate periodontal wounds and reside on tooth surfaces as plaque-associated biofilms. .

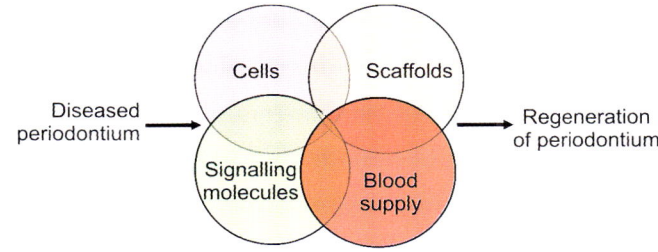

Fig. 62. 5: Periodontal tissue engineering

SCAFFOLDS FOR TISSUE ENGINEERING

Scaffolds act as a delivery vehicle for cell transplantation and as a three-dimensional template for tissue regeneration. It also provide specific clues to regulate bone formation. Naturally derived and synthetic scaffold materials have been used to exploit the regenerative capacities of host tissues or transplanted cells. The specific requirements for scaffold material include biocompatibility, mechanical support, controlled degradation and adequate interstitial fluid flow. Scaffold characteristics, such as porosity, topography and material composition, dictate certain of these features. Matrices that resemble the extracellular matrix of the tissue to be engineered can be used as scaffolds.

Types of Scaffolds

Nonresorbable (ePTFE)	Expanded polytetrafluoroethylene Ceramic, Titanium mesh
Resorbable	Alpha-hydroxyacids
	• Polyglycolic acid
	• Poly(L-lactic acid)
	• Copolymers of poly(lactic-co-glycolic acid)
	Amino acid-based polymers
	• Collagen-like proteins
	• Elastin-like proteins
	Natural products
	• Collagen
	• Hyaluronan
	• Chitosan
	• Gelatin
	• Fibrin
	• Alginate
	Synthetic hydrogels
	• Poly ethylene glycol
	• Poly ethylene oxide
	Matrix extracts
	• Matrigel

PERIODONTICS REVISITED

Nonresorbable membranes: Membranes made from expanded polytetrafluoroethylene could be used to nurture specific cells that are expanded *ex vivo* and then delivered to a defect site. Some ceramic materials have also been used as a scaffold. These ceramics have good biocompatibility, are porous and possess osseointegrative capabilities. Hydroxyapatite is a ceramic material with good mechanical properties. Porous hydroxyapatite lacking interconnectivity of the pores, makes neovascularization of any implant almost impossible. Biodegradable porous ceramic materials have also been developed and investigated. One of these, is beta-tricalcium phosphate which possesses high biocompatibility and biodegradability. This material has good mechanical properties regarding stiffness and elasticity and is relatively easy to handle during surgical placement. Another nonresorbable material with promising outcome is titanium mesh. The lack of bioresorbability of this material can be beneficial for the management of large osseous defects.

Resorbable materials: The alpha-hydroxy acid polymers include polyglycolic acid, poly L-lactic acid and copolymers of poly lactic-co-glycolic acid which are used for cell seeding. These polymers degrade by non enzymatic means and do not generally elicit a foreign body response resulting in massive macrophage infiltration and chronic inflammation. These materials can also be improved chemically to modify its period of degradation depending on clinical need. The seven disadvantage of these material is difficult attachment or entrapment of cell due to their hydrophobic nature and processing under stringent conditions.

Alginate beads can also serve as a cell carrier for tissue engineering. The technique is based on entrapment of individual cells and tissues into an alginate droplet that is transformed into a rigid bead by gelation in a divalent cation-rich solution. In this way transplanted cells are immune-protected and isolated from host tissue via a nondegradable, selectively permeable barrier.

Due to the significant role of Hyaluronate in development and organogenesis, it has considerable potential for tissue engineering. Hyaluronate can be modified with esterification and cross linking to provide structure and rigidity to gel for cell seeding purpose. Another biopolymer chitosan that structurally resembles naturally occurring glycosaminoglycans can also be used as tissue engineering scaffold. Collagen scaffolds also offer several advantages such as excellent biocompatibility, safety and easy seeding of cells.

Synthetic hydrogels, such as polyethylene glycol and polyethylene oxide, can be used as a 3D scaffold for cell delivery. Polyethylene oxide is currently approved by the U.S. Food and Drug Administration for several applications in medicine and, together with polyglycolic acid, is one of the most common synthetic materials used for tissue engineering.

Extracellular matrix extracts or derivatives have been developed as commercial products for cell delivery, such as Matrigel™, Dermagraft™ and Epidex™ have been developed to allow the incorporation of ex vivo-expanded cells. Main disadvantage of using these materials is that they are animal-derived products and/or allogenic tissues and thus, constitute a potential source of pathogens and therefore unlikely to be routinely used as cell delivery devices in the longer term.

CELLS FOR TISSUE ENGINEERING

Cells harvested for tissue engineering may be heterologous (different species), allogenic (same species, different individual), or autologous (same individual). When cells are used for tissue engineering, a small piece of donor tissue is dissociated into individual cells. These cells are either implanted directly into the host or are expanded in culture, attached to a support matrix and then reimplanted into the host after expansion. Autologous cells are preferred because they will not evoke an immunologic response and thus, the deleterious side effects of immunosuppressive agents can be avoided.

Stem cells therapy has introduced a new source for harvesting cells for tissue engineering. Stem cells have the ability to self replicate for indefinite periods. Under right conditions or given right signals stem cells can differentiate into many cell types. Stem cells can be grouped into either embryonic or the adult. Embryogenic stem cells are derived from the blastocyst stage of the embryonic development prior to implantation in uterine wall. These cells are clonogenic that is they are capable of unlimited self renewal by symmetric division, one daughter cell resembling its mother and other daughter giving rise to multiple types of differentiated cell representing all three germ layers. Incorporating these stem cells in a bioengineered matrix with appropriate mediators can be used for filling periodontal defects.

BIOLOGICAL MEDIATORS AND SIGNALING MOLECULES FOR TISSUE ENGINEERING

In order to enhance the *in vivo* efficacy, incorporation of bioactive molecules into scaffolding materials may facilitate sustained factor release for period of time. Bioactive molecules incorporated directly into a bioresorbable scaffold are generally released by a diffusion controlled mechanism that is regulated by the pore sizes. The rate of growth factor release depends on the type and rate of degradation of the delivery device and the rate of growth factor diffusion through pores of the scaffolds.

Several bioactive molecules have demonstrated strong effects in promoting periodontal wound repair in preclinical and clinical studies. These bioactive molecules include PDGF, IGF-I, FGF-2, TGF-1, BMP-2, -4, -7 and -12 and enamel matrix derivative (EMD). These molecules that have shown positive results in stimulating periodontal regeneration.

REQUIREMENT FOR SUCCESSFUL PERIODONTAL TISSUE ENGINEERING

A. Biomechanical requirements
  * *Space maintenance*: Bone grows into an adjacent tissue space provided the space is maintained and soft tissue ingrowth is prevented. This can be used when bio-engineered matrices are placed for regeneration. The scaffold should have the ability of easy molding and consistency compatible with easy handling.

Also, it should be of sufficient rigidity to withstand soft tissue collapse into the defect.
  * *Barrier or exclusionary function*: The engineered tissue should act as a barrier to the ingrowth of unwanted tissues and selectively permit the ingrowth of regenerative tissues. To achieve this, the external surface should be scaffold exclusionary yet the internal scaffold is still conducive to new tissue ingrowth. The principle aim of tissue engineering for peridontium is the total exclusion of epithelium yet encouraging it to form a rapid and successful biological seal.

B. Biological requirements
  * *Biocompatibility*: The bioengineered tissue should be either biocompatible with the tissues to be regenerated or biodegradable allowing for gradual replacement with regenerated tissue. Also, the porosity and pore size of the scaffold material should allow migration of cells and regeneration of tissues.
  * *Incorporation of cells*: It should be possible that the cells with periodontal regenerative phenotype be cultured and subsequently incorporated into a scaffold for immediate incorporation into periodontal defect. Likely source for these cells can be progenitor cells harvested from the host site i.e. cementum, periodontal ligament or bone.
  * *Incorporation of instructive messages*: The synthetic matrix should be able to adsorb appropriate growth factors and other instructive molecules normally found in regenerating tissues. These materials will later release slowly from the matrix and initiate and propagate regenerative events.

GENE THERAPY

INTRODUCTION

Periodontitis is a complex disease which affects the human population worldwide. Over the years many treatment modalities have been suggested to control this disease. Recently, new treatment modalities to regenerate lost peridontium have been developed like guided tissue regeneration with newer materials like Emdogain and rh-BMP, etc. With a better understanding of disease progression and new advancement in biological science, gene therapy has emerged to enhance existing therapy and radically recast approaches to the management of periodontal disease. Here we discuss the gene therapy and its impact on periodontium.

Gene therapy is a technique for correcting defective genes responsible for disease development. Gene therapy uses purified preparations of a gene or a fraction of a gene, to treat diseases. A common approach in gene therapy is to identify a malfunctioning gene and supply the patient with functioning copies of that gene. Whichever approach is used, the aim of gene therapy is to introduce therapeutic material into the target cells, where it becomes active and exerts the intended therapeutic effect.

APPROACHES FOR GENE THERAPY

For correcting faulty genes one of the following approaches may be employed:
• A normal gene may be inserted into a nonspecific location within the genome to replace a nonfunctional gene; this is the most common approach.
• An abnormal gene may be swapped for a normal gene through homologous recombination.
• The abnormal gene could be repaired through selective reverse mutation, which returns the gene to its normal functional status.
• The regulation (the degree to which a gene is turned on or off) of a particular gene could be altered.
• Somatic and Germ Line Gene Therapy—Gene therapy can target somatic (body) or germ (egg and sperm) cells. In somatic gene therapy the recipient's genome is changed, but the change is not passed on to the next generation; whereas with germ line gene therapy the newly introduced gene is passed on to the offspring.

GENE TRANSFER TECHNIQUES

1. *In vivo:* During *in vivo* gene transfer, the foreign gene is injected into the patient by viral and nonviral methods.
    a. Viral
    b. Non-viral
        i. Cationic liposomes
        ii. Microseeding
        iii. Gene activated matrices
        iv. Macromolecular conjugate
2. *Ex-vivo:* The *ex vivo* gene transfer involves a foreign gene transduced into cells of a tissue biopsy, outside the body and then resulting genetically modified cells, which are transplanted back into the patient.

Viral Methods

Viral approach is quite efficient method of gene transfer. A vector is used to introduce therapeutic gene into patient's target cell. Virus serves as the vector. These are

natural infectious agents for transferring genetic information.

Some of the viruses that can be used as vector are:
    i. Retrovirus: Their genetic material is RNA through which they can create DNA that can be integrated into chromosomes.
    ii. Adenoviruses are viruses with double stranded DNA genomes
    iii. Herpes Simplex viruses are double stranded virus that can infect a particular cell.
    iv. Adeno associated viruses are single stranded DNA viruses that insert genetic material at specific site on chromosome 19.
    v. Lenti viruses or hybrid viruses combine the traits of two or more viruses.

These vectors can be given intravenously or injected directly into a specific tissue in the body. The culture cells are exposed to the vector and then reintroduced into the patient.

Non-Viral Approaches

    i. *Cationic liposomes:* In this technique, artificial lipid spheres are created with an aqueous core. The liposome which carries the therapeutic DNA, is capable of passing the DNA through the target cell's membrane.
    ii. *Micro-seeding Gene Therapy:* This is the simplest method of gene therapy. It is the direct introdu-ction of therapeutic DNA into target cells using a gene gun. But, it requires large amount of DNA to bring out desired effect and can be used only with certain tissues, hence restricting its use.
    iii. *Gene activated matrices:* It employs polymer matrix sponges to deliver naked DNA to the target cells.
    iv. *Macromolecular conjugates:* In this technique, DNA is linked to a molecule that binds to special cell receptors. Once bound, the therapeutic DNA is engulfed by the cell membrane and passed into interior of target cell. This delivery system is less effective than others.

APPLICATION OF GENE THERAPY IN PERIODONTICS

1. **In prevention of periodontal disease**
    • *Periodontal vaccination:* Research is going on for vaccination techniques to prevent periodontal diseases. Gene transfer research has also started contributing to achieve vaccination against

periodontal disease. In this technique, plasmids containing DNA encoding antigens of periodontal pathogens can be injected to the host which results in production of immunoglobulins against the pathogens as a host response thus, preventing periodontal disease. For example: haemagglutinin is an important virulence factor of *Porphyromonas gingivalis*. It's gene has been identified, coded, cloned and expressed in *Escherichia coli*. This recombinant gene when injected in rats showed increased serum IgG antibody response against *P. gingivalis* and gave protection against bone loss.

- *Control of biofilm antibiotic resistance:* It has been observed that biofilm bacteria are 1000 fold more resistant to antibiotics compared to planktonic counterpart, making them hard to control. Recently, a gene has been identified in *Pseudomonas aeuroginosa* encoding for glycosyl-transferase required for synthesis of periplasmic glucans which protects it from effects of antibiotics. With the help of gene therapy, researchers have developed mutant of this gene capable of forming a biofilm but lacking periplamic glucans, therfore rendering biofilm more susceptible to antibiotic therapy.
- Alveolar remodelling: Periodontal tissues react to stimuli such as stress and inflammation by active remodelling with the expression of various molecules. Using a transfer gene responsible for various remodelling molecules (Lac Z gene) along with electroporation (electric impulse) for driving gene into cell, predictable alveolar bone remodelling can be achieved.

2. **To control periodontal disease progression**
   - *Antimicrobial gene therapy:* If a gene which encodes for an antimicrobial peptide is inserted into the host, it can drastically enhance the host defence mechanism. It was shown that when host cells were infected in vivo with α-defensin-2 gene via a retro viral vector, there was a potent antimicrobial activity.
   - *Tight adherence gene: Aggregatibacter actinomy-cetemcomitans* is a potent perio pathogen which expresses a 'tight adherence gene' for its adherence to host tissue and virulence. Researchers have developed a mutant strain of this pathogen lacking this gene, which could predictably control periodontal disease progression by limiting colonization and pathogenesis of *A. actinomy- cetemcomitans*.

3. **In treatment of periodontal disease**
   - *Gene enhanced tissue engineering:* Tissue engineering in general, supplements the regenerative site with therapeutic protein like growth factor. However, the problem with this technique is the short life of this growth factor because of proteolytic breakdown and solubility of delivery vehicle. To overcome this problem, gene therapy has been developed that provides long term exposure of the growth factor (at least two weeks) to the periodontal wound. Genetically engineered mesenchymal stem cell, when placed into an osseous defect, induced new bone and blood vessels formation by expressing BMP- 2. These cells were able to engraft, differentiate and display regulatory behaviours.
   Similarly, Platelet derived growth factor (PDGF) has been used for tissue engineering because of its potent effect on regeneration of hard and soft tissues.

DIFFICULTIES IN APPLICATION OF GENE THERAPY IN PERIODONTICS

- Gene therapy is still in infancy and has its own substantial problems, thus has not been applied to periodontics with success.
- Periodontal disease is multifactorial in origin comprising microbial challenge, variable host response modified by genetic and environmental factors.
- There are genetic variations in different populations like involvement of multiple genes, interaction between gene and environment. To complicate further, no single gene has been universally accepted as a causative factor for periodontitis.

LIMITATION AND DIFFICULTIES OF GENE THERAPY

- *Gene delivery:* Successful gene delivery is not easy or predictable, even in single-gene disorders. For example, although the genetic basis of cystic fibrosis is well known, the presence of mucus in the lungs makes it physically difficult to deliver genes to the target lung cells.
- *Durability and integration:* Some gene therapy approaches aim at long-term effects. Two possible ways of achieving this are to either use multiple

PERIODONTICS REVISITED

rounds of gene therapy or integrate the therapeutic genes so that they remain active for some time. Integrating therapeutic DNA may cause possible undesirable side effects.

- *Immune response:* Viral vector may be recognized as foreign and mobilize the immune system to attack it. This may hamper the efficacy of gene therapy or induce serious side effects.
- *Safety of vectors:* Viruses present a variety of potential problems to the patient, e.g. toxicity, immune and inflammatory responses, gene control and targeting issues. In addition, viral vector may recover its ability to cause disease.
- *Cost factor:* At present, gene therapy is very expensive. This may restrict its use and benefits in only a class of patients and not to wider population.
- *Ethical restrictions:* Applying gene therapy to protect from disabilities or diseases definitely pose a ethical problem. Also, the question that till where and how we can restrict gene therapy is a serious one.

NANOTECHNOLOGY

1. Introduction
2. Definitions
3. Four Generations of Nanotechnology Development
4. Properties of Nanomaterials
5. Nanomaterial Assemblies
6. Application in Periodontics
7. Other Applications

INTRODUCTION

With an escalating trend in increasing survival age of the population, scientists are now looking for options to construct biologic substitute with the help of regenerative medicine and tissue engineering. The ultimate endpoint in this field would be complete regeneration of human tissues. In recent years various biomaterials have been structured at nano scales that form ideal interfaces with tissues. One such example is the fabrication of nano fiber material for three dimensional cell cultures. Apart from tissue engineering, nanotechnology is finding application in various other diagnostic, therapeutic and preventive aspects of dentistry.

DEFINITIONS

The term "nanotechnology" was first defined by Norio Taniguchi of the Tokyo Science University in a paper in 1974 as follows: Nanotechnology mainly consists of the processing of, separation, consolidation, and deformation of materials by one atom or one molecule. Since that time the definition of nanotechnology has generally been extended to include features as large as 100 nm. Additionally, the idea that nanotechnology embraces structures exhibiting quantum mechanical aspects, such as quantum dots, has further evolved its definition. Later, the term "nanotechnology" was independently coined and popularized by Eric Drexler.

According to definition provided by National Nanotechnology Initiative, nanotechnology is the research and development of materials, devices and system exhibiting physical, chemical and biological properties that are different from those found on a larger scale.

Molecular nanotechnology (MNT) is the concept of engineering functional mechanical systems at the molecular scale designed and built atom-by-atom. It would make use of positionally-controlled mechanosynthesis guided by molecular machine systems. MNT involves combining physical principles demonstrated by chemistry, other nanotechnologies, and the molecular machinery of life with the systems engineering principles found in modern macroscale factories.

FOUR GENERATIONS OF NANOTECHNOLOGY DEVELOPMENT

Mike Roco of the US National Nanotechnology Initiative has described four generations of nanotechnology development **(Fig. 62.6)**. The first era is that of passive nanostructures, materials designed to perform one task. The second phase introduces active nanostructures for multitasking; for example, drug delivery devices and sensors. The third generation is expected to begin emerging around 2010 and will feature nanosystems with thousands of interacting components. A few years after

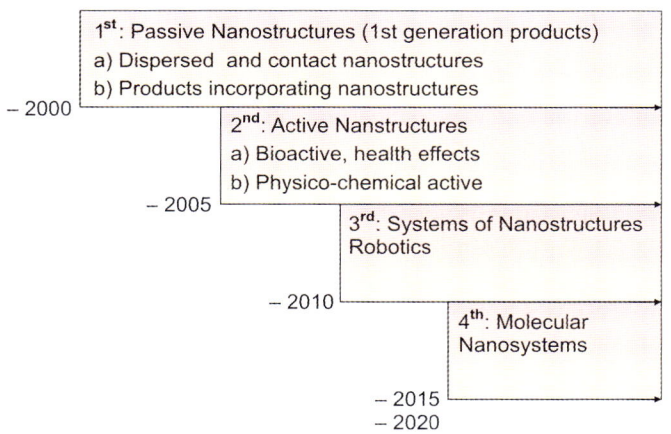

Fig. 62. 6: Generations of nanotechnology

that, the first integrated nanosystems, functioning much like a mammalian cell with hierarchical systems within systems, are expected to be developed.

PROPERTIES OF NANOMATERIALS

- Nanomaterials are those materials with components less than 100 nm in at least one dimension.
- Nanoparticles have significant surface effects, size effects and quantum effects and show better performance properties than traditional materials.
- They have special chemical, optical, magnetic and electro-optical properties that are different from similar material either individual molecule or at larger scale.
- Nanomaterials have an important property of self – assembly. They autonomously organize themselves in to patterns or structures without intervention. This can be manipulated and facilitated through correct setting of conditions. The driving forces for self assembly are electrostatic attractive interactions between positive and negative charges.

NANOMATERIAL ASSEMBLIES

- *Multilayer assemblies:* It is the layer by layer adsorption of individual atoms to form multilayered structures of various shapes and sizes.
- *Core shell assemblies:* Core shells can be formed of given size, topology and composition followed by removal of core by either dissolution to produce hollow particles or decomposition to give hollow shells.

- *Nanorods/Nanowires/Nanofibers:* These are linear structures with a very small diameter formed by linear arrangement of atoms.
- *Nanotubes:* Carbon nanotubes are the most researched nanomaterial. A sheet of carbon atoms can be rolled into a tube forming a carbon nanotube. Carbon nanotube properties depend on how sheet is rolled. With the right arrangement of atoms, a carbon nanotube can be created that is hundreds of time stronger than steel, but six times lighter.
- *Nanobuds:* Carbon nanobuds are a newly created material combining two previously discovered allotropes of carbon; carbons nanotubes and fullerene buckyball. A fullerene buckyball is a molecule composed entirely of carbon in the form of a hollow sphere. In Nanobuds fullerene buckyball – like buds are covalently bonded to the outer sidewalls of the underlying carbon nanotube.
- *Nanotorus:* A nanotorus is described as carbon nanotube bent into a torus (doughnut shape). Nanotori are predicted to have many unique properties, such as magnetic moments 1000 times larger than previously expected for certain specific radii.

APPLICATION IN PERIODONTICS

- *Treatment of dentin hypersensitivity:* Reconstructive dental nanorobots, using native biological materials, could selectively and precisely occlude specific tubules within minutes, offering patients a quick and permanent cure.
- *Nanorobotic dentifrices (Dentifrobots):* These nanorobots could be delivered by mouthwash or toothpaste. They could patrol all supragingival and subgingival surfaces at least once a day, metabolizing trapped organic matter into harmless and odorless vapours and performing continuous calculus debridement. They would also identify and destroy pathogenic bacteria in plaque where as allowing harmless bacteria to flourish. Dentifrobots would also be able to cure halitosis by preventing putrefaction of organic material in oral cavity.
- *Nanofibers:* Nanotechnology is producing nanofibers that have much better properties than conventional fibers. These nanofibers possess a larger surface area per unit mass and permit an easier addition of surface functionalities than polymer microfibers. These nanofibers have been used for drug delivery systems and tissue engineering scaffolds.

PERIODONTICS REVISITED

- *Nano Biomineralization*: Biomineralization refers to minerals formed biologically, which differ in structure and properties from laboratory formed materials, for example that in bone. Bone formation and structure is also being analyzed at nano level to construct a synthetic bone graft substitute with a nano structured architecture that resembles natural bone. Crystals are manipulated at nanolevels and embedded in to collagen fibers to create an organic-inorganic composite with unique mechanical properties. Such synthetic grafts would be accepted by the body very well and will guide body cells for mending of bone defects.
- *Tooth repair (Biomimicry)*: Nanotechnology can also be applied to synthesize both mineral and cellular components of tooth. Such a technique has been developed by Chen et al to form dental enamel. They used highly organized micro-architectural units of nanorod like calcium hydroxyapatite crystals arranged roughly parallel to each other. It is expected that within a span of time we would be able to mimic the periodontal tissues also and would be able to repair them in a natural way with the help of nanotechnology.
- Tissue engineering scaffold.
- Nano textured Implant surface.

OTHER APPLICATIONS

- *Inducing anesthesia*: For this, a colloidal solution of millions of dental nanorobots will be instilled on the patient's gingiva. These nanorobots will reach dentin by migrating into gingival sulcus and passing through cementoenamel junction. Through dentin they proceed towards the pulp either by biological guides or through instructions from outside computers. Inside pulp they control nerve impulse traffic inducing anesthesia. These robots will then come out after completion of task through natural pathways. Such a technique will offer more patient comfort, greater selectivity, a faster complete and reversible analgesic effect.
- *Tooth repositioning*: Orthodontic nanorobots will be able to manipulate the periodontal tissues, allowing rapid and painless tooth movements within hours.
- *Nano composites*: It is one of the dental products designes with nanotechnology which is commercially available today. It contains non-agglomerated discrete nanoparticles that are homogenously mixed in resins or coatings to produce nanocomposites. Their advantages being superior hardness, flexible strength, modulous of elasticity, high esthetic appeal, excellent finish and long standing polish.
- *Nanosolutions*: Nanoparticles homogeneously dispersed in to various solvents and polymers form nanosolutions. Such solutions provide superior properties than the parent materials. This technique is being applied in bonding agents to provide superior hold of filling materials.
- *Femto lasers*: Femto-lasers are like a pair of nanoscissors producing sharp cuts in the tissue. They act by vaporizing tissue locally while leaving adjacent tissue unharmed. This technique is being applied in plastic and ophthalmic surgery as well as individual chromosome surgery. In near future we can hope for its use in periodontal plastic surgery.
- *Nano-medical tests*: Chris Backous is developing a Lab-on-chip to give doctor immediate results for medical tests. It will also be able to analyze genetic information of individual cells. This will provide instant results and would be able to help with the diagnosis. Similar chips could also be designed for diagnosis of periodontal diseases in near future.

PERIODONTAL VACCINE

1. Introduction
2. Active Immunization
3. Passive Immunization

INTRODUCTION

The invention and development of periodontal vaccine to prevent periodontal disease is a big advancement in the field of preventive dentistry. It is administered either parenterally, intramuscularly, subcutaneously, intradermally or orally by which the host accepts well and the antibodies reach the destined target areas. The vaccine is tested in canine-bearers and other mammals for the immune response and the inflammatory inhibition. Periodontal disease leads to destruction of the tissues and later tooth loss at an early or middle age and bone loss reduces the chances of replacement with a proper prosthesis. Administering the vaccine, in early adolescent age before there is any sign of periodontitis, helps in prolonging the healthy life of the periodontium and risk of any inflammation is reduced.

The vaccine development program involves identifying the bacterial peptides and proteins that trigger the immune response, and using these as the basis of vaccines. The vaccines are being trialled in mouse models of periodontal disease and following a positive response, a vaccine will progress to clinical trials.

Due to the prevalence of periodontitis in the populations, particularly in the developing countries, vaccines for periodontitis would be expected to be administered to large numbers of people. To limit the transmission and or intraoral dissemination of periodontopathic bacteria, it would appear advantageous for an effective vaccine to induce immunity at three levels:
- Local mucosal secretory IgA
- Local draining lymph nodes
- Circulating specific T and B cell responses

ACTIVE IMMUNIZATION

Active immunity is induced by exposure to a foreign antigen. This activates lymphocytes to produce antibodies against the antigen. The immune system of the host plays an active role in responding to the antigen. Studies in non-human primate models using ligature-induced experimental periodontitis suggest that antibody responses by active immunization against *Porphyromonas gingivalis* can safely be induced, enhanced, and obtained over time. Immune responses to whole bacterial cell and purified protein preparations considered as vaccine candidates have been evaluated in different animal models demonstrating that there are several valid vaccine candidates. Data suggest that immunization reduces the rate and severity of bone loss. It is also, temporarily, possible to alter the composition of the subgingival microflora. Natural active immunization by therapeutic interventions results in antibody titre enhancement and potentially improves treatment outcomes.

Three types of vaccines were employed for the control of periodontal disease:
- Vaccines prepared from pure cultures of *streptococci*, and other oral organism
- Autogenous vaccines were prepared fom the dental plaque of patients with destructive periodontal diseases. Plaque samples were removed and sterilized by heat by immersion in formalin solution and reinjected into same patient.
- Stock vaccines, e.g. Inava Endocorps vaccine, Goldenberg's vaccine, VanCott's vaccine.

Inava Endocarps vaccine was made of mixture of 7 microorganisms.

The future vaccine of periodontal disease will likely contain a mixture of adhesins from the most prominent periodonto – pathogens. Inhibition of the lectin results in loss of ability of the bacteria to adhere to various surfaces. The lectin is a potent immunogen but it is not known if antibodies against the lectin prevent *streptococcal* adhesion in experimental animals.

PASSIVE IMMUNIZATION

Passive immune response can be achieved by transfer of antibodies via serum, lymphocytes from immunized individuals or monoclonal antibodies against specific pathogen. Passive immunization is short-lived and remains effective only as long as the injected antibody persists. Passive immunization is thought to be comparatively safer than active immunization. Passive immunization of humans using *P. gingivalis* monoclonal antibodies temporarily prevents colonization of *P. gingivalis*. Probiotic therapy may be an alternative approach. Regulatory and safety issues for human periodontal vaccine trials must be considered. Shared infectious etiology between periodontitis and systemic diseases may enhance vaccine effort developments.

MINIMALLY INVASIVE SURGERY

1. Historical Perspective
2. Rationale of Minimally Invasive Surgical Techniques
3. Minimally Invasive Surgery (MIS)

HISTORICAL PERSPECTIVE

The need for a non instrument based description of surgical procedures was recognized in 1990 by Wickham and Fitzpatric who described techniques of using smaller incisions as "minimally invasive surgery". The term periodontal minimally invasive surgery describes a smaller more precise surgical technique for periodontal

PERIODONTICS REVISITED

surgery. Minimally invasive surgery (MIS) for periodontal bone grafting was first described by Harrel in 1999. This technique utilizes very small incisions with minimal reflection to achieve pocket depth reduction, attachment level gain with minimal recession in operated site. In 2007, Cortellini and Tonetti gave a modified surgical approach to minimally invasive surgical technique (MIST) in treating isolated intrabony defects with periodontal regeneration. Later, in 2008 they described a MIST in treatment of multiple adjacent deep intrabony defects. More recently, in 2009 Trombelli et al has described a single flap approach (SFA) in conjunction with guided tissue regeneration (GTR) for intraosseous defects characterized by an extension prevalent either on buccal or lingual side. These techniques have so far shown promising results with GTR procedures and use of materials like Emdogain.

RATIONALE OF MINIMALLY INVASIVE SURGICAL TECHNIQUES

- Reduction of surgical trauma
- Increase in flap/wound stabilization
- Improvement of primary closure of wound
- Reduction of surgical chair time
- Minimization of intraoperative and postoperative patient discomfort and morbidity
- Prevention of postoperative gingival recession

MINIMALLY INVASIVE SURGERY (MIS)

Harrel in 1999 described a technique for periodontal bone grafting using a minimally invasive surgical approach. The difference in this technique and traditional approaches was the use of much smaller incisions to gain surgical access and debride the periodontal defect prior to placing bone graft and membrane. MIS was found to be effective in terms of mean clinical attachment gain and minimal recession. Later this technique was used by same author with emdogain giving similar results. The difference of MIS from traditional approach is the technique of accessing the periodontal defect, the handling of the soft tissue flaps, the method of debridement and wound closure. The technical skills and instruments necessary to handle MIS for soft tissue access, debridement of the periodontal defect and root surfaces are different from those associated with traditional periodontal surgery.

Indications

- The ideal site for bone grafting using a MIS is usually an isolated interproximal defect that does not extend significantly beyond the interproximal site.
- Another site well suited is a periodontal defect that borders on an edentulous area.
- A less ideal site but where this technique can be used is a defect that extends to the buccal and lingual from the interproximal area.
- Can also be used for many isolated defects as long as the incision at one site does not connect with incision at other site to become a continuous incision.

Contraindications

- Generalized horizontal bone loss
- Multiple interconnected vertical defects.

Surgical Procedure

- The area intended for surgery is anesthetized with local anesthesia with epinephrine 1:100000.
- *Incisions:* Intrasulcular incisions are made on teeth adjacent to defect. These incisions should be made separately incisions and should not be continuous across the interproximal tissue. By not making these incisions continuous more interproximal papillary tissue and tissue height could be retained. Two intrasulcular incisions were connected with a single horizontal incision that is placed 2 to 3 mm from the crest of the papilla. If the surgery is being performed in an esthetic area the horizontal incision is placed in the palatal aspect of the papilla so that the shape of the papilla is preserved and the graft site is covered by soft tissue. In non-esthetic area, horizontal incision can be given either of the buccal or lingual side which ever better covers the grafted site with soft tissue.
- *Tissue reflection:* Tissue is elevated using sharp dissection with a smaller sized Orban's knife. Sharp dissection minimizes trauma to flap and preserves blood supply to the tissues. The lack of embarrassment of blood supply is reason for improved soft tissue healing and minimal post operative soft tissue changes.
- *Visualization:* Visualization of field during MIS requires some form of magnification for which surgical telescopes with magnification of minimum 3.5x are recommended. During MIS it is necessary to visualize the defect from several angles which makes the use of an operating microscope cumbersome.

- *Defect debridement:* Granulation tissue removal in MIS is significantly different from traditional surgery. Following minimal flap reflection, tip of the curette is inserted vertically into the defect with the shank held parallel to long axis of the tooth and the tip is used to remove the granulation tissue. If the curette is used in usual manner that is, with shank horizontal to long axis of the tooth, the shank will impinge and fold the small gingival flap, which may traumatize them. Remaining granulation tissue is fragmented with use of ultrasonic scaler and then removed with degranulator, a mechanical granulation tissue removal instrument. It consists of a sharpened tube that can be used as curette, a vacuum which pulls the fragmented granulation tissue and a rotating bur which cuts the granulation tissue. Vacuum removes the granulation tissue and keeps the surgical field free of blood providing better visualization. Smoothing of the root surface is accomplished in a manner similar to closed root planing. Final root planing and smoothing can be accomplished with a high speed surgical length finishing bur.

- *Placement of grafting material:* Root conditioning is optional before placing a bone graft. Any combination of grafting material with GTR membrane can be used to regenerate the defect. The graft can be placed into the defect with a modified amalgam gun. The curved tip of the amalgam gun makes it easier to enter the defect through the MIS opening. A trimmed membrane is laid over the bone graft and margins of the membrane are placed under the buccal and lingual flap. This stabilizes the graft and keeps it from escaping through incisions. Membranes that are stiff or non resorbable are probably contraindicated due to difficulty of adapting the material and the need for second stage procedure.

- *Wound closure:* A vertical mattress suture can be used to close the interproximal site. Any type of suture material can be used but 4-0 plain gut suture is usually used. The suture is placed in the body of the papilla well away from the tip of the papilla. This suture will pull the buccal and lingual tissue together at the base of the flaps. Dressing is not routinely used with MIS.

- *Postoperative care:* Postoperative instructions are given thereafter. It includes antibiotic coverage and chlorhexidine mouthwash for 1 week.

Advantages:

- MIS yields improvement in probing depths and attachment levels that are similar to those obtained with regenerative procedures utilizing a traditional surgical approach.
- There is improvement in the rate of healing since smaller incision will heal faster.
- A lesser postoperative pain and discomfort than that with a larger incision.
- Improved retention of soft tissue height and contour.
- Excellent patient acceptance to the procedure.

BIBLIOGRAPHY

Lasers

1. Bader HI. Use of lasers in periodontics. Dent Clin North Am 2000;44(4):779-91.
2. Cobb CM, Low SB, Coluzzi DJ. Lasers and the treatment of chronic periodontitis. Dent Clin North Am 2010;54(1):35-53
3. Cobb CM. Lasers in periodontics: A Review of the literature. J Periodontol 2006;77:545-64.
4. Coleton S. Lasers in surgical periodontics and oral medicine. Dent Clin North Am 2004;48(4):937-62.
5. Gimbel CB. Hard tissue laser procedures. Dent Clin North Am 2000;44(4):931-53.
6. Ishikawa I, Aoki A, Takasaki AA, Mizutani K, Sasaki KM, Izumi Y. Application of lasers in periodontics: True innovation or myth? Periodontol 2000 2009;50:90-126.
7. Midda M. The use of lasers in periodontology. Curr Opin Dent 1992;2:104-8.
8. Rossmann JA, Cobb CM. Lasers in periodontal therapy. Periodontol 2000 1995;9:150-64.
9. Schwarz F, Arweiler N, Georg T, Reich E. Desensitising effects of an Er: YAG laser on hypersensitive dentin, a controlled, prospective clinical study. J Clin Periodontol 2002;29:211-15.
10. Slot DE, Kranendonk AA, Paraskevas S, Van der Weijden F. The effect of a pulsed Nd:YAG laser in non-surgical periodontal therapy. J Periodontol 2009;80:1041-56.
11. Sun G. The role of lasers in cosmetic dentistry. Dent Clin North Am 2000;44(4):831-50.

Photodynamic Therapy

1. Dortbudak O, Haas R, Bernhart T, Mailath-Pokorny G. Lethal photosensitization for decontamination of implant surfaces in the treatment of peri-implantitis. Clin Oral Implants Res 2001;12(2):104-8.
2. Komerik N, Nakanishi H, MacRobert AJ, Henderson B, Speight P, Wilson M. *In vivo* killing of *Porphyromonas gingivalis* by toluidine blue-mediated photosensitization in an animal model. Antimicrob Agents Chemother 2003;47(3):932-40.

Tissue Engineering

1. Bartold PM, Mcculloch CAG, Narayanan AS, Pitaru S. Tissue engineering: a new paradigm for periodontal regeneration based on molecular and cell biology. Periodontol 2000 2000;24:253-69.

PERIODONTICS REVISITED

2. Bartold PM, Xiao Y, lyngstaadas SP, Paine MI, Snead MI. Principles and applications of cell delivery systems for periodontal regeneration. Periodontol 2000 2006;41:123-35.
3. Hsiong SX, Mooney DJ. Regeneration of vascularized bone. Periodontol 2000 2006;41:109-22.
4. Lynch SE, Genco RJ, Marx RE. Tissue Engineering. Applications in Maxillofacial Surgery and Periodontics. Quintessence Publishing Co. Inc. Carol Stream, IL, 1999.

Gene Therapy in Periodontics

1. Karthikeyan BV, Pradeep AR. Gene Therapy in Periodontics: A review and future implications. J Contemp Dent Pract 2006;3:83-91.
2. Lin Z, Sugai JV, Jin Q, Chandler LA, Giannobile WV. Platelet-derived growth factor-B gene delivery sustains gingival fibroblast signal transduction. J Periodont Res 2008;43:440-9.
3. Mammen B, Ramakrishnan T, Sudhakar U, Vijayalakshmi. Principles of gene therapy. Indian J Dent Res, 2007;18(4):196-200.
4. Mahale S, Dani N, Ansari SS, Kale T. Gene therapy and its implications in periodontics. J Indian Soc Periodontol 2009;13(1):1-5.
5. Wikesjö UM, Sorensen RG, Kinoshita A, Jian Li X, Wozney JM. Periodontal repair in dogs: effect of recombinant human bone morphogenetic protein-12 (rhBMP-12) on regeneration of alveolar bone and periodontal attachment. J Clin Periodontol 2004;31(8):662-70.

Nanotechnology in Periodontics

1. Mitra SB, Wu D, Holmes BN. An application of nanotechnology in advanced dental materials. J Am Dent Assoc 2003;134:1382-90.
2. Nano A. The A to Z of nanotechnology and nanomaterials. The institute of nanotechnology, Azom Co Ltd; 2003.
3. Patil M, Mehta DS, Guvva S. Future Impact of nanotechnology on medicine and dentistry. J Indian Soc Periodontol 2008;12(2):34-40.

Periodontal Vaccine

1. Booth V, Ashley FP, Lehner T. Passive immunization with monoclonal antibodies against *Porphyromonas gingivalis* in patients with periodontitis. Infect immune 1996; 64: 422-27.
2. Grant DA, Stern IB, Listgarten MA. Microbiology (Plaque). In, Periodontics CV Mosby Company 6th ed 1988;147-97.
3. Nakagawa T, Saito A, Hosaka Y, Ishihara K. Gingipains as candidate antigens for *Porphyromonas gingivalis* vaccine. Keio J Med 2003;52(3):158-62.
4. Page RC. Vaccination and periodontitis: Myth or reality. J Int Acad Periodontol 2000;2:31-43.
5. Passive immunization against dental caries and periodontal disease: Development of recombinant and human monoclonal antibodies. Crit Rev Oral Biol Med 2000;11(2):140-58.
6. Persson GR. Immune responses and vaccination against periodontal infections. J Clin Periodontol 2005;32:54-56.

Minimally Invasive Surgery

1. Cortellini P, Nieri M, Prato GP, Tonetti MS. Single minimally invasive surgical technique with an enamel matrix derivative to treat multiple adjacent intrabony defects: Clinical outcomes and patient morbidity. J Clin Periodontol 2008;35(7):605-13.
2. Cortellini P, Tonetti MS. A minimally invasive surgical technique with an enamel matrix derivative in the regenerative treatment of intra-bony defects: a novel approach to limit morbidity. J Clin Periodontol 2007;34(1):87-93.
3. Harrel SK. A minimally invasive surgical approach for periodontal regeneration: Surgical technique and observations. J Periodontol 1999;70(12):1547-57.
4. Harrel SK, Nunn ME, Belling CM. Long-term results of a minimally invasive surgical approach for bone grafting. J Periodontol 1999;70(12):1558-63.
5. Trombelli L, Farina R, Franceschetti G, Calura G. Single-flap approach with buccal access in periodontal reconstructive procedures. J Periodontol 2009;80(2):353-60.

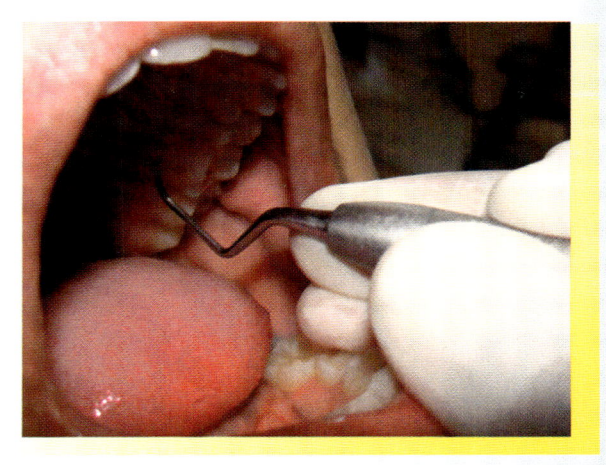

MAINTENANCE PHASE

CHAPTER 63

Supportive Periodontal Therapy (Maintenance Phase)

Shalu Bathla

INTRODUCTION

After Phase I therapy is completed, patients are placed on a schedule of periodic recall visits for maintenance care to prevent recurrence of the disease. Transfer of the patient from active treatment status to a maintenance program is a definitive step in total patient care that requires time and effort on the part of the dentist, staff and patient **(Fig. 63.1)**. Thus, the maintenance phase has been described as the cornerstone of successful periodontal therapy.

The continuing, periodic assessment and prophylactic treatment of the periodontal structures permitting early detection and treatment of new and recurring disease has been commonly referred to as periodontal maintenance or recall. The 3rd World Workshop of the American Academy of Periodontology (1989) has renamed this treatment phase as "supportive periodontal therapy" (SPT). This term expresses the essential need for therapeutic measures to support the patient's own efforts to control the periodontal infections and to avoid reinfection. Supportive periodontal therapy is considered more descriptive and, currently, is the accepted term.

AIMS OF SUPPORTIVE PERIODONTAL THERAPY

Two major aims of supportive periodontal therapy are to prevent the occurrence of new disease and to prevent the recurrence of previous disease. More specifically, the American Academy of Periodontology position paper on supportive periodontal therapy lists three goals of supportive periodontal therapy.

They are:

- to prevent or minimize the recurrence and progression of periodontal disease in patients who have been previously treated for gingivitis, periodontitis and peri-implantitis.
- to prevent or reduce the incidence of tooth loss by monitoring the dentition and any prosthetic replacements of the natural teeth.
- to increase the probability of locating and treating, in a timely manner, other diseases or conditions found within the oral cavity.

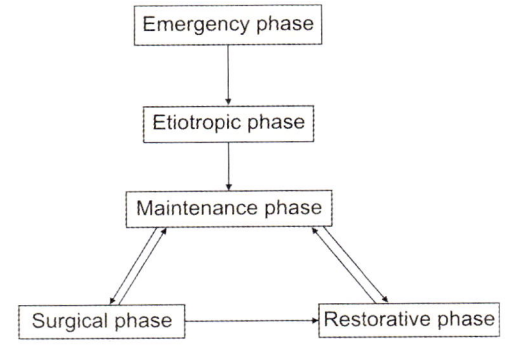

Fig. 63.1: Sequence of periodontal therapy

TABLE 63.1: Recall intervals for various classes of recall patients

Merin Classification	Characteristics	Recall interval
First year	First year patient: Routine therapy and uneventful healing or	3 months
	First year patient: Difficult case with complicated prosthesis, furcation involvement, poor crown-to-root ratios, or questionable patient cooperation.	1-2 months
Class A	Excellent results well maintained for 1 year or more.	
	Patient displays good oral-hygiene, minimal occlusal, no occlusal problems, no complicated prosthesis, no remaining pockets, and no teeth with less than 50% of alveolar bone remaining.	6 months to 1 year
Class B	Generally good results maintained reasonably well for 1 year or more, but patient displays some of the following: 1. Inconsistent or poor oral hygiene 2. Heavy calculus formation 3. Systemic disease that predisposes to periodontal breakdown 4. Some remaining pockets 5. Occlusal problems 6. Complicated prosthesis 7. Ongoing orthdontics therapy 8. Recurrent dental caries. 9. Some teeth with less than 50% of alveolar bone support 10. Smoking 11. Positive family history or genetic test	3-4 months
Class C	Generally, poor results after periodontal therapy and/or several negative factors from the following: 1. Inconsistent or poor oral hygiene 2. Heavy calculus formation 3. Systemic disease that predisposes to periodontal breakdown 4. Many remaining pockets 5. Occlusal problems 6. Complicated prosthesis 7. Recurrent dental caries 8. Periodontal surgery indicated but not performed for medical, psychologic, or financial reasons 9. Many teeth with less than 50% of alveolar bone support 10. Condition which cannot be improved by periodontal surgery 11. Smoking 12. Positive family history or genetic test 13. More than 20% of pockets bleed on probing.	1-3 months

MAINTENANCE INTERVAL

Various methods of determining maintenance intervals have been investigated. The 3-month interval is the most frequently used, but can be shortened or lengthened based on an individual patient's clinical parameters and needs (**Table 63.1**) The 3- month rationale is based on the time required for bacterial repopulation of the subgingival environment after mechanical debridement and multiple studies that have shown clinical success with this interval. A regular schedule of periodontal maintenance thus, appears critical for sustaining health.

MAINTENANCE COMPLIANCE

Patient compliance with maintenance program is an ongoing problem in dental practices and thus, various strategies for improvement have been investigated. Reasons for noncompliance have been varied and include fear, cost of therapy, type of treatment received, lack of patient motivation and smoking.

MAINTENANCE PROGRAM

The recall hour should be planned to meet the patient's individual needs. The time required for a recall visit for patients with multiple teeth in both arches is approximately 1 hour comprising of three parts **(Fig. 63.2)**.

- The first part is concerned with examination and re-evaluation of the patient's current oral health.
- The second part includes the necessary motivation, reinstructions and maintenance treatment.
- The third part involves scheduling the patient for the next recall appointment, additional periodontal treatment (polishing), or restorative dental procedures (fluoride application).

First Part (approx.10-15 min)

Examination: Periodontal examination includes an evaluation of the probing depths, bleeding on probing, mobility, the health of the gingival tissues, amount of additional recession, furcation involvement and incidence of suppuration. Determining the percentage of sites with bleeding on probing can be helpful and repeated site-specific bleeding on probing may indicate an individual area of periodontal breakdown. Any desired microbial monitoring can be accomplished at this stage of the appointment. The therapist is continually re-evaluating the success of the periodontal therapy and determining future maintenance procedures with the assessment of these clinical parameters.

Radiographs: Periodic vertical bitewing radiographs are taken to monitor for any radiographic bone loss or caries; these radiographs are compared with previous radiographs. During maintenance therapy, a full mouth series of radiographs may be beneficial approximately every 5 years to be able to accomplish a complete radiographic evaluation. If general periodontal deterioration is noted from the clinical parameters, then radiographs can be ordered at any appointment. Conversely, if the patient maintains excellent periodontal stability, a full-mouth series of radiographs may not be needed every 5 years.

A plaque assessment using disclosing solution can indicate areas that the patient consistently misses in their daily hygiene regimen and may indicate a needed change in patient hygiene techniques or instrumentation.

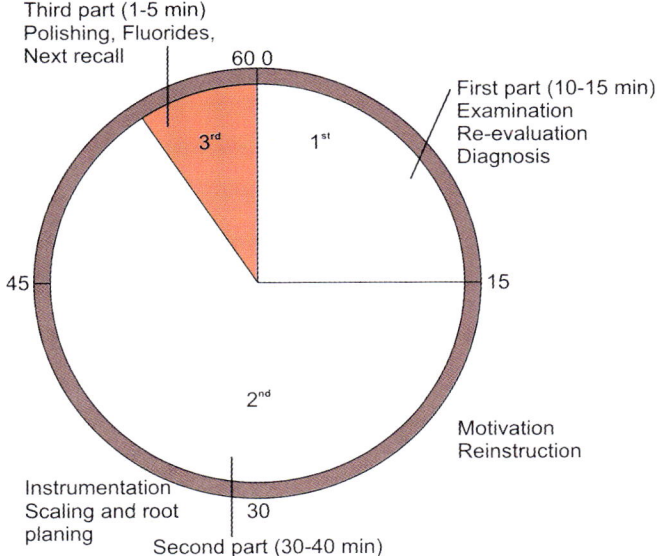

Fig. 63.2: Maintenance program SPT recall hours divided into three parts

Second Part (approx. 30-40 min)

Patients frequently need reinforcement of instructions and motivation to continue diligent oral hygiene. An overall increase in gingival inflammation with a generalized increase in the bleeding index may indicate continual poor patient oral hygiene efficiency. A significant increase in the bleeding index with an acceptable plaque index at the maintenance appointment may indicate that the patient had performed adequate oral hygiene for only a few days before the appointment.

Debridement procedures including scaling, root planing, and polishing vary depending on the clinical parameters and any presence of deteriorating sites. If significant deposits of subgingival calculus are detected, this may indicate a need for nonsurgical retreatment of selected areas. If multiple sites are found to need additional scaling and root planing, the patient may need to be re-appointed for additional treatment because the actual time for debridement during a maintenance visit is limited.

In some instances, a locally delivered antimicrobial agent may be indicated. Topical fluoride treatment for caries prevention is often indicated. Caries and restoration assessments are accomplished at every appointment because exposed root surfaces resulting from periodontal disease can be at risk for root caries.

PERIODONTICS REVISITED

Third Part (approx. 1-5 min)

Scheduling the patient for the next recall must be based on the patient's risk assessment. Polishing the entire dentition to remove all remaining soft deposits and stains provides freshness to the patient and facilitates the diagnosis of early carious lesions. Following polishing, fluorides should be applied in high concentration in order to replace the fluorides which might have been removed by instrumentation from the superficial layers of the teeth. Fluoride or chlorhexidine varnishes may also be applied to prevent root surface caries, especially in areas with gingival recession.

RETREATMENT OF SELECTED AREAS

During the maintenance visit, areas of periodontal breakdown may be indicated by increasing probing depth, increased attachment loss, increase in bleeding on probing, radiographic bone loss, progressing mobility. The various causes for recurrence of periodontal disease are:

- Inadequate plaque control on the part of the patient or failure to comply with recommended SPT schedules
- Inadequate or insufficient treatment that has failed to remove all the potential factors favoring plaque accumulation
- Inadequate restorations placed after the periodontal treatment was completed
- Failure of the patient to return for periodic checkup
- Presence of some systemic diseases that may affect host resistance to previously acceptable levels of plaque.

Treatment schedule vary depending on the following findings:

- If the cause of the generalized breakdown is poor patient plaque control, then surgical therapy should be delayed until nonsurgical therapy is reaccomplished and an adequate plaque control level is maintained by the patient.
- Retreatment of a single failing site will generally include scaling and root planing, with or without local drug delivery. If the area has not responded by the next maintenance appointment, localized surgical therapy may be necessary.

- If health of multiple adjacent sites is not improving, surgical therapy in the area often is indicated.
- If there is a generalized loss of attachment detected, a thorough analysis for any possible systemic disease should be accomplished. At this retreatment, systemic antibiotics may be considered as an adjunct to the scaling and root planing of the affected areas, with reevaluation for any possible surgical intervention
- If increasing mobility is detected, a thorough occlusal evaluation should be done to determine if any occlusal adjustment is necessary.

MAINTENANCE FOR IMPLANT PATIENT

Explained in Chapter no. 61 Peri-implantitis.

PONITS TO PONDER

✓ The goals of periodontal and maintenance therapies are identical i.e healthy, comfortable, esthetic and functional dentition with stable probing depths.
✓ The maintenance appointment consists of data collection and the re-evaluation of all clinical parameters.
✓ Retreatment is needed at times and is considered a part of the maintenance phase of periodontal therapy.

BIBLIOGRAPHY

1. Axelson P, Lindhe J. The significance of maintenance care in the treatment of periodontal disease. J Clin Periodontol 1981;8:281-84.
2. Becker W, Berg L, Becker B. Untreated periodontal disease: a longitudinal study. J Periodontol 1979; 50:234-44.
3. Lang NP, Bragger U, Salvi G, Tonetti MS. Supportive Periodontal Therapy. In, Lindhe J, Karring T, Lang NP. Clinical Periodontology and Implant dentistry. 4th ed Blackwell Munksgaard 2003;781-808.
4. Merin RL. Supportive Periodontal Treatment. In, Newman, Takei, Carranza. Clinical Periodontology 9th ed WB Saunders 2003;966-77.
5. Rapley JW. Periodontal and Dental Implant Maintenance. In, Rose LF, Mealey BL, Genco RJ, Cohen DW. Periodontics, Medicine, Surgery and Implants. Elsevier Mosby 2004;263-275.
6. The American Academy of Periodontology: Supportive periodontal therapy (AAP Position Paper). J Periodontol 1998; 69:502-06.

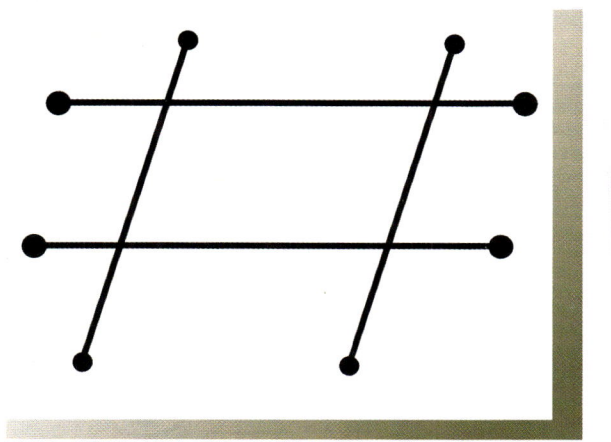

SECTION ELEVEN

MISCELLANEOUS

Miscellaneous

Shalu Bathla

STERILIZATION

BASIC PERSONAL PROTECTIVE BARRIER EQUIPMENTS

Basic personal protective barrier equipment (PPE) include face mask, protective eyewear, gloves and clinical gown (Fig. 64.1). Facemask should be positioned first when preparing for clinical care procedure, then the protective eyewear and after that hands are washed/scrubbed prior to gloving.

PPE application sequence	PPE removal sequence
1. Eye wear	1. Gloves
2. Facemask	2. Facemask
3. Gloves	3. Eye wear

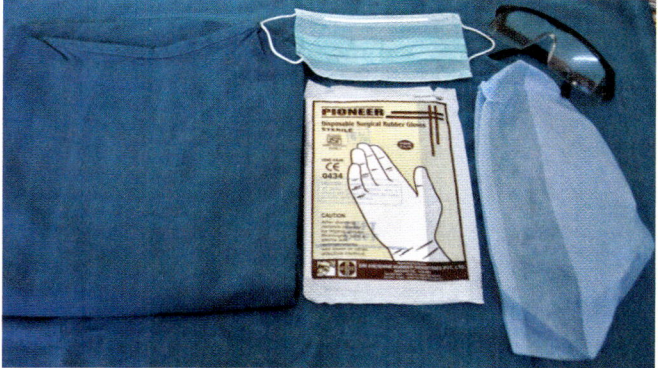

Fig. 64.1: Personal protective equipments

Facemask

Do's and Do not's while wearing facemask

Do's
- ✓ Adjust the mask and position the eyewear before scrub/handwash
- ✓ Should fit snugly with no gaps
- ✓ Change mask each hour or more frequently when it becomes wet
- ✓ Use fresh mask for each patient
- ✓ Grasp side elastic or tie strings to remove.

Do not's
- × Do not wear mask only over mouth (but also on nose)
- × Never place the mask under chin
- × Never handle the outside of a contaminated mask with gloved/barehands
- × Mask should not be worn longer than 1 hour
- × Should not leave the treatment area with the mask hanging around the neck.

Handwashing

Three methods: Short scrub, short standard handwash and surgical scrub.

Jewellery should be removed. Brushes should be used for cleaning finger nails. A scrubbing up time of 3–5 minutes with chlorhexidine soap or povidone iodine soap is utilized; the former is a broad spectrum rapidly active agent with persistent activity, whereas the latter has a relatively short duration. The technique should include a thorough washing of hands up to the elbows, with removal of the soap in the direction hand to elbow. Excess soap is not required but a steady and methodical method of massage is important, and adequate drying is again essential.

Gloves

The various types of gloves are:
i. *Examination or procedure gloves:* Available as:
   a. Sterile or non-sterile latex.
   b. Vinyl latex–free synthetic.
ii. *Over gloves:* These are thin vinyl or copolymer gloves placed over examination glove to prevent cross contamination, e.g. to retrieve additional supplies from a drawer, use a pen to make treatment notation or press button during X-ray taking.

iii. *Utility gloves:* These are heavy gloves worn during handling of any chemicals or infectious waste; cleaning of contaminated surfaces instruments or materials and environmental surface. Gloves made of nitrite rubber have an increased resistance to instrument punctures and can be autoclaved.
iv. *Dermal under gloves:* These gloves are worn to reduce irritation from latex or non-latex.

Procedure of wearing gloves **(Figs 64.2A to G)**
  i. Right hand grasps inside cuff surface of left glove.
  ii. Left glove is pulled into place.
 iii. Gloved fingers of left hand are inserted into cuff (outer surface) of right glove
 iv. Right glove is pulled into place.
  v. Cuff of left glove is unfolded.

Procedure of removal of gloves **(Figs 64.3A and B)**
  i. Use left fingers to pinch right glove near edge to fold back.

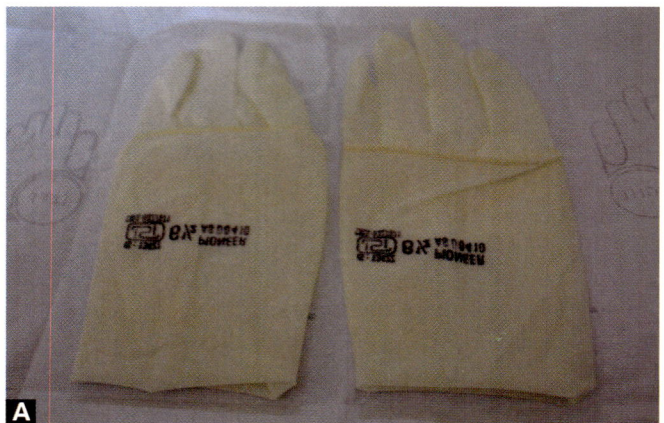

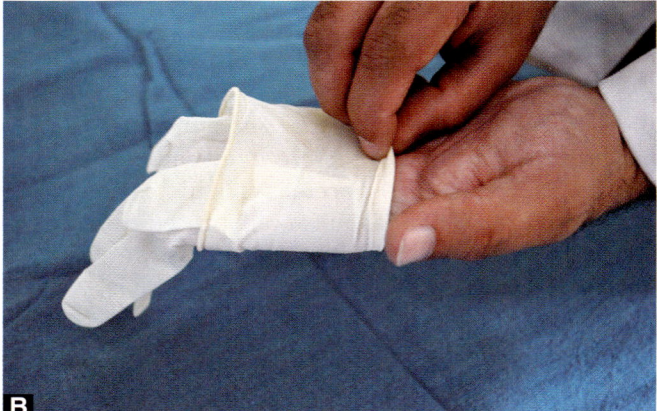

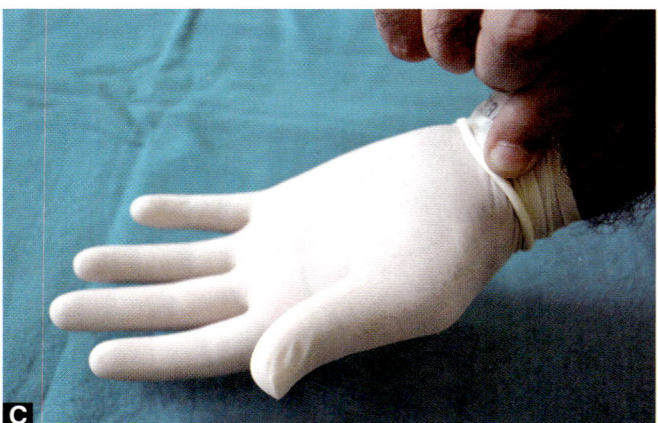

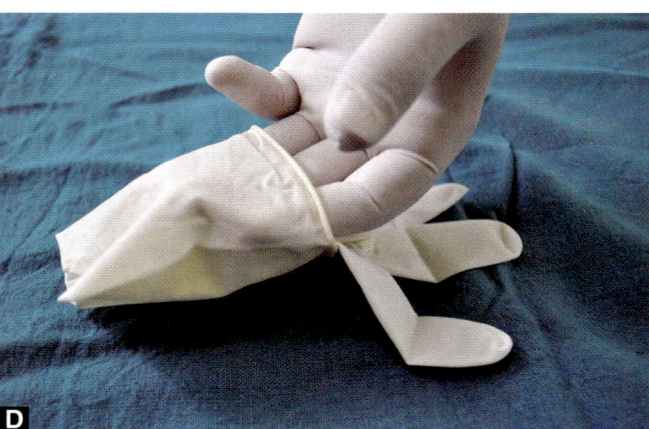

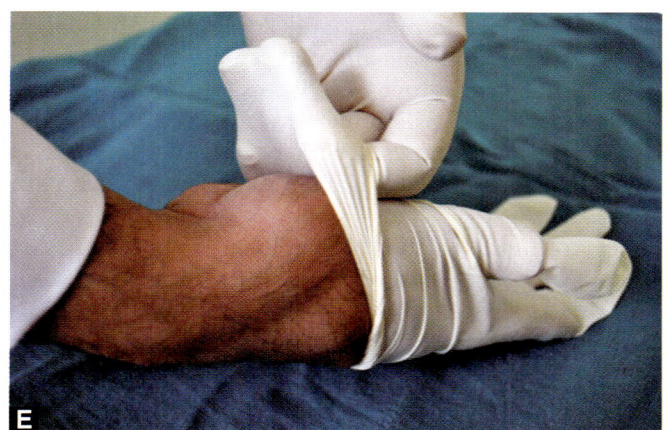

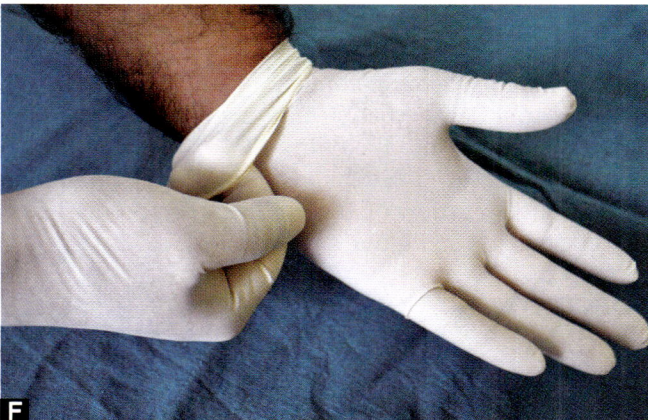

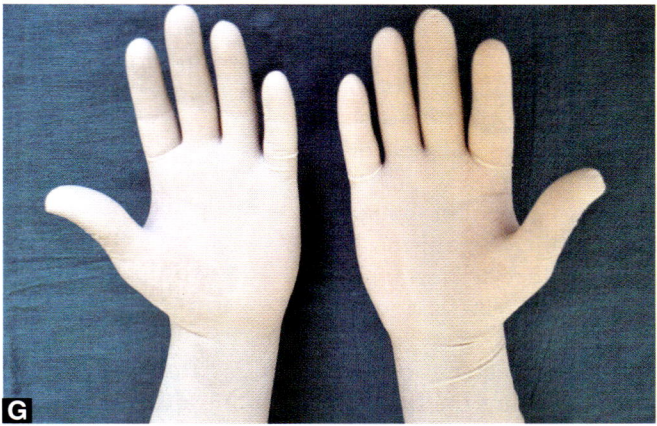

Figs 64.2A to G: Wearing of gloves

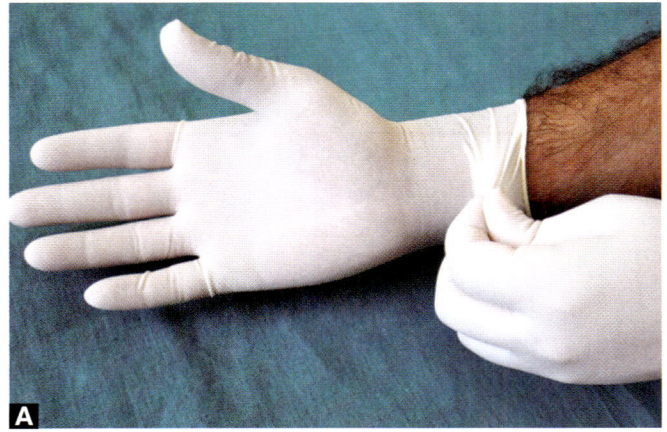

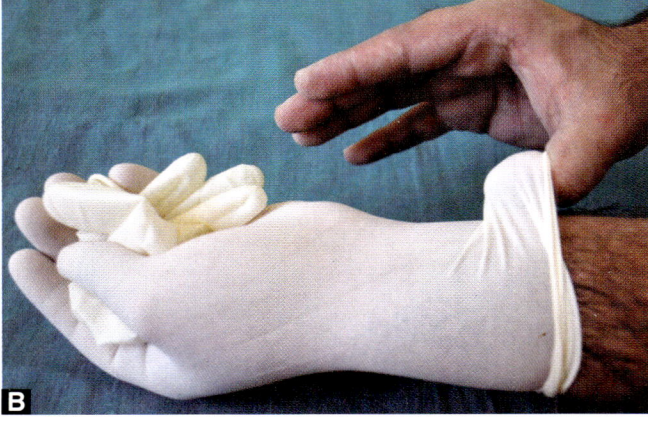

Figs 64.3A and B: Removing of gloves

ii. Fold edge back without contact with clean inside surface.
iii. Use right fingers to contact outside of left glove at the wrist to invert and remove.
iv. Bunch glove into the palm.
v. With ungloved left hand, grasp inner noncontaminated portion of the right glove to peel it off, enclosing other glove as it is inverted.

DECONTAMINATION OF DENTAL INSTRUMENTS (FIG. 64.4)

Dental instruments that are laid out for use during the day must be cleaned and sterilized at the end of the day, whether or not they are actually used. Just by placing out the instruments in a dental office, they can collect bacteria and other contaminants that could spread to a patient if they are used without proper cleaning and treatment. They must be properly cleaned, sterilized and stored in order to prepare them for future use.

- Cleaning is a process which removes contamination but does not necessarily destroy microorganisms. It is an essential prerequisite of decontaminating equipment before sterilization or disinfection is undertaken.
- Sterilization results in complete destruction or removal of all viable microorganisms including spores and viruses. In practice, it may be difficult to establish. The term is usually applied to solid objects, such as instruments and equipment, but not to skin.
- Disinfection reduces the number of viable microorganisms but will not necessarily inactivate viruses and bacterial spores. It may be classified into:
  a. *High level:* which is cidal to spores, bacteria and viruses;
  b. *Medium:* which is cidal to bacteria and viruses;
  c. *Low:* which is cidal to only bacteria and viruses of low resistance.

It is applicable to delicate instruments that will be damaged by sterilization.

The efficiency of decontamination depends on:
a. The nature of microorganisms
b. The load of microorganisms
c. The duration of exposure to the agent
d. The temperature

Steps to Sterilize Dental Instruments

Step 1: Clean the dental instruments manually or through mechanical means like a thermal washer disinfector or an ultrasonic bath. They should be immersed in lukewarm water, scrubbed below the water surface and then rinsed.

Step 2: Afterward cleaning through either manual or mechanical means, the dental instruments should be dried with a disposable cloth.

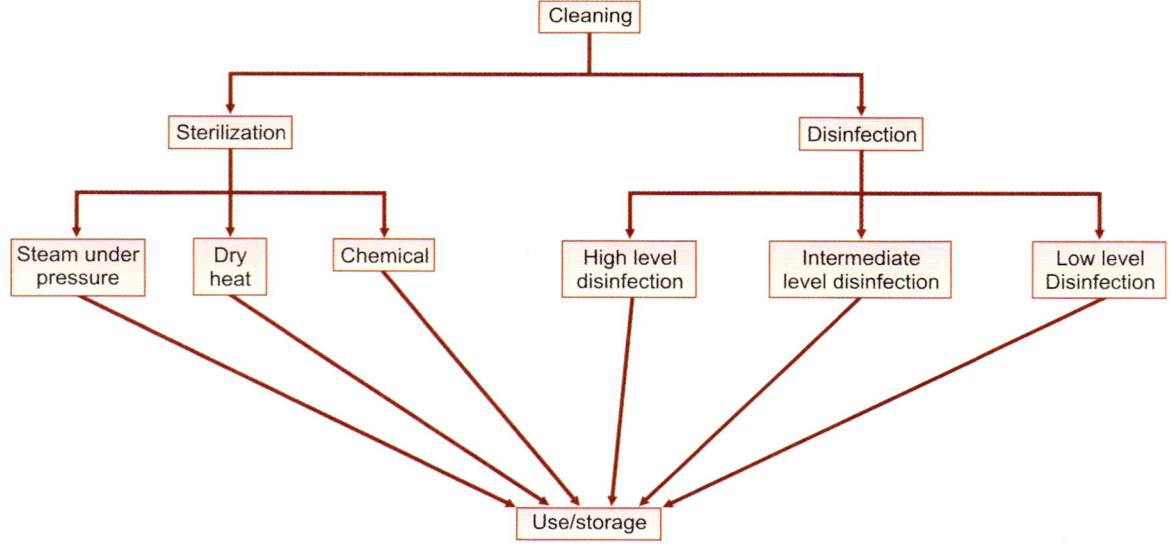

Fig. 64.4: Decontamination steps

Step 3: Pack the dried items into medical grade sterilization wraps or sterilization cassettes to prepare them for sterilization. They must be properly packed before they are loaded into the heat sterilization unit.

Step 4: Sterilize the instruments using a heat, steam, or chemical process. Heat is the usual method used in a dental setting. Use sterilization equipment that is approved by the Food and Drug Administration for dental sterilization work and operate it according to the manufacturer's specific instructions.

Step 5: Store the sterilized instruments in their intact packaging. According to the Centers for Disease Control, the packaging must remain sealed and undamaged in order to retain sterile nature of the instrument. If the packaging gets wet, tears or is damaged in some way, the instrument should be sterilized again through the same process.

Dental assistants are often responsible for preparing treatment rooms before and after each patient, by cleaning and disinfecting surfaces and for instrument cleaning, disinfection and sterilization. Unless the appropriate product for the task is selected, the results can potentially be damaging to instruments and equipment and dangerous for both health care workers and their patients.

Patient care items are categorized as critical, semicritical and noncritical **(Fig. 64.5)**.

a. *Critical objects:* These items penetrate or contact soft tissue, bone and bloodstream. They are sterilized or disposed. Examples, include periodontal scalers, forceps, scalpels and surgical burs.

b. *Semi-critical objects:* These items typically contact mucous membranes and non-intact skin. They are sterilized or high level disinfected. Examples include such items as handpieces, mouth mirrors, reusable impression trays, ultrasonic handpiece and radiographic biteblock.

c. *Noncritical objects:* These objects do not touch mucous membrane, e.g. light handles, safety eyewear, X-ray machine parts. They are disinfected.

Sterilization Methods and their Applications

Objects	Methods of sterilization
1. Disposable syringes	Gamma radiations Ethylene oxide
2. Nondisposable syringes	Autoclave Hot air oven Infrared radiation
3. Glasswares	Autoclave Hot air oven
4. Metal instruments (Scalers, curettes)	Autoclave Hot air oven Infrared radiation
5. Operation theatre, inoculation hood and cubical entrance	Ultraviolet radiation

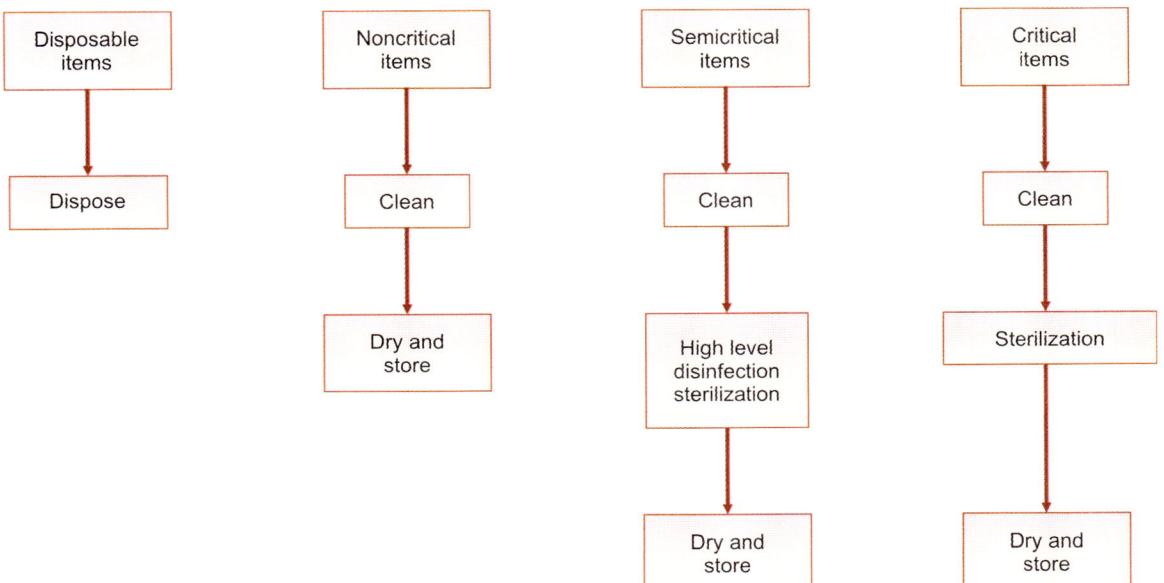

Fig. 64.5: Sterilization of critical, semicritical and noncritical items

DISCOVERIES IN PERIODONTICS

	Year		*Discovery/Invention*
1.	1535	Paracelsus	Introduced the term tartar and developed doctrine of calculus
2.	1815	Levi Spear Parmly	Invented dental floss
3.	1823	Alphonse Toirac	Gave the term Pyorrhea alveolaris
4.	1844	Gunnel	First reported Pericoronitis
5.	1846	William Sharpey	Described Sharpey's fibers
6.	1868	Paul Langerhan	Described Langerhans cell
7.	1875	Friedrich Sigmund	Described merkel cells.
8.	1877	Wilkerson	First hydraulic dental chair
9.	1882	Metchnikoff	Discovered the mechanism of phagocytosis
10.	1884	Robiecsek	Gingivectomy with straight incision
11.	1885	Malassez	First described epithelial rests of Malassez cell
12.	1897	Vincentini	Described Corncob structure of plaque
13.	1898	GV Black	First used the term plaque in dental context
14.	1899	Talbot	Intially proposed Bass method of toothbrushing
15.	1914	Grace Rogers Splading and Gillette Hayden	Founded American Academy of Periodontology
16.	1918	Leonard Widman	Described original Widman flap procedure
17.	1918	Zentler	Described gingivectomy with scalloped incision
18.	1923	Hegedus	First used bone grafts for reconstruction of bone defects produced by periodontal disease
19.	1923	Dr Abraham Wesley Ward	Introduced Periodontal dressing Wonder Pack
20.	1923	Gottlieb	Introduced the term diffuse atrophy of alveolar bone
21.	1928	Gottlieb	Introduced the term deep cementopathia
22.	1931	Kirkland	Described modified flap operation
23.	1932	Prinz	Coined the term chronic desquamative gingivitis
24.	1932	Paul R Stillman	Described Stillman toothbrushing technique
25.	1934	Alfred Fones	Described circular toothbrushing technique known as Fones method
26.	1935	William J Charters	Described Charters toothbrushing method
27.	1938	Dupont	Created nylon toothbrush bristle
28.	1938	Wannenmacher	Introduced the term Periodontitis marginalis progressive
29.	1940	Thoma and Goldman	Introduced the term Paradontosis
30.	1942	Orban and Weinmann	Introduced the term Periodontosis
31.	1950	Nathan Friedman	Gave the term Mucogingival surgery
32.	1951	Goldman	Introduced the term Gingivoplasty
33.	1954	Nabers	Developed Apically repositioned flap
34.	1955	Friedman	Introduced the term Osteoplasty
35.	1956	Grupe and Warren	Originally described Laterally displaced flap
36.	1956	Russell	Developed Periodontal index
37.	1957	Ariaudo and Tyrrell	Later modified the apically repositioned flap
38.	1959	Ramfjord	Introduced Periodontal disease index
39.	1959	Cohen	First described Col

40.	1960	Green and Vermillion	Developed Oral hygiene index
41.	1961	Garguilo	Found biologic width to be 2.04 mm
42.	1962	Friedman	Proposed the term Apically repositioned flap
43.	1962	Schroder	Described antiplaque property of chlorhexidine
44.	1962	Gross Lapiere	Discovered MMPs in the tail of metamorphosing tadpole
45.	1963	Bjorn	Intially described free gingival autograft
46.	1963	Brannstrom	Gave Hydrodynamic theory of Dentin hypersensitivity
47.	1964	Silness and Loe	Developed Plaque index
48.	1964	Green and Vermillion	Gave Simplified oral hygiene index (OHI-S)
49.	1964	Simring and Goldberg	First described relationship between periodontal and pulpal disease
50.	1965	Ewen	Introduced bone swaging as autogenous bone grafting
51.	1966	Nabers	Introduced gingival grafts
52.	1967	Marshall Urist	Discovered bone morphogenetic protein (BMP)
53.	1967	Chaput et al	Introduced the term Juvenile periodontitis
54.	1968	Cohen and Ross	First described Double papilla procedure
55.	1968	Podshadley and Haley	Developed Patient hygiene performance (PHP) index
56.	1969	Robinson	Devised Osseous coagulum technique as autogenous bone grafting
57.	1969	L Hench	Invented Bioactive glass
58.	1971	Jones	Coined the term Corncob structure of plaque
59.	1971	Muhlemann and son	Developed Sulcus bleeding index (SBI)
60.	1972	Diem et al	Described Bone Blend as autogenous bone grafting technique
61.	1972	O'Leary, Drake and Naylor	Developed Plaque control record index
62.	1974	Ramfjord and Nissle	Modified Widman Flap procedure
63.	1974	Ingber	Gave the concept of forced orthodontic eruption for treatment of one wall and two wall osseous defects
64.	1975	Bernimoulin	Gave two step procedure free gingival graft followed by coronally positioned flap
65.	1975	Ainamo and Bay	Developed Gingival bleeding index (GBI)
66.	1978	Dr Paul	Gave Keyes technique/Keyes salt – out technique
67.	1979	Max Goodson et al	Developed controlled intrapocket antimicrobial drug deliveries
68.	1979	Maynard andWilson	Coined the term marginal tissue recession
69.	1979	Jan Lindhe et al	First introduced the concept of host modulation therapy
70.	1982	Nyman et al	Pioneered GTR technique
71.	1985	Langer and Langer	Described Subepithelial connective tissue graft
72.	1985	Takei	Gave Papilla Preservation technique
73.	1986	Gottlow	Coined the term GTR
74.	1986	Tarnow	Described Semilunar coronally positioned flap
75.	1987	Nelson	Described Subpedicle connective tissue graft
76.	1993	Miller	Proposed Periodontal plastic surgery
77.	1999	Prosser	Discovered Quorum sensing in biofilms
78.		McCall and Box	Introduced the term Periodontitis
79.		WH Hanford and CO Patten	Invented periodontal probe
80.		Gibbon and Nygaard	Discovered Interspecies coaggregation of plaque
81.		PiniPrato	Described GTR for root coverage in recession
82.		Edel	Originally described free connective tissue autograft

PERIODONTICS REVISITED

83.	Klingsberg	Reported the application of Sclera as nonbone graft material
84.	Kwan and Lekovic	Described periosteum as GTR material
85.	Rateitschak	Described Accordion technique of free gingival autografts
86.	Han and associates	Developed Strip technique of free gingival autografts
87.	Friedman	Described Beveled flap
88.	Edlan and Mejchar	Described Vestibular extension technique
89.	David Sackett	Gave the term Evidence based dentistry
90.	Scandinavian group	Jens Waerhaug and coworkers
91.	Michigan group	Ramfjord and coworkers
92.	Gothenburg group	Lindhe and coworkers

WORDS WITH PREFIX "PERIO" USED IN PERIODONTICS

1. *Perio-Aid:* It is a toothpick holder, which is one of the most effective aids available for cleaning exposed furcation after periodontal therapy.

2. *Perioalert:* Immunoassay to detect serum antibodies to specific bacterial pathogens, monocytes response to LPS and peripheral neutrophil function. Site of sample is peripheral blood.

3. *Periocare:* It is a zinc oxide noneugenol periodontal dressing available in the form of paste - gel and setting occurs by chemical reaction. Paste consists of zinc oxide, calcium hydroxide, magnesium oxide and vegetable oils; Gel consists of resins, fatty acid, ethyl cellulose, lanolin and calcium hydroxide.

4. *Periocheck:* It is rapid chair side test kit developed to detect neutral proteases in GCF.

5. *Periochip:* Periochip is a small, pale orange chip of baby's thumb nail 4 mm x 5 mm x 350 µm size, weighing 7.4 mg. The prescription chip contains 2.5 mg of Chlorhexidine gluconate, of a biodegradable hydrolyzed gelatin matrix, cross linked with glutaraldehyde and also containing glycerin and water.

6. *PerioCline:* It is subgingival delivery system of 2% Minocycline hydrochloride in syringable gel suspension formulation.

7. *Periodex:* 0.12% Chlorhexidine gluconate.

8. *Periodontometer:* Instrument used for detecting tooth mobility.

9. *Periogard:* Rapid chair side test kit for Aspartate aminotransferase (AST). GCF collected is placed in Tromethamine hydrochloride buffer is allowed to react with mixture of L-aspartic and α-Ketoglutaric acids for 10 minutes. If AST is present the aspartate and α-glutarate are catalyzed to oxalacetate and glutamate.

10. *PerioGard:* 0.12% Chlorhexidine gluconate.

11. *PerioGlass:* Bioactive glass alloplast consisting of sodium and calcium salts, phosphates, silicon dioxide of irregular particles of 90-170 µm.

12. *Periograft:* Nonporous hydroxyapatite alloplast.

13. *Periopac:* It is premixed zinc oxide non-eugenol dressings. It contains calcium phosphate, zinc oxide, acrylate, organic solvents, flavouring and coloring agents, when this material is exposed to air or moisture, it sets by the loss of organic solvents.

14. *Periopaper:* It is blotter on which GCF is collected.

15. *PerioPik:* Tip used for subgingival irrigation. It is a rigid metal cannula inserted into the pocket to release irrigant for subgingival irrigation performed by an oral health professional before scaling, simultaneously with scaling or directly after scaling.

16. *Perioplaner/Periopolisher:* Powered devices for removal of plaque and calculus with reciprocating motion.

17. *Perio-probe:* Electronic probe with a tip diameter of 0.5 mm and uses standardized probing force of 0.3-0.4 N.

18. *Perioscan:* It is chair side diagnostic kit using BANA reaction to identify *Tannerella forsythia*, *P.gingivalis*, *Treponema denticola* and *Capnocytophaga species*.

19. *Perioscopy:* It consists of 0.99 mm-diameter reusable fiber optic endoscope over, which is, fitted a disposable sterile sheath. The new fiber optic endoscope instrument fits into specially designed periodontal explorers with 24-46 power magnification and fiber optic illumination, this device allows clear visualization into deep subgingival pockets and in furcations.

20. *Periostat:* It is subantimicrobial dose of Doxycycline hyclate capsule of 20 mg prescribed for patients with chronic periodontitis twice daily.

21. *PerioTemp:* It is probe, which detects pocket temperature differences of 0.1°C from a referenced subgingival temperature. It consists of copper-nickel thermocouple connected to a digital thermometer attached to metal probe.

22. *Periotest:* It is device for determining tooth mobility by measuring the reaction of the periodontium to a defined percussion force which is applied to the tooth and delivered by a tapping instrument. Periotest scale ranges from − 8 to + 50:

PERIODONTICS REVISITED

- − 8 to 9 —— Clinically firm teeth
- 10 to 19 —— First distinguishable sign of movement
- 20 to 29 —— Crown deviates within 1 mm of its normal position
- 30 to 50 —— Mobility is readily observed

23. *PERIO-TOR:* These are the instrument tips for scaling and root planing causing minimal removal of tooth structures.
24. *Periotriever:* Highly magnetized instruments designed for retrieval of broken instrument tips from the periodontal pocket.
25. *Periotron:* It is the electronic machine used for measuring the amount of fluid or GCF collected on filter paper.
26. *Perio 2000 System:* Diamond probe is a recently developed instrument, which combines the features of a periodontal probe with the Silver sulfide sensor for detection of volatile sulphur compounds.
27. *Periowave™:* It is a photodynamic disinfection system developed by Ondine Biopharma Corporation that utilizes low intensity lasers and wavelength-specific, light-activated compounds to specifically target and destroy microbial pathogens and reduce the symptoms of disease. The photosensitive compounds are topically applied in the gingival sulcus and the laser is used to activate the compounds and complete the disinfection.
28. *Periodontology:* The science that deals with the structures and behavior of the periodontium in health and disease.
29. *Periodontics:* The branch of dentistry concerned with prevention and treatment of periodontal diseases.

Annexures

ANATOMICAL FEATURES OF NORMAL GINGIVA

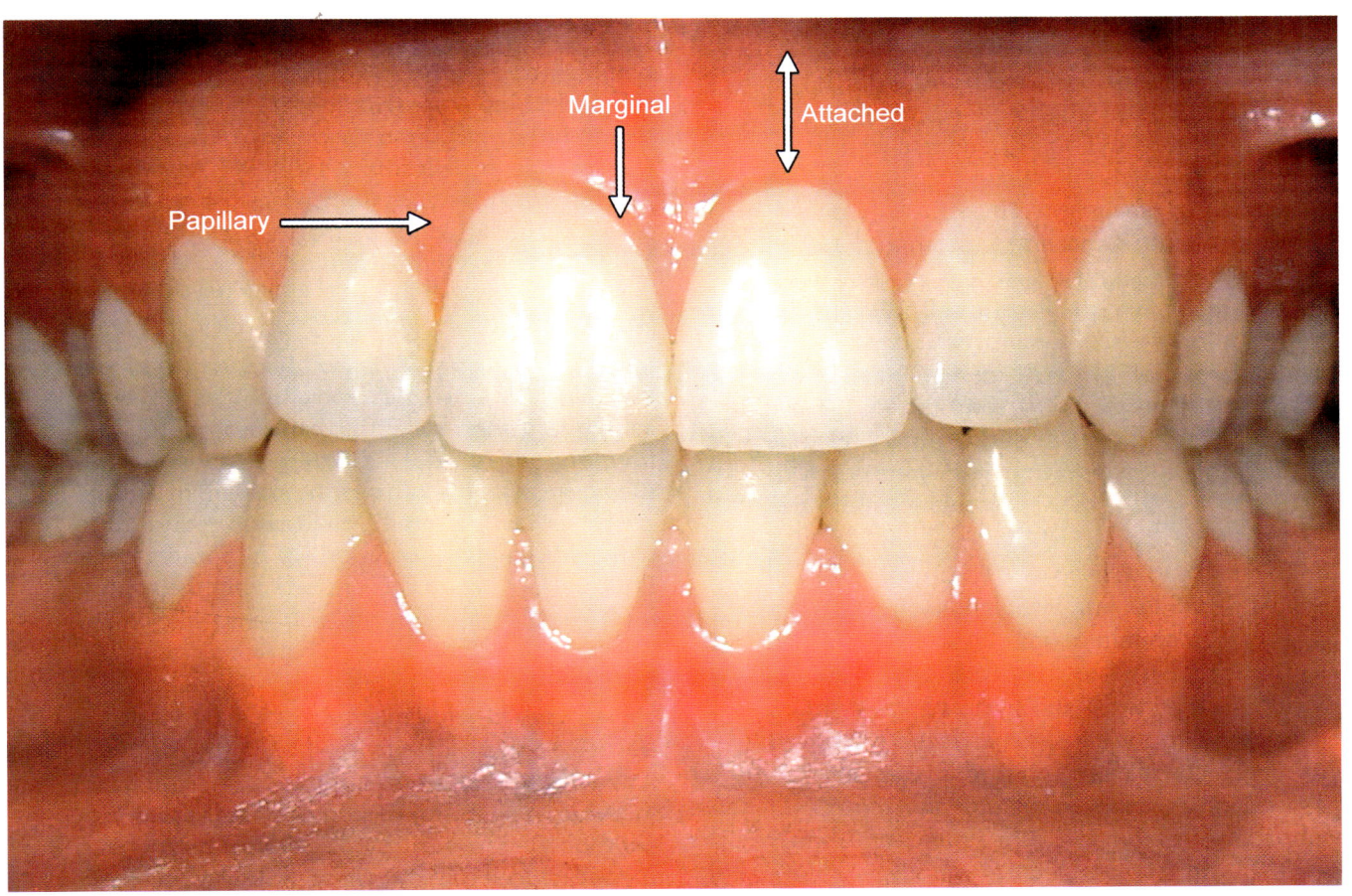

1. Marginal Gingiva
2. Papillary/Interdental Gingiva
3. Attached Gingiva

PREPARING THE SURGICAL PERIODONTAL PACK

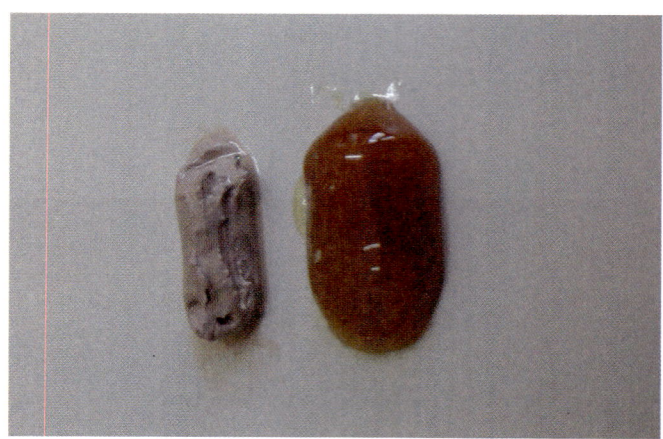

Fig. 1: Equal lengths of two pastes are placed on paper pad

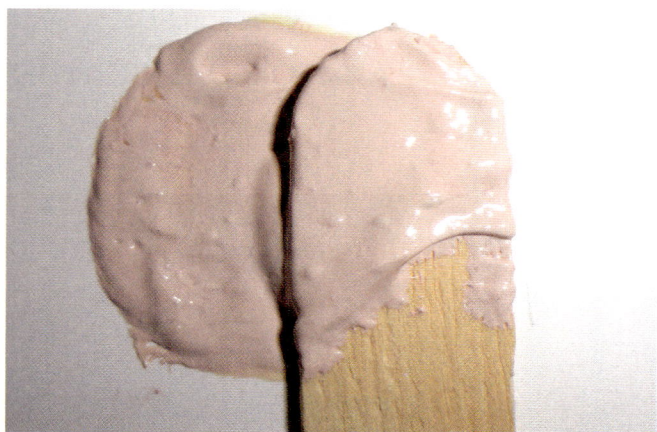

Fig. 2: Pastes are uniformly mixed with wooden tongue depressor

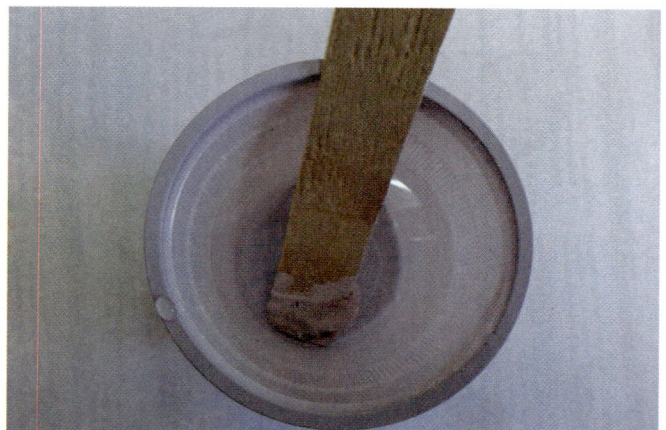

Fig 3: Paste is placed in a cup of water at room temperature to lose its tackiness

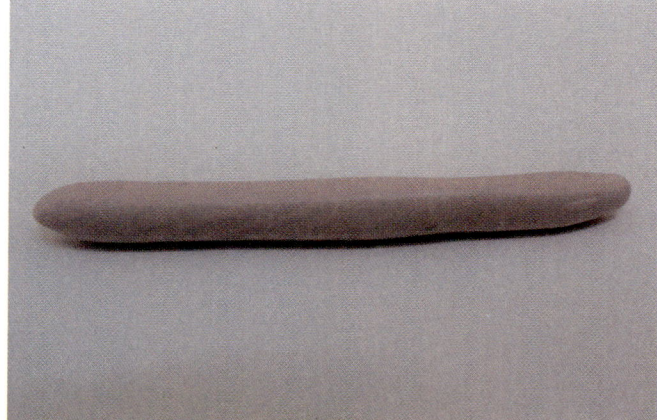

Fig. 4: Paste is rolled into cylinder with lubricated fingers

GINGIVECTOMY PROCEDURE

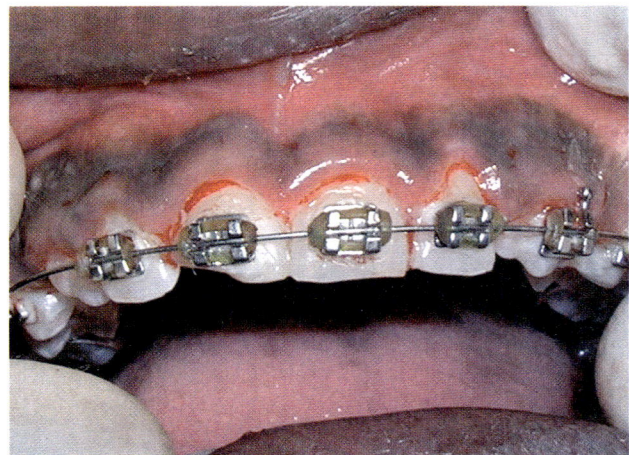

Fig. 1: Bleeding points marked

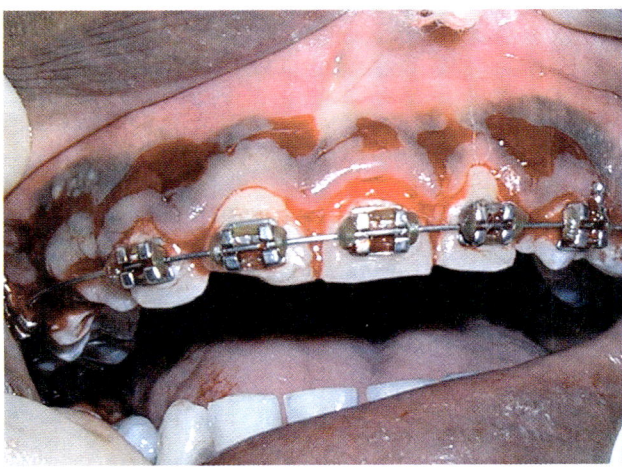

Fig. 2: External bevel incision given

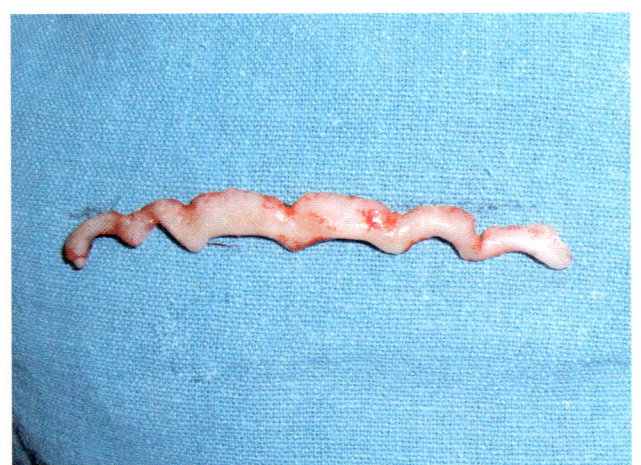

Fig. 3: Cervical wedge tissue removed

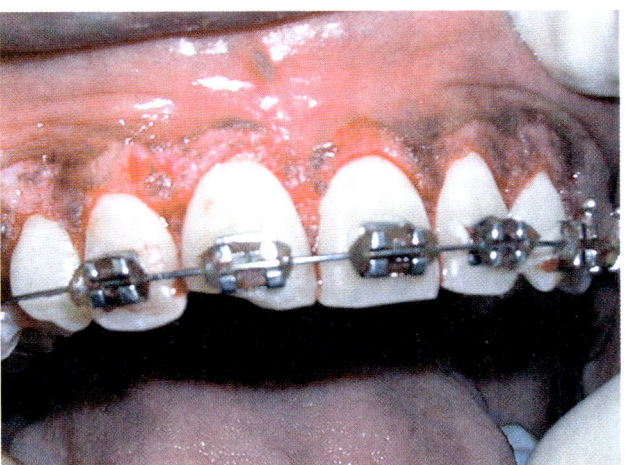

Fig. 4: After removal of excess tissue and gingivoplasty

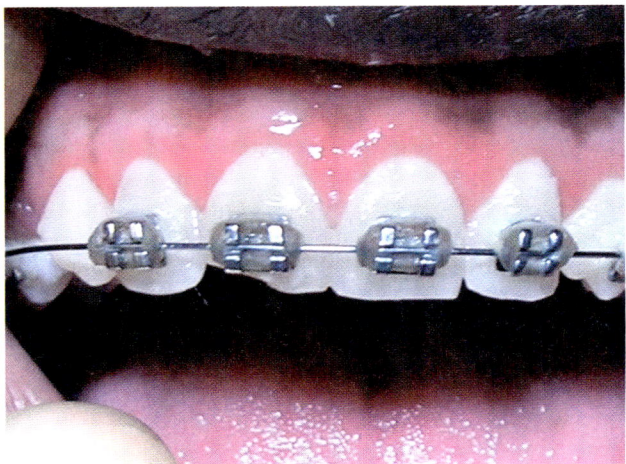

Fig. 5: Postoperatively after 2 weeks of gingivectomy procedure

PAPILLA PRESERVATION FLAP PROCEDURE

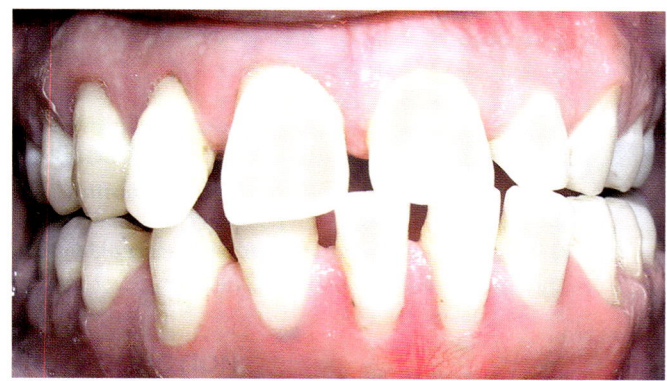

Fig. 1: Preoperative photograph showing diastema

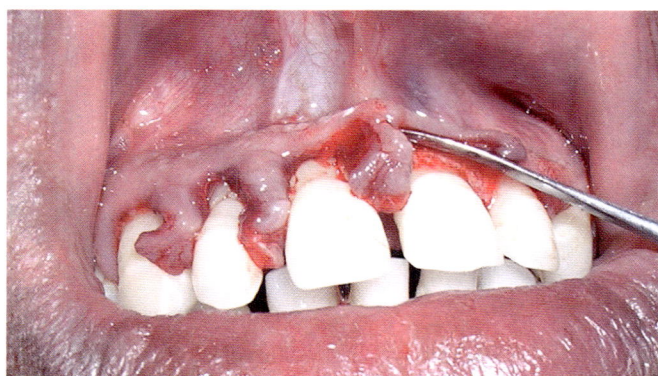

Fig. 2: Facial view after flap reflection

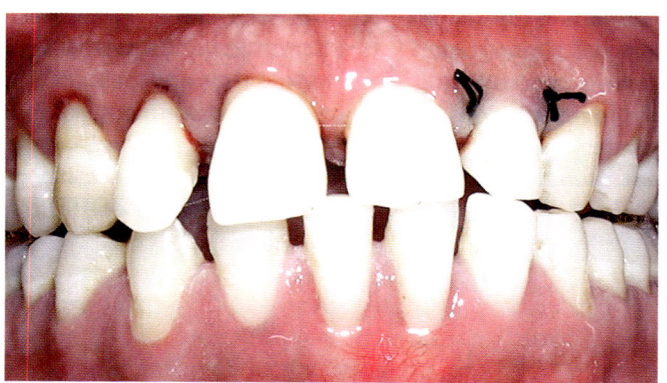

Fig. 3: Facial view after suturing

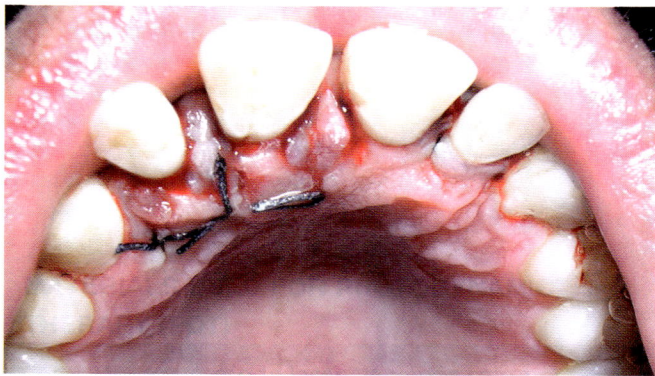

Fig. 4: Palatal view after suturing

LATERAL PEDICLE FLAP PROCEDURE

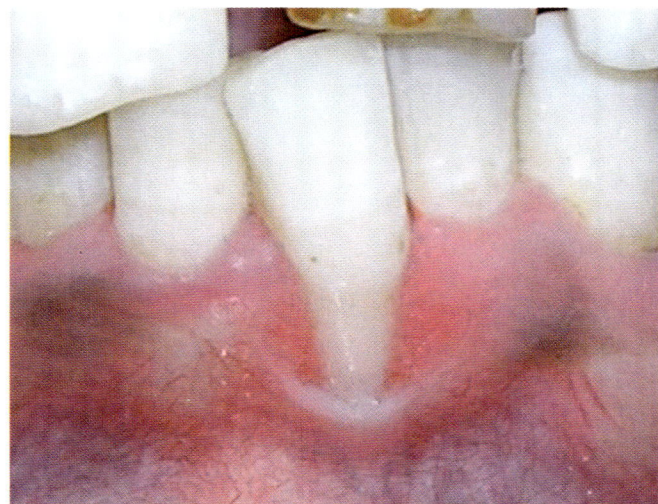

Fig. 1: Preoperative photograph showing gingival recession around 41 (recipient site)

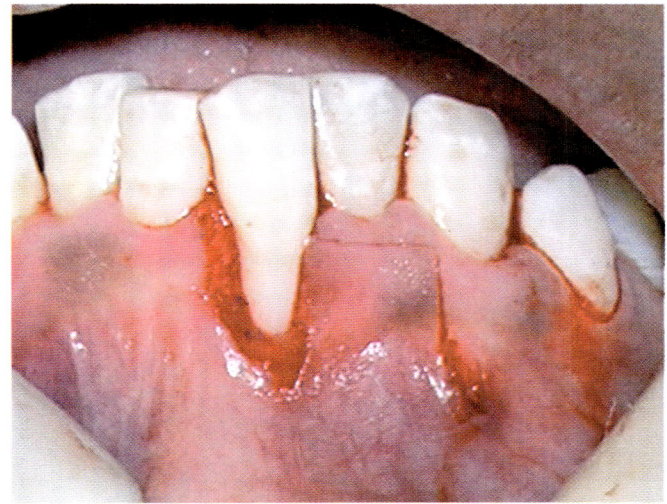

Fig. 2: Horizontal and vertical incisions given on 31 and 32 (donor site)

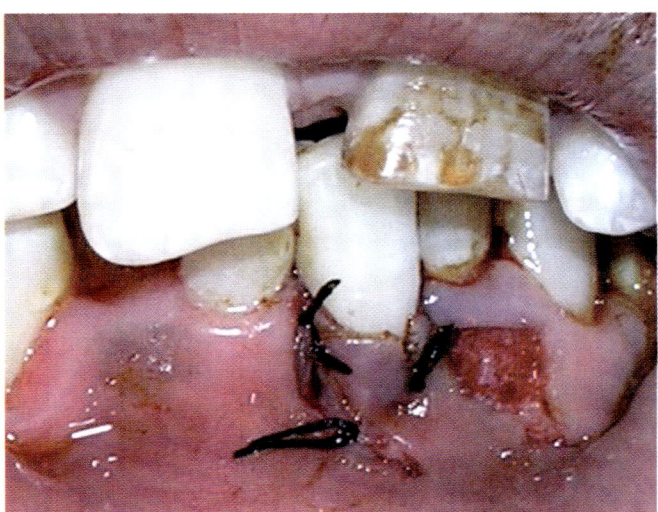

Fig. 3: Partial thickness flap is laterally displaced and sutured on 41(recipient site)

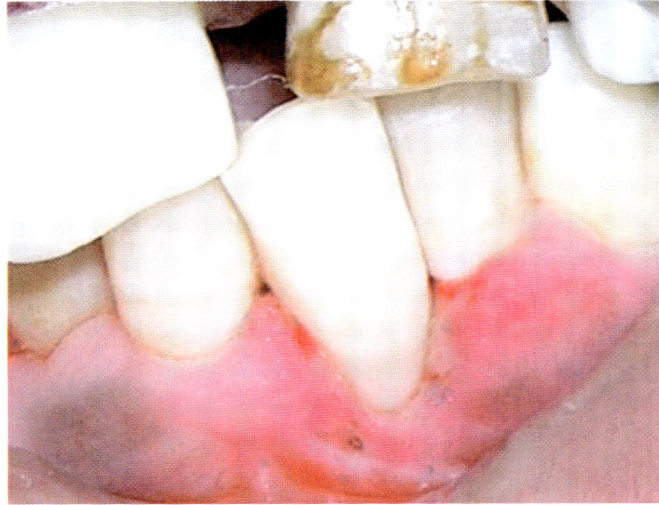

Fig. 4: Postoperative photograph showing root coverage

FREE EPITHELIAL GRAFT

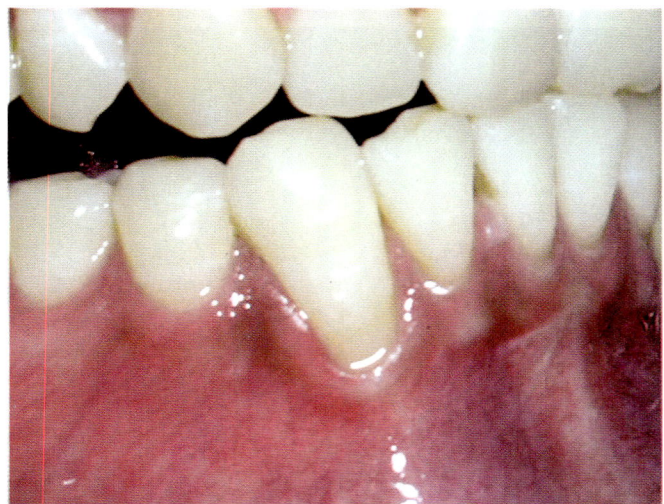

Fig. 1: Preoperative photograph showing lack of attached gingiva on 43 (recipient site)

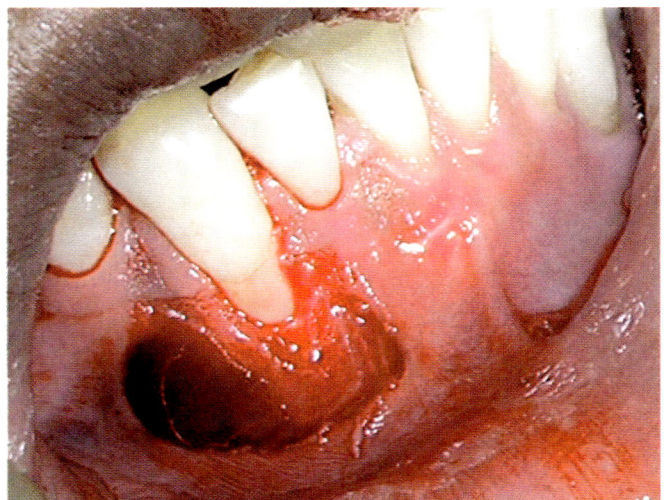

Fig. 2: Surgical recipient bed prepared

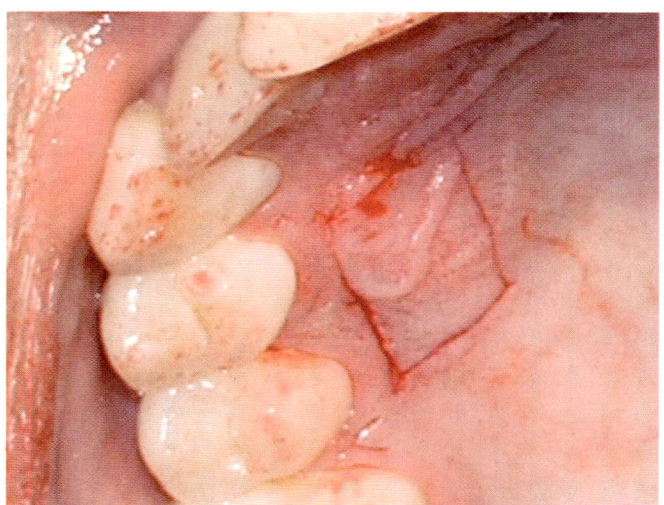

Fig. 3: Incision at the donor site

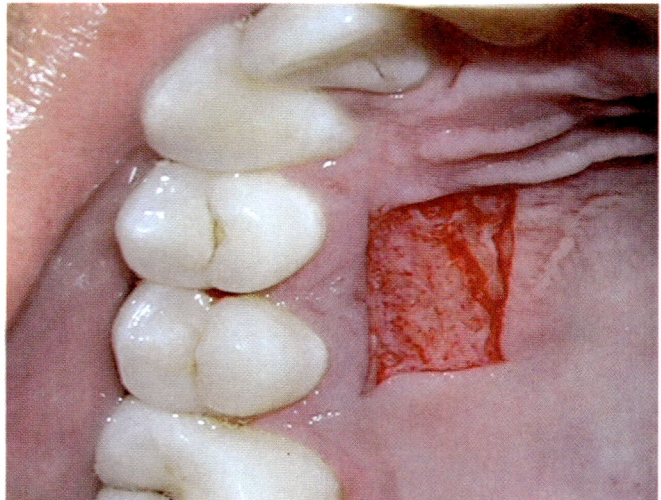

Fig. 4: Donor site in the palatal area immediately after removal of tissue for grafting

FREE EPITHELIAL GRAFT

Contd.

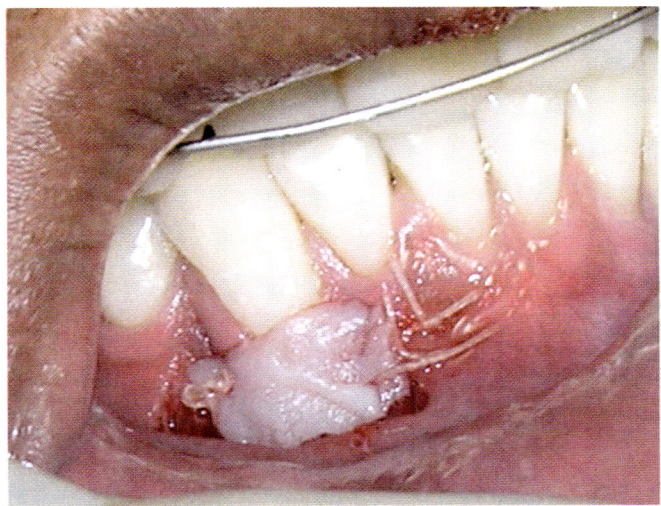

Fig. 5: Donor tissue placed and sutured at the recipient site

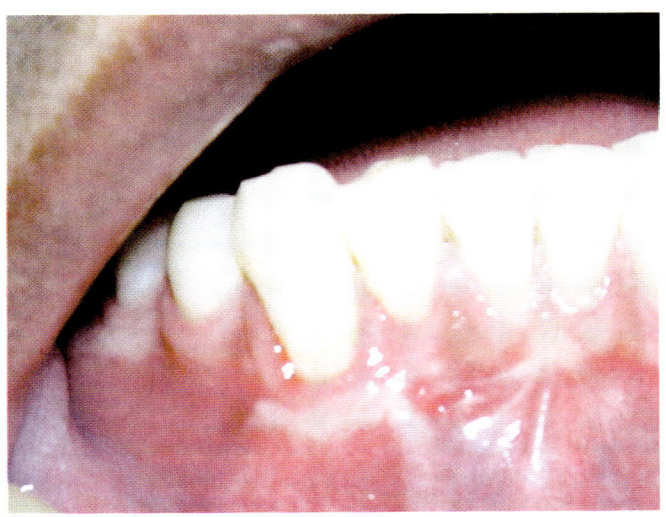

Fig. 6: Recipient site showing increased width of attached gingiva one month postoperatively

SUBEPITHELIAL CONNECTIVE TISSUE GRAFT (*Courtesy:* Dr Alka)

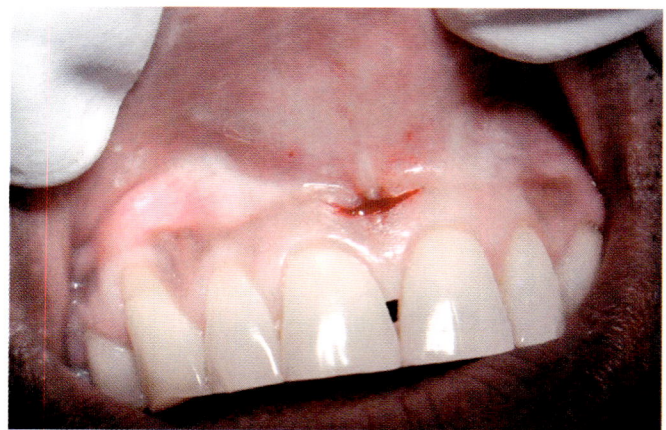

Fig. 1: Incision given at the recipient site

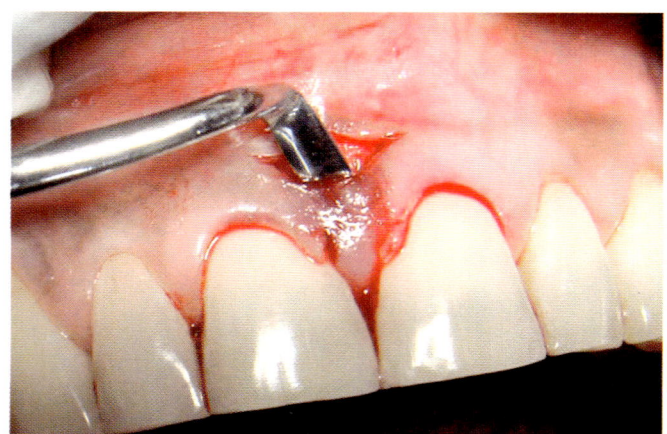

Fig. 2: Recipient bed prepared for subepithelial connective tissue graft

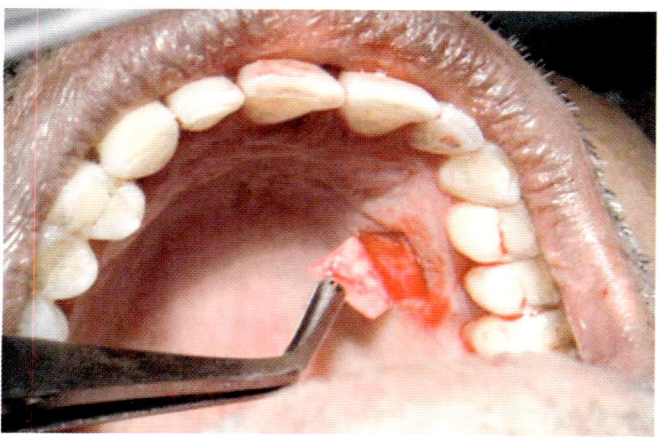

Fig. 3: Flap is raised and underlying connective tissue to be used as donor tissue

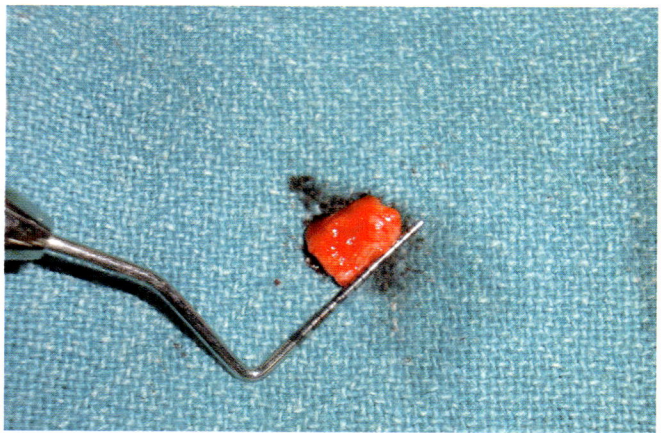

Fig. 4: Donor connective tissue

Contd.

SUBEPITHELIAL CONNECTIVE TISSUE GRAFT (*Courtesy:* Dr Alka)

Contd.

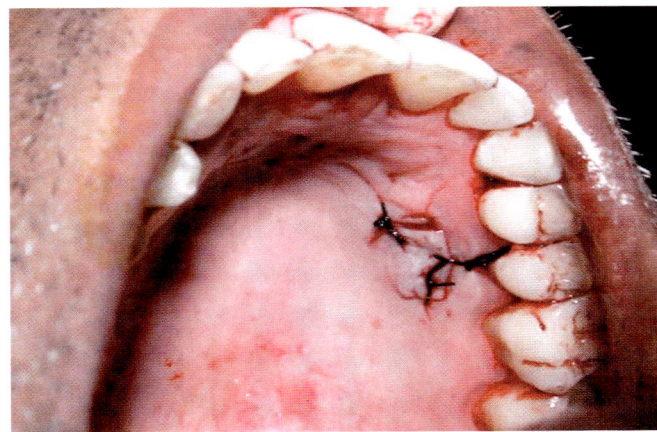

Fig. 5: Overlying flap is sutured back after taking the donor connective tissue

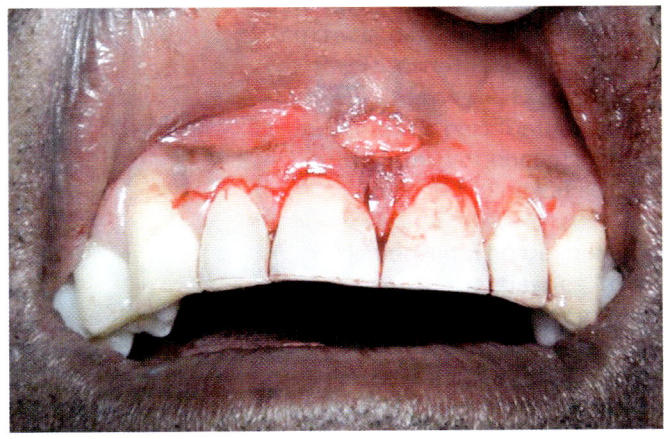

Fig. 6: Donor connective tissue placed on the recipient site

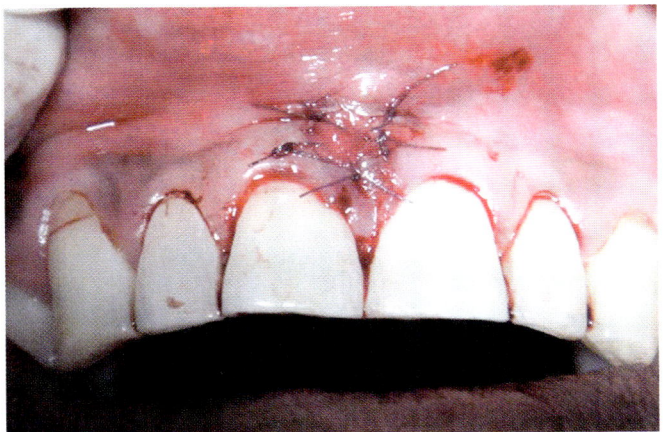

Fig. 7: Donor connective tissue sutured on the recipient site

Index